D1664872

Hemangiomas and Vascular Malformations

Raul Mattassi • Dirk A. Loose
Massimo Vaghi

Editors

Hemangiomas and Vascular Malformations

An Atlas of Diagnosis and Treatment

Second Edition

Foreword by J. Leonel Villavicencio

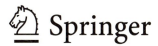

Editors

Raul Mattassi
Center for Vascular Malformations
"Stefan Belov"
Department of Vascular Surgery
Clinical Institute Humanitas
"Mater Domini"
Castellanza (Varese)
Italy

Dirk A. Loose
Vascular Malformations
Facharztklinik Hamburg
Hamburg
Germany

Massimo Vaghi
Department of Vascular Surgery
"G. Salvini" Hospital
Garbagnate Milanese (Milan)
Italy

ISBN 978-88-470-5672-5   ISBN 978-88-470-5673-2   (eBook)
DOI 10.1007/978-88-470-5673-2
Springer Milano Heidelberg New York Dordrecht London

Library of Congress Control Number: 2014959862

Printed on acid-free paper

Springer is part of Springer Science+Business Media (www.springer.com)

Foreword to the Second Edition

In the preface to the first edition of this atlas, the authors mentioned the role of a tourist guide in a foreign land and his/her importance in enticing the visitor to return by making the tour interesting, attractive, and useful. The authors have clearly succeeded in their endeavor since it has been only 6 years that we all embarked on this trip and it seems that we liked it enough to merit our return to this land, where we will find plenty of reasons to justify the trip.

It is indeed fortunate that the interest in the field of congenital vascular anomalies has grown enough to merit, for the first time, a full-day program dedicated to them in the largest vascular meeting of the world, held in November 2013 in New York City. Many of the contributing authors to this atlas participated in that meeting. It was evident during that program that there are still many unknowns in the field and that many areas of controversy remain. But what was also evident was the noble, genuine desire to help the unfortunate patients suffering from these diseases. The effort, sacrifice, tenacity, and dedication of the editors and contributors to this new edition of *Hemangiomas and Vascular Malformations* will undoubtedly be reflected in better care and benefit to their patients.

Every new edition of an important book brings new advances and examines the progress made in the care of a group of enigmatic diseases that are not the favorite among many of our colleagues. Refinements in contrast-enhanced MR imaging have served as a stepping-stone to guide the approach to the endovascular management of vascular malformations. New and improved catheters and embolizing materials, and increasing experience with the use of lasers in either localized or extensive lesions, have played an important role in the management of complex malformations that, not long ago, were considered incurable. All these improvements and many others have been beautifully and elegantly treated in this new edition. I am genuinely impressed by the quality of the paper and the clarity and sharpness of the photographic illustrations that undoubtedly contribute to the reading pleasure of this fine new edition. I am sure that Professor Stefan Belov, a true pioneer in the study and management of congenital vascular anomalies, teacher and friend of the editors, and a respected friend of mine, wherever he is, will be pleasantly smiling while reading this book.

April 2015   J. Leonel Villavicencio, MD, FACS
                                              Distinguished Professor of Surgery,
                        Uniformed Services University School of Medicine,
                              Walter Reed National Military Medical Center,
                                                         Bethesda, MD, USA

Foreword to the First Edition

The field of congenital vascular malformations and the unfortunate patients that suffer from them will welcome this truly multidisciplinary international contribution to the study and treatment of a group of diseases that is gradually becoming better known, but not better liked, by the majority of our colleagues. Without question, the power of the Internet with its access to worldwide medical literature and the publication of complete issues of medical journals devoted to the subject of vascular malformations have contributed to expanding knowledge and eliciting curiosity among physicians who, some decades ago, would not have wanted to deal with unusual, poorly understood, and challenging diseases. A group of authors from 10 different countries, experts in their respective medical and surgical specialties who have felt the pain of the many patients afflicted by vascular malformations, have made a combined effort to increase and update the growing knowledge of these diseases. The tremendous technological advances in noninvasive as well as invasive diagnostic techniques, imaging, genetics, and therapeutic surgical and endovascular procedures have given us new weapons with which to treat and improve the lives of many desperate patients afflicted by diseases that, some years ago, produced only sorrow, compassion, and despair in their families and in the rare physicians who dared to tackle their problems. Congenital vascular malformations exert a powerful and fascinating attraction in a small group of dedicated and compassionate physicians, who see in these problems a challenge that is difficult to overcome. Often, the magnitude of the problem incites us to seek new avenues to solve it or, at least, to improve our patients' suffering. A great deal of progress has been made in the understanding and management of congenital vascular anomalies. These new advances are shared with other physicians so that they can find, through the pages of this book, new ideas on how to treat their patients and, hopefully, the solution to their patients' problems.

Bethesda, MD, USA   J. Leonel Villavicencio, MD, FACS

Preface to the Second Edition

After 6 years from the first edition of this atlas, we felt the necessity to update the concepts discussed in the extensive field of vascular anomalies and tumors. Several new data have thrown new lights in vascular pathologies, and new roads were opened in these years. The introduction of propranolol in the treatment of infantile hemangiomas, new concepts of classification, and the description of different types of arteriovenous malformations, among others, have significantly changed the comprehension and approach to these diseases.

The second edition has been extensively reviewed and extended in order to cover several new topics. The number of chapters has been increased from 38 to 53; much more space has been reserved for the discussion of the treatment of specific locations of the disease as specific sites require specific treatment. The chapters dedicated to the approach on different locations have been increased from 8 to 16. Collaborators to the book have also increased from 32 to 62, demonstrating how many new data have been included.

This volume is not a textbook but an atlas centered mainly on a practical approach to the topics. The goal of this book is to offer information on the management of hemangiomas and vascular malformations, with a short and precise text supported by pictures. Theory, although present, has been reduced to essential concepts in order to devote more space to practical descriptions to help the reader find out how to manage specific cases. As vascular malformations may be variable, often general concepts and extensive discussions of theory may not be helpful to solve some specific, uncommon conditions. For this reason, chapter authors have been selected especially because of their practical and direct experience in the specific argument.

Moreover, as opinions may vary among experts, we tried to involve authors from different countries and groups in order to offer a wide overview and different opinions.

We are all curious travelers in the world of science, and we are aware that as science fellows, our task is to share knowledge.

We are well aware that even a published book can be improved still: in this light, any input or comment from readers is welcome and will help us to update future editions.

Castellanza, Italy	Raul Mattassi
Hamburg, Germany	Dirk A. Loose
Garbagnate Milanese, Italy	Massimo Vaghi

Preface to the First Edition

When a curious tourist travels through an unknown country following a guidebook, at the end of his trip he may have a number of different feelings. If the land he visited was interesting and the guidebook brought him to the remarkable places and clearly explained the meaning of what he was seeing and how to move through the country, he may remain interested in his trip, love the new country, and want to return in order to explore it more in detail. If the guidebook was unclear, did not give him the correct explanations, or did not guide him to the best places, he will leave without an interest in the land, will lay down his guidebook, and will not come back. The goal of this atlas is to guide the reader through the difficult field of hemangiomas and vascular malformations, help him to understand them, and give him answers to questions mainly about practical approaches to these diseases. All the authors have made an effort to explain their topics in the simplest way with text and pictures. If we succeed in our effort and this small atlas is appreciated by readers, we will be happy that we have accomplished the goal given to us by our teacher and friend, Professor Stefan Belov, who dedicated his life to the study of these diseases and strongly desired to publish an atlas to help colleagues understand hemangiomas and vascular malformations in order to propagate knowledge and possibilities for treatment. He passed away before he could see his idea become a reality, but we hope that our efforts fulfill his wishes. We thank all the authors who spent their time making this book a reality. Special thanks to all our friends at Springer-Verlag in Milan and particularly Antonella Cerri and Alessandra Born.

Castellanza, Italy   Raul Mattassi
Hamburg, Germany   Dirk A. Loose
Garbagnate Milanese, Italy   Massimo Vaghi

Acknowledgments

This atlas, as the former edition, is dedicated to our beloved teacher and friend, Stefan Belov, under whose guidance we approached the mysterious field of vascular malformations.

Step by step, he taught us how to manage one of the most difficult challenges in angiology. He showed us how to apply techniques and encouraged us to change our approach. Only by humbly recognizing one's errors and accepting the knowledge and experiences of others can vascular malformations be managed. Through him, we learned that with courage, perseverance, and true caring of the suffering patient, a solution can be found even in apparently untreatable cases.

His greatest dream was to spread the knowledge he acquired when working all by himself in a very difficult condition. This stimulated us to prepare an atlas on this special topic. Thanks to him, first an Italian edition and later two English editions of this book appeared.

We hope that we made a contribution to realizing his dream: to expand knowledge and to extract vascular malformations from the niche of rare and untreatable diseases. We are also indebted to our patients, who showed us how living with a vascular malformation that no one is willing to treat can be heavy with suffering and frustration but full of love and meaning.

Our deepest gratitude goes to all authors for their enormous efforts to prepare high-quality chapters, and our sincere thanks go to the Springer editorial team in Milano for their help and support throughout the publishing process of the second edition.

And last but not least, a heartfelt thanks to our wives for their constant support and understanding.

Raul Mattassi
Dirk A. Loose
Massimo Vaghi

Contents

Part I   Introduction and General Overview

1   **Vascular Embryology**.................................   3
Jörg Wilting and Jörg Männer

2   **Molecular and Genetic Aspects of Hemangiomas
and Vascular Malformations**...........................   21
Nisha Limaye and Miikka Vikkula

3   **Historical Background**...............................   39
Raul Mattassi

4   **Coagulation Disorders Associated with
Vascular Anomalies**   45
Anne Dompmartin, Morgane Barreau, Yohann Repessé,
and Agnès Le Querrec

Part II   Hemangiomas and Vascular Tumors

5   **Hemangiomas of Infancy: Epidemiology**.................   55
Maria Rosa Cordisco

6   **Classification of Vascular Tumors**   59
Juan Carlos Lopez Gutierrez

7   **Hemangiomas: Clinical Picture**   67
Maria Rosa Cordisco

8   **Diagnosis of Hemangiomas**.............................   77
Juan Carlos Lopez Gutierrez

9   **Diagnostics of Infantile Hemangiomas Including
Visceral Hemangioma**   81
Josee Dubois and Francoise Rypens

10 **Principles of Treatment of Hemangiomas**   89
Hans-Peter Berlien and Carsten Philipp

11 **Propanolol and Beta-Blockers in the Medical Treatment
of Infantile Hemangiomas**...............................   97
Christine Léauté-Labrèze

**12 Other Medical Treatments for Infantile Hemangioma
       and Congenital Vascular Tumors** 103
      Jochen Rössler

13 Laser Treatment of Hemangiomas 109
      Hans-Peter Berlien and Margitta Poetke

14 Surgery of Hemangiomas 123
      Gianni Vercellio and Vittoria Baraldini

15 Treatment of Hemangiomas by Embolization 131
      Patricia E. Burrows and David J.E. Lord

**16 Treatment of Infantile Hemangiomas
       of the Head and Neck** 137
      Milton Waner and Teresa O

17 Treatment of Visceral Hemangiomas 145
      Juan Carlos Lopez Gutierrez

18 Treatment of Genital Infantile Hemangiomas 151
      Rainer Grantzow

**19 Management of Syndromes Related
       to Infantile Hemangiomas** 155
      Carlo Mario Gelmetti, Riccardo Cavalli, and Marco Rovaris

Part III   Vascular Malformations

20 Epidemiology of Vascular Malformations 165
      Byung-Boong Lee, James Laredo, Richard F. Neville,
      Young-Wook Kim, and Young Soo Do

21 Histology of Vascular Malformations 171
      Paula E. North

22 Classification of Vascular Malformations 181
      Raul Mattassi and Dirk A. Loose

23 Principles of Diagnostics 187
      Raul Mattassi, Dirk A. Loose, and Massimo Vaghi

24 Clinical Aspects in Vascular Malformations 189
      Byung-Boong Lee, James Laredo, and Richard F. Neville

**25 Dermatological Manifestations
       of Vascular Malformations** 199
      Kurosh Parsi

26 Ultrasound Diagnostics 207
      Massimo Vaghi

27 Role of MR and CT in Diagnostics 213
      Josee Dubois and Gilles Soulez

28 **Nuclear Medicine Diagnostics**. 223
Roberto Dentici and Raul Mattassi

29 **Imaging of Vascular Malformations**. 237
Andrea Ianniello, Roberta Giacchero, Massimo Vaghi,
Alberto Cazzulani, and Gianpaolo Carrafiello

30 **Principles of Treatment**. 245
Raul Mattassi, Dirk A. Loose, and Massimo Vaghi

31 **Surgical Techniques in Vascular Malformations** 249
Raul Mattassi, Dirk A. Loose, and Massimo Vaghi

32 **Interventional Treatment in AVM** 255
Friedhelm Brassel, Dan Meila, and Martin Schlunz-Hendann

33 **Classification of Arteriovenous Malformation
and Therapeutic Implication** 263
Wayne F. Yakes and Alexis M. Yakes

34 **Sclerotherapy in Vascular Malformations
with Polidocanol Foam** 277
Juan Cabrera Garrido, Maria V. Rubia, and Dirk A. Loose

35 **Laser Treatment in Vascular Malformations** 291
Hans-Peter Berlien

36 **Possibilities and Limits of Medical Treatment** 307
Jennifer Fahrni and Iris Baumgartner

37 **Definition and Correlation of Syndromes Related
to Congenital Vascular Malformations** 313
Massimo Vaghi, and Vittoria Baraldini

Part IV Treatment of Problems According to Specific Localizations

38 **Introduction** 325
Raul Mattassi, Dirk A. Loose, and Massimo Vaghi

39 **Surgical Management of Head and Neck Vascular
Malformations** 327
Graham M. Strub and Jonathan A. Perkins

40 **Head and Neck Congenital Vascular Malformations:
Sclerosis Treatment** 337
Francesco Stillo and Giuseppe Bianchini

41 **Upper Airway Congenital Vascular Lesions** 343
Teresa O and Milton Waner

42 **Vascular Malformations of the Orbit**. 357
Aaron Fay, Vicky Massoud, and Milton Waner

43 **Orthopedic Problems**. 369
Jürgen Hauert and Dirk A. Loose

44 **Treatment of Vascular Malformations in the Hand** 379
Piero Di Giuseppe

45 **Thorax Wall** 387
Francesco Stillo and Giuseppe Bianchini

46 **Vascular Malformations in the Viscera** 393
Nader Ghaffarpour

47 **Pelvic Vascular Malformations** 407
Raul Mattassi and Massimo Vaghi

48 **Vascular Malformations of the Limbs: Treatment
of Venous and Arteriovenous Malformations** 417
Raul Mattassi

49 **Lymphatic Vascular Malformations of the Limbs:
Treatment of Extratruncular Malformations** 431
Byung-Boong Lee, James Laredo, and Richard F. Neville

50 **Veno-lymphatic Vascular Malformations:
Medical Therapy** 445
Sandro Michelini and Marco Cardone

51 **Lymphatic Truncular Malformations of the Limbs:
Surgical Treatment** 451
Corradino Campisi, Melissa Ryan, Caterina Sara Campisi,
Francesco Boccardo, and Corrado Cesare Campisi

52 **Thoracic Duct Dysplasias and Chylous Reflux** 463
Corradino Campisi, Melissa Ryan, Caterina Sara Campisi,
Francesco Boccardo, and Corrado Cesare Campisi

53 **Conclusions** 475
Raul Mattassi, Dirk A. Loose, and Massimo Vaghi

Index 477

Contributors

Vittoria Baraldini Hemangioma and Vascular Malformations Centre – "V.Buzzi" Children's Hospital, Milan, Italy

Morgane Barreau Department of Dermatology, Hospital Center of Caen, University of Caen Basse-Normandie, Caen Cedex 9, France

Iris Baumgartner Department of Angiology, Swiss Cardiovascular Center, Bern, Switzerland

Hans-Peter Berlien Center for Laser Medicine, Elisabeth Hospital, Berlin, Germany

Giuseppe Bianchini Division of Vascular Surgery, Istituto Dermopatico dell'Immacolata, Center of Vascular Anomalies, Rome, Italy

Francesco Boccardo Operative Unit of General and Lymphatic Surgery, Section & Research Center of Lymphatic Surgery, Lymphology, and Microsurgery, Department of Surgery (DISC), IRCCS University Hospital San Martino – IST National Institute for Cancer Research, Genoa, Italy

Friedhelm Brassel Department of Radiology and Neuroradiology, Klinikum Duisburg GmbH, Duisburg, Germany

Patricia E. Burrows Department of Radiology, Children's Hospital of Wisconsin, Medical College of Wisconsin, Milwaukee, WI, USA

Juan Cabrera Garrido Surgical Unit, Dr JC Cabrera Vascular Clinics, Granada, Spain

Corradino Campisi Operative Unit of General and Lymphatic Surgery, Section & Research Center of Lymphatic Surgery, Lymphology, and Microsurgery, Operative Unit of General and Lymphatic Surgery, Department of Surgery (DISC), IRCCS University Hospital San Martino – IST National Institute for Cancer Research, Genoa, Italy

Postgraduate School of Alimentary Tract Surgery, Siena, Italy

Corrado Cesare Campisi Operative Unit of Plastic, Reconstructive and Aesthetic Surgery, Department of Surgery (DISC), IRCCS University Hospital San Martino – IST National Institute for Cancer Research, Genoa, Italy

Caterina Sara Campisi Operative Unit of Dermatology, Department of Health Sciences (DISSAL), IRCCS University Hospital San Martino – IST National Institute for Cancer Research, Genoa, Italy

Marco Cardone Department of Rehabilitation Medicine, San Giovanni Battista Hospital– ACISMOM – Rome, Rome, Italy

Gianpaolo Carrafiello Department of Interventional Radiology, Macchi Foundation Hospital, University of Insubria, Varese, Italy

Riccardo Cavalli Foundation Ca' Granda "Ospedale Maggiore Policlinico", Milano, Italy

Alberto Cazzulani Department of Radiology, "G. Salvini" Hospital, Milan, Italy

Maria Rosa Cordisco Department of Dermatology, Strong Memorial Hospital/Golisano Children Hospital, University of Rochester, NY, USA

Roberto Dentici Nuclear Medicine Service, Hospital "Caduti Bollatesi", Bollate (Milan), Italy

Piero Di Giuseppe Unit of Plastic and Hand Surgery, Hospital of Magenta, A.O. Ospedale Civile di Legnano, Magenta, MI, Italy

Young Soo Do Department of Radiology, Samsung Medical Center, Sungkyunkwan University School of Medicine, Seoul, Republic of Korea

Anne Dompmartin Department of Dermatology, Hospital Center of Caen, University of Caen Basse-Normandie, Caen, France

Josee Dubois Department of Medical Imaging, CHU Sainte-Justine, Montreal, QC, Canada

Jennifer Fahrni Department of Angiology, Swiss Cardiovascular Center, Bern, Switzerland

Aaron Fay Department of Ophthalmology, Harvard Medical School, Boston, MA, USA

Carlo Mario Gelmetti Department of Pathophysiology and Transplantation, University of Milan, Milan, Italy
IRCCS Fondazione Ca' Granda "Ospedale Maggiore Policlinico" di Milano, Milan, Italy

Nader Ghaffarpour Department of Pediatric Surgery Q3:03, Astrid Lindgren Children's Hospital, Karolinska University Hospital, Stockholm, Sweden

Roberta Giacchero Department of Pediatrics, San Paolo Hospital, Milan, Italy

Rainer Grantzow Department of Pediatric Surgery, Ludwig-Maximilians-Universität, Munich, Germany

Jürgen Hauert Department of Orthopedics and Emergency Surgery, Hospital "Dr.Guth" and Facharztklinik Hamburg, Hamburg, Germany

Andrea Ianniello Department of Radiology, "G. Salvini" Hospital, Milan, Italy

Young-Wook Kim Division of Vascular Surgery, Cardiac and Vascular Center, Samsung Medical Center, Sungkyunkwan University School of Medicine, Seoul, Korea

James Laredo Division of Vascular Surgery, Department of Surgery, George Washington University Medical Center, Washington, DC, USA

Agnès Le Querrec Department of Hematology, Hospital Center of Caen, University of Caen Basse-Normandie, Caen, France

Christine Léauté-Labrèze Unit of Pediatric Dermatology, Reference Center for Rare Skin Diseases, CHU Bordeaux-Pellegrin-Enfants Hospital, Bordeaux, France

Byung-Boong Lee Division of Vascular Surgery, Department of Surgery, George Washington University Medical Center, Washington, DC, USA

Nisha Limaye Laboratory of Human Molecular Genetics, de Duve Institute, Université catholique de Louvain, Brussels, Belgium

Dirk A. Loose Section Vascular Surgery and Angiology, Facharztklinik Hamburg, Hamburg, Germany

Juan Carlos Lopez Gutierrez Department of Pediatric Surgery, Vascular Anomalies Center, La Paz Children's Hospital, Madrid, Spain

David J.E. Lord Department of Radiology, Children's Hospital at Westmead, The University of Sydney, Westmead, Sydney, NSW, Australia

Jörg Männer Institute of Anatomy and Embryology, University Medical Center Goettingen, Goettingen, Germany

Vicky Massoud Department of Otolaryngology, Massachusetts Eye and Ear Infirmary, Boston, MA, USA

Raul Mattassi Center for Vascular Malformations "Stefan Belov", Department of Vascular Surgery, Clinical Institute Humanitas "Mater Domini", Castellanza (Varese), Italy

Dan Meila Department of Radiology and Neuroradiology, Klinikum Duisburg GmbH, Duisburg, Germany

Institute for Diagnostic and Interventional Neuroradiology, Medical School Hannover, Hannover, Germany

Sandro Michelini Department of Rehabilitation Medicine, San Giovanni Battista Hospital– ACISMOM – Rome, Rome, Italy

Richard F. Neville Division of Vascular Surgery, Department of Surgery, George Washington University Medical Center, Washington, DC, USA

Paula E. North Department of Pathology, Medical College of Wisconsin, Milwaukee, WI, USA

Department of Pathology and Laboratory Medicine, Children's Hospital of Wisconsin, Milwaukee, WI, USA

Teresa O Department of Otolaryngology, Center for Vascular Birthmarks, Vascular Birthmark Institute, New York Head and Neck Institute, Lenox Hill Hospital and Manhattan Eye, Ear, and Throat Hospital, New York, NY, USA

Jonathan A. Perkins Department of Otolaryngology/Head and Neck Surgery, University of Washington, Seattle, WA, USA

Children's Hospital and Regional Medical Center, Seattle, WA, USA

Carsten Philipp Center for Laser Medicine, Elisabeth Hospital, Berlin, Germany

Margitta Poetke Center for Laser Medicine, Elisabeth Hospital, Berlin, Germany

Yohann Repessé Department of Hematology, Hospital Center of Caen, University of Caen Basse-Normandie, Caen Cedex 9, France

Jochen Rössler Pediatric Hematology/Oncology, Center of Pediatrics and Adolescent Medicine, University Medical Center Freiburg, Freiburg, Germany

Marco Rovaris Department of Pathophysiology and Transplantation, University of Milan, Milan, Italy

Maria Rubia Unit of Phlebology and Intensive Care, Dr JC Cabrera Vascular Clinics, Barcelona, Spain

Melissa Ryan Operative Unit of General and Lymphatic Surgery, Section & Research Center of Lymphatic Surgery, Lymphology, and Microsurgery, Department of Surgery (DISC), IRCCS University Hospital San Martino – IST National Institute for Cancer Research, Genoa, Italy

Francoise Rypens Department of Radiology, Radio-Oncology and Nuclear Medicine, CHU Sainte-Justine, Montreal, QC, Canada

Martin Schlunz-Hendann Department of Radiology and Neuroradiology, Klinikum Duisburg GmbH, Duisburg, Germany

Gilles Soulez Department of Radiology, CHUM Notre-Dame (University of Montreal), Montreal, QC, Canada

Francesco Stillo Casa di Cura Guarnieri, Center of Vascular Anomalies, Rome, Italy

Graham M. Strub Otolaryngology/Head and Neck Surgery, University of Washington, Seattle, WA, USA

Kurosh Parsi Department of Dermatology, St. Vincent's Hospital, Darlinghurst, Sydney, Australia

Massimo Vaghi Department of Vascular Surgery, A.O.G. Salvini Hospital, Garbagnate Milanese, Italy

Gianni Vercellio Vascular Malformations Centre – "V.Buzzi" Children's Hospital, Milan, Italy

Miikka Vikkula Laboratory of Human Molecular Genetics, de Duve Institute, Université catholique de Louvain, Brussels, Belgium

Milton Waner Department of Otolaryngology, Center for Vascular Birthmarks, Vascular Birthmark Institute, New York Head and Neck Institute, Lenox Hill Hospital and Manhattan Eye, Ear, and Throat Hospital, New York, NY, USA

Jörg Wilting Institute of Anatomy and Cell Biology, University Medical Center Goettingen, Goettingen, Germany

Alexis M. Yakes Department of Neuroradiology and Radiology, Vascular Malformation Center, Englewood, CO, USA

Wayne F. Yakes Department of Neuroradiology and Radiology, Vascular Malformation Center, Englewood, CO, USA

Part I

Introduction and General Overview

Vascular Embryology

1

Jörg Wilting and Jörg Männer

Introduction

The circulation of immune cells and nutrients and the clearance of pathogens and metabolites are of utmost importance for homeostasis and health. In higher vertebrates and in man, these functions are fulfilled by the cardiovascular system and the lymphatic system, with their major routes, the blood vessels, and the lymphatics. In general, the histological structure of blood vessels and lymphatics consists of three layers: (1) an inner layer, the *tunica interna* (intima), comprising a single layer of flattened endothelial cells (ECs) supported – in most blood vessels but not the initial lymphatics – by a basement membrane and subendothelial connective tissue; (2) an intermediate muscular layer, the *tunica media* (media), comprising smooth muscle cells (SMCs) and fibrocytes intermingled with networks of elastin and collagen; and (3) an outer layer of connective tissue, the *tunica externa* (adventitia), containing *vasa vasorum* (blood vessels and lymphatics), immune cells, and nerves. The media is

reduced with the size of the vessels and finally absent in the capillaries, which can be associated with pericytes in the blood vascular but not in the lymphatic system. In contrast to the conductive blood vessels, lymphatic collectors and trunks contain phasic SMCs and pacemaker cells that induce and transmit autonomous peristaltic contractions for the centripetal transport of lymph. Below the level of the heart, veins contain valves, which are even more numerous in lymphatic collectors. Valves are formed solely by intimal cells and specialized extracellular matrix (ECM) [1–3].

Focus on the Human Circulatory System

The cardiovascular system is the first organ system to form and function in vertebrate embryos. In human beings, the first contractions of the heart can be detected by ultrasound around the 21st day of embryonic development (days post conception), which is only 7 days after the first missed menstrual period [4–6]. At this early stage of development, the human embryo is only 2–3 mm long, and the length of his heart is about 0.5 mm. The beginning of cardiac pumping action coincides with the establishment of the first closed vascular circuit, which connects the embryo proper with the developing placenta [7]. The components of this vascular circuit are (1) a valveless tubular heart, which contracts in a

J. Wilting (✉)
Institute of Anatomy and Cell Biology,
University Medical Center Goettingen,
Goettingen, Germany
e-mail: joerg.wilting@med.uni-goettingen.de

J. Männer
Institute of Anatomy and Embryology,
University Medical Center Goettingen,
Goettingen, Germany

R. Mattassi et al. (eds.), *Hemangiomas and Vascular Malformations: An Atlas of Diagnosis and Treatment*,
DOI 10.1007/978-88-470-5673-2_1, © Springer-Verlag Italia 2009, 2015

peristaltic fashion and pumps the blood from its venous inflow into a common arterial root [8] termed (2) the *aortic sac*; (3) a bilaterally symmetric pair of *pharyngeal arch arteries*, which connects the aortic sac with (4) a bilaterally symmetric pair of *dorsal aortae*; (5) a bilaterally symmetric pair of *umbilical arteries*, which connects the paired dorsal aortae with (6) the *placental vasculature*; and (7) a bilaterally symmetric pair of *umbilical veins*, which connects the placental vasculature to the venous inflow of the embryonic heart tube [9].

The abovementioned anatomical design of the cardiovascular system of 3-week-old human embryos differs considerably from the well-known anatomy of the fetal and postnatal cardiovascular system of the human body. During the following 5 weeks of development, however, the circulatory system of human embryos loses its initially simple design and assumes all of the well-known anatomical features (e.g., four-chambered heart, pulmonary and systemic circulations) characterizing the fetal circulation. Thus, the embryonic cardiovascular system is a highly dynamic system, which continuously changes its morphological and physiological features (e.g., size, vascular branching patterns, vessel wall structure) concomitant with the continuously changing functional demands of the embryo.

General Schedule for the Development of Embryonic Blood Vessels

Formation of "Primary Vascular Plexuses" and "Primary Plexiform Vascular Channels"

The wall of early embryonic blood vessels consists only of endothelial cells so that the initial structure of embryonic arteries and veins resembles the structure of capillaries in the mature organism [10]. Thus, endothelial cells and their precursors – the so-called angioblasts – are the fundamental cellular building blocks from which early embryonic blood vessels are assembled, and the commitment of angioblasts may be regarded as the initial

step in the formation of embryonic blood vessels. Blood vessel angioblasts (BV-angioblasts) derive from undifferentiated mesenchymal cells and their assemblage to primitive endothelial blood vessels occurs in spaces filled with mesenchyme [11]. The process of de novo formation of endothelial blood vessels via the assemblage of BV-angioblasts within the primary avascular mesenchyme is named "vasculogenesis" [12, 13]. In the implanted human egg, mesenchyme first appears in the extra-embryonic compartments such as the placenta (chorion mesenchyme) and the yolk sac (yolk sac mesenchyme) by the end of the 2nd week of development (4th post-menstrual week). The first intra-embryonic mesenchyme appears during the 3rd week of development (5th post-menstrual week). It stems from primitive streak-derived mesoderm. Corresponding to the extraembryonic to intraembryonic sequence of mesenchyme formation, extraembryonic vasculogenesis precedes intraembryonic vasculogenesis.

The precondition for vasculogenesis is the presence of scattered BV-angioblasts within the local mesenchyme. In a given subcompartment of the extra- or intraembryonic mesenchyme, BV-angioblasts may derive (1) from local mesenchymal cells that are competent to develop into BV-angioblasts or (2) from an extrinsic source, which provides migratory BV-angioblasts that colonize distant mesenchymal compartments [14]. In the yolk sac mesenchyme and in the mesenchymal layer covering of the primitive gut endoderm (the so-called splanchnopleura), BV-angioblasts derive from local mesenchymal cells, while the local mesenchyme of the developing body wall (the so-called somatopleura) becomes colonized by BV-angioblasts derived from the somites [11, 15]. The origin of BV-angioblasts found within the chorion mesenchyme has not been clarified up to now.

The first visible sign for the onset of vasculogenesis is the coalescence of primary scattered BV-angioblasts to solid cell aggregates or cell cords termed "angioblastic aggregates" or "angioblastic cords" (Fig. 1.1). During subsequent development, a fluid-filled lumen is formed within these primary solid structures [16]. The primitive vascular anlagen thereby assume the

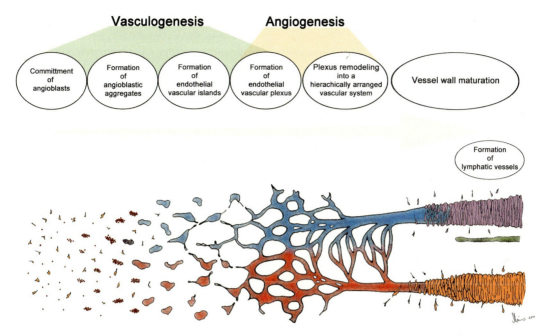

Fig. 1.1 Schematic illustration of the general principles of the stepwise development of a local vascular circuit within extensive mesenchymal spaces. The main steps are (1) formation of a primary vascular plexus, (2) plexus remodeling, and (3) maturation of the vessel wall

phenotype of endothelium-lined vesicles, which may be termed "blood vessel islands" (BV-islands). In the yolk sac mesenchyme and in the chorion mesenchyme, the lumen of BV-islands is filled with nucleated erythrocytes [17, 18]. Extraembryonic BV-islands are the first sites of "embryonic" hematopoiesis, and there is good evidence that the erythrocytes found in these vesicles derive from local endothelial progenitor cells, which are named "hemogenic endothelial cells" [19].

During subsequent development, the originally isolated BV-islands fuse with neighboring BV-islands. Consequently, a primitive vascular plexus is formed, which is frequently named the "capillary vascular plexus" since the wall of its vascular meshes consists only of endothelial cells. We should note, however, that the vessel diameters found in primitive embryonic vascular plexuses are larger than the diameters of most of the mature capillaries. Therefore, if we compare such plexuses with vascular beds of the mature human body, we will find that they have more resemblance with the sinusoidal vessels of the

adult spleen or bone marrow than with typical capillary beds. We, therefore, think that the term *capillary vascular plexus* is a misnomer that may provide a wrong picture of important components of the embryonic vasculature. We prefer usage of the term "primary vascular plexus."

The extent and configuration of a given primary vascular plexus seem to correspond to the spatial configuration of the local mesenchymal space. In cases of extensive mesenchymal spaces, such as the yolk sac mesenchyme, we usually find extensive vascular networks that do not show main vascular channels before the onset of blood flow (Fig. 1.1). In cases of narrow mesenchymal spaces, such as the pharyngeal arches, we usually find narrow vascular plexuses (Fig. 1.2). The anatomy of such plexuses is best described as a "primary plexiform vascular channel" rather than a vascular network. Primary plexiform vascular channels represent the direct forerunners of some of the main arterial or venous trunks of the embryo (e.g., pharyngeal arch arteries, cranial portions of the paired dorsal aortae), while primary vascular plexuses become remodeled into

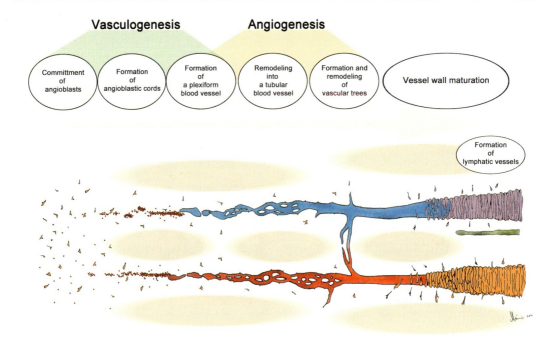

Fig. 1.2 Schematic illustration of the general principles of the formation of arterial and venous channels within narrow mesenchymal spaces. The main steps are (1) for-mation of primary plexiform vascular channels, (2) channel remodeling, and (3) maturation of the vessel wall

hierarchically arranged local vascular circuits consisting of arteries, veins, and capillaries.

In the initial state, primary vascular plexuses are not perfused with blood, and visual examina-tion does not facilitate the identification of the future course of arterial or venous trunks within the meshes of the vascular network. However, molecular biological analyses have shown that the endothelial cells of the plexuses are already specified for arterial and venous fates. However, the factors causing the arterial-venous pre-patterning of primary vascular plexuses are unknown at the present time [20, 21].

Remodeling of Primary Vascular Plexuses into Hierarchically Arranged Vascular Circuits

As already noted, primary vascular plexuses lack externally visible signs for a hierarchical arrange-ment of their vascular meshes. The situation changes, however, when a primary vascular plexus becomes connected to already perfused blood vessels. Subsequent to the establishment of permanent blood flow through a primary vascular plexus, the plexus undergoes a process of vascular remodeling, which leads to the establishment of a hierarchically arranged vascular bed consisting of large vascular channels, representing arteries and veins, and of small vascular channels repre-senting capillaries. The wall of all these vessels still consists only of endothelial cell, but their arterial, venous, or capillary identities can be deduced from their topography and the direction of blood flow. During remodeling, the arterial and venous channels first appear as plexiform vascular channels before they assume the pheno-type of tubular vessels (Figs. 1.1 and 1.3).

Experimental studies on avian embryos (chick, quail) and zebrafish mutants have shown that the prevention of blood flow through pri-mary vascular plexuses prevent the remod-eling of such plexuses into hierarchically arranged vascular systems [22–24]. Moreover, experimentally induced changes in the normal blood flow changed the initial arterial-venous pre-patterning of the plexuses [23, 25]. These data suggest that hemodynamic factors play fundamental roles in the remodeling of primary vascular plexuses as well as in the specification of arteries and veins [24, 25].

Fig. 1.3 Schematic illustration of the development of a hierarchical vascular tree. (1) Remodeling of the primary vascular plexus into a hierarchically arranged vascular circuit consisting of arteries, capillaries, and veins. (2) Four distinct morphogenetic mechanisms contributing to the remodeling process

Angiogenesis + Plexus Remodeling

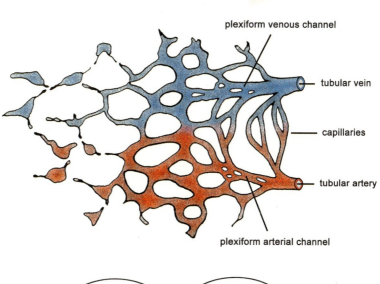

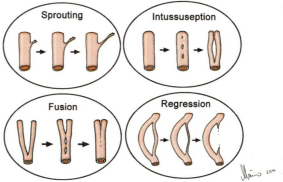

Remodeling of primary vascular plexuses is accomplished by a set of various morphogenetic mechanisms, which facilitate locally confined changes in size and number of the vascular meshes (Fig. 1.3). The number of originally existing vascular meshes is reduced either by fusion of two neighboring vessels or by the regression of vessels. Vasculogenesis may still contribute to an increase in the number of vascular meshes of the plexus. However, the majority of new blood vessels that become added to a plexus now are generated either by the formation of vascular sprouts that grow out from already existing vessels or from the splitting of already existing vessels. The formation of new blood vessels from preexisting vessels is generally termed "angiogenesis" [12, 13]. Consequently, the abovementioned mechanisms have been named "sprouting angiogenesis," "splitting angiogenesis," and "intussusceptive angiogenesis."

Vessel Wall Maturation

The formation of primary vascular plexuses (Fig. 1.1), primary plexiform vascular channels (Fig. 1.2), as well as plexus remodeling (Fig. 1.3) is induced and controlled by an interplay of genetic factors, such as the expression of regulatory genes and signaling molecules [21, 26–28], and epigenetic factors, such as oxygen [29], metabolites [30], and hemodynamic loads [24, 25, 31]. During embryonic development, all these factors continuously change in a highly dynamic fashion. Corresponding to the continuously changing genetic and epigenetic landscape of the embryo, the developing cardiovascular system undergoes continuous growth and remodeling, which is facilitated by the primary endothelial structure of its vessel walls. At a certain size, however, purely endothelial vessel walls cannot withstand the continuously increasing hemodynamic loads (e.g., blood pressure) acting on the walls of main vascular channels. At this stage of blood vessel development, the walls of the main arterial and venous channels become reinforced by the recruitment of vascular smooth muscle cells (VSMCs) and fibroblasts as well as by the synthesis of extracellular matrix components such as collagen and elastin [32]. This leads to the establishment of the well-known, multilayered wall structure of mature arteries and veins. The establishment of the mature arterial wall structure generally proceeds in a proximal-to-distal direction suggesting that hemodynamic factors play fundamental roles in the maturation of blood vessels [24, 31, 32].

Fate mapping studies on avian (chick, quail) and mammalian (mouse) embryos have shown that the VSMCs forming the tunica media of the aorta and its main branches derive from various embryonic sources (Fig. 1.4) [33, 34]: (1) The so-called secondary heart field provides VSMCs that colonize the roots of the aorta and pulmonary trunk [35]. (2) The "cephalic neural crest" provides VSMCs forming the tunica media of the pulmonary trunk and ductus arteriosus, the ascending aorta and aortic arch, and the brachiocephalic trunk and common carotid arteries [36–39]. (3) The ventral portions of the "somites" provide VSMCs forming the tunica media of the descending and abdominal aorta as well as internal carotid, subclavian, and iliac arteries [39–41]. (4) The mesenchyme of the embryonic body wall – the so-called somatopleura – provides VSMCs forming the media of the limb arteries [15]. (5) The "visceral mesothelium" of the heart, lungs, and intraperitoneal organs provide VSMCs forming the media of the coronary arteries [42, 43], pulmonary arteries [44], and unpaired visceral branches of the abdominal aorta [45].

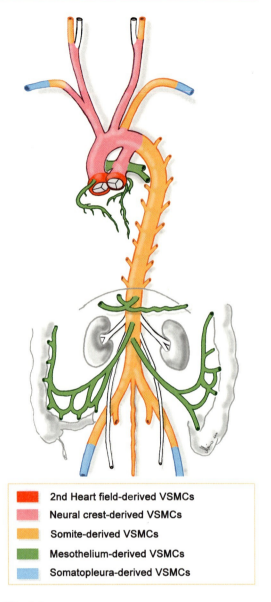

	2nd Heart field-derived VSMCs
	Neural crest-derived VSMCs
	Somite-derived VSMCs
	Mesothelium-derived VSMCs
	Somatopleura-derived VSMCs

Fig. 1.4 Embryonic origin of vascular smooth muscle cells. Scheme showing the various embryonic origins of vascular smooth muscle cells forming the tunica media of the aorta and its main branches

Cellular and Molecular Mechanisms of Blood Vascular Development

In embryos, blood vascular development occurs a considerable time before development of lymphatics. Blood vessels develop by a number of different mechanisms involving the emergence of endothelial cells (ECs) from mesodermal angioblasts and hemangioblasts, followed by proliferation and coalescence of the cells to form a primary vascular plexus, as well as remodeling and differentiation of this plexus into maturing vascular networks, as outlined above. The initial phases of vascular development have been defined as vasculogenesis and angiogenesis [12, 13].

Vasculogenesis

Originally, the term "angioblast" was introduced by His [46], and the terms angiogenesis and vasculogenesis were used as synonyms that time with the general meaning of blood vessel development. The terms were then newly defined, unfortunately neglecting the existence of the second vascular system, the lymphatic vascular system. Thus, the blood vessels were the main focus, and vasculogenesis was defined as in situ differentiation of angioblasts or hemangioblasts into blood vessels [47, 48]. The growth of blood vessels from preexisting ones was called angiogenesis, but the two mechanisms cannot be clearly separated temporally and spatially [10, 49].

Already Sabin [17] proposed a subdivision of embryonic angiogenesis into three phases. Firstly, ECs are derived from precursor cells. These are either unipotent angioblasts (giving rise to endothelial cells) or bipotent hemangioblasts (giving rise to ECs and hematopoietic cells (HCs)) [18, 50]. The development of both ECs and HCs from a single precursor cell has not been shown unequivocally but was suggested because of their simultaneous development in blood islands. Evidence for the existence of hemangioblasts was provided mainly by in vitro studies in mice [51]. Here, it was shown that vascular endothelial growth factor receptor-2 (VEGFR-2)-positive embryonic stem (ES) cells are able to generate ECs as well as HCs. In accordance, VEGFR-2 null mice lack yolk sac blood islands and ECs [52]. In the chick, a single VEGFR-2$^+$ cell can only give rise to either an EC or a HC colony [53]. Thereby, the emergence of ECs in vertebrates does not depend on normal mesoderm formation and can even be observed when gastrulation is prevented [54, 55], but, nevertheless, ECs and HCs are usually regarded as mesodermal cells. Secondly, endothelial cells are derived from precursor cells and simultaneously from ECs that are already integrated into the primary vascular plexus of the embryo. Thirdly, new endothelial cells solely emerge from already existing ones. This aspect has been challenged by the finding of circulating angioblasts in adults [56], which may, however, be of greater importance in pathologic angiogenesis than in embryonic angiogenesis.

There are two sources for blood vascular endothelial cells: mesodermal precursor cells (angioblasts and hemangioblasts) and proliferation-competent endothelial cells that exist as endothelial progenitor cells (EPCs) in vascular niches, which have not been defined unequivocally [57]. Angioblasts and EPCs possess high migratory potential. They migrate as single cells through the ECM or within the endothelial lining – preferentially against the blood stream [58, 59]. Angioblasts aggregate, flatten, and form tubes, so that the intercellular space becomes the lumen of the vessel [60]. However, intracellular lumen formation by confluence of vacuoles has also been described [61, 62], but live imaging studies in zebrafish again support the original view of lumen formation by expansion of the luminal cell membrane [63].

Angiogenesis

In earlier studies on embryonic angiogenesis, the term angiogenesis was used heterogeneously but was then commonly defined in a broad sense as the development of blood vessels from preexisting one, irrespective of the mechanisms involved in this process such as sprouting, intussusceptive vascular growth, splitting of vessels, and circumferential growth of vessels [13, 64]. In differentiated organisms, circumferential growth of arterioles and small arteries into larger arteries has been termed arteriogenesis [65]. In the early embryo, the initial (primitive) vascular plexus is made up of sinusoidal vessels lined solely by ECs. This early plexus has often been called "capillary plexus," which is wrong because

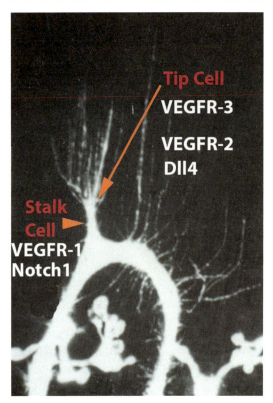

Fig. 1.5 Molecular characteristics of tip cells and stalk cells in vascular sprouts. Tip cells have long filopodia, are highly migratory, and express high levels of VEGFR-3, VEGFR-2, and Dll4. Stalk cells are highly proliferative, start forming a lumen, and express high levels of VEGFR-1 and Notch1 (Modified from Wilting et al. [49])

capillaries are organo-typically differentiated vessels with small lumen and often invested by a basal lamina and pericytes. Further growth of the initial vascular plexus is by integration of angioblasts and by a variety of mechanisms: mainly by sprouting and intussusceptive growth.

Sprouting

During sprouting the ECs extend long filopodia into their environment (Fig. 1.5). The leading cell of the sprout is called tip cell, while the more proximal cells are called stalk cells [66]. Tip cells and stalk cells communicate with each other as outlined below. The process of sprouting has been subdivided into sequential steps [67]: Firstly, there is local degradation of the vascular basement membrane by endothelial proteases [68]. This step, however, may not be of greatest

importance in early embryos, since the extracellular matrix (ECM) is only just being produced, but is of great importance when ECs invade epithelial tissues such as the neural tube. Then, tip cells migrate toward angiogenic stimuli, which are presented as diffusible gradients, bound to the ECM or to neighboring cells. The short, intermediate, and long splice variants of VEGF fulfill these requirements: The short forms (121 amino acids) are highly diffusible, the intermediate forms (165aa) bind to the ECM, and the long forms (209aa) stick to the cell membrane of the secreting cell [63]. Then, lumen formation starts proximally in the sprout as a continuation of the lumen of the preexisting vessel. Lumen formation by confluence of intraendothelial vacuoles has been reported in intersomitic vascular sprouts of zebrafish embryos [69], but this finding was challenged as noted above. While tip cells usually do not proliferate, stalk cells undergo mitosis [70]. Proliferation studies with BrdU have shown that in the aorta of avian embryos, the labeling index of ECs declines from 30 % at stage 17 (HH) to 10 % at stage 29 (HH) [71]. Finally, adjacent sprouts anastomose, form loops, and become perfused with blood. The question how individual sprouts find each other has been resolved to some extent, when it was shown that angiogenic macrophages can regulate sprout anastomosis [72]. The Notch1 signaling pathway is active in these macrophages [73].

Interaction of Tip Cells and Stalk Cells

Angiogenesis proceeds by various mechanisms; however, most of our knowledge about the molecular control of this process has been discovered in sprouting angiogenesis. Sprouting is an important mechanism during the development of the central nervous system. There, the leading cell of the sprout, the "tip cell," forms filopodia of up to 60 μm length [74]. The tip cell is a polarized migratory cell, which sits on a "stalk cell" that has proliferative potential and starts forming the lumen. The phenotypes of tip and stalk cells are transient and convertible. The Notch signaling pathway is high in stalk cells and low in tip cells (Fig. 1.5). The Notch ligand Dll4 is highly expressed in tip cells and suppresses tip cell behavior in stalk cells via Notch1 signaling. Notch1 upregulates VEGFR1 in stalk cells. This receptor acts as a trap for VEGF-A and thereby reduces tip cell characteristics. The main function of tip cells is the guidance of the sprout by filopodia. Tip cells express high levels of VEGFR-2 and VEGFR-3 and have low levels of Notch signaling activity. They migrate along a gradient of VEGF-A. Thereby, VEGF-A induces expression of Dll4 in tip cells, which by this means inhibit stalk cells from becoming a tip cell. Dll4-induced Notch signaling in stalk cells reduces expression of VEGFR-2 and VEGFR-3, but VEGFR-2 signaling is still sufficient to induce proliferation and lumen formation in stalk cells [66, 70].

Intussusceptive Microvascular Growth

The massive increase of the volume of developing organs by intercalation of cells is reflected by an overall expansion of the embryonic vascular plexus by a mechanism that has been called intussusceptive microvascular growth (IMG). The advantage of IMG is the possibility of a constant perfusion of the growing network. A detailed ultrastructural description of this process was provided by Burri and Tarek [75] and Patan et al. [76] for the developing lung and the avian chorioallantoic membrane. However, IMG can be observed in almost all parenchymal organs. In large sinusoidal capillaries, ECs form protrusions that "sprout" into the vascular lumen and make contact with the opposite luminal cell membrane. Intercellular junctions are formed and the endothelial cells become perforated centrally. Thereby, transluminal pillars are produced, which become invaded by mesenchymal cells and ECM. The pillars increase in diameter, thereby remodeling the sinusoidal vessel into a loop.

Circulating Endothelial Progenitor Cells

It was thought that the pool of angioblasts and hemangioblasts is completely used up during embryonic development, and in the adult new vessels are derived exclusively from preexisting ones. However, EPCs were identified in bone marrow and peripheral blood of adults on the basis of their expression of VEGFR-2 and CD34 [77]. However, these antigens are shared by angioblasts and hematopoietic cells (HCs). EPCs express VE-cadherin and AC133, which are lost once the cells differentiate into ECs [78]. Circulating EPCs seem to be of relevance during pathologic angiogenesis. They are recruited into sites of neovascularization in ischemic hind limbs, ischemic myocardium, injured corneas, cutaneous wounds, and tumor vessels [56, 77]. Data suggest that the circulating EPCs are of bone marrow origin and contribute to vasculogenesis mainly in the adult [79].

Remodeling of the Blood Vascular System: Arteriogenesis and Venogenesis

Soon after the formation of the initial vascular plexus, conduit vessels are formed. The first larger vessels are the aorta and the cardinal veins. In higher vertebrates and man, but not in fish, the aorta is initially formed from paired vessels, which fuse in the midline [80]. The specification of arterial and venous endothelium takes place in very early stages. The term arteriogenesis, however, has originally been proposed for the establishment of collateral arteries in ischemia [65]. The term "collateral formation" may be better suited to describe this process, and the terms arterio- and venogenesis seem to be more appropriate to describe the embryonic development of these vessel types.

The first markers that were found to differentiate between arterial and venous ECs were the juxtacrine signaling molecules EphrinB2 in arterial ECs and EphB4 in venous ECs [81]. Ephrins and Ehps are transmembrane molecules that bind to each other and induce signaling in both directions, forward and backward. EphrinB2 and EphB4 are expressed in arterial and venous ECs even before the onset of circulation but mainly appear to be functional during the remodeling of embryonic vascular networks [82]. The high plasticity of ECs has been demonstrated in grafting experiments that showed the capability of venous ECs to integrate into embryonic arteries during development, thereby adopting the arterial marker EphrinB2 [83]. Aberrant expression of the arterial marker EphrinB2 was observed in ECs of venous malformations [84]. Differentiation of embryonic arteries is accomplished by high expression of members of the Notch signaling pathway (Notch1, Notch4, Jag1, Jag2, Dll4, Hey2) and the upstream regulators sonic hedgehog (Shh) and VEGF-A.

Development of veins had been regarded as kind of a default pathway of vessel differentiation; however, the transcription factor COUP-TFII (nr2f2), an orphan nuclear receptor, was shown to induce venous specification. Disruption of its expression in murine ECs results in the upregulation of the arterial markers EphrinB2, Jag1, Notch1, and NP1 [80]. Development of veins is the prerequisite for the subsequent development of lymphatics.

Mechanisms of Lymphatic Vascular Development (Lymphangiogenesis)

Structure and Function of Lymphatics

Due to the pressure produced by the heart, 20–30 l of plasma leak each day from the blood vessels into the interstitium [85]. Ninety percent of the extravasated fluid is reabsorbed into the blood at the venous end of the capillaries and the post-capillary venules due to osmotic forces [86]. The remaining 10 % is taken up by initial lymphatics (lymphatic capillaries) and drained centripetally in lymphatic precollectors, collectors, and trunks [1]. Initial lymphatics are formed by only one cell type: lymphatic endothelial cells (LECs). A continuous basal lamina and pericytes are missing [87]. The diameter of initial lymphatics measures about 50 μm and is significantly larger than that of blood capillaries. LECs of initial lymphatics are interconnected by overlapping junctions, which, more appropriately, should be named "overlapping leaflets," as they represent valves (first valve system), which allow the influx of fluid and hinder the efflux [88].

Precollectors measure about 100 μm in diameter. Their intermediate morphology still allows uptake of interstitial fluid, but occasionally they possess a muscular wall and a "second valve system." This is made up of leaflets, formed by the intima in a comparable manner as in the veins. Next, collectors of up to 600 μm in width transfer lymph centrally. They possess numerous valves. Their wall is made up of three layers: intima, media, and adventitia. As a result of endogenous pacemaker cell activity and vegetative innervation, the nonstriated myocytes of the media contract spontaneously approximately 6–12 times per minute, which is of great importance for the lymph flow [2]. Collectors often drain the lymph over long distances (30–40 cm) into the first regional lymph node. Via lymphatic trunks and lymphatic ducts, such as the thoracic duct, the lymph is transported into the jugulo-subclavian junction [89].

Formation of Lymph Sacs and Primary Lymphatic Vessels

In the human, the heart starts pumping around the 21st developmental day, when blood vessels are already present [90]. Development of lymphatics starts considerably later. Lymph sacs, which are the first lymphatic anlagen detectable by routine histology, have been found in embryos of 10–14 mm total length, corresponding to developmental week 6 or 7 [91]. However, with specific markers LECs can be detected in earlier stages of development. Studies on mammalian embryos have shown that there are three paired and two unpaired lymph sacs, which will later give rise to primary lymph nodes [92]. The consecutive development of BECs and LECs has led to the hypothesis that LECs are derived from BECs, specifically from segments of adjacent veins [93]. This has been supported on the basis of the expression pattern of the homeobox transcription factor Prox1, which is indispensible for LEC development [94]. Direct proof for the development of LECs from venous ECs came from in vivo cell lineage tracing studies in zebrafish embryos. Cells delaminating from a parachordal vein assembled into the thoracic duct-homolog lymphatic vessel [95]. Budding and migration of lymphangioblasts from multiple vessels was observed during development of facial lymphatics using similar techniques in zebrafish [96]. In mice, too, the major source for the developing lymphatics is the embryonic veins [97]. Delamination from the endothelial lining and migration of mesenchymal lymphangioblasts, in combination with sprouting phenomena, then give rise to early lymphatic networks [98, 99]. In larger animals, e.g., chicken, indications for direct differentiation of LECs from mesenchymal lymphangioblasts have been found [100]. In the human, circulating lymphangioblasts were found to contribute to inflammation-induced lymphangiogenesis in patients suffering from kidney transplant rejection [101], but it is unknown if integration of mesenchymal lymphangioblasts is an important mechanisms of embryonic lymphangiogenesis in the human. Growth and expansion of lymphatics is preferentially along embryonic arteries, which obviously secret lymphangiogenic growth factors effectively, as well as chemokines, which orchestrate the patterning of lymphatic trunks [102].

Molecular Control of Lymphangiogenesis

Commitment of LECs starts in specific segments of early embryonic veins, probably induced by adjacent mesenchymal cells and the regulation of retinoic acid concentrations [103]. Committed LECs express the transcription factor SOX18 [104], VEGFR-3, and the hyaluronan receptor Lyve-1 [105]. Upregulation of the homeobox transcription factor Prox1, which is a master regulator of LEC development, is a crucial step for the development of the lymphatic vascular network [94], and maintenance of Prox1 expression is found in lymphatics of aged humans [106]. Transcriptional profiling of LECs identified a large number of genes with high specificity for LECs, such as *PDPN* (podoplanin), *RELN* (reelin), *WNT5A*, and others [107–109]. High levels of VEGFR-3 expression were found in LECs of lymphangiomas [110], showing that fine tuning of the VEGF-C signaling is of major importance

for tissue specific forming of lymphatics. This is underlined by the observation of lymphatic hyperplasia in mice after downregulation of soluble VEGFR-2 (esVEGFR-2), the endogenous inhibitor of VEGF-C signaling [111]. A soluble splicing variant of VEGFR-3 (esVEGFR-3) with anti-lymphangiogenic activity has been found recently [112]. The majority of familial cases of lymphedema seem to be due to mutations in the VEGFR-3 gene [113]. Molecules that regulate LEC development and the differentiation of lymphatic networks are shown in Fig. 1.6, taken from the review by Tammela and Alitalo [105]. For a detailed description of the molecular interactions, we recommend reading of this review. Not only cell-cell interactions but also the ECM controls lymphangiogenesis. Mutations of the CCBE1 protein (collagen and calcium-binding EGF domain-containing protein 1), which seems to control the composition of the ECM, cause lymphatic dysplasia in man, and functional analyses in animals have confirmed the importance of CCBE1 in embryonic lymphangiogenesis [114]. Important interactions of LECs with the ECM are mediated by integrin receptors, predominantly by integrin α9, which forms heterodimers with integrin β1. Inactivation of integrin α9 causes fatal chylothorax in mice [115].

Development of Lymphatic Collectors and Valves

The primary lymphovascular network differentiates into initial lymphatics, precollectors, collectors, and trunks. Starting with the precollectors, recruitment of smooth muscle cells (SMCs) and the formation of valves are important characteristics of the differentiation process. The ECM protein reelin, secreted by LECs, seems to be an important attractant for SMCs toward the collecting lymphatics [116]. The angiopoietin (Ang) growth factors and their receptor tyrosine kinases Tie1 and Tie2 regulate lymphatic collector formation and stabilization, as evidenced by mice with defects in this signaling system. Mice that have mutations in the ephrinB2 tyrosine kinase are characterized by insufficient valve

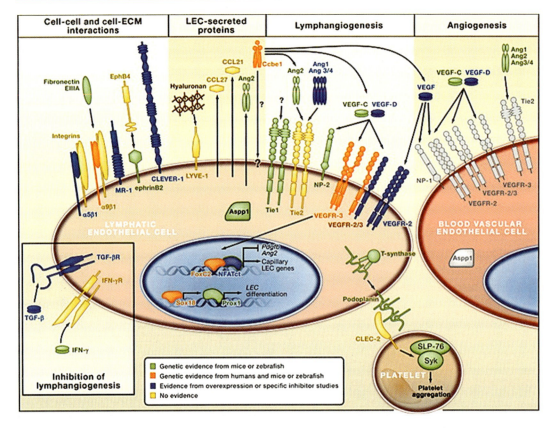

Fig. 1.6 Molecular control of the development and differentiation of lymphatic endothelial cells (LECs) and blood vascular endothelial cells (BECs). In adults, the transforming growth factor-β (TGF-β) induces ECM formation and inhibits lymphangiogenesis. The ECM component fibronectin, which binds to integrins in the cell membrane, is an important regulator of both hemangiogenesis and lymphangiogenesis. Ephrins and Ephs regulate vascular development via cell-cell contact. Angiopoietins (Ang1, Ang2) regulate vascular differentiation and stability via the Tie2 (Tie1 also?) receptors. Vascular endothelial growth factor-C (VEGF-C), and, to a lesser extent, VEGF-D control lymphangiogenesis mainly by binding to the receptor VEGFR-3 and the co-receptor neuropilin-2 (NP-2). The transcription factors Sox18 and Prox1 determine the early embryonic specification of the LEC fate. The transcription factors FoxC2 and NFATct control differentiation and valve formation of collectors. (Further details see Tammela and Alitalo [105]. Reproduced with permission of Elsevier license number 3337740261947)

formation, and similar defects are found when the forkhead transcription factor FOXC2 is not functional [105]. In the lymphovascular system, development of valves precedes the development of a SMC coverage of the collectors and starts with the onset of lymph flow. In contrast, in veins, valves develop after the vessels have acquired a SMC coverage [3]. In both types of vessels, morphogenesis of valves is regulated by almost identical patterns of gene expression, including the transcription factors GATA2, PROX1, NFAT (nuclear factor of activated T-cells), and FOXC2, the gap junction component connexin-37, and the

ECM component integrin α5 [3]. Directed growth of LECs into the vascular lumen is regulated by signals that regulate "planar cell polarity" [117], a mechanism controlling laterality in epithelial sheets.

Maturation of Lymphatic Vessels

Maturation of the initial lymphatics is accompanied by the development of "overlapping leaflets" with specialized junctions, which allow the influx of interstitial fluid [88]. A continuous basement membrane does not develop, but the LECs are embedded in the ECM by anchoring filaments that contain the protein Emilin1, which is of functional importance for fluid homeostasis [118]. Recruitment of smooth muscle cells (SMCs) to lymphatic collectors and trunks stabilizes these vessels. Mice that are deficient for the growth factor angiopoietin 2 (Ang2), which binds the receptor tyrosine kinase Tie2 on ECs, are characterized by an impaired recruitment of SMCs to the lymphatics, resulting in dysplastic collectors [119].

References

1. Wilting J (2002) Integrated anatomy of the vascular system. In: Lanzer P, Topol EJ (eds) Panvascular medicine. Springer, Heidelberg, pp 50–75
2. Witte MH, Jones K, Wilting J, Dictor M, Selg M, McHale N, Gershenwald JE, Jackson D (2006) Structure-function relationships in the lymphatic system and implications for cancer biology. Cancer Metastasis Rev 25:159–184
3. Bazigou E, Makinen T (2013) Flow control in our vessels: vascular valves make sure there is no way back. Cell Mol Life Sci 70:1055–1066
4. Britten S, Soenksen DM, Bustillo M, Coulam CB (1994) Very early (24–56 days from the last menstrual period) embryonic heart rate in normal pregnancies. Hum Reprod 9:2424–2426
5. Wisser J, Dirschedl P (1994) Embryonic heart rate in dated human embryos. Early Hum Dev 37:107–115
6. Coulam CB, Britten S, Soenksen DM (1996) Early (34–56 days from last menstrual period) ultrasonographic measurements in normal pregnancies. Hum Reprod 11:1771–1774
7. Eternod ACF (1898) Premiers stades de la circulation sanguine dans l'oeuf et l'embryon humains. Anat Anz 15:181–189
8. Männer J, Wessel A, Yelbuz TM (2010) How does the tubular embryonic heart work? Looking for the physical mechanism generating unidirectional blood flow in the valveless embryonic heart tube. Dev Dyn 239:1035–1046
9. Payne F (1925) General description of a seven somite embryo. Contr Embryol Carnegie Inst 16:115–124
10. Wilting J, Brand-Saberi B, Kurz H, Christ B (1995) Development of the embryonic vascular system. Cell Mol Biol Res 41:219–232
11. Evans HM (1911) Die Entwicklung des Blutgefäßsystems. In: Keibel F, Mall FP (eds) Handbuch der Entwicklungsgeschichte des Menschen, Bd 2. Hirzel Verlag, Leipzig, pp 551–688
12. Risau W, Flamme I (1995) Vasculogenesis. Ann Rev Cell Dev Biol 11:73–91
13. Risau W (1997) Mechanisms of angiogenesis. Nature 386:671–674
14. Schmidt A, Brixius K, Bloch W (2007) Endothelial precursor cell migration during vasculogenesis. Circ Res 101:125–136
15. Yvernogeau L, Auda-Boucher G, Fontaine-Perus J (2012) Limb bud colonization by somite-derived angioblasts is a crucial step for myoblast emigration. Development 139:277–287
16. Xu K, Cleaver O (2011) Tubulogenesis during blood vessel formation. Semin Cell Dev Biol 22:993–1004
17. Sabin FR (1917) Preliminary note on the differentiation of angioblasts and the method by which they produce blood-vessels, blood-plasma and red blood-cells as seen in the living chick. Anat Rec 13:199–204
18. Sabin FR (1920) Studies on the origin of blood-vessels and of red blood corpuscles as seen in the living blastoderm of chicks during the second day of incubation. Carnegie Contrib Embryol 272:214–262
19. Hirschi KK (2012) Hemogenic endothelium during development and beyond. Blood 119:4823–4827
20. Eichmann A, Yuan L, Moyon D, Le Noble F, Pardanaud L, Breant C (2005) Vascular development: from precursor cells to branched arterial and venous networks. Int J Dev Biol 49:259–267
21. Ribatti D (2006) Genetic and epigenetic mechanisms in the early development of the vascular system. J Anat 208:139–152
22. Männer J, Seidl W, Steding G (1995) Formation of the cervical flexure: an experimental study on chick embryos. Acta Anat 152:1–10
23. Le Noble F, Moyon D, Pardanaud L, Yuan L, Djonov V, Matthijsen R, Breant C, Fleury V, Eichmann A (2004) Flow regulates arterial-venous differentiation in the chick embryo yolk sac. Development 131:361–375
24. Culver JC, Dickinson ME (2010) Effects of hemodynamic force on embryonic development. Microcirculation 17:164–178
25. Jones EAV, Le Noble F, Eichmann A (2006) What determines blood vessel structure? Genetic prespecification vs hemodynamics. Physiology 21:388–395
26. Ribatti D, Nico B, Crivellato E (2009) Morphological and molecular aspects of physiological vascular morphogenesis. Angiogenesis 12:101–111
27. Hoffmann JJ, Iruela-Arispe ML (2007) Notch signaling in blood vessels. Who is talking to whom about what? Circ Res 100:1556–1568
28. Udan RS, Culver JC, Dickinson ME (2013) Understanding vascular development. Dev Biol 2:327–346
29. Fraisl P, Mazzone M, Schmidt T, Carmeliet P (2009) Regulation of angiogenesis by oxygen and metabolism. Dev Cell 16:167–179
30. Murray B, Wilson DJ (2001) A study of metabolites as intermediate effectors in angiogenesis. Angiogenesis 4:71–77
31. Roman BL, Pekkan K (2012) Mechanotransduction in embryonic vascular development. Biomech Model Mechanobiol 11:1149–1168

32. Hungerford JE, Little CD (1999) Developmental biology of the vascular smooth muscle cell: building a multilayered vessel wall. J Vasc Res 36:2–27

33. Majesky MW (2007) Developmental basis of vascular smooth muscle diversity. Arterioscler Thromb Vasc Biol 27:1248–1258

34. Majesky MW, Dong XR, Regan JN, Hoglund VJ (2011) Vascular smooth muscle progenitor cells: building and repairing blood vessels. Arterioscler Circ Res 108:365–377

35. Waldo KL, Hutson MR, Ward CC, Zdanowicz M, Stadt HA, Kumiski D, Abu-Issa R, Kirby ML (2005) Secondary heart field contributes myocardium and smooth muscle to the arterial pole of the developing heart. Dev Biol 281:78–90

36. Le Lievre CS, Le Douarin NM (1975) Mesenchymal derivatives of the neural crest: analysis of chimeric quail and chick embryos. J Embryol Exp Morphol 34:125–154

37. Kirby ML, Waldo KL (1995) Neural crest and cardiovascular patterning. Circ Res 77:211–215

38. Bergwerff M, Verberne ME, De Ruiter MC, Poelmann RE, Gittenberger-de Groot AC (1998) Neural crest contribution to the developing circulatory system: implications for vascular morphology? Circ Res 82:221–231

39. Jiang X, Rowitch DH, Soriano P, McMahon AP, Sucov HM (2000) Fate of the mammalian cardiac neural crest. Development 127:1607–1616

40. Wiegreffe C, Christ B, Huang R, Scaal M (2009) Remodeling of aortic smooth muscle during avian embryonic development. Dev Dyn 238:624–631

41. Sato Y (2013) Dorsal aorta formation: separate origins, lateral-to-medial migration and of remodeling. Dev Growth Differ 55:113–129

42. Dettman RW, Denetclaw W, Ordahl CP, Bristow J (1998) Common epicardial origin of coronary vascular smooth muscle, perivascular fibroblasts, and intermyocardial fibroblasts in the avian heart. Dev Biol 193:169–181

43. Männer J (1999) Does the subepicardial mesenchyme contribute myocardioblasts to the myocardium of the chick embryo heart? A quail-chick chimera study tracing the fate of the epicardial primordium. Anat Rec 255:212–226

44. Que J, Wilm B, Hasegawa H, Wang F, Bader DM, Hogan BLM (2008) Mesothelium contributes to vascular smooth muscle and mesenchyme during lung development. Proc Natl Acad Sci U S A 105:16626–16630

45. Wilm B, Ipenberg A, Hastie ND, Burch JB, Bader DM (2005) The serosal mesothelium is a major source of smooth muscle cells of the gut vasculature. Development 132:5317–5328

46. His W (1900) Lecithoblast und Angioblast der Wirbeltiere. Abhandl Math Naturwiss Kl sächs Akad Wiss (Wien) 26:171–328

47. Risau W, Sariola H, Zerwes HG, Sasse J, Ekblom P, Kemler R, Doetschman T (1988) Vasculogenesis and angiogenesis in embryonic-system-cell-derived embryoid bodies. Development 102:471–478

48. Pardanaud L, Yassine F, Dieterlen-Lievre F (1989) Relationship between vasculogenesis, angiogenesis and haemopoiesis during avian ontogeny. Development 105:473–485

49. Wilting J, Kurz H, Oh S-J, Christ B (1998) Angiogenesis and lymphangiogenesis: analogous mechanisms and homologous growth factors. In: Little C, Mironov V, Sage H (eds) Vascular morphogenesis: in vivo, in vitro and in mente. Birkhäuser, Boston, pp 21–34

50. Pardanaud L, Luton D, Prigent M, Bourcheix LM, Catala M, Dieterlen-Lievre F (1996) Two distinct endothelial lineages in ontogeny, one of them related to hemopoiesis. Development 122:1363–1371

51. Kubo H, Alitalo K (2003) The bloody fate of endothelial stem cells. Genes Dev 17:322–329

52. Shalaby F, Rossant J, Yamaguchi TP, Gertsenstein M, Wu XF, Breitman ML, Schuh AC (1995) Failure of blood-island formation and vasculogenesis in Flk-1-deficient mice. Nature 376:62–66

53. Eichmann A, Pardanaud L, Yuan L, Moyon D (2002) Vasculogenesis and the search for the hemangioblast. J Hematother Stem Cell Res 11:207–214

54. Azar Y, Eyal-Giladi H (1979) Marginal zone cells - the primitive streak-inducing component of the primary hypoblast in the chick. J Embryol Exp Morphol 52:79–88

55. Christ B, Grim M, Wilting J, von Kirschhofer K, Wachtler F (1991) Differentiation of endothelial cells in avian embryos does not depend on gastrulation. Acta Histochem 91:193–199

56. Asahara T, Masuda H, Takahashi T, Kalka C, Pastore C, Silver M, Kearne M, Magner M, Isner JM (1999) Bone marrow origin of endothelial progenitor cells responsible for postnatal vasculogenesis in physiological and pathological neovascularization. Circ Res 85:221–228

57. Tilki D, Hohn HP, Ergün B, Rafii S, Ergün S (2009) Emerging biology of vascular wall progenitor cells in health and disease. Trends Mol Med 15:501–509

58. Noden DM (1988) Interactions and fates of avian craniofacial mesenchyme. Development 103 Suppl: 121–140

59. Wilms P, Christ B, Wilting J, Wachtler F (1991) Distribution and migration of angiogenic cells from grafted avascular intraembryonic mesoderm. Anat Embryol 183:371–377

60. Hirakow R, Hiruma T (1983) TEM-studies on development and canalization of the dorsal aorta in the chick embryo. Anat Embryol 166:307–315

61. Benninghoff A, Hartmann A, Hellmann T (1930) Blutgefäß- und Lymphgefäßapparat, Atmungsapparat und Innersekretorische Drüsen. In: von Möllendorff W (ed) Handbuch der mikroskopischen Anatomie des Menschen. Springer, Berlin, pp 1–160

62. Wolff JR, Bär T (1972) Nahtlose cerebrale Capillarendothelien während der Cortexentwicklung der Ratte. Brain Res 41:17–24

63. Wacker A, Gerhardt H (2011) Endothelial development taking shape. Curr Opin Cell Biol 23:676–685

64. Yancopoulos GD, Davis S, Gale NW, Rudge JS, Wiegand SJ, Holash J (2000) Vascular-specific growth factors and blood vessel formation. Nature 407:242–248

65. Schaper W, Buschmann I (1999) Arteriogenesis, the good and bad of it. Cardiovasc Res 43:835–837

66. Potente M, Gerhardt H, Carmeliet P (2011) Basic and therapeutic aspects of angiogenesis. Cell 146: 873–887

67. Folkman J (1985) Tumor angiogenesis. Adv Cancer Res 43:175–203

68. Moscatelli D, Rifkin DB (1988) Membrane and matrix localization of proteases: a common theme in tumor invasion and angiogenesis. Biochem Biophys Acta 948:67–85

69. Kamei M, Saunders WB, Bayless KJ, Dye L, Davis GE, Weinstein BM (2006) Endothelial tubes assemble from intracellular vacuoles in vivo. Nature 442:453–456

70. Ribatti D, Crivellato E (2012) "Sprouting angiogenesis", a reappraisal. Dev Biol 372:157–165

71. Seifert R, Zhao B, Christ B (1992) Cytokinetic studies on the aortic endothelium and limb bud vascularization in avian embryos. Anat Embryol 186:601–610

72. Fantin A, Vieira JM, Gestri G, Denti L, Schwarz Q, Prykhozhij S, Peri F, Wilson SW, Ruhrberg C (2010) Tissue macrophages act as cellular chaperones for vascular anastomosis downstream of VEGF-mediated endothelial tip cell induction. Blood 116: 829–840

73. Outtz HH, Tattersall IW, Kofler NM, Steinbach N, Kitajewski J (2011) Notch1 controls macrophage recruitment and Notch signaling is activated at sites of endothelial cell anastomosis during retinal angiogenesis in mice. Blood 118:3436–3439

74. Kurz H, Gärtner T, Christ B (1996) The first blood vessels in the avian neural tube are formed by a combination of dorsal immigration and ventral sprouting of endothelial cells. Dev Biol 173:133–147

75. Burri PH, Tarek MR (1990) A novel mechanism of capillary growth in the rat pulmonary microcirculation. Anat Rec 228:35–45

76. Patan S, Haenni B, Burri PH (1993) Evidence for intussusceptive capillary growth in the chicken chorioallantoic membrane. Anat Embryol 187:121–130

77. Luttun A, Carmeliet G, Carmeliet P (2002) Vascular progenitors: from biology to treatment. Trends Cardiovasc Med 2(2):88–96

78. Peichev M, Naiyer AJ, Pereira D, Zhu Z, Lane WJ, Williams M, Oz MC, Hicklin DJ, Witte L, Moore MA, Rafii S (2000) Expression of VEGFR-2 and AC133 by circulating human CD34(+) cells identifies a population of functional endothelial precursors. Blood 95:952–958

79. Lyden D, Hattori K, Dias S, Costa C, Blaikie P, Butros L, Chadburn A, Heissig B, Marks W, Witte L, Wu Y, Hicklin D, Zhu Z, Hackett NR, Crystal RG, Moore MA, Hajjar KA, Manova K, Benezra R, Rafii S (2001) Impaired recruitment of bone-marrow-derived endothelial and hematopoietic precursor cells blocks tumor angiogenesis and growth. Nat Med 7:1194–1201

80. Swift MR, Weinstein BM (2009) Arterial-venous specification during development. Circ Res 104: 576–588

81. Gale NW, Holland SJ, Valenzuela DM, Flenniken A, Pan L, Ryan TE, Henkemeyer M, Strebhardt K, Hirai H, Wilkinson DG, Pawson T, Davis S, Yancopoulos GD (1996) Eph receptors and ligands comprise two major specificity subclasses and are reciprocally compartmentalized during embryogenesis. Neuron 7:9–19

82. Kullander K, Klein R (2002) Mechanisms and functions of Eph and ephrin signalling. Nat Rev Mol Cell Biol 3:475–486

83. Othman-Hassan K, Patel K, Papoutsi M, Rodriguez-Niedenführ M, Christ B, Wilting J (2001) Arterial identity of endothelial cells is controlled by local cues. Dev Biol 237:398–409

84. Diehl S, Bruno R, Wilkinson GA, Loose DA, Wilting J, Schweigerer L, Klein R (2005) Altered expression patterns of EphrinB2 and EphB2 in human umbilical vessels and congenital venous malformations. Pediatr Res 57:537–544

85. Landis EM, Pappenheimer JR (1963) Exchange of substances through the capillary wall. In: Pow P (ed) Handbook of physiology. American Physiological Society, Washington, pp 961–1073

86. Starling EH (1896) On the absorption of fluids from the connective tissue spaces. J Physiol 19:312–326

87. Casley-Smith JR (1980) The fine structure and functioning of tissue channels and lymphatics. Lymphology 13:177–183

88. Baluk P, Fuxe J, Hashizume H, Romano T, Lashnits E, Butz S, Vestweber D, Corada M, Molendini C, Dejana E, McDonald DM (2007) Functionally specialized junctions between endothelial cells of lymphatic vessels. J Exp Med 204:2349–2362

89. Berens von Rautenfeld D, Drenckhahn D (1994) Bau der Lymphgefäße. In: Drenckhahn D, Zenker W (eds) Benninghoff Anatomie: Makroskopische Anatomie, Embryologie und Histologie des Menschen. Urban & Schwarzenberg, München, pp 756–761

90. Wilting J, Männer J (2013) Development and patterning of the cardiac lymphatic network. In: Karunamuni G (ed) The cardiac lymphatic system. Springer, Heidelberg/New York, pp 17–31

91. Van der Putte SCJ (1975) The development of the lymphatic system in man. Adv Anat Embryol Cell Biol 51:1–60

92. Sabin FR (1909) The lymphatic system in human embryos, with consideration of the system of a whole. Am J Anat 9:43–91

93. Sabin FR (1902) On the origin and development of the lymphatic system from the veins and the development of the lymph hearts and the thoracic duct in the pig. Am J Anat 1:367–389

94. Wigle JT, Oliver G (1999) Prox1 function is required for the development of the murine lymphatic system. Cell 98:769–778

95. Yaniv K, Isogai S, Castranova D, Dye L, Hitomi J, Weinstein BM (2006) Live imaging of lymphatic development in the zebrafish. Nat Med 12:711–716

96. Okuda KS, Astin JW, Misa JP, Flores MV, Crosier KE, Crosier PS (2012) Lyve1 expression reveals novel lymphatic vessels and new mechanisms for lymphatic vessel development in zebrafish. Development 39:2381–2391

97. Srinivasan RS, Dillard ME, Lagutin OV, Lin FJ, Tsai S, Tsai MJ, Samokhvalov IM, Oliver G (2007) Lineage tracing demonstrates the venous origin of the mammalian lymphatic vasculature. Genes Dev 21:2422–2432

98. Buttler K, Kreysing A, von Kaisenberg CS, Schweigerer L, Gale N, Papoutsi M, Wilting J (2006) Mesenchymal cells with leukocyte and lymphendothelial characteristics in murine embryos. Dev Dyn 235:1554–1562

99. Pollmann C, Hägerling R, Kiefer F (2014) Visualization of lymphatic vessel development, growth, and function. Adv Anat Embryol Cell Biol 214:167–186

100. Papoutsi M, Tomarev SI, Eichmann A, Pröls F, Christ B, Wilting J (2001) Endogenous origin of the lymphatics in the avian chorioallantoic membrane. Dev Dyn 222:238–251

101. Kerjaschki D, Huttary N, Raab I, Regele H, Bojarski-Nagy K, Bartel G, Kröber SM, Greinix H, Rosenmaier A, Karlhofer F, Wick N, Mazal PR (2006) Lymphatic endothelial progenitor cells contribute to de novo lymphangiogenesis in human renal transplants. Nat Med 12:230–234

102. Cha YR, Fujita M, Butler M, Isogai S, Kochhan E, Siekmann AF, Weinstein BM (2012) Chemokine signaling directs trunk lymphatic network formation along the preexisting blood vasculature. Dev Cell 22:824–836

103. Bowles J, Secker G, Nguyen C, Kazenwadel J, Truong V, Frampton E, Curtis C, Skoczylas R, Davidson TL, Miura N, Hong YK, Koopman P, Harvey NL, François M (2014) Control of retinoid levels by CYP26B1 is important for lymphatic vascular development in the mouse embryo. Dev Biol 386:25–33

104. François M, Caprini A, Hosking B, Orsenigo F, Wilhelm D, Browne C, Paavonen K, Karnezis T, Shayan R, Downes M, Davidson T, Tutt D, Cheah KS, Stacker SA, Muscat GE, Achen MG, Dejana E, Koopman P (2008) Sox18 induces development of the lymphatic vasculature in mice. Nature 456:643–647

105. Tammela T, Alitalo K (2010) Lymphangiogenesis: molecular mechanisms and future promise. Cell 140:460–476

106. Wilting J, Papoutsi M, Christ B, Nicolaides KH, von Kaisenberg CS, Borges J, Stark GB, Alitalo K, Tomarev SI, Niemeyer C, Rössler J (2002) The transcription factor Prox1 is a marker for lymphatic endothelial cells in normal and diseased tissues. FASEB J 16:1271–1273

107. Podgrabinska S, Braun P, Velasco P, Kloos B, Pepper MS, Skobe M (2002) Molecular characterization of lymphatic endothelial cells. Proc Natl Acad Sci U S A 99:16069–16074

108. Becker J, Fröhlich J, Perske C, Pavlakovic H, Wilting J (2012) Reelin signalling in neuroblastoma: migratory switch in metastatic stages. Int J Oncol 41:681–689

109. Buttler K, Becker J, Pukrop T, Wilting J (2013) Maldevelopment of dermal lymphatics in Wnt5a-knockout-mice. Dev Biol 381:365–376

110. Norgall S, Papoutsi M, Rössler J, Schweigerer L, Wilting J, Weich HA (2007) Elevated expression of VEGFR-3 in lymphatic endothelial cells from lymphangiomas. BMC Cancer 7:105

111. Albuquerque RJ, Hayashi T, Cho WG, Kleinman ME, Dridi S, Takeda A, Baffi JZ, Yamada K, Kaneko H, Green MG, Chappell J, Wilting J, Weich HA, Yamagami S, Amano S, Mizuki N, Alexander JS, Peterson ML, Brekken RA, Hirashima M, Capoor S, Usui T, Ambati BK, Ambati J (2009) Alternatively spliced vascular endothelial growth factor receptor-2 is an essential endogenous inhibitor of lymphatic vessel growth. Nat Med 15:1023–1030

112. Singh N, Tiem M, Watkins R, Cho YK, Wang Y, Olsen T, Uehara H, Mamalis C, Luo L, Oakey Z, Ambati BK (2013) Soluble vascular endothelial growth factor receptor 3 is essential for corneal alymphaticity. Blood 121:4242–4249

113. Mendola A, Schlögel MJ, Ghalamkarpour A, Irrthum A, Nguyen HL, Fastré E, Bygum A, van der Vleuten C, Fagerberg C, Baselga E, Quere I, Mulliken JB, Boon LM, Brouillard P, Vikkula M, Lymphedema Research Group (2013) Mutations in the VEGFR3 signaling pathway explain 36 % of familial lymphedema. Mol Syndromol 4:257–266

114. Alders M, Hogan BM, Gjini E, Salehi F, Al-Gazali L, Hennekam EA, Holmberg EE, Mannens MM, Mulder MF, Offerhaus GJ, Prescott TE, Schroor EJ, Verheij JB, Witte M, Zwijnenburg PJ, Vikkula M, Schulte-Merker S, Hennekam RC (2009) Mutations in CCBE1 cause generalized lymph vessel dysplasia in humans. Nat Genet 41:1272–1274

115. Huang XZ, Wu JF, Ferrando R, Lee JH, Wang YL, Farese RV Jr, Sheppard D (2000) Fatal bilateral chylothorax in mice lacking the integrin alpha9beta1. Mol Cell Biol 20:5208–5215

116. Lutter S, Xie S, Tatin F, Makinen T (2012) Smooth muscle-endothelial cell communication activates Reelin signaling and regulates lymphatic vessel formation. J Cell Biol 197:837–849

117. Tatin F, Taddei A, Weston A, Fuchs E, Devenport D, Tissir F, Makinen T (2013) Planar cell polarity protein Celsr1 regulates endothelial adherens junctions and directed cell rearrangements during valve morphogenesis. Dev Cell 26:31–44

118. Danussi C, Spessotto P, Petrucco A, Wassermann B, Sabatelli P, Montesi M, Doliana R, Bressan GM,

Colombatti A (2008) Emilin1 deficiency causes structural and functional defects of lymphatic vasculature. Mol Cell Biol 28:4026–4039

119. Gale NW, Thurston G, Hackett SF, Renard R, Wang Q, McClain J, Martin C, Witte C, Witte MH, Jackson D, Suri C, Campochiaro PA, Wiegand SJ, Yancopoulos GD (2002) Angiopoietin-2 is required for postnatal angiogenesis and lymphatic patterning, and only the latter role is rescued by Angiopoietin-1. Dev Cell 3:411–423

Molecular and Genetic Aspects of Hemangiomas and Vascular Malformations

2

Nisha Limaye and Miikka Vikkula

Introduction

Vascular anomalies are localized, structural irregularities of the vasculature, which occur during vasculogenesis, angiogenesis, and lymphangiogenesis, the major processes that give rise to and maintain the adult lymphatic and vascular systems [1]. Vascular anomalies include vascular tumors, which consist mainly of infantile hemangiomas and vascular malformations that are divided according to the component on which they arise: capillary, lymphatic, venous, arterial, and combined malformations [2].

Infantile Hemangioma

Hemangiomas are benign vascular tumors that occur in 10–12 % of Caucasian infants, with a sex bias of 3:1 in females vs. males. Most often, they appear on the head or neck, proliferate rapidly over the first 6–12 months of life, and then spontaneously and gradually regress over a period of several years. Rare congenital forms that involute rapidly (rapidly involuting congenital hemangioma, RICH) or fail to involute (non-involuting congenital hemangioma, NICH) are also known.

N. Limaye • M. Vikkula (✉)
Laboratory of Human Molecular Genetics,
de Duve Institute, Université catholique de Louvain,
Brussels, Belgium
e-mail: miikka.vikkula@uclouvain.be

While most hemangiomas are sporadic, rare familial cases allowed for linkage to a locus on *5q31–33*, the causative gene within which remains to be identified [3]. Heterozygous missense substitutions in the endothelial cell (EC) tyrosine kinase receptor for vascular endothelial growth factor VEGF-A/VEGFR2 (KDR; p. Cys482Arg) and the anthrax receptor ANTXR1 (TEM8; p.Ala326Thr) have been shown to be enriched in patients with infantile hemangioma [4]. The two receptors form a complex with β1-integrin on the surface of ECs, which acts through the transcription factor NFATc1 to produce VEGFR1 (FLT1). VEGFR1 in turn competes for VEGF-A, thereby controlling the level of ligand-stimulated VEGFR2 signaling. The changes identified in hemangioma destabilize this receptor complex, resulting in a reduction in the level of VEGFR1 and a concomitant increase in VEGFR2 signaling [4]. While the genetic changes have only been identified in a fraction of samples, all hemangioma-derived ECs seem to be characterized by increased VEGFR2 signaling, which contributes to their proliferative nature, making it a promising target for therapy [4]. The generation of a mouse model using hemangioma-derived stem cells implanted into immunocompromised mice results in the formation of lesions that mimic those observed in patients, in appearance as well as the evolution from proliferative to spontaneously involuting tumors [5]. The model promises to be useful in furthering our understanding of the underlying disease processes and in testing the means by which to block them.

Vascular Malformations

Vascular malformations are rare, with an estimated overall incidence of about 0.3 % [6]. Unlike hemangiomas, they are present at birth, grow proportionately with the individual, and do not spontaneously regress. They show no sex preponderance and have normal EC turnover, in contrast to hemangiomas in their proliferative phase. Malformations are further subdivided on the basis of the particular vascular component involved and their flow characteristics as detected by techniques such as Doppler ultrasound. Thus, they include the slow-flow capillary, venous, and lymphatic malformations and the fast-flow arterial malformations, as well as combinations of these (Table 2.1). Lesions vary widely in terms of their number (single or multiple, the latter more commonly observed in hereditary forms), extensiveness (isolated or large and diffuse), and localization (cutaneous, mucocutaneous, or deep, involving the viscera, nerve, bone, or muscle). They can sometimes occur in association with other sign and symptoms, i.e., in syndromes (for a detailed review see [6, 7]).

Major advances have been made in identifying the genetic bases of several vascular malformations (Table 2.1; reviewed in [8]). This has allowed for more accurate "molecular" diagnosis and therefore appropriate treatment of diseases with overlapping symptoms. In addition, knowledge of the genetic bases of pathology has led to insights into the pathways and mechanisms dysregulated downstream, which may be targeted for therapy.

Capillary Malformation (CM)

CMs (OMIM 163000) are the most frequently occurring vascular malformations, with an incidence of about 0.3 % in the population. They appear flat, reddish to purple, and irregular, giving them the name "port-wine stain." Sometimes quite extensive, they are most frequently found in the face and neck regions but can also occur on the trunk and limbs. Histologically, they consist of dilated capillary-like channels, usually within the dermis. CMs are predominantly sporadic in nature, although rare autosomal-dominant hereditary forms, such as capillary malformation-arteriovenous malformation (CM-AVMs), have been observed in some families.

Capillary Malformation-Arteriovenous Malformation (CM-AVM)

CM-AVM (OMIM 608354) is characterized by small, multifocal, pink-red CMs, often with a pale halo. In about a third of cases, these are accompanied by AVMs, AVFs, or Parkes Weber syndrome (PWS; OMIM 608355), characterized by large cutaneous stains on an extremity, which also shows soft tissue and skeletal hypertrophy, and AV micro-fistulas. Mutations in p120Ras-GAP (*RASA1*), which encodes a Ras GTPase-activating protein (RasGAP), have been identified to cause the autosomal-dominant disorder [9–11]. The changes primarily cause premature truncation and loss of function of the protein. The reduced penetrance and phenotypic heterogeneity observed in affected families suggest that a somatic second hit may be required to locally inactivate the second allele of the gene. In support of this hypothesis, Revencu et al. identified a somatic loss of chromosome 5q that includes *RASA1*, in a neurofibroma that developed (during adulthood) on a congenital Parkes Weber lesion, in one individual with a germ line RASA1 mutation. Two somatic hits to *NF1* were in addition identified in the tissue [11]. Loss of p120RasGAP would be expected to lead to chronic Ras activation. *RASA1* may also be able to act in a Ras-independent manner through its interaction with *p190RhoGAP*, which seems to play a role in cell movement [12, 13], or through its ability to promote pro-survival *Akt* activation [14]. While mice that are heterozygous for a deletion of *Rasa1* appear normal, homozygous deletion of the gene is embryonic lethal

Table 2.1 Genes and loci implicated in vascular malformations, classified by vascular compartment

Malformation	Chr region (locus)	Gene	Inheritance pattern(s)	Mutation type(s)
Arterial and capillary anomalies				
Arteriovenous malformations (AVM)	?	?	Sporadic	?
Ataxia-telangiectasia (AT)	*11q23 (AT1)*	*ATM*	Autosomal recessive	Germline
Capillary malformation-arteriovenous malformation (CM-AVM)	*5q14.3 (CMC1)*	*RASA1*	Autosomal dominant	Germline, somatic 2nd hit
Cerebral cavernous malformation (CCM)	*7q21.2 (CCM1)*	*KRIT1*	Autosomal dominant	Germline, somatic 2nd hit
	7p13 (CCM2)	*CCM2/malcavernin*	Autosomal dominant	Germline, somatic 2nd hit
	3q26.1 (CCM3)	*PDCD10*	Autosomal dominant	Germline, somatic 2nd hit
	3q26.3–27.2 (CCM4)	?	Autosomal dominant	?
Hereditary hemorrhagic telangiectasia or Rendu-Osler-Weber (HHT/ROW)	*9q33–34 (HHT1)*	*ENG*	Autosomal dominant	Germline
	12q11–14 (HHT2)	*ALK1*	Autosomal dominant	Germline
	5q31.3–32 (HHT3)	?	Autosomal dominant	?
	7p14 (HHT4)	?	Autosomal dominant	?
Juvenile polyposis-HHT (JPHT)	*18q21.1 (JPHT)*	*SMAD4/MADH4*	Autosomal dominant	Germline
HHT-like	*10q11.22*	*GDF2/BMP9*	?	Germline
Isolated capillary malformation (CM)	*1q21.2*	*GNAQ*	Sporadic	Somatic mosaic
Sturge-Weber syndrome (SWS)	*1q21.2*	*GNAQ*	Sporadic	Somatic mosaic
Microcephaly-capillary malformation syndrome (MICCAP)	*2p13.1*	*STAMBP*	Autosomal recessive	Germline
Venous anomalies				
Glomuvenous malformation (GVM)	*1p22.1 (VMGLOM)*	*GLMN*	Autosomal dominant	Germline, somatic 2nd hit
Cutaneomucosal venous malformation (VMCM)	*9p21 (VMCM1)*	*TEK/TIE2*	Autosomal dominant	Germline, somatic 2nd hit
Unifocal sporadic venous malformation (VM)	*9p21*	*TEK/TIE2*	Sporadic	Somatic mosaic
Blue rubber bleb nevus syndrome (BRBN)	*9p21*	*TEK/TIE2*	Sporadic	Somatic mosaic
Lymphatic anomalies				
Lymphatic malformation (LM)	?	?	Sporadic	?
Primary lymphedema (LE)				
Primary congenital LE (Nonne-Milroy disease)	*5q35.3 (PCL1)*	*FLT4/VEGFR3*	Autosomal dominant	Germline
	5q35.3	*FLT4/VEGFR3*	Sporadic	De novo germline
	5q35.3	*FLT4/VEGFR3*	Autosomal recessive	Germline
	4q34.3	*VEGFC*	Autosomal dominant	Germline
LE-choanal atresia	*1q32.2*	*PTPN14*	Autosomal recessive	Germline

(continued)

Table 2.1 (continued)

Malformation	Chr region (*locus*)	*Gene*	Inheritance pattern(s)	Mutation type(s)
LE-lymphangiectasia-mental retardation (Hennekam syndrome)	*18q21.32*	*CCBE1*	Autosomal recessive	Germline
LE-distichiasis/ptosis/yellow nail	*16q24.3 (LD)*	*FOXC2*	Autosomal dominant	Germline
Hypotrichosis-LE-telangiectasia (HLT)	*20q13.33 (HLT)*	*SOX18*	Autosomal dominant	Germline
	20q13.33	*SOX18*	Autosomal recessive	Germline
LE-myelodysplasia (Emberger syndrome)	*3q21.3*	*GATA2*	Autosomal dominant	Germline
Four-limb LE	*1q42.13*	*GJC2/CX47*	Autosomal dominant	Germline
Oculodentodigital syndrome-LE	*6q22.31*	*GJA1/CX43*	Autosomal dominant	Germline
LE-microcephaly-chorioretinopathy (MLCRD)	*10q24.1*	*KIF11/EG5*	Autosomal dominant	Germline
Osteoporosis-LE-anhidrotic ectodermal-dysplasia-immunodeficiency (OLEDAID)	*Xq28 (IP2)*	*NEMO/IKBKG*	X-linked recessive	Germline
LE-hereditary cholestasis (Aagenaes syndrome)	*15q (LCS1)*	?	Autosomal recessive	?
Combined vascular malformations				
CLOVES	*3q26.3*	*PIK3CA*	Sporadic	Somatic mosaic
Klippel-Trenaunay syndrome (KTS)	*5q13.3*	*AGGF1/VG5Q*	Sporadic	Germline
PTEN hamartoma tumor syndrome (PHTS) (including Cowden, Bannayan-Riley-Ruvalcaba, and "Proteus" syndromes)	*10q23.3 (PHTS)*	*PTEN*	Autosomal dominant	Germline
Cowden, Cowden like syndrome	*3q26.3*	*PIK3CA*	Autosomal dominant	Germline
	14q32.3	*AKT1*	Autosomal dominant	Germline
"Proteus" syndrome	*14q32.3*	*AKT1*	Sporadic	Somatic mosaic
Congenital lipomatous overgrowth with vascular, epidermal, and skeletal anomalies (CLOVES)	*3q26.3*	*PIK3CA*	Sporadic	Somatic mosaic

(at E10.5), due to defects in the development of the blood vasculature and increased apoptosis [15]. In support of the second hit hypothesis, mice that are mosaic for Rasa1$^{+/-}$ and Rasa1$^{-/-}$ cells develop localized vascular defects [15]. Homozygous deletion of Rasa1, whether ubiquitous or lymphatic endothelial cell (LEC)-specific, results in defects in the lymphatic rather than the blood vasculature when induced in adult mice; lymphatic defects have also been observed in certain patients with PWS and CM-AVM [16].

Isolated and Syndromic Sporadic Capillary Malformations

The presence of deeper vascular anomalies in association with CMs is also observed in sporadic syndromes, such as Sturge-Weber syndrome (SWS, OMIM 185300; characterized in addition by leptomeningeal and ocular vascular malformations) and Klippel-Trenaunay syndrome (KTS, OMIM 149000; in which an affected extremity shows, in addition, hypertrophy of soft tissue and bone, varicose veins, deep venous defects, and venolymphatic malformation). While its symptoms overlap with those of PWS, KTS does not appear to be part of the spectrum of phenotypes mediated by germline mutations in RASA1 [17]. The genetic basis of KTS is not known, although a balanced translocation ((5;11) (q13.3;p15.1)) with a breakpoint in the AGGF1 (angiogenic factor with G patch and FHA, previously VG5Q) gene promoter has been identified in one patient [18, 19]. AGGF1, upregulation of which is associated with KT, plays a role in endothelial cell proliferation and in the establishment of venous identity in zebra fish, which may account for the occurrence of venous malformations in KT [20]. The somewhat overlapping CLOVES syndrome, characterized by congenital lipomatous overgrowth, vascular malformations, and epidermal nevi (OMIM 612918), is caused by somatic activating mutations in PIK3CA, the p110 subunit of PI3kinase [21]; some proportion of Klippel-Trenaunay syndrome likely has a similar basis.

The use of whole-genome sequencing comparing paired affected and normal tissues from patients with SWS recently resulted in the identification of a somatic mutation in GNAQ (guanine nucleotide-binding protein G (q) subunit alpha; p.Arg183Gln) [22]. Targeted deep sequencing revealed that this change was present in affected (skin or brain) tissues from 88 % of SWS patients and 92 % of patients with isolated CM. Mutant allele frequency ranged from 1 to 18 %, highlighting the importance of high depth of coverage in the discovery of mosaic mutations. The change was also present at a frequency of 1–1.5 % in 5 of 669 control blood samples, hypothesized to correlate with the incidence of CM in the general population. The pathogenic effects of this mutation, which induces mild activation of p42/44 MAPK but not JNK, p38, or AKT in vitro, remain to be elucidated [22].

Whole-exome sequencing revealed recessive germline mutations in STAMBP in microcephaly-capillary malformation syndrome (OMIM 614261), in which cortical atrophy, epilepsy, and profound developmental delay are accompanied by multiple cutaneous capillary malformations

[23]. STAMBP is a deubiquitinating isopeptidase that plays a role in endosomal sorting and trafficking of ubiquitinated proteins. Reduced levels of STAMBP in patient cells are associated with an accumulation of ubiquitinated proteins and activation of the RAS-MAPK and PI3K-Akt pathways [23].

Cerebral Cavernous Malformation (CCM)

CCM (OMIM 116860) occurs as a sporadic or autosomal-dominantly inherited cerebral vascular anomaly with incomplete penetrance. It is characterized by enlarged capillary-like channels lined with a single layer of endothelial cells lacking tight junctions, within a dense collagenous matrix with no intervening brain parenchyma. Lesions occur predominantly in the brain but have also been observed in the retina, spinal cord, and skin, as crimson, irregular hyperkeratotic cutaneous capillary-venous malformations (HCCVMs). Symptoms of CCM include headaches, seizures, and cerebral hemorrhage, but while the anomaly has an estimated prevalence of 0.5 % based on large-scale magnetic resonance scanning (MRI) and autopsies, the clinical incidence is much lower, since it is often asymptomatic. Truncating mutations and/or large genomic deletions in three different genes have so far been identified to cause the disease, *CCM1* (*KRIT1* [24, 25]), *CCM2* (*malcavernin* or *MGC4607*; [26]), and *CCM3* (*PDCD10*; [27]), with a fourth locus suggested on *3q26.3–27.2* [28]. Cutaneous HCCVMs are mostly due to mutations in CCM1/KRIT1 [29, 30]. It has become evident that somatic "2nd-hit" mutations that are allelic to the inherited change and cause complete localized loss of function cause lesion formation [31, 32].

CCM 1, CCM2, and CCM3 have been found to interact with each other [33, 34] and form a complex with the kinase MEKK3, the small GTPase RAC1, and integrin cytoplasmic domain-associated protein-1 α (ICAP-1α), which function in integrin and the MAP-kinase pathway [35, 36]. CCM1 also interacts with Rap1, which stabilizes EC junctions [37, 38] and promotes DLL4-Notch signaling through Akt while inhibiting ERK [39]. In vitro, knockdown of any of the three CCM proteins decreases tube formation and invasion by ECs [40, 41]. In vivo, $CCM1^{-/-}$ mice die at mid-gestation with abnormal differentiation of arteries. This raises the possibility that it is important in arterial development, failing which, a default venous phenotype results in the CCM sinusoids [42]. The absence of the tumor suppressor in $Trp53^{-/-}$ $Ccm1^{+/-}$ mice results in the formation of vascular lesions in the brain [43]. $CCM1^{+/-}$ mice, on the other hand, fail to show any CCM-like lesions. Similarly, homozygous $CCM2$ deletion causes embryonic lethality at mid-gestation, while heterozygous mice appear healthy [44]. Morpholino-mediated inactivation of the CCM genes results in vessel dilation and embryonic death in zebra fish [45, 46].

Venous Anomalies

Venous anomalies [6] are a group of slow-flow malformations, with an estimated incidence of about 1 in 10,000, primarily comprising of venous malformations (VMs), which account for about 95 % of patients. These are primarily sporadic in nature (sporadic venous malformation or VM) but can also occur in the autosomal-dominantly inherited form, cutaneomucosal venous malformation (VMCM; about 1 %). About 5 % of venous anomalies are glomuvenous malformations (GVM), typically dominantly inherited.

Glomuvenous Malformation (GVM)

GVMs (OMIM 138000) consist of raised, nodular, pink to blue-purple cutaneous lesions, often multifocal and hyperkeratotic. Histologically, they appear as distended venous channels, their hallmark being the presence of rounded "glomus" mural cells, lacking the spindle shape of normal vSMCs as well as certain developmental markers. Unlike VMs, these malformations do not infiltrate deeply, are often painful upon palpation, cannot

be completely emptied upon compression, and do not cause the coagulation abnormalities that can be observed in VMs [47, 48].

Most GVMs (about 70 %) are autosomal-dominantly inherited, showing incomplete penetrance that increases with age and wide heterogeneity even among members of the same family. Mutations in the glomulin ($GLMN$) gene mediate the anomaly [49], with >30 loss-of-function changes identified in >100 families. 11 of these mutations account for >80 % of families, allowing for relatively efficient screening of the gene [50, 51]. The mutations occur across the entire gene, with no genotype-phenotype correlation. Glomus cells in GVMs lack expression of $GLMN$, explained by the fact that somatic 2nd hits to gene have been identified in the majority of tissues [49, 52]. Interestingly, uniparental isodisomy of the entire 1p arm, which results in the replacement of the normal allele with a second defective copy of $GLMN$, is the predominant somatic change [52].

$GLMN$ is observed primarily in vascular SMCs, which fail to differentiate appropriately in its absence [53]. GLMN has been found to be able to bind FKBP12, which in turn impairs TGF-β signaling by binding TGF-β RI and inhibiting its phosphorylation by TGF-β RII [54, 55]. Thus, by competing for binding with FKBP12, GLMN could play a role in promoting TGF-β signaling, known to be important in SMC development. GLMN can also bind the inactive form of c-MET [56], the tyrosine kinase receptor for hepatocyte growth factor (HGF), which participates in cell proliferation, tube formation by ECs, and SMC migration [57]. Upon ligand binding and phosphorylation of c-MET by HGF, GLMN undergoes phosphorylation and is released, accompanied by activation of the kinase p70S6K and its downstream target PI3-K [56]. TGF-β regulates the expression of HGF as well as c-MET [58, 59], and thus, GLMN may act in a coordinated manner in the two pathways.

GLMN also binds Cul7 and Rbx1, subunits of the cullin RING ligase 1 (CRL1) complex [60]. It inhibits the E3 ubiquitin ligase activity of the complex, which is responsible for the recruitment and transfer of ubiquitin to protein substrates destined for ubiquitination and degradation [61]. Lack of GLMN results in a decrease in Fbw7, a substrate receptor for CRL1 that targets cyclin E and c-Myc for degradation, therefore leading to increased levels of these pro-oncogenic proteins [62]. This would suggest that their increase contributes to GVM, possibly accounting for the accumulation of large numbers of rounded GLMN-negative glomus cells.

Venous Malformation (VM)

VMs consist of expanded venous-like channels, with a thin, flat endothelial cell layer, and sparse, patchy areas of vascular smooth muscle cells (vSMCs). They are usually located in the skin or mucosa but can infiltrate deeper into the muscles, nerves, bones, and viscera [47, 48]. VMs are congenital and appear flat or raised and bluish purple, ranging from small blebs to extensive lesions. Localized intravascular coagulation (LIC) in VMs causes increased D-dimer products in 40 % of patients, and soluble fibrin and decreased fibrinogen are associated with more extreme lesions [63, 64]. VMs can be part of combined lesions in the context of more complex syndromes such as KTS, described earlier, or occur along the GI tract, as seen in the blue rubber bleb nevus syndrome.

Cutaneomucosal Venous Malformation (VMCM)

The autosomal-dominant VMCM (OMIM 600195) is characterized by multiple small, raised cutaneous lesions that seldom infiltrate deeply. The presence of oral mucosal lesions along with family history is typical, although the anomaly can often be asymptomatic. Activating mutations in *TIE2* (*TEK*), the endothelial cell-specific tyrosine kinase receptor for the angiopoietins (*ANG-1*, *ANG-2*, and *ANG-4* in human or *ANG-3* in mouse; [65–67]), have been found to mediate the disease [68–70].

TIE2 plays an important role in microvascular sprouting, maturity, stability, and integrity (reviewed in [71]). Upon ligand binding with

multimeric forms of its activating ligand *ANG-1*, TIE2 forms homodimers and undergoes phosphorylation. ANG-2, on the other hand, is generally considered to be an antagonist; its effects however seem to be strongly context dependent. TIE2 has also been found to heterodimerize with TIE1, a close paralogue, with the latter being able to modulate TIE2 signaling [72, 73].

Deletions of the *TIE1*, *TIE2*, or *ANG-1* or *ANG-2* genes all result in severe defects in vascular development and embryonic lethality in mice. *Tie2*^{-/-} mice have defects in primary capillary plexus formation due to a deficiency of ECs, as well as incomplete cardiac development, and hemorrhage [74, 75]. While *Ang1*^{-/-} mice show a similar, overlapping phenotype [65], *Ang2-overexpressing* transgenics are similar to *TIE2-defective* mice [66].

TIE2 activation results in the phosphorylation and activation of a variety of downstream signaling intermediates, including PI3K and Akt, which have an anti-apoptotic effect [76]. PI3K can also activate focal adhesion kinase (FAK) and the endothelial-specific nitric oxide synthase (eNOS), which participate in cell migration and sprouting. Other signaling molecules that can interact with TIE2 include Dok-R, which can affect cell migration, Grb2, 7, and 14, and the protein tyrosine phosphatase Shp2, which can in turn associate with FAK and activate the mitogen activated protein kinase (MAPK) pathway, influencing EC migration and survival [77, 78]. By interacting with ABIN-2, an inhibitor of NFkB, TIE2 may exert anti-inflammatory effects on ECs, reducing leukocyte extravasation and promoting vessel stability and integrity [79].

Eight *TIE2* mutations have been identified in VMCM. Of these, p.Arg849Trp (R849W) is recurrent, having been reported in 10/17 families [68–70, 80]. All VMCM-associated mutations are intracellular, located in the 1st tyrosine kinase, kinase insert, and C-terminal tail domains of the receptor. They cause ligand-independent *TIE2* hyperphosphorylation when overexpressed in vitro [68–70]. The R849W mutation has been found to have a strong Akt and ShcA-dependent anti-apoptotic effect [81, 82] but does not cause proliferation. It also causes hyperphosphorylation of the transcription factor STAT1 in human umbilical vein endothelial cells (HUVECs) in vitro, inhibiting VEGF-A-mediated angiogenesis by competing with STAT3 for its promoter targets [83, 84]. A somatic 2nd-hit mutation has been identified in one patient with the inherited R849W change, indicating that VMCM, like CCM and GVM, has a paradominant mode of inheritance [85]. The somatic mutation deletes most of the extracellular *Ig2* ligand-binding domain of the wild-type allele, resulting in a loss of its function. This would suggest that the presence of the wild-type receptor exerts an as-yet-undefined protective or competitive effect on the mutant receptor.

Sporadic Venous Malformation (VM)

Somatic mutations in TIE2 also cause common sporadic VM, characterized by the presence of single large lesions, although multifocal lesions can in rare cases occur [85, 86]. A recurrent p. Leu914Phe (L914F) has been identified in affected tissues from >75 % of patients. Almost all of the remainder carry double mutations in cis (on the same allele), commonly combining modifications of p.Tyr897 (to Cys, His, Phe, or Ser) with a second change in the kinase insert or C-terminal tail domains [85, 86]. All of the mutations cause ligand-independent receptor phosphorylation when overexpressed. This is also true for certain mutations that cause premature truncation of TIE2 in the C-terminal tail region, which is otherwise held in an inhibitory conformation. The relatively strong phosphorylation caused by L914F as compared to R849W is echoed by a stronger effect on downstream AKT and STAT1 phosphorylation [87].

In addition to a pro-survival effect on ECs, Akt phosphorylation causes phosphorylation and inactivation of transcription factors FOXO1 and 4. The major vascular smooth muscle cell-attractant PDGFB is among the FOXO1 target genes downregulated as a result in vitro as well as in vivo around malformed veins in patient tissues [87]. This is hypothesized to account for the paucity

and irregularity of the mural cell layer observed in VM. Angpt1 ligand activation of TIE2 similarly results in downregulation of PDGFB, suggesting that it does not play a role in the recruitment of vSMCs to nascent vessels, but in the stabilization and homeostasis of established ones [87].

Blue Rubber Bleb Nevus Syndrome (BRBN)

Blue rubber bleb nevus syndrome (OMIM 112200) is a rare congenital disorder characterized by the presence of a few to hundreds of cutaneous and internal VMs, with gastrointestinal lesions being pathognomonic. Somatic activating mutations in the intracellular region of the TIE2 receptor have been identified in the lesions from a large (>80 %) percentage of patients with BRBN [88]. Double (cis) mutations seem to predispose to multifocal lesions and are significantly enriched in BRBN as compared to common unifocal VM. As in rare multifocal sporadic VM, multiple lesions from the same patient bear the same mutations, undetected in blood, suggesting they arise from common cellular progenitors [88].

Lymphatic Malformations (LM)

LMs are defects in lymphatic structure characterized by no-flow microcystic or macrocystic lesions, lacking connections with the lymphatic vessel system. They consist of dilated channels lined by a flat endothelium, filled with a clear fluid, but no blood except when intracystic bleeding occurs. This can cause the malformations, which otherwise appear to be of normal skin color, to appear bluish purple to red. LMs can be secondary, due to infection or trauma, or primary, in which case they are usually congenital or appear in infancy, growing with the individual. The etiology of these sporadic malformations remains unknown, with major controllers of lymphatic development, such as those implicated in lymphedema, remaining good candidates.

Lymphedema

Lymphedema is a diffuse lymphatic anomaly, characterized by swelling caused by fluid accumulation due to defective lymphatic drainage, usually of the lower extremities. Lymphedema can be primary or secondary due to infection or trauma. Primary lymphedema, which can occur in sporadic as well as incompletely penetrant, inherited forms, can either be isolated or form part of syndromes, such as Turner syndrome (short stature, estrogen deficiency, and cardiac and other problems caused by partial or complete chromosome X-monosomy) and Noonan syndrome (short stature, facial dysmorphism, and cardiac defects, for which gain-of-function mutations in genes in the *MAPK* kinase pathway including *PTPN11*, *KRAS*, *SOS1*, and *RAF1* have been identified). Primary lymphedema is further subdivided according to age at onset of the disease into: type I congenital lymphedema, usually present at birth, which can sometimes cause prenatal pleural effusion and hydrops fetalis; type II praecox lymphedema or Meige disease (OMIM 153200), which occurs between puberty and 35 years of age; and lymphedema tarda, which occurs later in life.

Eleven genes have been identified to cause different forms of lymphedema, several of which modulate, or respond to, VEGFR3 signaling [89]. These account for only a small proportion of the disease, however, an indication of the high level of genetic heterogeneity underlying the phenotype when defined broadly. An autosomal-dominant inherited form of congenital primary lymphedema called Nonne-Milroy disease (OMIM 153100) can be caused by phosphorylation-inhibitory mutations in the tyrosine kinase domain of the vascular endothelial growth factor receptor 3 (*VEGFR-3* or *FLT-4*) [90, 91]. De novo mutations in the gene have been identified in sporadic cases [92], and a homozygous change creating a hypomorphic allele was identified in a recessive case [93]. *VEGFR3* expression is found to be elevated in lymphatic ECs; *Vegfr3* mutant (*Chy*) and receptor-deficient mice show a very similar phenotype to the human, supporting its role in lymphangiogenesis and lymphedema pathogenesis [94, 95].

Exome sequencing identified a small frame-shifting deletion in the VEGFR3 ligand VEGFC in one family with a phenotype similar to that associated with VEGFR3 mutations [96]. *Chy-3* mice, which are lack one copy of the *VEGFC* gene, have chylous ascites and lymphedema. Homozygous knockout mice are unable to form lymphatics, while heterozygotes show lymphatic hypoplasia [97, 98].

A homozygous frame-shifting deletion of exon 7 has been identified in PTPN14, a non-receptor type protein tyrosine phosphatase, in a family with lymphedema with choanal atresia (OMIM 608911) [99]. PTPN14 was shown to interact with VEGFR3, and complex formation was increased by stimulation with VEGFC. Mice lacking the phosphatase develop lymphatic hyperplasia and lymphedema by about 5 months of age [99].

Homozygous and compound-heterozygous mutations in collagen and calcium-binding protein with EGF domain 1 (CCBE1) cause Hennekam syndrome (lymphedema, lymphangiectasia-mental retardation; OMIM 235510) [100–102]. CCBE1 has been found to amplify VEGFC-mediated lymphangiogenesis [103]. Both mouse and zebra fish embryos lacking the protein develop edema due to the failure to develop lymphatic vessels [103, 104].

Mutations in the transcription factors FOXC2, SOX18, and GATA2 have been implicated in forms of primary lymphedema. Loss of function and missense mutations in *FOXC2* can cause inherited lymphedema associated with distichiasis (OMIM 153400), ptosis (OMIM 153000), and yellow nail syndrome (OMIM 153300) [105–107]. Foxc2-deficient mice have abnormally patterned lymphatics with increased pericyte coverage and fail to develop lymphatic valves [108].

The causative gene in some inherited cases of hypotrichosis-lymphedema-telangiectasia syndrome (HLTS; OMIM 607823), characterized by sparse hair and lymphedema and, sometimes, cutaneous telangiectasias, has been identified as *SOX18* [109]. Mutations can act in either a dominant or a recessive manner, and the dominant truncating mutation is associated with progressive renal failure [110]. *Ragged (Ra)* mice have a very similar phenotype to the human, caused by four different (probably dominant-negative) mutations in *Sox-18*, which impair its transactivation and interaction with partner *MEF2C* [111, 112].

Whole-exome sequencing was instrumental in the discovery that mutations in GATA2 can cause Emberger syndrome (OMIM 614038) [113, 114], in which myelodysplastic syndromes occur with lymphedema. No obvious lymphatic phenotypes were observed in GATA2-deficient mice [115]; however, the protein is highly expressed in lymphatic valves and controls the expression of genes involved in their development [114]. Certain connexins also play important roles in the lymphatic valves, and missense mutations in two members of this family of gap junction proteins can cause lymphedema: GJC2 (CX47), which causes lymphedema of all four limbs [116, 117], and GJA1 (CX43), which causes oculodentodigital syndrome (OMIM 164200) with which lymphedema was associated in one family [118].

Whole-exome sequencing identified heterozygous mutations in the kinesin KIF11 (EG5) in lymphedema associated with microcephaly with or without chorioretinopathy and mental retardation (MLCRD; OMIM 152950) [119]. The kinesins are involved in spindle formation, chromosome arrangement, and centrosome separation during cell division. While homozygous KIF11 knockout mice show preimplantation lethality, heterozygotes appear normal, suggesting the mutations that occur in humans may exert dominant-negative effects [120]. Finally, the rare osteoporosis, lymphedema, anhidrotic ectodermal dysplasia with immunodeficiency (OLEDAID; OMIM 308300) syndrome, in which lymphedema occurs in early childhood, has been found to be caused by loss-of-function mutations in IKBKG (NEMO) [121–124]. IKBKG is a component of the IKB kinase (IKK) complex, which activates the transcription factor NFkB by phosphorylating the inhibitor IKB, causing the ubiquitination and degradation of the latter. Loss of NEMO therefore decreases the activation of NFkB in response to inflammatory cytokines [125]. Autosomal recessive Aagenaes syndrome or hereditary cholestasis with lymphedema (OMIM 214900), which shows, among other symptoms, growth retardation, rickets, jaundice, and lymphedema, may be caused by an as-yet unidentified gene on 15q [126].

Arteriovenous Malformation (AVM)

AVMs are fast-flow lesions in which a direct connection is made between arteries and veins (AV fistulas or AVF), or the capillary bed interconnecting them is replaced by a "nidus," in which many arteries connect with and empty directly into draining veins, accompanied by fibrosis and thickened muscle walls. The genetic bases of sporadic AVM are unknown, and molecules that participate in AV differentiation, such as those involved in the Notch signaling pathway, are considered to be good candidates (as reviewed in [127]). Genes for various inherited syndromes associated with AVMs, such as CM-AVM and hereditary hemorrhagic telangiectasia (HHT), have on the other hand been successfully identified.

Hereditary Hemorrhagic Telangiectasia (HHT)

HHT (Rendu-Osler-Weber or ROW; OMIM 187300), an autosomal-dominant disorder characterized by epistaxis, telangiectasias, and AVMs in the brain, lung, or liver, has an estimated incidence of about 1–2 in 10,000. Telangiectasias, which are local dilations of postcapillary venules with increased SMC layers, are also observed in other syndromes including ataxia-telangiectasia (Louis Bar syndrome; OMIM 208900), a recessive disorder with neurovascular symptoms including cerebellar ataxia, caused by inactivating mutations in the nuclear protein kinase *ATM* [128], which activates cellular responses to double-stranded breaks in DNA.

At least four different genes can mediate the disease: HHT1 is caused by mutations in endoglin

(*ENG*) [129], and HHT2 by those in activin receptor-like kinase 1 (*ALK1*) [130]. The hundreds of mutations identified in both genes seem to cause haploinsufficiency (reviewed in [131]). Loci on *5q31.3–32* and *7p14* are linked to HHT3 and HHT4, respectively [132, 133], although the causative genes remain to be identified. HHT1 and HHT2 have similar phenotypes, although cerebral and pulmonary AVMs are more common in HHT1, which shows earlier onset and a lower penetrance than HHT2, in which hepatic AVMs are more frequent [134]. Autosomal-dominant juvenile (gastrointestinal) polyposis-HHT syndrome (JPHT; OMIM 175050) is caused by *MADH4/SMAD4* [135].

Both the *HHT1* and *HHT2* genes, as well as *SMAD4*, belong to the TGF-β pathway, known to be extremely important in regulating cell proliferation, migration, and differentiation, as well as the extracellular matrix composition in the vascular (and many other) systems (reviewed in [127]). Ligands of the TGF superfamily, which include the TGF-βs, activin, and bone morphogenetic proteins (BMPs), bind heteromeric receptor complexes consisting of the type 1 (binding) receptors and the type II (signaling) receptors. ALK1 is a type I serine-threonine kinase receptor, activated by BMPs 9 and 10 [136, 137]. ENG is a homodimeric transmembrane glycoprotein that interacts with the heteromeric receptors for the TGF-β family (including *ALK1* in vECs), modulating cellular responses to these ligands [138, 139]. In vECs, TGF-β signaling through ALK1 is mediated by the receptor-regulated (R-)SMADs 1, 5, and 8. Ubiquitously expressed SMAD4 hetero-oligomerizes with activated R-SMADs, which then translocate to the nucleus and transcriptionally activate gene expression [140, 141].

Alk1$^{-/-}$ mice die at mid-gestation, with few capillaries, AVMs between major vessels, and defective vSMC recruitment. *Alk1*$^{+/-}$ heterozygous deletion mutants do have an HHT-like phenotype, with mucocutaneous and visceral lesions [142, 143]. *Eng*$^{-/-}$ mice also show embryonic lethality, with vascular and cardiac defects, and the presence of AVMs between major vessels with *Eng*$^{+/-}$ mice showing HHT phenotypes like cerebral AVMs and telangiectasias [144].

Deletion of the murine version *Dpc4* causes embryonic death, with significantly smaller size, low levels of proliferation, lack of a mesoderm, and disorganized endoderm; heterozygous mutants however seem normal [145].

A recent study employed exome sequencing on probands diagnosed with HHT but with no mutation identified in the known genes and identified mutations in BMP9 in a small proportion of cases [146]. Careful examination revealed that the dermal lesions in these individuals more closely resembled those of CM-AVM. BMP9 is a ligand that binds the ENG and ALK1 receptors on endothelial cells; it therefore belongs to the pathway previously implicated in HHT pathogenesis. The mutations identified seem to reduce processing of the protein into the mature, secreted form. Morpholino-mediated knockdown of BMP9 in zebra fish resulted in subtle defects in venous remodeling, suggesting other ligands may compensate for its absence in this system [146].

Overgrowth Syndromes

Mutations in the tumor suppressor gene phosphatase and tensin homolog (*PTEN*) have been identified in a group of complex tumor-susceptibility syndromes often associated with fast-flow vascular anomalies, collectively termed PTEN hamartoma tumor syndrome or PHTS (reviewed in [147]). They include Cowden syndrome (CS; OMIM 158350), with mucocutaneous lesions, GI hamartomas, and increased risk of carcinomas; Bannayan-Riley-Ruvalcaba syndrome (BRRS; OMIM 153480) which shows macrocephaly, lipomas, GI polyps, thyroiditis, and vascular malformations; and Proteus syndrome (PLS; OMIM 176920), with hand and foot overgrowth, limb asymmetry, and cranial hyperostosis. PTEN, a lipid and protein (tyrosine and serine-threonine) phosphatase, inhibits the PI3K-Akt survival pathway [148]. EC-specific deletion of *PTEN* is embryonic lethal due to cardiac and vascular anomalies, increased EC proliferation, drop in the number of vessels, which are dilated, and defective vSMC recruitment; heterozygous knockouts do not manifest vascular abnormalities [149].

More recently, mutations in other components of the PI3K-Akt pathway have been implicated in overgrowth syndromes: germline activating mutations in PIK3CA and AKT1 were identified in Cowden and Cowden-like syndrome [150], while next-generation exome sequencing of patient tissues revealed somatic mosaic activating mutations in AKT1 in Proteus syndrome [151] and PIK3CA in CLOVES syndrome (congenital lipomatous overgrowth with vascular, epidermal, and skeletal anomalies; OMIM 612918) [21].

Concluding Remarks

The genetic etiology and pathogenic mechanisms underlying the wide variety of vascular malformations that occur in humans represent a complex problem. Studies have begun to reveal certain common themes, however. While vascular malformations are more commonly sporadic than inherited, factors such as incomplete penetrance and the presence of small or asymptomatic lesions can make it difficult to rule out any family history of these anomalies. The sporadic forms are sometimes caused by somatic mosaic mutations in the same genes and/or pathways implicated in their rare, inherited counterparts. Somatic mutations also play an important role both in the inherited forms, with local 2nd hits compounding the effects of inherited pathogenic alleles. This is corroborated by data from animal models: homozygous gene deletions typically cause profound vascular defects and embryonic lethality, while heterozygous deletion mutants fail to exhibit any vascular phenotypes; the use of conditional, cell-specific mutants with localized (homozygous) defects in gene function can be more useful in recapitulating and unraveling the effects of disease mutations. In this context, it is interesting to note that endothelial cells seem to be the primary cell type affected by most of the disease-causative mutations identified thus far. The detection of somatic mosaic mutations can be hampered by tissue heterogeneity and inadequate sensitivity of screening methods. Enrichment of affected cells by careful resection of affected tissue areas and/or laser microdissection, and the use of deep sequencing that allows for the detection of variants across the genome, even when present at low frequencies, has led to an explosion in the number of disease-causative changes identified.

References

1. Adams RH, Alitalo K (2007) Molecular regulation of angiogenesis and lymphangiogenesis. Nat Rev Mol Cell Biol 8:464–478
2. Mulliken JB, Glowacki J (1982) Hemangiomas and vascular malformations in infants and children: a classification based on endothelial characteristics. Plast Reconstr Surg 69:412–422
3. Walter JW, Blei F, Anderson JL, Orlow SJ, Speer MC, Marchuk DA (1999) Genetic mapping of a novel familial form of infantile hemangioma. Am J Med Genet 82:77–83
4. Jinnin M, Medici D, Park L, Limaye N, Liu Y, Boscolo E, Bischoff J, Vikkula M, Boye E, Olsen BR (2008) Suppressed NFAT-dependent VEGFR1 expression and constitutive VEGFR2 signaling in infantile hemangioma. Nat Med 14:1236–1246
5. Khan ZA, Boscolo E, Picard A, Psutka S, Melero-Martin JM, Bartch TC, Mulliken JB, Bischoff J (2008) Multipotential stem cells recapitulate human infantile hemangioma in immunodeficient mice. J Clin Invest 118:2592–2599
6. Boon LM, Vikkula M (2007) Vascular malformations. In: Fitzpatrick's dermatology in general medicine. McGraw-Hill Professional Publishing, Maidenhead
7. Boon LM, Vikkula M (2013) Molecular genetics of vascular malformations. In: Mulliken JB, Burrows PE, Fishman SJ, (eds) Mulliken and Young's Vascular Anomalies: Hemangiomas and Malformations. 2nd ed. New York, NY: Oxford University Press
8. Uebelhoer M, Boon LM, Vikkula M (2012) Vascular anomalies: from genetics toward models for therapeutic trials. Cold Spring Harb Perspect Med 2. doi:10.1101/cshperspect.a009688
9. Eerola I, Boon LM, Mulliken JB, Burrows PE, Dompmartin A, Watanabe S, Vanwijck R, Vikkula M (2003) Capillary malformation-arteriovenous malformation, a new clinical and genetic disorder caused by RASA1 mutations. Am J Hum Genet 73:1240–1249
10. Revencu N, Boon LM, Mulliken JB, Enjolras O, Cordisco MR, Burrows PE, Clapuyt P, Hammer F, Dubois J, Baselga E et al (2008) Parkes Weber syndrome, vein of Galen aneurysmal malformation, and other fast-flow vascular anomalies are caused by RASA1 mutations. Hum Mutat 29:959–965
11. Revencu N, Boon LM, Mendola A, Cordisco MR, Dubois J, Clapuyt P, Hammer F, Amor DJ, Irvine AD, Baselga E et al (2013) RASA1 mutations and associated phenotypes in 68 families with capillary malformation-arteriovenous malformation. Hum Mutat 34:1632–1641

12. Hu KQ, Settleman J (1997) Tandem SH2 binding sites mediate the RasGAP-RhoGAP interaction: a conformational mechanism for SH3 domain regulation. EMBO J 16:473–483

13. Kulkarni SV, Gish G, van der Geer P, Henkemeyer M, Pawson T (2000) Role of p120 Ras-GAP in directed cell movement. J Cell Biol 149:457–470

14. Yue Y, Lypowy J, Hedhli N, Abdellatif M (2004) Ras GTPase-activating protein binds to Akt and is required for its activation. J Biol Chem 279:12883–12889

15. Henkemeyer M, Rossi DJ, Holmyard DP, Puri MC, Mbamalu G, Harpal K, Shih TS, Jacks T, Pawson T (1995) Vascular system defects and neuronal apoptosis in mice lacking ras GTPase-activating protein. Nature 377:695–701

16. Burrows PE, Gonzalez-Garay ML, Rasmussen JC, Aldrich MB, Guilliod R, Maus EA, Fife CE, Kwon S, Lapinski PE, King PD et al (2013) Lymphatic abnormalities are associated with RASA1 gene mutations in mouse and man. Proc Natl Acad Sci U S A 110:8621–8626

17. Revencu N, Boon LM, Dompmartin A, Rieu P, Busch WL, Dubois J, Forzano F, van Hagen JM, Halbach S, Kuechler A et al (2013) Germline mutations in RASA1 are not found in patients with Klippel-Trenaunay syndrome or capillary malformation with limb overgrowth. Mol Syndromol 4:173–178

18. Whelan AJ, Watson MS, Porter FD, Steiner RD (1995) Klippel-Trenaunay-Weber syndrome associated with a 5:11 balanced translocation. Am J Med Genet 59:492–494

19. Tian XL, Kadaba R, You SA, Liu M, Timur AA, Yang L, Chen Q, Szafranski P, Rao S, Wu L et al (2004) Identification of an angiogenic factor that when mutated causes susceptibility to Klippel-Trenaunay syndrome. Nature 427:640–645

20. Chen D, Li L, Tu X, Yin Z, Wang Q (2013) Functional characterization of Klippel-Trenaunay syndrome gene AGGF1 identifies a novel angiogenic signaling pathway for specification of vein differentiation and angiogenesis during embryogenesis. Hum Mol Genet 22:963–976

21. Kurek KC, Luks VL, Ayturk UM, Alomari AI, Fishman SJ, Spencer SA, Mulliken JB, Bowen ME, Yamamoto GL, Kozakewich HP et al (2012) Somatic mosaic activating mutations in PIK3CA cause CLOVES syndrome. Am J Hum Genet 90:1108–1115

22. Shirley MD, Tang H, Gallione CJ, Baugher JD, Frelin LP, Cohen B, North PE, Marchuk DA, Comi AM, Pevsner J (2013) Sturge-Weber syndrome and port-wine stains caused by somatic mutation in GNAQ. N Engl J Med 368:1971–1979

23. McDonell LM, Mirzaa GM, Alcantara D, Schwartzentruber J, Carter MT, Lee LJ, Clericuzio CL, Graham JM Jr, Morris-Rosendahl DJ, Polster T et al (2013) Mutations in STAMBP, encoding a deubiquitinating enzyme, cause microcephaly-capillary malformation syndrome. Nat Genet 45:556–562

24. Laberge-le Couteulx S, Jung HH, Labauge P, Houtteville JP, Lescoat C, Cecillon M, Marechal E,

Joutel A, Bach JF, Tournier-Lasserve E (1999) Truncating mutations in CCM1, encoding KRIT1, cause hereditary cavernous angiomas. Nat Genet 23: 189–193

25. Sahoo T, Johnson EW, Thomas JW, Kuehl PM, Jones TL, Dokken CG, Touchman JW, Gallione CJ, Lee-Lin SQ, Kosofsky B et al (1999) Mutations in the gene encoding KRIT1, a Krev-1/rap1a binding protein, cause cerebral cavernous malformations (CCM1). Hum Mol Genet 8:2325–2333

26. Liquori CL, Berg MJ, Siegel AM, Huang E, Zawistowski JS, Stoffer T, Verlaan D, Balogun F, Hughes L, Leedom TP et al (2003) Mutations in a gene encoding a novel protein containing a phosphotyrosine-binding domain cause type 2 cerebral cavernous malformations. Am J Hum Genet 73:1459–1464

27. Bergametti F, Denier C, Labauge P, Arnoult M, Boetto S, Clanet M, Coubes P, Echenne B, Ibrahim R, Irthum B et al (2005) Mutations within the programmed cell death 10 gene cause cerebral cavernous malformations. Am J Hum Genet 76:42–51

28. Liquori CL, Berg MJ, Squitieri F, Ottenbacher M, Sorlie M, Leedom TP, Cannella M, Maglione V, Ptacek L, Johnson EW et al (2006) Low frequency of PDCD10 mutations in a panel of CCM3 probands: potential for a fourth CCM locus. Hum Mutat 27:118

29. Eerola I, Plate KH, Spiegel R, Boon LM, Mulliken JB, Vikkula M (2000) KRIT1 is mutated in hyperkeratotic cutaneous capillary-venous malformation associated with cerebral capillary malformation. Hum Mol Genet 9:1351–1355

30. Sirvente J, Enjolras O, Wassef M, Tournier-Lasserve E, Labauge P (2009) Frequency and phenotypes of cutaneous vascular malformations in a consecutive series of 417 patients with familial cerebral cavernous malformations. J Eur Acad Dermatol Venereol 23:1066–1072

31. Kehrer-Sawatzki H, Wilda M, Braun VM, Richter HP, Hameister H (2002) Mutation and expression analysis of the KRIT1 gene associated with cerebral cavernous malformations (CCM1). Acta Neuropathol 104:231–240

32. Gault J, Shenkar R, Recksiek P, Awad IA (2005) Biallelic somatic and germ line CCM1 truncating mutations in a cerebral cavernous malformation lesion. Stroke 36:872–874

33. Zawistowski JS, Stalheim L, Uhlik MT, Abell AN, Ancrile BB, Johnson GL, Marchuk DA (2005) CCM1 and CCM2 protein interactions in cell signaling: implications for cerebral cavernous malformations pathogenesis. Hum Mol Genet 14:2521–2531

34. Voss K, Stahl S, Schleider E, Ullrich S, Nickel J, Mueller TD, Felbor U (2007) CCM3 interacts with CCM2 indicating common pathogenesis for cerebral cavernous malformations. Neurogenetics 8:249–256

35. Zhang J, Clatterbuck RE, Rigamonti D, Chang DD, Dietz HC (2001) Interaction between krit1 and icap1alpha infers perturbation of integrin beta1-mediated

angiogenesis in the pathogenesis of cerebral cavernous malformation. Hum Mol Genet 10:2953–2960

36. Uhlik MT, Abell AN, Johnson NL, Sun W, Cuevas BD, Lobel-Rice KE, Horne EA, Dell'Acqua ML, Johnson GL (2003) Rac-MEKK3-MKK3 scaffolding for p38 MAPK activation during hyperosmotic shock. Nat Cell Biol 5:1104–1110

37. Serebriiskii I, Estojak J, Sonoda G, Testa JR, Golemis EA (1997) Association of Krev-1/rap1a with Krit1, a novel ankyrin repeat-containing protein encoded by a gene mapping to 7q21-22. Oncogene 15:1043–1049

38. Glading A, Han J, Stockton RA, Ginsberg MH (2007) KRIT-1/CCM1 is a Rap1 effector that regulates endothelial cell cell junctions. J Cell Biol 179:247–254

39. Wustehube J, Bartol A, Liebler SS, Brutsch R, Zhu Y, Felbor U, Sure U, Augustin HG, Fischer A (2010) Cerebral cavernous malformation protein CCM1 inhibits sprouting angiogenesis by activating DELTA-NOTCH signaling. Proc Natl Acad Sci U S A 107:12640–12645

40. Borikova AL, Dibble CF, Sciaky N, Welch CM, Abell AN, Bencharit S, Johnson GL (2010) Rho kinase inhibition rescues the endothelial cell cerebral cavernous malformation phenotype. J Biol Chem 285:11760–11764

41. Stockton RA, Shenkar R, Awad IA, Ginsberg MH (2010) Cerebral cavernous malformations proteins inhibit Rho kinase to stabilize vascular integrity. J Exp Med 207:881–896

42. Whitehead KJ, Plummer NW, Adams JA, Marchuk DA, Li DY (2004) Ccm1 is required for arterial morphogenesis: implications for the etiology of human cavernous malformations. Development 131:1437–1448

43. Plummer NW, Gallione CJ, Srinivasan S, Zawistowski JS, Louis DN, Marchuk DA (2004) Loss of p53 sensitizes mice with a mutation in Ccm1 (KRIT1) to development of cerebral vascular malformations. Am J Pathol 165:1509–1518

44. Plummer NW, Squire TL, Srinivasan S, Huang E, Zawistowski JS, Matsunami H, Hale LP, Marchuk DA (2006) Neuronal expression of the Ccm2 gene in a new mouse model of cerebral cavernous malformations. Mamm Genome 17:119–128

45. Hogan BM, Bussmann J, Wolburg H, Schulte-Merker S (2008) ccm1 cell autonomously regulates endothelial cellular morphogenesis and vascular tubulogenesis in zebrafish. Hum Mol Genet 17:2424–2432

46. Voss K, Stahl S, Hogan BM, Reinders J, Schleider E, Schulte-Merker S, Felbor U (2009) Functional analyses of human and zebrafish 18-amino acid in-frame deletion pave the way for domain mapping of the cerebral cavernous malformation 3 protein. Hum Mutat 30:1003–1011

47. Boon LM, Mulliken JB, Enjolras O, Vikkula M (2004) Glomuvenous malformation (glomangioma) and venous malformation: distinct clinicopathologic and genetic entities. Arch Dermatol 140:971–976

48. Dompmartin A, Vikkula M, Boon LM (2010) Venous malformation: update on aetiopathogenesis, diagnosis and management. Phlebology 25:224–235

49. Brouillard P, Boon LM, Mulliken JB, Enjolras O, Ghassibe M, Warman ML, Tan OT, Olsen BR, Vikkula M (2002) Mutations in a novel factor, glomulin, are responsible for glomuvenous malformations ("glomangiomas"). Am J Hum Genet 70:866–874

50. Brouillard P, Ghassibe M, Penington A, Boon LM, Dompmartin A, Temple IK, Cordisco M, Adams D, Piette F, Harper JI et al (2005) Four common glomulin mutations cause two thirds of glomuvenous malformations ("familial glomangiomas"): evidence for a founder effect. J Med Genet 42:e13

51. Brouillard P, Boon LM, Revencu N, Berg J, Dompmartin A, Dubois J, Garzon M, Holden S, Kangesu L, Labreze C et al (2013) Genotypes and phenotypes of 162 families with a glomulin mutation. Mol Syndromol 4:157–164

52. Amyere M, Aerts V, Brouillard P, McIntyre BA, Duhoux FP, Wassef M, Enjolras O, Mulliken JB, Devuyst O, Antoine-Poirel H et al (2013) Somatic uniparental isodisomy explains multifocality of glomuvenous malformations. Am J Hum Genet 92:188–196

53. McIntyre BA, Brouillard P, Aerts V, Gutierrez-Roelens I, Vikkula M (2004) Glomulin is predominantly expressed in vascular smooth muscle cells in the embryonic and adult mouse. Gene Expr Patterns 4:351–358

54. Chambraud B, Radanyi C, Camonis JH, Shazand K, Rajkowski K, Baulieu EE (1996) FAP48, a new protein that forms specific complexes with both immunophilins FKBP59 and FKBP12. Prevention by the immunosuppressant drugs FK506 and rapamycin. J Biol Chem 271:32923–32929

55. Chen YG, Liu F, Massague J (1997) Mechanism of TGFbeta receptor inhibition by FKBP12. EMBO J 16:3866–3876

56. Grisendi S, Chambraud B, Gout I, Comoglio PM, Crepaldi T (2001) Ligand-regulated binding of FAP68 to the hepatocyte growth factor receptor. J Biol Chem 276:46632–46638

57. Taher TE, Derksen PW, de Boer OJ, Spaargaren M, Teeling P, van der Wal AC, Pals ST (2002) Hepatocyte growth factor triggers signaling cascades mediating vascular smooth muscle cell migration. Biochem Biophys Res Commun 298:80–86

58. Harrison P, Bradley L, Bomford A (2000) Mechanism of regulation of HGF/SF gene expression in fibroblasts by TGF-beta1. Biochem Biophys Res Commun 271:203–211

59. Zhang X, Yang J, Li Y, Liu Y (2005) Both Sp1 and Smad participate in mediating TGF-beta1-induced HGF receptor expression in renal epithelial cells. Am J Physiol Renal Physiol 288:F16–F26

60. Arai T, Kasper JS, Skaar JR, Ali SH, Takahashi C, DeCaprio JA (2003) Targeted disruption of p185/Cul7 gene results in abnormal vascular morphogenesis. Proc Natl Acad Sci U S A 100:9855–9860

61. Duda DM, Olszewski JL, Tron AE, Hammel M, Lambert LJ, Waddell MB, Mittag T, DeCaprio JA, Schulman BA (2012) Structure of a glomulin-RBX1-CUL1 complex: inhibition of a RING E3 ligase through masking of its E2-binding surface. Mol Cell 47:371–382

62. Tron AE, Arai T, Duda DM, Kuwabara H, Olszewski JL, Fujiwara Y, Bahamon BN, Signoretti S, Schulman BA, DeCaprio JA (2012) The glomuvenous malformation protein Glomulin binds Rbx1 and regulates cullin RING ligase-mediated turnover of Fbw7. Mol Cell 46:67–78

63. Dompmartin A, Acher A, Thibon P, Tourbach S, Hermans C, Deneys V, Pocock B, Lequerrec A, Labbe D, Barrellier MT et al (2008) Association of localized intravascular coagulopathy with venous malformations. Arch Dermatol 144:873–877

64. Dompmartin A, Ballieux F, Thibon P, Lequerrec A, Hermans C, Clapuyt P, Barrellier MT, Hammer F, Labbe D, Vikkula M et al (2009) Elevated D-dimer level in the differential diagnosis of venous malformations. Arch Dermatol 145:1239–1244

65. Suri C, Jones PF, Patan S, Bartunkova S, Maisonpierre PC, Davis S, Sato TN, Yancopoulos GD (1996) Requisite role of angiopoietin-1, a ligand for the TIE2 receptor, during embryonic angiogenesis. Cell 87:1171–1180

66. Maisonpierre PC, Suri C, Jones PF, Bartunkova S, Wiegand SJ, Radziejewski C, Compton D, McClain J, Aldrich TH, Papadopoulos N et al (1997) Angiopoietin-2, a natural antagonist for Tie2 that disrupts in vivo angiogenesis. Science 277:55–60

67. Valenzuela DM, Griffiths JA, Rojas J, Aldrich TH, Jones PF, Zhou H, McClain J, Copeland NG, Gilbert DJ, Jenkins NA et al (1999) Angiopoietins 3 and 4: diverging gene counterparts in mice and humans. Proc Natl Acad Sci U S A 96:1904–1909

68. Vikkula M, Boon LM, Carraway KL 3rd, Calvert JT, Diamonti AJ, Goumnerov B, Pasyk KA, Marchuk DA, Warman ML, Cantley LC et al (1996) Vascular dysmorphogenesis caused by an activating mutation in the receptor tyrosine kinase TIE2. Cell 87:1181–1190

69. Calvert JT, Riney TJ, Kontos CD, Cha EH, Prieto VG, Shea CR, Berg JN, Nevin NC, Simpson SA, Pasyk KA et al (1999) Allelic and locus heterogeneity in inherited venous malformations. Hum Mol Genet 8:1279–1289

70. Wouters V, Limaye N, Uebelhoer M, Irrthum A, Boon LM, Mulliken JB, Enjolras O, Baselga E, Berg J, Dompmartin A et al (2010) Hereditary cutaneomucosal venous malformations are caused by TIE2 mutations with widely variable hyper-phosphorylating effects. Eur J Hum Genet 18:414–420

71. Limaye N, Uebelhoer M, Boon LM, Vikkula M. TIE2 and cutaneomucosal venous malformation. In: Epstein CJ, Erickson RP, Wynshaw-Boris A (ed) Inborn errors of development. Oxford University Press, Oxford (in press)

72. Hansen TM, Singh H, Tahir TA, Brindle NP (2010) Effects of angiopoietins-1 and −2 on the receptor tyrosine kinase Tie2 are differentially regulated at the endothelial cell surface. Cell Signal 22:527–532

73. Seegar TC, Eller B, Tzvetkova-Robev D, Kolev MV, Henderson SC, Nikolov DB, Barton WA (2010) Tie1-Tie2 interactions mediate functional differences between angiopoietin ligands. Mol Cell 37:643–655

74. Dumont DJ, Gradwohl G, Fong GH, Puri MC, Gertsenstein M, Auerbach A, Breitman ML (1994) Dominant-negative and targeted null mutations in the endothelial receptor tyrosine kinase, tek, reveal a critical role in vasculogenesis of the embryo. Genes Dev 8:1897–1909

75. Sato TN, Tozawa Y, Deutsch U, Wolburg-Buchholz K, Fujiwara Y, Gendron-Maguire M, Gridley T, Wolburg H, Risau W, Qin Y (1995) Distinct roles of the receptor tyrosine kinases Tie-1 and Tie-2 in blood vessel formation. Nature 376:70–74

76. Kontos CD, Stauffer TP, Yang WP, York JD, Huang L, Blanar MA, Meyer T, Peters KG (1998) Tyrosine 1101 of Tie2 is the major site of association of p85 and is required for activation of phosphatidylinositol 3-kinase and Akt. Mol Cell Biol 18:4131–4140

77. Jones N, Master Z, Jones J, Bouchard D, Gunji Y, Sasaki H, Daly R, Alitalo K, Dumont DJ (1999) Identification of Tek/Tie2 binding partners. Binding to a multifunctional docking site mediates cell survival and migration. J Biol Chem 274:30896–30905

78. Jones N, Chen SH, Sturk C, Master Z, Tran J, Kerbel RS, Dumont DJ (2003) A unique autophosphorylation site on Tie2/Tek mediates Dok-R phosphotyrosine binding domain binding and function. Mol Cell Biol 23:2658–2668

79. Hughes DP, Marron MB, Brindle NP (2003) The antiinflammatory endothelial tyrosine kinase Tie2 interacts with a novel nuclear factor-kappaB inhibitor ABIN-2. Circ Res 92:630–636

80. Shu W, Lin Y, Hua R, Luo Y, He N, Fang L, Tan J, Lu J, Hu Z, Yuan Z (2012) Cutaneomucosal venous malformations are linked to the TIE2 mutation in a large Chinese family. Exp Dermatol 21:456–457

81. Morris PN, Dunmore BJ, Brindle NP (2006) Mutant Tie2 causing venous malformation signals through Shc. Biochem Biophys Res Commun 346:335–338

82. Morris PN, Dunmore BJ, Tadros A, Marchuk DA, Darland DC, D'Amore PA, Brindle NP (2005) Functional analysis of a mutant form of the receptor tyrosine kinase Tie2 causing venous malformations. J Mol Med 83:58–63

83. Hu HT, Huang YH, Chang YA, Lee CK, Jiang MJ, Wu LW (2008) Tie2-R849W mutant in venous malformations chronically activates a functional STAT1 to modulate gene expression. J Invest Dermatol 128:2325–2333

84. Huang YH, Wu MP, Pan SC, Su WC, Chen YW, Wu LW (2013) STAT1 activation by venous malformations mutant Tie2-R849W antagonizes

VEGF-A-mediated angiogenic response partly via reduced bFGF production. Angiogenesis 16:207–222

85. Limaye N, Wouters V, Uebelhoer M, Tuominen M, Wirkkala R, Mulliken JB, Eklund L, Boon LM, Vikkula M (2009) Somatic mutations in angiopoietin receptor gene TEK cause solitary and multiple sporadic venous malformations. Nat Genet 41:118–124

86. Soblet J, Limaye N, Uebelhoer M, Boon LM, Vikkula M (2013) Variable somatic TIE2 mutations in half of sporadic venous malformations. Mol Syndromol 4:179–183

87. Uebelhoer M, Natynki M, Kangas J, Mendola A, Nguyen HL, Soblet J, Godfraind C, Boon LM, Eklund L, Limaye N et al (2013) Venous malformation-causative TIE2 mutations mediate an AKT-dependent decrease in PDGFB. Hum Mol Genet 22:3438–3448

88. Soblet J, Kangas J, Nätynki M, Mendola A, Helaers R, Uebelhoer M, Kaakinen M, Cordisco M, Dompmartin A, Enjolras O et al. Somatic Gain-of-function TIE2 Mutations cause Blue Rubber Bleb Nevus Syndrome and Multifocal Sporadic Venous Malformation. In Preparation.

89. Mendola A, Schlögel MJ, Ghalamkarpour A, Irrthum A, Nguyen HL, Fastré E, Bygum A, van der Vleuten C, Fagerberg C, Baselga E et al (2013) Mutations in the VEGFR3 signaling pathway explain 36% of familial lymphedema. Mol Syndromol 4:257–266

90. Irrthum A, Karkkainen MJ, Devriendt K, Alitalo K, Vikkula M (2000) Congenital hereditary lymphedema caused by a mutation that inactivates VEGFR3 tyrosine kinase. Am J Hum Genet 67:295–301

91. Karkkainen MJ, Ferrell RE, Lawrence EC, Kimak MA, Levinson KL, McTigue MA, Alitalo K, Finegold DN (2000) Missense mutations interfere with VEGFR-3 signalling in primary lymphoedema. Nat Genet 25:153–159

92. Ghalamkarpour A, Morlot S, Raas-Rothschild A, Utkus A, Mulliken JB, Boon LM, Vikkula M (2006) Hereditary lymphedema type I associated with VEGFR3 mutation: the first de novo case and atypical presentations. Clin Genet 70:330–335

93. Ghalamkarpour A, Holnthoner W, Saharinen P, Boon LM, Mulliken JB, Alitalo K, Vikkula M (2009) Recessive primary congenital lymphoedema caused by a VEGFR3 mutation. J Med Genet 46:399–404

94. Karkkainen MJ, Saaristo A, Jussila L, Karila KA, Lawrence EC, Pajusola K, Bueler H, Eichmann A, Kauppinen R, Kettunen MI et al (2001) A model for gene therapy of human hereditary lymphedema. Proc Natl Acad Sci U S A 98:12677–12682

95. Dumont DJ, Jussila L, Taipale J, Lymboussaki A, Mustonen T, Pajusola K, Breitman M, Alitalo K (1998) Cardiovascular failure in mouse embryos deficient in VEGF receptor-3. Science 282:946–949

96. Gordon K, Schulte D, Brice G, Simpson MA, Roukens MG, van Impel A, Connell F, Kalidas K, Jeffery S, Mortimer PS et al (2013) Mutation in vascular endothelial growth factor-C, a ligand for vascu-

lar endothelial growth factor receptor-3, is associated with autosomal dominant milroy-like primary lymphedema. Circ Res 112:956–960

97. Karkkainen MJ, Haiko P, Sainio K, Partanen J, Taipale J, Petrova TV, Jeltsch M, Jackson DG, Talikka M, Rauvala H et al (2004) Vascular endothelial growth factor C is required for sprouting of the first lymphatic vessels from embryonic veins. Nat Immunol 5:74–80

98. Dellinger MT, Hunter RJ, Bernas MJ, Witte MH, Erickson RP (2007) Chy-3 mice are Vegfc haploinsufficient and exhibit defective dermal superficial to deep lymphatic transition and dermal lymphatic hypoplasia. Dev Dyn 236:2346–2355

99. Au AC, Hernandez PA, Lieber E, Nadroo AM, Shen YM, Kelley KA, Gelb BD, Diaz GA (2010) Protein tyrosine phosphatase PTPN14 is a regulator of lymphatic function and choanal development in humans. Am J Hum Genet 87:436–444

100. Alders M, Hogan BM, Gjini E, Salehi F, Al-Gazali L, Hennekam EA, Holmberg EE, Mannens MM, Mulder MF, Offerhaus GJ et al (2009) Mutations in CCBE1 cause generalized lymph vessel dysplasia in humans. Nat Genet 41:1272–1274

101. Connell F, Kalidas K, Ostergaard P, Brice G, Homfray T, Roberts L, Bunyan DJ, Mitton S, Mansour S, Mortimer P et al (2010) Linkage and sequence analysis indicate that CCBE1 is mutated in recessively inherited generalised lymphatic dysplasia. Hum Genet 127:231–241

102. Alders M, Mendola A, Ades L, Al Gazali L, Bellini C, Dallapiccola B, Edery P, Frank U, Hornshuh F, Huisman SA et al (2013) Evaluation of clinical manifestations in patients with severe lymphedema with and without CCBE1 mutations. Mol Syndromol 4:107–113

103. Bos FL, Caunt M, Peterson-Maduro J, Planas-Paz L, Kowalski J, Karpanen T, van Impel A, Tong R, Ernst JA, Korving J et al (2011) CCBE1 is essential for mammalian lymphatic vascular development and enhances the lymphangiogenic effect of vascular endothelial growth factor-C in vivo. Circ Res 109:486–491

104. Hogan BM, Bos FL, Bussmann J, Witte M, Chi NC, Duckers HJ, Schulte-Merker S (2009) Ccbe1 is required for embryonic lymphangiogenesis and venous sprouting. Nat Genet 41:396–398

105. Fang J, Dagenais SL, Erickson RP, Arlt MF, Glynn MW, Gorski JL, Seaver LH, Glover TW (2000) Mutations in FOXC2 (MFH-1), a forkhead family transcription factor, are responsible for the hereditary lymphedema-distichiasis syndrome. Am J Hum Genet 67:1382–1388

106. Bell R, Brice G, Child AH, Murday VA, Mansour S, Sandy CJ, Collin JR, Brady AF, Callen DF, Burnand K et al (2001) Analysis of lymphoedema-distichiasis families for FOXC2 mutations reveals small insertions and deletions throughout the gene. Hum Genet 108:546–551

107. Finegold DN, Kimak MA, Lawrence EC, Levinson KL, Cherniske EM, Pober BR, Dunlap JW, Ferrell

RE (2001) Truncating mutations in FOXC2 cause multiple lymphedema syndromes. Hum Mol Genet 10:1185–1189

108. Petrova TV, Karpanen T, Norrmén C, Mellor R, Tamakoshi T, Finegold D, Ferrell R, Kerjaschki D, Mortimer P, Ylä-Herttuala S et al (2004) Defective valves and abnormal mural cell recruitment underlie lymphatic vascular failure in lymphedema distichiasis. Nat Med 10(9):974–981

109. Irrthum A, Devriendt K, Chitayat D, Matthijs G, Glade C, Steijlen PM, Fryns JP, Van Steensel MA, Vikkula M (2003) Mutations in the transcription factor gene SOX18 underlie recessive and dominant forms of hypotrichosis-lymphedema-telangiectasia. Am J Hum Genet 72:1470–1478

110. Moalem S, Brouillard P, Kuypers D, Legius E, Harvey E, Taylor G, Francois M, Vikkula M, Chitayat D (2014) Hypotrichosis-lymphedema-telangiectasia-renal defect associated with a truncating mutations in the SOX18 gene. Clin Genet (Epub ahead of print) doi:10.1111/cge.12388

111. Pennisi D, Gardner J, Chambers D, Hosking B, Peters J, Muscat G, Abbott C, Koopman P (2000) Mutations in Sox18 underlie cardiovascular and hair follicle defects in ragged mice. Nat Genet 24:434–437

112. James K, Hosking B, Gardner J, Muscat GE, Koopman P (2003) Sox18 mutations in the ragged mouse alleles ragged-like and opossum. Genesis 36:1–6

113. Ostergaard P, Simpson MA, Connell FC, Steward CG, Brice G, Woollard WJ, Dafou D, Kilo T, Smithson S, Lunt P et al (2011) Mutations in GATA2 cause primary lymphedema associated with a predisposition to acute myeloid leukemia (Emberger syndrome). Nat Genet 43:929–931

114. Kazenwadel J, Secker GA, Liu YJ, Rosenfeld JA, Wildin RS, Cuellar-Rodriguez J, Hsu AP, Dyack S, Fernandez CV, Chong CE et al (2012) Loss-of-function germline GATA2 mutations in patients with MDS/AML or MonoMAC syndrome and primary lymphedema reveal a key role for GATA2 in the lymphatic vasculature. Blood 119:1283–1291

115. Tsai FY, Keller G, Kuo FC, Weiss M, Chen J, Rosenblatt M, Alt FW, Orkin SH (1994) An early haematopoietic defect in mice lacking the transcription factor GATA-2. Nature 371:221–226

116. Ferrell RE, Baty CJ, Kimak MA, Karlsson JM, Lawrence EC, Franke-Snyder M, Meriney SD, Feingold E, Finegold DN (2010) GJC2 missense mutations cause human lymphedema. Am J Hum Genet 86:943–948

117. Ostergaard P, Simpson MA, Brice G, Mansour S, Connell FC, Onoufriadis A, Child AH, Hwang J, Kalidas K, Mortimer PS et al (2011) Rapid identification of mutations in GJC2 in primary lymphoedema using whole exome sequencing combined with linkage analysis with delineation of the phenotype. J Med Genet 48:251–255

118. Brice G, Ostergaard P, Jeffery S, Gordon K, Mortimer PS, Mansour S (2013) A novel mutation in GJA1 causing oculodentodigital syndrome and primary lymphoedema in a three generation family. Clin Genet 84:378–381

119. Ostergaard P, Simpson MA, Mendola A, Vasudevan P, Connell FC, van Impel A, Moore AT, Loeys BL, Ghalamkarpour A, Onoufriadis A et al (2012) Mutations in KIF11 cause autosomal-dominant microcephaly variably associated with congenital lymphedema and chorioretinopathy. Am J Hum Genet 90:356–362

120. Chauviere M, Kress C, Kress M (2008) Disruption of the mitotic kinesin Eg5 gene (Knsl1) results in early embryonic lethality. Biochem Biophys Res Commun 372:513–519

121. Smahi A, Courtois G, Vabres P, Yamaoka S, Heuertz S, Munnich A, Israel A, Heiss NS, Klauck SM, Kioschis P et al (2000) Genomic rearrangement in NEMO impairs NF-kappaB activation and is a cause of incontinentia pigmenti. The International Incontinentia Pigmenti (IP) Consortium. Nature 405:466–472

122. Doffinger R, Smahi A, Bessia C, Geissmann F, Feinberg J, Durandy A, Bodemer C, Kenwrick S, Dupuis-Girod S, Blanche S et al (2001) X-linked anhidrotic ectodermal dysplasia with immunodeficiency is caused by impaired NF-kappaB signaling. Nat Genet 27:277–285

123. Roberts CM, Angus JE, Leach IH, McDermott EM, Walker DA, Ravenscroft JC (2010) A novel NEMO gene mutation causing osteopetrosis, lymphoedema, hypohidrotic ectodermal dysplasia and immunodeficiency (OL-HED-ID). Eur J Pediatr 169:1403–1407

124. Carlberg VM, Lofgren SM, Mann JA, Austin JP, Nolt D, Shereck EB, Davila-Saldana B, Zonana J, Krol AL (2013) Hypohidrotic ectodermal dysplasia, osteopetrosis, lymphedema, and immunodeficiency in an infant with multiple opportunistic infections. Pediatr Dermatol. Epub ahead of print. doi:10.1111/pde.12103

125. Schmidt-Supprian M, Bloch W, Courtois G, Addicks K, Israel A, Rajewsky K, Pasparakis M (2000) NEMO/IKK gamma-deficient mice model incontinentia pigmenti. Mol Cell 5:981–992

126. Bull LN, Roche E, Song EJ, Pedersen J, Knisely AS, van Der Hagen CB, Eiklid K, Aagenaes O, Freimer NB (2000) Mapping of the locus for cholestasis-lymphedema syndrome (Aagenaes syndrome) to a 6.6-cM interval on chromosome 15q. Am J Hum Genet 67:994–999

127. Atri D, Larrivée B, Eichmann A, Simons M (2013) Endothelial signaling and the molecular basis of arteriovenous malformation. Cell Mol Life Sci 71(5):867–883

128. Savitsky K, Bar-Shira A, Gilad S, Rotman G, Ziv Y, Vanagaite L, Tagle DA, Smith S, Uziel T, Sfez S et al (1995) A single ataxia telangiectasia gene with a product similar to PI-3 kinase. Science 268: 1749–1753

129. McAllister KA, Grogg KM, Johnson DW, Gallione CJ, Baldwin MA, Jackson CE, Helmbold EA, Markel DS, McKinnon WC, Murrell J et al (1994) Endoglin, a TGF-beta binding protein of endothelial

cells, is the gene for hereditary haemorrhagic telangiectasia type 1. Nat Genet 8:345–351

130. Johnson DW, Berg JN, Baldwin MA, Gallione CJ, Marondel I, Yoon SJ, Stenzel TT, Speer M, Pericak-Vance MA, Diamond A et al (1996) Mutations in the activin receptor-like kinase 1 gene in hereditary haemorrhagic telangiectasia type 2. Nat Genet 13: 189–195

131. Govani FS, Shovlin CL (2009) Hereditary haemorrhagic telangiectasia: a clinical and scientific review. Eur J Hum Genet 17:860–871

132. Cole SG, Begbie ME, Wallace GM, Shovlin CL (2005) A new locus for hereditary haemorrhagic telangiectasia (HHT3) maps to chromosome 5. J Med Genet 42:577–582

133. Bayrak-Toydemir P, McDonald J, Akarsu N, Toydemir RM, Calderon F, Tuncali T, Tang W, Miller F, Mao R (2006) A fourth locus for hereditary hemorrhagic telangiectasia maps to chromosome 7. Am J Med Genet A 140:2155–2162

134. Revencu N, Boon LM, Vikkula M (2008) Arteriovenous malformation in mice and men. In: Marmé D, Fusenig N (eds) Tumor angiogenesis: mechanisms and cancer therapy. Springer, Heidelberg, pp 363–374

135. Gallione CJ, Repetto GM, Legius E, Rustgi AK, Schelley SL, Tejpar S, Mitchell G, Drouin E, Westermann CJ, Marchuk DA (2004) A combined syndrome of juvenile polyposis and hereditary haemorrhagic telangiectasia associated with mutations in MADH4 (SMAD4). Lancet 363:852–859

136. Goumans MJ, Valdimarsdottir G, Itoh S, Rosendahl A, Sideras P, ten Dijke P (2002) Balancing the activation state of the endothelium via two distinct TGF-beta type I receptors. EMBO J 21:1743–1753

137. David L, Mallet C, Mazerbourg S, Feige JJ, Bailly S (2007) Identification of BMP9 and BMP10 as functional activators of the orphan activin receptor-like kinase 1 (ALK1) in endothelial cells. Blood 109: 1953–1961

138. Barbara NP, Wrana JL, Letarte M (1999) Endoglin is an accessory protein that interacts with the signaling receptor complex of multiple members of the transforming growth factor-beta superfamily. J Biol Chem 274:584–594

139. Lebrin F, Goumans MJ, Jonker L, Carvalho RL, Valdimarsdottir G, Thorikay M, Mummery C, Arthur HM, ten Dijke P (2004) Endoglin promotes endothelial cell proliferation and TGF-beta/ALK1 signal transduction. EMBO J 23:4018–4028

140. Lagna G, Hata A, Hemmati-Brivanlou A, Massague J (1996) Partnership between DPC4 and SMAD proteins in TGF-beta signalling pathways. Nature 383:832–836

141. Zhang Y, Musci T, Derynck R (1997) The tumor suppressor Smad4/DPC 4 as a central mediator of Smad function. Curr Biol 7:270–276

142. Bourdeau A, Dumont DJ, Letarte M (1999) A murine model of hereditary hemorrhagic telangiectasia. J Clin Invest 104:1343–1351

143. Oh SP, Seki T, Goss KA, Imamura T, Yi Y, Donahoe PK, Li L, Miyazono K, ten Dijke P, Kim S et al (2000) Activin receptor-like kinase 1 modulates transforming growth factor-beta 1 signaling in the regulation of angiogenesis. Proc Natl Acad Sci U S A 97:2626–2631

144. Bourdeau A, Faughnan ME, Letarte M (2000) Endoglin-deficient mice, a unique model to study hereditary hemorrhagic telangiectasia. Trends Cardiovasc Med 10:279–285

145. Sirard C, de la Pompa JL, Elia A, Itie A, Mirtsos C, Cheung A, Hahn S, Wakeham A, Schwartz L, Kern SE et al (1998) The tumor suppressor gene Smad4/Dpc4 is required for gastrulation and later for anterior development of the mouse embryo. Genes Dev 12:107–119

146. Wooderchak-Donahue WL, McDonald J, O'Fallon B, Upton PD, Li W, Roman BL, Young S, Plant P, Fulop GT, Langa C et al (2013) BMP9 mutations cause a vascular-anomaly syndrome with phenotypic overlap with hereditary hemorrhagic telangiectasia. Am J Hum Genet 93:530–537

147. Mester J, Eng C (2013) When overgrowth bumps into cancer: the PTEN-opathies. Am J Med Genet C Semin Med Genet 163C:114–121

148. Stambolic V, Suzuki A, de la Pompa JL, Brothers GM, Mirtsos C, Sasaki T, Ruland J, Penninger JM, Siderovski DP, Mak TW (1998) Negative regulation of PKB/Akt-dependent cell survival by the tumor suppressor PTEN. Cell 95:29–39

149. Hamada K, Sasaki T, Koni PA, Natsui M, Kishimoto H, Sasaki J, Yajima N, Horie Y, Hasegawa G, Naito M et al (2005) The PTEN/PI3K pathway governs normal vascular development and tumor angiogenesis. Genes Dev 19:2054–2065

150. Orloff MS, He X, Peterson C, Chen F, Chen JL, Mester JL, Eng C (2013) Germline PIK3CA and AKT1 mutations in Cowden and Cowden-like syndromes. Am J Hum Genet 92:76–80

151. Lindhurst MJ, Sapp JC, Teer JK, Johnston JJ, Finn EM, Peters K, Turner J, Cannons JL, Bick D, Blakemore L et al (2011) A mosaic activating mutation in AKT1 associated with the Proteus syndrome. N Engl J Med 365:611–619

Historical Background

3

Raul Mattassi

Visible abnormal vascular masses were the first congenital vascular malformations (CVM) reported in the literature. Probably the first report was that of Guido Guidi, personal physician of King Francis I of France in the sixteenth century. He described a young Florentine man with extremely dilated vessels of the scalp, which looked like enormous varices. He sent this patient to the famous surgeon Gabriele Falloppio who refused to operate on such a difficult case [1]. This case and several others were considered to represent abnormal dilated vessels because the concept of hemodynamics was not understood.

In 1628 William Harvey published his famous book *Excercitatio anatomica de motu cordis et sanguinis in animalibus* in Frankfurt, Germany, in which he explained blood circulation [2]. This discovery provided the basis upon which to understand abnormal circulation, such as arterio-venous (AV) connections. The first description of an AV fistula was by Lealis Lealis in 1707, in an uncommon site, between the spermatic artery and vein [3]. Between 1719 and 1721, Winslow described AV fistulas between the esophageal artery and left pulmonary vein, between the left bronchial artery and vein, and between the bronchial artery and azygos vein. In 1739 he also described a case of transposition of pulmonary veins [4]. Stenzel (1723) and Morgagni (1761) first described congenital stenosis of the aortic isthmus [5, 6].

In 1757 William Hunter described typical signs of AV communications, such as the bruit that disappears by compression of the feeding artery or at the site of communication [7]. In 1827 George Bushe reported a congenital temporal AV fistula treated by ligation of the external carotid artery because of hemorrhage [8]. Sir Prescott Hewitt (1867) clearly described a congenital AV malformation of a lower limb with "heating" in the leg, vibratory thrill, and superficial dilated veins [9]. In the same year, an Italian doctor, Gerini, reported at the French Society of Surgery at Paris on a case of a congenital pulsating tumor of the hand treated successfully by ligation of the radial and later of the ulnar artery [10].

In 1843 Norris performed a successful surgical treatment of an acquired AV fistula by double ligature of the artery [11], but later Breschet (1883) described two cases of ligature of the proximal artery in an AV fistula, followed by gangrene [12]. Nicoladoni in 1875 [13] and Branham in 1890 [14] described the pulse frequency reduction by compression of the fistula or the feeding artery, giving their name to this sign. A review of 447 published cases of AV fistulas was presented by Halsted to the American Surgical Association in 1889. This concluded that the great majority of AV fistulas were acquired [15]; but Rienhoff in another review

R. Mattassi
Center for Vascular Malformations "Stefan Belov",
Department of Vascular Surgery,
Clinical Institute Humanitas "Mater Domini",
Castellanza (Varese), Italy
e-mail: raulmattassi@gmail.com

R. Mattassi et al. (eds.), *Hemangiomas and Vascular Malformations: An Atlas of Diagnosis and Treatment*,
DOI 10.1007/978-88-470-5673-2_3, © Springer-Verlag Italia 2009, 2015

found mainly congenital cases [16]. Other main reviews were carried out at the Mayo Clinic by Ward and Horton [17].

In the nineteenth century, many descriptions of cases of visible diffuse venous anomalies appeared. Von Pitha (1869) [18] described dilated superficial veins in the upper limb which Bockenheimer later called "diffuse phlebectasia" (1907) [19]. In 1869 Weber reported "diffuse phlebarteriectasia" [20].

The first descriptions of segmentary somatic hypertrophy coupled with vascular anomalies were published by Geoffroy Saint-Hilaire in 1832 in his great teratological work *Histoire generale et particuliere des anomalies de l'organisation chez l'homme et les animaux* [21]. Later, other cases were described, such as the case of Foucher (1850), Broca (1859) [22], Krause [23], Friedberg [24], and others (Figs. 3.1 and 3.2). In 1869 Trélat and Monod

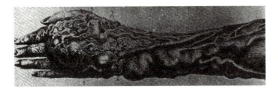

Fig. 3.1 Case described by Krause in 1862. Elongated left arm with visible pulsating "angiomata," present since the age of 7. At the age of 45, the arm was amputated after appearance of ulcers on the fingers (Reproduced with permission from Krause [23])

described a patient with hypertrophy of leg bones, nevus, and varicose veins and reviewed different published cases. They expressed the opinion that this pathology was congenital and that the cause of the hypertrophy is the venous stasis [25]. The same concepts were presented 31 years later in the best known paper of the French neurologists Klippel and Trenaunay (1900). These authors noticed that the vascular defect involved only veins and capillaries, but not arteries. They also described "incomplete and subclinical forms" without the three signs, including only bone hypertrophy without nevus and varices, nevus without bone hypertrophy and varices, and bone hypertrophy with nevus and no varices. They considered an infection of the embryo during pregnancy the cause of the defect [26].

Between 1907 and 1918, F. Parkes-Weber published different cases of limb hypertrophy and described signs of AV fistulas as "...a definite thrill or pulsation... is transmitted to the veins." He put together different vascular dysplasias, ranging from lymphangioma, nevus, and cirsoid aneurysm to diffuse AV fistulas, and labeled all these cases as "hemangiectatic hypertrophy of limbs" [27–29].

The efforts of all these authors were limited by the lack of diagnostic technology and were therefore only based on clinical data.

The year 1923 marked a new step in diagnostics after the introduction of arteriography by

Fig. 3.2 Case described by Friedberg in 1867. A girl aged 10 with a hypertrophy of the right leg with a limb length discrepancy of 18 cm. This patient had also lymphangiomas on the left arm and hand with repeated episodes of phlebitis and lymphangitis, treated by wet packs and digitalis. She died of tuberculosis few years later (Reproduced with permission from Friedberg [24])

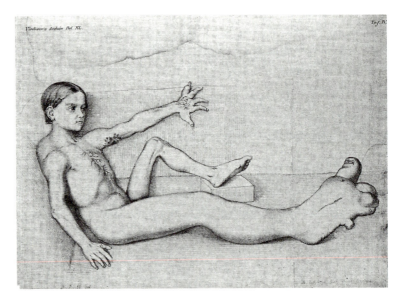

Sicard and Forestier [30] using Lipiodol in France and by Berberich and Hirsch in Germany, injecting strontium bromide [31]. Arteriography made it possible to better study the hemodynamic of vascular malformations.

Dysplasias of the deep veins of the lower limbs were studied by Servelle with phlebographies. In 1962 he described stenosis of the popliteal vein due to compression of fibrous bands [32], but this data was not confirmed by others. Pathogenesis of limb overgrowth was considered to be due to the venous stasis. Soltesz demonstrated experimentally with angiography that AV shunts open by performing ligature of popliteal veins in young animals; he concluded that limb hypertrophy is always due to AV fistulas [33].

A significant contribution toward comprehension of the different types of CVM was the paper of de Takats [34]; he made a clear distinction between AV malformations and other vascular defects, such as pure venous malformations and venous "angioma." Differentiation between hemangioma and vascular malformation was difficult. Even though Ewing in 1940 defined the hemangioma as a vascular tumor, different from a vascular malformation [35], only the publication of Mulliken and Young in 1988 was able to definitively clarify the difference [36].

Reports of cases with CVM of the limbs and limb shortening instead of hypertrophy were described later. In 1948 Servelle and Trinquecoste described two cases of venous hamartoma of the limbs with phleboliths and bone hypotrophy [37]. Martorell described a similar case in 1949 with "angiocavernomas" and severe bone destruction; he called this syndrome "angiomatosis braquial osteolitica" [38]. In 1957 Olivier distinguished two different types of "varicose angiomatosis," one superficial and one with deep-sited "angiomas" [39]. The opinion that even these venous-appearing malformations had AV communications was expressed by Pratt (1949) and Piulachs and Vidal Barraquer (1953) [40, 41].

Lymphatic dysplasia was described clearly in the nineteenth century. Cystic hygroma was first described by Wernher in 1843 [42]. Wegener (1877) divided lymphatic dysplasias or lymphangiomas into simplex, cavernosum, and cysticum types, a classification which is accepted even today [43]. Extensive studies on diagnosis and treatment of lymphatic malformations were carried out by Kinmonth [44] and Servelle [45]. The rare condition of chylus reflux was first reported clearly by Servelle and Deysson in 1949 [46]. Reports of combination of peripheral vascular malformations and lymphatic dysplasia were still included in some historical papers, like those of Klippel and Trenaunay and Parkes-Weber, but clear recognition of the lymphatic component was not achieved. Better data appeared only recently due to Pierer [47], Lindemayr et al. [48], and Partsch (1968) and also in the cited work of Kinmonth, among others.

In 1965 Malan published two papers in which he extensively analyzed all types of CVM, trying to clear problems of classification, diagnostics, and treatment [49, 50].

The first monograph, *Abnormal Arteriovenous Communications*, was published by Holman in 1968 [51] and was followed by the books of Belov in 1971 [52] and those of Giampalmo in 1972 [53]; the latter two had little diffusion because of their languages (Bulgarian and Italian). In 1974 Malan published his monograph in English with a report of 451 cases [54], followed by those of Schobinger [55]. Other remarkable works were due to Dean and O'Neal (1983) [17], Belov et al. [56], and Mulliken and Young [36].

Surgical treatment of CVM had been attempted for many years. Sometimes results were disappointing, as reported by Szilagyi et al. in 1976 [57]; however, other authors, like Vollmar [58], Malan [59], and Belov [60], had better results. Belov was the first person to put surgery into a systematic level.

Endovascular treatment was attempted first by Brooks in 1930: the author embolized a traumatic carotido-cavernous fistula with muscle fragments attached to a silver clip [61]. In 1960 Lussenhop and Spence embolized an intracranial AV malformation with spheres of methyl methacrylate through a surgically exposed common carotid artery [62]. Development of catheter technology and embolizing materials after 1970 increased the interest in these techniques. Zanetti and Sherman reported embolization with isobutyl

2-cyanoacrylate [63] and Carey and Grace with Gelfoam particles [64], while Gianturco created the coil in 1975 [65]. Yakes proposed the occlusion of CVM by alcohol injection through a direct puncture [66].

Recent progress was the publication of an international consensus, led by BB Lee with a selected group of international experts about venous malformations in 2009 [67] and about arteriovenous defects in 2013 [68].

In 1976, Anthony Young (London) and John Mulliken (Boston) organized a small meeting with other colleagues interested in these problems, in order to exchange experiences and discuss difficult cases. Meetings were held every 2 years as interest in them increased. During the congress held in 1990 in Amsterdam, organized by Jan Kromhout, a group of experts agreed to find a scientific society to convene all the physicians interested in vascular malformations and hemangiomas, in order to obtain international acceptance. During the meeting held in Denver in 1992, organized by Wayne Yakes, the new society was founded. The first assembly agreed on the name International Society for the Study of Vascular Anomalies (ISSVA). The first president was Robert Schobinger (Switzerland). Today, ISSVA meets every 2 years. It brings together a multidisciplinary group of experts from all over the world dedicated to approaching these difficult topics. Interest in these diseases is growing and progress is on its way.

References

1. Guido G, cited by Vichow R (1876) Pathologie des Tumeurs. Germer-Balliére, Paris
2. Whitterige G (1966) The anatomical lectures of William Harvey. E & S Livingstone, Edimburg and London
3. Lealis L, cited by Malan E, Puglionisi A (1965) Congenital angiodysplasias of the extremities (note II: arterial, arterial and venous and hemolymphatic dysplasias). J Cardiovasc Surg 6:255–345 (reference 50)
4. Winslow GB, cited by Malan E, Puglionisi A (1965) Congenital angiodysplasias of the extremities (note II: arterial, arterial and venous and hemolymphatic dysplasias). J Cardiovasc Surg 6:255–345 (reference 50)
5. Stenzel ZG (1723) Dissertatio anatomico-pathologica de steatomatibus in principio aortae repertis. Vittembergae 4
6. Morgagni GB (1761) De sedibus et causis morborum. Typografia Remondiniana, Venezia
7. Hunter W, cited by Fairbairn JF, Bernatz PE (1972) Arteriovenous fistulas. In: Fairbairn GF, Juergens JL, Spittel JA (eds) Peripheral vascular diseases. Saunders, Philadelphia
8. Bushe G (1827–1928) Temporal aneurysm: a case where, after an excision of an anastomoting aneurysm from the right temple, ligature of the external carotid became necessary to restrain hemorrhage. Lancet 2:413
9. Hewitt P (1867) A case of congenital aneurismal varix. Lancet 1:146
10. Gerini C (1867) Societé Imperial de Chirurgie. Séance du Juin 1867. Gas d. Hosp de Paris, p 303
11. Norris cited by Fairbairn JF, Bernatz PE (1972) Arteriovenous fistulas. In: Fairbairn GF, Juergens JL, Spittel JA (eds) Peripheral vascular diseases. Saunders, Philadelphia
12. Brechet G, cited by Malan E, Puglionisi A (1965) Congenital angiodysplasias of the extremities (note II: arterial, arterial and venous and hemolymphatic dysplasias). J Cardiovasc Surg 6:255–345 (reference 50)
13. Nicoladoni C (1875) Phlebarteriectasie der rechten oberen Extremität. Arch Klin Chir 18:252–274
14. Branham HH (1890) Aneurismal varix of the femoral artery and vein following a gunshot wound. Int J Surg 3:250–251
15. Callander CL (1920) Study of arteriovenous fistula with analysis of 447 cases (relation about the report of Halsted in 1889). John Hopkins Hosp Rep 19:259
16. Rienhoff WF Jr (1924) Congenital arterio-venous fistula. An embryological study with the report of a case. John Hopkins Hosp Bull 35:271
17. Ward CE, Horton BT (1940) Congenital arteriovenous fistula in children. J Pediatr 16:763
18. von Pitha F. Die Krankheiten der Extremitäten. In: Von Pitha F, Billroth T (eds) Handbuch der allgemeinen und speciellen Chirurgie, mit Einschluss der topographischen Anatomie und Verbandlehre. Erlangen, 1869
19. Bockenheimer P (1970) Über der genuine diffuse Phlebektasie der oberen Extremität. Festschrift f, vol 38. G.E. von Rindfleisch, Leipzig, p 311
20. Weber KO, cited by Malan E, Puglionisi A (1965) Congenital angiodysplasias of the extremities (note II: arterial, arterial and venous and hemolymphatic dysplasias). J Cardiovasc Surg 6:255–345
21. Geoffroy Saint Hilaire I: Histoire générale et particulière des anomalies de l´organisation ches l´homme et les animaux. Bailliere, Paris; 1832
22. Broca P (1856) Des aneurysmes et de leur traitement. Labé, Paris
23. Krause W (1862) Traumatische angiectasis des linken Armes. Arch Klin Chir 2:143, Published in: Deutsche Gesellschaft für Chirurgie (1947) Langenbecks Archiv für klinische Chirurgie … vereinigt mit Deutsche Zeitschrift für Chirurgie. Springer, Germany
24. Friedberg H (1867) Riesenwuchs des rechten Beines. Virchows Arch 40(3–4):343–379
25. Trelat U, Monod A (1869) De l'hypertrophie unilatérale ou totale du corps. Arch Gen de Med 13:536–558

26. Klippel M, Trenaunay I (1900) Du noevus variqueux et ostéohypertrophique. Arch Gen Med 3:641–672

27. Weber FP (1907) Angioma formation in connection with hypertrophy of limbs and hemihypertrophy. Br J Dermatol Syph 19:231–235

28. Weber FP (1908) Haemangiectatic hypertrophies of the foot and lower extremity, congenital or acquired, vol 136. Med Press, London, p 261

29. Weber FP (1918) Haemangiectatic hypertrophy of limbs – congenital phlebarteriectasis and so-called congenital varicose veins. Br J Chil Dis 15:13–17

30. Sicard JA, Forestier G (1923) Injections intravasculaires d'huile iodeé sous control radiologique. CR Soc Biol 88:1200–1202

31. Berberich J, Hirsch S (1923) Die roenthgenographische Darstellung der Arterien und Venen am Lebenden. Munch Klin Wochenschr 49:2226

32. Servelle M (1962) Oedémes chroniques des members chez l'enfant et l'adulte. Masson, Paris

33. Soltez L (1965) Contribution of clinical and experimental studies of the hypertrophy of the extremities in congenital arteriovenous fistulae. J Cardiovasc Surg (Suppl) 260–261

34. de Takats G (1932) Vascular anomalies of the extremities. Report of five cases. Surg Gynecol Obstet 55:227

35. Ewing J (1940) Neoplastic diseases: a treatise on tumors. Saunders, Philadelphia, p 1160

36. Mulliken JB, Young AE (1988) Vascular birthmarks: hemangiomas and malformations. Saunders, Philadelphia

37. Servelle M, Trinquecoste D (1948) Des angiomes veineux. Arch Mal Coeur 41:436

38. Martorell F (1949) Hemangiomatosis braquial osteolìtica. Angiologia 1(4):219–123

39. Olivier CL (1957) Maladies des veins. Masson, Paris

40. Pratt GH (1949) Arterial varices. A syndrome. Am J Surg 77(4):456–460

41. Piulachs P, Vidal Barraquer F (1953) Pathogenetic study of varicose veins. Angiology 4:59–99

42. Wernher A (1843) Die angeborenen Kysten-hygrome und die ihnen verwandten Genschwulste in anatomischer, diagnostischer und therapeutischer Beziehung. GF Heyer, Vater, Giessen

43. Wegener G (1877) Über Lymphangiome. Arch Klin Chir 20:641–707

44. Kinmonth JB (1972) The lymphatics. Diseases, lymphography and surgery. Edward Arnold, London

45. Servelle M (1975) Pathologie vasculaire, vol 3, Pathologie lymphatique. Masson, Paris

46. Servelle M, Deysson H (1949) Reflux du chyle dans les lymphatiques jambieres. Arch Mal Coeur 12:1181

47. Pierer H (1965) Klippel-Trenaunay-Weber syndrome from the surgical viewpoint. Klin Med Osterr Z Wiss Prakt Med 20(6):265–272

48. Lindemayr W, Lofferer O, Mostbeck A, Partsch H (1967) Lymphatic system in Klippel-Trenaunay-Weber's phakomatosis. Z Haut Geschlechtskr 43(5):183–188

49. Malan E, Puglionisi A (1964) Congenital angiodysplasias of the extremities (note I: generalities and classification; venous dysplasias). J Cardiovasc Surg 5:87–130

50. Malan E, Puglionisi A (1965) Congenital angiodysplasias of the extremities (note II: Arterial, arterial and venous and hemolymphatic dysplasias). J Cardiovasc Surg 6:255–345

51. Holman E (1968) Abnormal arteriovenous communications. Charles C Thomas, Springfield

52. Belov S (1971) Congenital angiodysplasia and their surgical treatment. Medicina I Fizkultura, Sofia

53. Giampalmo A (1972) Patologia delle malformazioni vascolari. Società Editrice Universo, Roma

54. Dean RH, O'Neill JA Jr (1983) Vascular disorders of childhood. Lea & Febiger, Philadelphia

55. Schobinger RA (1977) Periphere angiodysplasien. Hans Huber, Bern

56. Belov S, Loose DA, Müller E (1985) Angeborene Gefäßfehler. Einhorn Presse, Reinbek

57. Szilagyi DE, Smith RF, Elliott JP, Hageman JH (1976) Congenital arteriovenous anomalies of the limbs. Arch Surg 11(4):423–429

58. Vollmar J (1963) Arteriovenous fistulae. Their patophysiology, clinical aspects and treatment. Med Welt 15:802–806

59. Malan E (1974) Vascular malformations (angiodysplasias). Carlo Erba Foundation, Milan

60. Belov S (1990) Surgical treatment of congenital vascular defects. Int Angiol 9(3):173–182

61. Brooks B (1930) The treatment of traumatic arteriovenous fistula. South Med J 23:100–106

62. Lussenhop AJ, Spence WT (1960) Artificial embolization of cerebral arteries: report of use in a case of arteriovenous malformation. JAMA 172: 1153–1155

63. Zanetti PH, Sherman FE (1972) Experimental evaluation of a tissue adhesive as an agent for the treatment of aneurysms and arteriovenous anomalies. J Neurosurg 36(1):72–79

64. Carey LS, Grace DM (1974) The brisk bleed: control by arterial catheterization and gelfoam plug. J Can Assoc Radiol 25(2):113–115

65. Gianturco C, Anderson JH, Wallace S (1975) Mechanical devices for arterial occlusion. Am J Roentgenol Radium Ther Nucl Med 124(3): 428–435

66. Yakes WF, Pervsner PH, Reed MD et al (1986) Serial embolizations of an extremity arteriovenous malformation with alcohol via direct percutaneous puncture. AJR Am J Roentgenol 146:1038–1040

67. Lee BB, Bergan J, Gloviczki P, Laredo J, Loose DA, Mattassi R, Parsi K, Villavicencio JL, Zamboni P (2009) Diagnosis and treatment of venous malformations. Consensus document of the International Union of Phlebology (IUP)-2009. Int Angiol 28(6): 434–451

68. Lee BB, Baumgartner I, Berlien HP, Bianchini G, Burrows P, Do YS, Ivancev K, Kool LS, Laredo J, Loose DA, Lopez-Gutierrez JC, Mattassi R, Parsi K, Rimon U, Rosenblatt M, Shortell C, Simkin R, Stillo F, Villavicencio L, Yakes W (2013) Consensus document of the International Union of Angiology (IUA)-2013. Current concept on the management of arterio-venous management. Int Angiol 32(1):9–36

Coagulation Disorders Associated with Vascular Anomalies

4

Anne Dompmartin, Morgane Barreau, Yohann Repessé, and Agnès Le Querrec

Introduction

Coagulation disorders have been associated with vascular anomalies. Kasabach–Merritt phenomenon (KMP) describes thrombocytopenia and consumptive coagulopathy in the presence of a kaposiform hemangioendothelioma (KHE) or a tufted angioma (TA). A variant of KMP is associated with multifocal lymphangioendotheliomatosis with thrombocytopenia (MLT). Localized intravascular coagulopathy (LIC) is encountered in 45 % of venous malformations, and it is characterized by high D-dimer level, low fibrinogen, and normal platelet count. All these patients are at risk of potential aggravation to disseminated intravascular coagulopathy (DIC). To avoid therapeutic mismanagement, interdisciplinary vascular anomalies centers need to collaborate with hematologists.

A. Dompmartin, MD, PhD (✉) • M. Barreau, MD
Department of Dermatology, Hospital Center of Caen,
University of Caen Basse-Normandie,
Caen Cedex 9, France
e-mail: dompmartin-a@chu-caen.fr;
barreau-m@chu-caen.fr

Y. Repessé, MD • A. Le Querrec, MPhSc
Department of Hematology, Hospital Center of Caen,
University of Caen Basse-Normandie,
Caen Cedex 9, France
e-mail: repesse-y@chu-caen.fr;
lequerrec-a@chu-caen.fr

Coagulation (Fig. 4.1)

The *coagulation process* involves successive protease reactions leading to the conversion of soluble fibrinogen into insoluble fibrin. Fibrin strands linked to aggregated platelets form a stable thrombus. The new cell-based model of coagulation explains the mechanism of hemostasis in vivo. This process is initiated when TF-bearing cells are exposed to blood at the site of endothelial injury or abnormal endothelium (vascular abnormalities). Briefly, the initiation of the coagulation leads to the production of small amounts of *thrombin* (FIIa) that amplify its own generation (amplification phase). The burst of thrombin induces the formation of cross-linked fibrin (FIa). Similarly, platelet activation on altered endothelium leads to platelet aggregation and subsequently to the formation of FIIa and fibrin clots. Fibrinolysis is essential for clot dissolution. Fibrin plug is cleaved by plasmin with the production of fibrin degradation products (FDP) and *D-dimers*.

KMP and Vascular Tumors

Introduction

In 1940, Kasabach and Merritt described an infant with a "capillary hemangioma" with extensive purpura and profound thrombocytopenia [1].

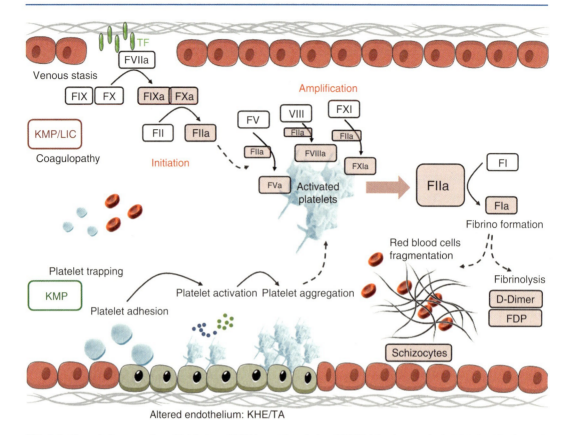

Fig. 4.1 Coagulation cascade and initiation of LIC (coagulopathy) and KMP (platelet trapping). *KMP* kasabach merrit phenomenom, *FDP* fibrin degradation product, *KHE* kaposiform hemangioendothelioma, *LIC* localized intravascular coagulopathy, *TA* tufted angioma

This type of coagulopathy was named Kasabach–Merritt phenomenon (KMP) and was assumed to be a complication of common infantile hemangioma. In 1980 and 1993, kaposiform hemangioendothelioma (KHE) and tufted angioma (TA) were differentiated from infantile hemangioma (Part II Chap. 7) [2–4]. Review of different cases presenting with KMP revealed that these children did not have classical infantile hemangioma but KHE or TA [5, 6]. TA and KHE are now considered as benign vascular tumors with similar presenting symptoms with a potential for developing KMP. Histologic examination usually can distinguish between KHE and TA but overlap of histologic characteristics can be observed especially on small biopsy specimens. KMP can be also associated with malignant vascular tumors such as angiosarcoma [7, 8].

Epidemiology and Predisposing Factors

Kasabach–Merritt phenomenon is very rare, occurring in 0.3 % of benign vascular tumors but in more than 50 % of the cases of *kaposiform hemangioendothelioma* and *tufted angioma* during the first year of life [9]. These tumors are either congenital or appear postnatally. There is no sex ratio and no familial cases or underlying genetic mutations. To date, in the largest cohort of 107 KHE patients, KMP developed in 71 % of the patients, and the greater risk factors were mediastinal or retroperitoneal involvement, deep infiltration of the tumor into muscle or fascia, and large cutaneous lesions (>5–8 cm) [10, 11]. Enjolras et al. found that histologic features of KHE were more common during the active phase of KMP compared with features of TA in the beginning of KMP or in the residual after cure [12]. In this chapter, we shall use KHE/TA as an all-encompassing term.

Clinical Features

KHE/TA is usually solitary tumor which develops on the lateral neck, axilla, groin, extremities, and trunk. When associated with KMP, it appears as an ecchymotic mass with centrifugal purpura. It can also occur in noncutaneous and sometimes hidden locations: retroperitoneum, mediastinum, or bones. Therefore, thrombocytopenia in a newborn unexplained by other routine tests (such as for sepsis) should prompt for occult vascular tumor. Multifocal lesions have rarely been reported [13, 14].

Laboratory Features and Pathogenesis (Fig. 4.1)

KMP is characterized by severe thrombocytopenia ($<20 \times 10^9$/L) associated with hypofibrinogenemia, increase of fibrin degradation products (PDF) and presence of schizocytes due to red cell fragmentation by fibrin filaments. Anemia is not a common presenting sign unless significant bleeding occurs within the tumor. As a consequence of platelet activation, platelet half-life is drastically shortened to 1–24 h.

KMP belongs to a spectrum of diseases characterized by a thrombotic microangiopathy (TMA). TMA results from red cell activation and platelet trapping with subsequent thrombocytopenia and microangiopathic hemolytic anemia with negative Coombs test [9]. Although the pathogenesis of this syndrome is not well elucidated, it is probable that the abnormal endothelium of the associated vascular tumors (KHE/TA) leads to platelet trapping and aggregation followed by activation of coagulation factors, fibrin deposition, and subsequently red blood cell damage and consumptive coagulopathy (DIC). Fibrinolysis occurs with consumption of clotting factors and intralesional bleeding with rapid enlargement of the tumor.

In addition, liver immaturity of the premature neonates may enhance impairment of coagulation because of low synthesis of clotting factors [15].

Treatment

Treatment is challenging without a consensus on the optimal medical management. There are no standardized protocols, no prospective studies, and no long-term follow-up published in the literature [16]. The goal of the treatment of KMP is to reduce the tumor size as it generates hematologic instability. In 2013, a multidisciplinary and multi-institutional expert panel published a standardized consensus-derived standard of practice for the treatment of KHE/TA with and without KMP [17]. Medical therapy is the first approach as KHE/TA with KMP is usually deep and infiltrative, and surgical excision is considered when the tumor can be safely and completely excised. There is a consensus on the fact that KHE/TA should be treated aggressively with a combination regimen administered as soon as possible. The first-line recommended pharmacologic protocol is intravenous *vincristine* (0.05 mg/kg) once weekly AND oral *prednisolone* 2 mg/kg/day OR intravenous methylprednisolone 1.6 mg/kg/day. However, if administration of vincristine is not immediately possible (lack of central venous access), treatment must not be delayed, and corticosteroid therapy should be started before the availability of vincristine. The duration of the treatment depends on the individual clinical response and stabilization of the coagulopathy. Corticosteroids can be weaned after 3–4 weeks of full-dose treatment. The average length of vincristine therapy is usually 20–24 weeks, but it depends on the shrinkage of the tumor, the stabilization of the hematologic status, and the toxicity of the drug. Complete clearance of the tumor is rare; residual fibrotic lesions can be visualized by follow-up imaging, and there is no point in prolonging therapy although these residua are considered as dormant vascular tumors and not scars [12]. Interferon alpha has been used with success but was associated with a risk of spastic diplegia in infants less than 8 months of age [18]. The use of propranolol cannot be recommended because varied responses to treatment have been observed [19, 20]. Sirolimus, a mammalian target of rapamycin (mTOR) inhibitor, is widely used in patients following organ transplantation. It also has an antiangiogenic activity and may have an application in the treatment of vascular lesions. Rapid improvement of hematologic disorders with no recurrence several years after treatment was reported in two patients with KHE/TA associated with KMP [21, 22]. It seems to be a promising treatment, and prospective studies are needed to evaluate safety and efficacy of this agent.

Adjuvant therapies are used to improve thrombocytopenia and diminish the risk of bleeding. Platelet transfusion increases platelet trapping and may induce enlargement of the tumor and increased pain. Moreover, local platelet activation leads to the release of proangiogenic factors and possible tumor proliferation [23]. Therefore, platelet transfusions are only indicated for active bleeding and/or immediately prior surgery. Inhibitors of platelets' function such as aspirin, *ticlopidine*, and clopidogrel have been used in combination with other therapies to prevent platelet activation. They are not effective in preventing platelet consumption, but aspirin may be successful in controlling pain [24, 25]. The use of antifibrinolytic agents such as ε-aminocaproic acid or tranexamic acid was proposed because it is considered that inhibition of fibrinolysis might delay fibrin lysis and reduce bleeding. However, in the published cases, when important bleeding occurred, these agents rarely reduced blood transfusions [26, 27]. When bleeding is associated with hypofibrinogenemia (<100 mg/dl), administration of fibrinogen or fresh frozen plasma is recommended to replace the consumed clotting factors. Heparin is not indicated because of absence of effect on platelets and bleeding risk.

Multifocal Lymphangioendotheliomatosis with Thrombocytopenia (MLT)

Introduction

Multifocal vascular lesions have recently been classified as *multifocal lymphangioendotheliomatosis with thrombocytopenia* (MLT) and mul-

tifocal infantile hemangiomatosis (IH) [28]. MLT has a much higher mortality compared to IH because of severe gastrointestinal (GI) bleeding.

Clinical and Histologic Features

Skin lesions in MLT range from 1 to 2 mm telangiectatic plaques to large exophytic hemorrhagic nodules. They are associated with similar GI lesions distributed diffusely throughout the GI tract. GI bleeding in MLT is often profuse causing significant morbidity or even death. Multifocal IH is clinically different as cutaneous lesions are small disseminated red papules which may occasionally be associated with segmental GI involvement, but the main extracutaneous site is the liver. MLT and IH have similar histopathologic findings with dilated vessels in the dermis and subcutis. To differentiate MLT from infantile hemangioma, relevant stains are necessary to confirm the absence of the specific marker of infantile hemangioma GLUT 1 and the positivity of a lymphatic endothelial cell-specific marker LYVE-1 (lymphatic endothelial receptor-1) or podoplanin (D2–40) on the lining of the dilated vessels. MLT's lesions co-express blood and lymphatic markers, like kaposiform hemangioendothelioma and angiosarcoma endothelial cells. Lesions are slowly progressive in the first years of life and remain stable, contrary to multifocal IH which are rapidly progressive in the first months of life and disappear within 1–5 years.

Laboratory Findings and Pathogenesis

Mild thrombocytopenia is reportedly associated with anemia due to GI bleeding. A consumptive coagulopathy is observed with elevated D-dimer levels.

Pathogenesis of MLT is unknown, but thrombocytopenia is probably also due to platelet destruction within the vascular lesions which have indeterminate blood/lymphatic vascular endothelial differentiation [29].

Treatment

Contrary to IH, MLT does not respond to usual treatments such as prednisone, propranolol, vincristine, and interferon. Bevacizumab, an antibody to the vascular endothelial factor, has been used with success in one case [30].

Localized Intravascular Coagulopathy (LIC) and Venous Malformations (VMs)

Clinical and Laboratory Features

Venous malformations (VMs) are associated with spontaneous thrombosis and thrombolysis. This is witnessed by elevated D-dimer levels in 42 % of patients and associated with size, deepness, and presence of palpable phleboliths [31–33]. This phenomenon is named *localized intravascular coagulopathy* (LIC). *D-dimer levels* are often very high (25 % of patients >1.0 mg/mL), even if these otherwise healthy patients do not have other conditions to increase D-dimer levels, e.g., cancer, inflammatory disease, thrombophilia, ischemic heart disease, arterial aneurysm or dissection, or pregnancy. In other conditions, such as oral contraception, ulceration, and old age, D-dimer levels can also mildly increase, but levels are much lower than that reported for VMs [33–35]. VM is the only disease that can permanently highly increase D-dimer levels in otherwise healthy patients. Thus, it is a biomarker helpful for diagnosis. When D-dimer levels are elevated in vascular anomaly patients with no associated pathology, a venous component is present in 96.5 % of patients. This is true for pure, isolated VMs (uni- or multifocal) as well as for combined and syndromic lesions (e.g., capillary venous malformation and Klippel–Trenaunay syndrome (KTS)) (Chaps. 22 and 23). In contrast, sensitivity is lower (42 %). Thus, when D-dimer levels are normal, a small VM cannot be ruled out.

Among all patients with vascular malformations, D-dimer levels are normal in all glomuvenous malformations (GVMs), lymphatic malformations (LMs), and Maffucci syndrome as well as in fast flow malformations such as arteriovenous malformations (AVMs) and Parkes Weber syndrome (Chaps. 22 and 23). Thus, D-dimer measurement is a useful biomarker for the differential diagnosis of VMs. It can help, e.g., in differentiating GVMs from other multifocal venous lesions. It can also detect a venous component in combined and syndromic malformations. Thus, this easy and cheap biomarker test must be used as a routine test in clinical evaluation of vascular anomaly patients [36].

Evolution

LIC is usually well tolerated during everyday life. However, a few patients with extensive VMs, mainly affecting an extremity, have a severe LIC with a very high D-dimer level (>1.8 mg/mL) and a low fibrinogen level. These patients are at risk of potential aggravation of LIC to disseminated intravascular coagulopathy (DIC) with dramatic bleeding during a surgical excision and marked consumption of platelets, coagulation factors, and fibrinogen [32]. Thus, measurement of D-dimer levels is mandatory for the management of VMs.

Patients with Klippel–Trenaunay syndrome (KTS) (Chap. 23) have elevated D-dimer levels in 70 % of cases. The main complication of KTS is thrombophlebitis which occurs in 20–40 % of patients and leads to pulmonary embolism in 4–25 % of cases [37]. Extensive VMs share the same risk, especially the "varicose-like" forms which have a close relationship with the venous system [38, 39]. Recurrent and unresolved pulmonary embolisms due to hypercoagulability can lead to the development of chronic thromboembolic pulmonary hypertension (CTEPH). There is probably an association between the risk of *pulmonary arterial hypertension* (PAH), the size and extent of venous malformations, and D-dimer levels. PAH leads to right ventricular insufficiency and can cause death [40].

Pathogenesis

Elevated D-dimer levels are the hallmark of an hypercoagulable/prothrombotic state of venous malformations, probably due to the venous stasis in numerous dilated abnormal venous channels. There is also a correlation between the importance of the D-dimer levels and the size and/or the deepness of the lesions [32]. However, this hypothesis does not explain why multifocal small lesions are often associated with elevated D-dimer levels. In a recent trial, Redondo demonstrated that several angiogenic factors and endothelial damage/dysfunction markers are elevated in patients with venous malformations, suggesting an abnormal disassembly level between endothelial cells and mesenchymal cells, leading to dilated vessels with insufficient mural components which promote coagulation and fibrinolysis [41]. Some evidence suggests that angiogenesis and thrombosis are closely linked and that platelets and local microthrombi may promote angiogenesis [42, 43]. Finally, the proinflammatory/prothrombotic profile of VMs probably influences the development of these vascular malformations.

DIC is a consumptive coagulopathy associated with generation of large amount of thrombin and monomers of fibrin, consumption of fibrinogen, and some clotting factors and increased risk of bleeding. Secondarily, *fibrinolysis* is activated and levels of D-dimer increase.

Treatment

Management of VMs associated with LIC needs interdisciplinary discussion. *Tailored compression* garment is the first-line treatment for symptomatic and extensive VMs of the extremities to reduce pain and thrombosis. Low-dose aspirin and/or anti-inflammatory drugs are proposed if pain is not relieved or if compression is not anatomically possible. When associated with elevated D-dimer levels, pain can be relieved with low-molecular-weight heparin 100 Anti-Xa/kg for 20 days, or longer if pain relapses. Patients with important or severe LIC need careful management to prevent severe bleeding during a surgical procedure. To improve the hematological status and to avoid DIC, preventive treatment with *enoxaparin* (100 Anti-Xa/kg) should be started 2 or 3 days before any surgical procedure for a total of 20 days [36]. New oral anticoagulants have not been assessed in this indication [44].

> ### Conclusion
>
> Initiation of the coagulation cascade is different in vascular tumors and venous malformations: KMP, characterized by a profound thrombocytopenia, is secondary to platelet activation initiated by the altered endothelium of KHE/TA. The coagulation disorder of MLT is close to KMP [28]. However, this multifocal hemangiomatosis, recently individualized, seems more chronic than KMP. Other studies are necessary to understand and treat it. In contrast, LIC is initiated by both the exposure of TF and venous stasis in abnormal dilated vessels associated with an increase of D-dimer levels. Clinicians and biologists must work in concert to diagnose the vascular anomaly and understand the pathophysiology of the coagulation disorder. Although the coagulation activation always generates thrombocytopenia and elevation of D-dimer levels, the targets of the treatment are different: tumor for KMP and consumption of the coagulation factors for LIC.

References

1. Kasabach HH, Merritt KK (1940) Capillary hemangioma with extensive purpura. Am J Dis Child 59:1063–1070
2. Zukerberg LR, Nickoloff BJ, Weiss SW (1993) Kaposiform hemangioendothelioma of infancy and childhood. An aggressive neoplasm associated with Kasabach–Merritt syndrome and lymphangiomatosis. Am J Surg Pathol 17:321–328
3. Alessi E, Bertani E, Sala F (1986) Acquired tufted angioma. Am J Dermatopathol 8:426–429
4. Jones EW, Orkin M (1989) Tufted angioma (angioblastoma). A benign progressive angioma, not to be confused with Kaposi's sarcoma or low-grade angiosarcoma. J Am Acad Dermatol 20:214–225

5. Enjorlas O, Wassef M, Mazoyer E et al (1997) Infants with Kasabach–Merritt syndrome do not have "true" hemangiomas. J Pediatr 130:631 640

6. Sarkar M, Mulliken JB, Kozakewich HP et al (1997) Thrombocytopenic coagulopathy (Kasabach–Merritt phenomenon) is associated with Kaposiform hemangioendothelioma and not with common infantile hemangioma. Plast Reconstr Surg 100:1377–1386

7. Salameh F, Henig I, Bar-Shalom R et al (2007) Metastatic angiosarcoma of the scalp causing Kasabach-Merritt syndrome. Am J Med Sci 333:293–295

8. Tan SM, Tay YK, Liu TT et al (2012) Cutaneous angiosarcoma associated with the Kasabach-Merritt syndrome. Ann Acad Med Singapore 39:941–942

9. Radhi M, Carpenter SL (2012) Thrombotic microangiopathies. IRSN Hematol 2012:310596

10. Gruman A, Liang MG, Mulliken JB et al (2005) Kaposiform hemangioendothelioma without Kasabach–Merritt phenomenon. J Am Acad Dermatol 52:616–622

11. Croteau SE, Liang MG, Kozakewich HP et al (2013) Kaposiform hemangioendothelioma: atypical features and risks of Kasabach–Merritt phenomenon in 107 referrals. J Pediatr 162:142–170

12. Enjorlas O, Mulliken JB, Wassef M et al (2000) Residual lesions after Kasabach–Merritt phenomenon in 41 patients. J Am Acad Dermatol 42:225–235

13. Gianotti R, Gelmetti C, Alessi E (1999) Congenital cutaneous multifocal kaposiform hemangioendothelioma. Am J Dermatopathol 21:557–561

14. Veening MA, Verbeke JI, Witbreuk MM et al (2010) Kaposiform (spindle cell) hemangioendotelioma in a child with an unusual presentation. J Pediatr Hematol Oncol 32:240–242

15. Hall GW (2001) Kasabach-Merritt syndrome: pathogenesis and management. Br J Haematol 112:851–862

16. Tlougan BE, Lee MT, Drolet BA et al (2013) Medical management of tumors associated with Kasabach-Merritt phenomenon: an expert survey. J Pediatr Hematol Oncol 35:618–622

17. Drolet BA, Trenor CC 3rd, Brandao LR et al (2013) Consensus-derived practice standards plan for complicated Kaposiform hemangioendothelioma. J Pediatr 163:285–291

18. Barlow CF, Priebe CJ, Mulliken JB et al (1998) Spastic diplegia as a complication of interferon Alfa-2a treatment of hemangiomas of infancy. J Pediatr 132:527–530

19. Hermans DL, van Beynum IM, van der Vijver RJ et al (2011) Kaposiform hemangioendothelioma with Kasabach-Merritt syndrome: a new indication for propranolol treatment. J Pediatr Hematol Oncol 33:171–173

20. Chiu YE, Drolet BA, Blei F et al (2012) Variable response to propranolol treatment of kaposiform hemangioendothelioma, tufted angioma, and Kasabach-Merritt phenomenon. Pediatr Blood Cancer 59:934–938

21. Blatt J, Stavas J, Moats-Staats B et al (2010) Treatment of childhood kaposiform hemangioendothelioma with sirolimus. Pediatr Blood Cancer 55:1396–1398

22. Hammill AM, Wentzel M, Gupta A et al (2011) Sirolimus for the treatment of complicated vascular anomalies in children. Pediatr Blood Cancer 57:1018–1024

23. Philips WG, Marsden JR (1993) Kasabach Merritt syndrome exacerbated by platelet transfusion. J R Soc Med 86:231–232

24. Fernandez-Pineda I, Lopez-Gutierrez JC, Chocarro G et al (2013) Long-term outcome of vincristine-aspirin-ticlopidine (VAT) therapy for vascular tumors associated with Kasabach-Merritt phenomenon. Pediatr Blood Cancer 60:1478–1481

25. Fernandez-Pineda I, Lopez-Gutierrez JC, Ramirez G et al (2010) Vincristine-ticlopidine-aspirin: an effective therapy in children with Kasabach-Merritt phenomenon associated with vascular tumors. Pediatr Hematol Oncol 27:641–645

26. Hanna BD, Bernstein M (1989) Tranexamic acid in the treatment of Kasabach-Merritt syndrome in infants. Am J Pediatr Hematol Oncol 11:191–195

27. Morad AB, McClain KL, Ogden AK (1993) The role of tranexamic acid in the treatment of giant hemangiomas in newborns. Am J Pediatr Hematol Oncol 15:383–385

28. Glick ZR, Frieden IJ, Garzon MC et al (2012) Diffuse neonatal hemangiomatosis: an evidence-based review of case reports in the literature. J Am Acad Dermatol 67:898–903

29. Esparza EM, Deutsch G, Stanescu L et al (2012) Multifocal lymphangioendotheliomatosis with thrombocytopenia: phenotypic variant and course with propranolol, corticosteroids, and aminocaproic acid. J Am Acad Dermatol 67:62–64

30. Kline RM, Buck LM (2009) Bevacizumab treatment in multifocal lymphangioendotheliomatosis with thrombocytopenia. Pediatr Blood Cancer 52:534–536

31. Mazoyer E, Enjolras O, Bisdorff A et al (2008) Coagulation disorders in patients with venous malformation of the limbs and trunk: a case series of 118 patients. Arch Dermatol 144:861–867

32. Dompmartin A, Acher A, Thibon P et al (2008) Association of localized intravascular coagulopathy with venous malformations. Arch Dermatol 144:873–877

33. Dompmartin A, Ballieux F, Thibon P et al (2009) Elevated D-dimer level in the differential diagnosis of venous malformations. Arch Dermatol 145:1239–1244

34. Kluft C, Meijer P, LaGuardia KD et al (2008) Comparison of a transdermal contraceptive patch vs. oral contraceptives on hemostasis variables. Contraception 77:77–83

35. Cuderman TV, Bozic M, Peternel P et al (2008) Hemostasis activation in thrombophilic subjects with or without a history of venous thrombosis. Clin Appl Thromb Hemost 14:55–62

36. Dompmartin A, Vikkula M, Boon LM (2010) Venous malformation: update on aetiopathogenesis, diagnosis and management. Phlebology 25:224–235

37. Samuel M, Spitz L (1995) Klippel-Trenaunay syndrome: clinical features, complications and management in children. Br J Surg 82:757–761

38. Berenguer B, Burrows PE, Zurakowski D et al (1999) Sclerotherapy of craniofacial venous

malformations: complications and results. Plast Reconstr Surg 104:1–11

39. Rodríguez-Mañero M, Aguado L, Redondo P (2010) Pulmonary arterial hypertension in patients with slow-flow vascular malformations. Arch Dermatol 146:1347–1352

40. van Beers EJ, Douma RA, Oduber CE et al (2010) Extensive slow-flow vascular malformations and pulmonary hypertension. Arch Dermatol 146:1416–1418

41. Redondo P, Aguado L, Marquina M et al (2010) Angiogenic and prothrombotic markers in extensive slow-flow vascular malformations. Implications for antiangiogenic/antithrombotic therapies. Br J Dermatol 162:350–356

42. Kisucka J, Butterfield CE, Duda DG et al (2006) Platelets and platelet adhesion support angiogenesis while preventing excessive hemorrhage. Proc Natl Acad Sci U S A 103:855–860

43. Moser M, Patterson C (2003) Thrombin and vascular development: a sticky subject. Arterioscler Thromb Vasc Biol 23:922–930

44. Bauer KA (2013) Pros and cons of new oral anticoagulants. Hematol Am Soc Hematol Educ Prog 2013:464–470

Part II

Hemangiomas and Vascular Tumors

Hemangiomas of Infancy: Epidemiology

Maria Rosa Cordisco

Infantile hemangioma (IH) or hemangioma of infancy (HOI) is the most common soft tissue tumor of infancy, but understanding of its etiology and pathogenesis is still under research. The true incidence of infantile hemangiomas is unknown [1]. No prospective studies have been published for several decades examining their incidence.

Hemangiomas of infancy may be visible at birth or may not be recognized until the first 2–3 weeks of age, or even months of life, and have a natural history of growth early in infancy followed by spontaneous involution. In addition, the word "hemangioma" has been used to describe a wide array of lesions. For these reasons, in reviewing the literature it is difficult to almost impossible to determine the true incidence due to a lack of a clear definition in the classification, study design, and population selection [1]. Although they are classically said to occur in up to 10 % of Caucasian infants, the estimated incidence is between 4 and 5 % [2, 3]. About 30 % of IH are noted at birth, and 70–90 % will appear during the first 4 weeks of life [4, 5].

Although IH can be seen in all races, it is more common in Caucasian infants and less common in those of African descent. The exact occurrence of IH in Asian infants has not been well studied but is predicted to be 1 % [6].

The majority of hemangiomas occur sporadically; nonetheless, familial occurrence of IH has been reported. Blei et al. documented the autosomal dominant transmission of IH and vascular malformations in six kindred, and the locus involved has been identified at 5q 31-33 [7, 8].

A recent study showed a third of the patients had a first-degree relative with a vascular anomaly, and 12 % had a first-degree relative with a hemangioma [9].

Risk factors for the development of infantile hemangioma include female gender (female-to-male ratio of 2.4:1), prematurity, low birth weight (especially in those weighing less than 1,500 g), multiple gestations, pre- eclampsia, placenta previa, and advanced maternal age [9–11]. Assisted reproductive technologies and strategies promoting ovulation also increased the incidence of hemangiomas [10, 12]. The cause for this female preponderance is unknown but may be related to hormonal differences.

Chorionic villous sampling (CVS) during pregnancy has been associated with a higher risk of hemangioma development, but this was not supported by a recent large prospective study [9, 13]. Amniocentesis and transabdominal CVS do not seem to produce a significant difference in hemangioma incidence [14]. Drolet et al. considerer that low birth weight (LBW) was the most significant risk factor; with less than 2,500 g for every 500 g decrease in birth weight, the risk of

M.R. Cordisco
Department of Dermatology, Strong Memorial Hospital/Golisano Children Hospital,
University of Rochester,
New York, USA
e-mail: mariacordisco2000@yahoo.com

IH increased 40 % [10]. These pregnancy-related morbidities could hypothetically lead to an imbalance toward proangiogenic factors as responses to a hypoxic environment, either via the expression of growth factors, such as insulin-like growth factor, or via hypoxia-inducible factor 1, which is unregulated in proliferating hemangiomas [2, 7, 15].

In a prospective cohort study conducted in the United States by members of the Hemangioma Investigator Group (HIG), demographic data in 1,058 patients with IH revealed that white non-Hispanic patients comprised 68.9 % of patients, while African–American and Hispanic patients represented 2.8 and 14.4 % of patients, respectively [9]. The authors found that infants with hemangiomas were more likely to be female, the product of premature birth, low birth weight, and multiple gestations. Preterm (defined as younger than 37 weeks gestational age) and very preterm (defined as younger than 32 weeks of gestational age) were frequent. There was no increased usage of prescription drugs and illicit drugs in this group. The majority of hemangiomas were classified as localized 66.8 %; whereas 13.1 % were segmental, 16.5 % were indeterminate, and 3.6 % were multifocal. Segmental hemangiomas were 11 times more likely to experience complications and eight times more likely to receive treatment than localized hemangiomas.

In a prospective cohort study of 252 patients that were followed up in the Department of Dermatology of Garrahan Hospital in Argentina, female predominance was noted (71.5 %), and males were 28.5 %. 39 % was Caucasian and 61 % were Latin Americans, 22.68 % presented low birth weight (defined as 1,500–2,499 g), while 7.5 % presented with very low birth weight (less than 1,500 g). A positive family history of vascular lesions was found in 16.6 % (87.5 % of them had hemangiomas), and 2.8 % were the product of multiple gestation [16].

Garzon et al. [17] and collaborative Hemangioma Investigator Group found that multiple hemangiomas were increased in preterm infants; however, female predominance was less than in term infants.

Localized hemangiomas were more common than either segmental or indeterminate subtypes in both preterm and term groups, but there is no significant difference in the incidence of segmental hemangiomas between term and preterm infants. The recent suggestion for a role of endothelial progenitor cells in IH development could help explain both the increase in frequency and numbers of hemangiomas in preterm infants because these progenitor cells might be more likely to be present and in higher numbers in an immature fetus than in a mature one [5].

Lopez Gutierrez et al. [18] found a high incidence of placental pathology in prematures less than 1,500 g who developed HI, and the authors speculated that ischemic changes in placental circulation could be related to hemangioma development.

A case–control study of 1,832 prospectively enrolled children with hemangiomas and 1,832 controls was held in two hospitals in China [19]. Risk factors for hemangiomas included lower level of maternal education, mother engaged in manual labor, multiple gestations, maternal medication use during the periconceptional, and a positive family history of hemangiomas.

Similar to previous studies, most of the IH were focal and located on the facial area [9, 20]. There were no differences in the incidence of complications or hemangioma behavior between preterm and term infants.

In opposition to the study by Garzon et al., an increased number of segmental hemangiomas was found in this preterm population [17].

Periconceptional use of drugs that includes prescription drugs and nonprescription drugs (ATB Chinese herbal medicines, antifungal drug, progesterone, and nonsteroidal antiinflammatory) was the strongest risk factor.

In another recently controlled study conducted at Vascular Anomaly Center in Shanghai, a total of 650 infants with IH were compared with 650 infants without IH. Female predominance, prematurity, LBW, and multiple gestation were found strongly associated with IH [21]. Diabetes, hypertension, preeclampsia and CVS, older maternal age, and multiple births were not significantly different in both groups, but they found that IVF showed a positive association with IH that were greater in the female subgroup.

Maternal vaginal bleeding and progesterone therapy during the first trimester of pregnancy were found to be independent risk factors for IH [22]. The role of vaginal bleeding and progesterone treatment in IH is unclear, but the timing coincides with the important phases of placental development. High concentrations of progesterone and local tissue ischemia could promote hypoxia-inducible growth factor (HIF-1alpha) and vascular endothelial growth factor activation, increasing the number of capillaries in the hemangioma tissue beds [23, 24].

Twins have a higher-than-expected risk of infantile hemangiomas, but the exact reasons for this association are not clear.

As evidenced by a review of the literature by Burns et al. and a study showing the incidence of IH in monozygotic and dizygotic twin pairs, it does not differ statistically [25, 26]. A recently multicenter prospective cohort study of 202 sets of twins conducted by members of the Hemangioma Investigator Group (HIG) and other pediatric dermatology centers at 12 different sites in the United States, Canada, Argentina, and Spain did confirm several previously reported findings that genetic predisposition is not the most potent risk factor for occurrence of IH [27]. Other known IH risk factors including advanced maternal age (mean and a median of 33 years), assisted reproduction, and maternal hypertension were also confirmed in our study [28]. In a retrospective cohort study of IH diagnoses before newborn hospital discharge during a period of 28 years was held by Amrock and colab. This study supports prior findings about female predominance and that whites received an IH diagnosis 3.6 times more than blacks, Asian, and American–Indian, respectively [29]. Given the high incidence of IH, all these findings suggest that the pathogenesis of IH is the result of the interaction between several different and common factors.

References

1. Kilcline C, Frieden IJ (2008) Infantile hemangiomas: how common are they? A systematic review of the medical literature. Pediatr Dermatol 25:168
2. Jacobs AH, Walton RG (1976) The incidence of birthmarks in the neonate. Pediatrics 58:218
3. Alper JC, Holmes LB (1983) The incidence and significance of birthmarks in a cohort of 4,641 newborns. Pediatr Dermatol 1:58
4. Pratt AG (1953) Birthmarks in infants. AMA Arch Derm Syphilol 67:302
5. Jacobs AH (1967) Strawberry hemangiomas; the natural history of the untreated lesion. Calif Med 86:8
6. Hohenleutner U, Landthaler M, Hamm H et al (2007) Hemangiomas of infancy and childhood. J Dtsch Dermatol Ges 5:334–338
7. Blei F, Walter J, Orlow SJ, Marchuk DA (1998) Familial segregation of hemangiomas and vascular malformations as an autosomal dominant trait. Arch Dermatol 134(6):718–722
8. Walter JW, Blei F, Anderson JL, Orlow SJ, Speer MC, Marchuk DA (1999) Genetic mapping of a novel familial form of infantile hemangioma. Am J Med Genet 82(1):77–83
9. Haggstrom AN, Drolet BA, Hemangioma Investigator Group et al (2007) Prospective study of infantile hemangiomas: demographic, prenatal, and perinatal characteristics. J Pediatr 150(3):291–294
10. Drolet BA, Swanson EA, Frieden IK et al (2008) Infantile hemangiomas: an emerging health issue linked to an increased rate of low birth weight infants. J Pediatr 153(5):712, No-715
11. Amir J, Metzker A, Krikler R, Reisner SH (1986) Strawberry hemangioma in preterm infants. Pediatr Dermatol 3:331–332
12. Dickison P, Christou E, Wargon O (2011) A prospective study of infantile hemangiomas with a focus on incidence and risk factors. Pediatr Dermatol 28: 663–669
13. Burton BK, Schulz CJ, Angle B, Burd LI (1995) An increased incidence of haemangiomas in infants born following chorionic villus sampling (CVS). Prenat Diagn 15:209–214
14. Van der Vleuten C, Bauland CG, Bartelink LR, Scheffers SM, Rieu PNMA, Spauwen PMH (2004) The effect of amniocentesis and choriovillus sampling on the incidence of haemangiomas. 15th International Society for the Study of Vascular Anomalies. Wellington, (abstract)
15. Kleinman ME, Grieves MR, Churgin SS et al (2007) Hypoxia-induced mediators of stem/progenitor cell trafficking are increase in children with hemangioma. Arterioscler Thromb Vasc Biol 27(12):2664–2670
16. Cordisco MR, Castro C, Pierini AM (2008) Hemangioma of infancy: a prospective study of 252 patients. 17th International Workshop on Vascular Anomalies. Boston (abstract)

17. Garzón MC et al., The Hemangioma Investigator Group (2008) Comparison of infantile hemangiomas in preterm and term infants. Arch Derm 144:1231–1232.
18. Lopez Gutierrez JC, Avila LF, Sosa G, Patron M (2007) Placental anomalies in children with infantile hemangiomas. Pediatr Dermatol 24:353
19. Li J, Chen X, Zhao Z, Hu X, Chen C, Ouyang F, Liu Q, Ding R, Shi O, Juan Su J, Kuang Y, Chang J, Li F, Xie H (2011) Demographic and clinical characteristics and risk factors for infantile hemangioma. A Chinese case-control study. Arch Dermatol 147(9): 1049–1056
20. Chiller KG, Passaro D, Frieden IJ (2002) Hemangiomas of infancy: clinical characteristics, morphologic subtypes, and their relationship to race, ethnicity, and sex. Arch Dermatol 138:1567–1576
21. Chen X, Ma G, Chen H, Ye X, Jin J, Lin X (2013) Maternal and perinatal risk factors for infantile hemangioma: a case–control study. Pediatr Dermatol 30(4):457–461
22. Speert H, Guttmacher A (1954) Frequency and significance of bleeding in early pregnancy. JAMA 155:712–715
23. North PE, Waner M, Mizeracki A et al (2001) A unique microvascular phenotype shared by juvenile hemangiomas and human placenta. Arch Dermatol 137:559–570
24. Chen D, Lin XX, Li W (2005) The relationship between the expression of HIF-1a and the angiogenesis in infantile hemangioma. Chin J Plast Surg 21:115–118
25. Cheung SM, Warman ML, Mulliken JB (1997) Hemangioma in twins. Ann Plast Surg 38:269–274
26. Burns AJ, Kaplan LC, Mulliken JB (1991) Is there an association between hemangioma and syndromes with dysmorphic features? Pediatrics 88(6):1257–1267
27. Greco MF, Drolet B, Garzon M, Mancini A, Chamlin S, Metry D, Lucky A, Horii KA, Baselga E, Powell J, Mc Cuaig C, Haggstrom A, Siegel D, Morel K, Cordisco MR, Frieden IJ, and the Hemangioma Investigator Group (2012) Infantile hemangiomas in twins: a prospective cohort study authors presented 19th International Workshop on Vascular Anomalies. Malmo, 16–19 June
28. Drolet B, Frieden IJ (2010) Characteristics of IH as clues to pathogenesis: does hypoxia connect the dots? Arch Dermatol 146:1295–1299
29. Amrock SM, Weitzman M (2013) Diverging racial trends in neonatal infantile hemangioma diagnoses 1979–2006. Pediatr Dermatol 30(4):493–507

Classification of Vascular Tumors

6

Juan Carlos Lopez Gutierrez

Many physicians are still confused by their pathologists in reports on excised specimens or biopsies because of the widespread use of the Enzinger's classification of vascular tumors of soft tissue, which employs the word hemangioma in a totally different way. Due to advances in nomenclature, diagnosis, and treatment, morbidity and mortality rates are progressively decreasing. Current vascular tumors classification (ISSVA) includes benign tumors (infantile hemangioma, congenital hemangioma, pyogenic granuloma, spindle cell hemangioma, and tufted angioma), borderline tumors (kaposiform hemangioendothelioma, retiform hemangioendothelioma, composite hemangioendothelioma, Dabska tumor, and Kaposi sarcoma), and malignant tumors (angiosarcoma and epithelioid hemangioendothelioma).

Hemangioma of Infancy/Infantile Hemangioma (IH)

Hemangioma is the most common tumor of infancy, but the understanding of its etiology and pathogenesis has lagged far behind other diseases. The incidence of IH may be as high as 25 % in premature infants of a low birth weight (fewer

J.C. Lopez Gutierrez, MD, PhD
Department of Pediatric Surgery,
Vascular Anomalies Center,
La Paz Children's Hospital, Madrid, Spain
e-mail: queminfantil.hulp@salud.madrid.org

than 1,000 g). The average age when hemangioma appears is 2 weeks. Hemangiomas never develop in an adult. Although the precise events leading to the formation of hemangiomas are not known, research in angiogenesis and blood vessel development has provided some clues. IH has a unique vascular phenotype which most closely resembles that of placental microvasculature, rather than ordinary cutaneous vasculature, demonstrated by staining markers such as glucose transporter 1 (GLUT-1) which is present in all phases of IH, merosin, and Lewis Y antigen [1].

Several clinical subtypes of hemangiomas (superficial, mixed, and deep or focal, segmental, and indeterminate) are recognized depending on factors as size and depth of skin penetration [2].

According to the growth phase, IH can be classified as early proliferative, late proliferative, plateau, involuting, or abortive (arrested growth). They deserve attention as they are difficult to recognize, mimicking a port-wine stain [3].

A distinct subset of IH consists of multiple small lesions varying in size from a few millimeters to 1–2 cm. This form of hemangioma (so-called diffuse hemangiomatosis) has a higher risk of visceral involvement, particularly in the liver and gastrointestinal tract [4].

One more uncommon variant is the reticular hemangioma, occurring in the extremity and associated with intractable ulceration, anogenito-urinary-sacral anomalies, and sometimes cardiac overload.

Infantile hepatic hemangiomas are classified into three types: focal (RICH analog), multifocal,

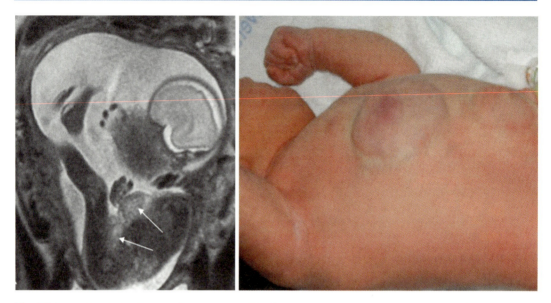

Fig. 6.1 Multiple RICH with prenatal diagnosis on MRI. Two arrows are remarking the presence of 2 RICH on MRI

and diffuse. Each type demonstrates different imaging appearances, pathologic features, and clinical behavior.

Congenital Hemangioma (CH)

Congenital hemangiomas are much more rare tumors than IH. They are clearly distinguished on the basis of their distinctive clinical, histological, and immunophenotypic features. Three main characteristics differentiate them from IH. CH are fully formed in utero, being noticeable immediately after birth, they never proliferate, and they show a lack of immunoreactivity for GLUT-1 marker.

Two types of congenital hemangiomas exist: rapidly involuting congenital hemangiomas (RICH) and noninvoluting congenital hemangiomas (NICH). Recently a different type has been described: partially involuting congenital hemangiomas (PICH).

RICH are round and usually large vascular tumors that are most commonly located close to a joint on the limbs or on the head. They undergo a postnatal involution commonly achieved in 6–12 months. After regression, two types of sequelae can occur: lipoatrophy or a telangiectatic plaque. In large tumors, transient

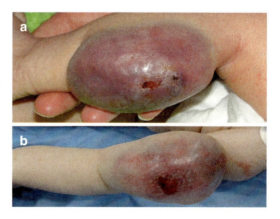

Fig. 6.2 Macroscopic similarity between RICH (**a**) and fibrosarcoma (**b**)

thrombocytopenia occurs in the first week of life: this should not be misdiagnosed as Kasabach-Merritt syndrome. Antenatal diagnosis of RICH during prenatal ultrasound or MRI follow-up is feasible as early as the 18th week of pregnancy [5, 6] (Fig. 6.1).

In some instances differential diagnosis with other congenital tumors is needed (Fig. 6.2).

RICH differs from rapidly involuting congenital hemangiomas because they do not undergo a postnatal involuting phase. They are mainly located on the head or neck and limbs. In contrast to RICH, prenatal color Doppler ultrasound or

MRI follow-up during pregnancy rarely leads to the detection of NICH [7].

PICH are congenital hemangiomas with a distinct behavior, evolving from RICH to persistent NICH-like lesions [8].

Tufted Angioma (TA)

TA is an uncommon vascular tumor that usually has its onset during infancy or early childhood but rarely can be congenital.

They had already been recognized half a century earlier by Japanese authors who referred to the tumors under the name of Nakagawa's angioblastoma. Various presentations have been described, including solitary tumors, large infiltrated plaques sometimes having increased lanugo hair, and "port-wine stain-like" areas with a cobblestone surface. The appearance of the lesions changes with time and they are sensitive upon palpitation or even painful if subjected to trauma. Tufted angiomas may be associated with Kasabach-Merritt syndrome (KMS), in which thrombocytopenia can be life-threatening [9].

Kaposiform Hemangioendothelioma (KHE)

KHE is a rare and locally aggressive vascular tumor that can occur in the skin, pleura, and retroperitoneum and may be associated with severe thrombopenia with consumption coagulopathy (Kasabach-Merritt syndrome) in pediatric patients. The use of the term "kaposiform" relates to its unmistakable resemblance to Kaposi's sarcoma, assumed by the compact spindled tumor cells characterized by the formation of slit-like lumen. KHE and TA have been viewed as two separate disease entities in past classifications of vascular tumors. However, the clinical similarities with TA, the association of both conditions with Kasabach-Merritt phenomenon, and the histological features of these syndromes have led to the suggestion that kaposiform hemangioendothelioma and tufted angioma are part of the same clinical spectrum of vascular tumors. In the largest reported case series of 107 patients, 71 %

developed KMP (11 % of patients lacked cutaneous findings). Retroperitoneal and intrathoracic lesions, though less common, were complicated by KMP in 85 and 100 % of cases, respectively [10]. Current multidisciplinary management protocols have dramatically reduced mortality rates [11].

Spindle Cell Hemangioma (SCH)

SCH is a rare, benign vascular tumor of the dermis and subcutis. The lesions can be multifocal and are overrepresented in Maffucci syndrome, in which patients also have multiple enchondromas. Somatic mosaic R132C IDH1 hotspot mutations were recently identified in Maffucci syndrome (71 % SCHs harbored mutations in exon 4 of IDH1 or IDH2). Although originally spindle cell hemangioendothelioma was proposed as a specific clinicopathologic variant of hemangioendothelioma, currently, it is considered as an entirely benign lesion, and thus, the name spindle cell hemangioma seems to be the most accurate for this lesion [12].

Pyogenic Granuloma (PG)

Pyogenic granuloma is a condition usually occurring in the skin or mucosa and often related to prior local trauma or pregnancy. However, the etiopathogenesis of pyogenic granuloma is poorly understood, and whether pyogenic granuloma is a reactive process or a tumor is unknown. Pyogenic granuloma seems to be a reactive lesion resulting from tissue injury, followed by an impaired wound healing response, during which vascular growth is driven by FLT4 and the nitric oxide pathway.

Retiform Hemangioendothelioma (RH)

RH is a very rare tumor of the blood vessels that occurs mainly in the limbs of young adults.

RH mostly occurs as an asymptomatic, slow-growing single lesion. Most cases are present as exophytic, dermal, or subcutaneous

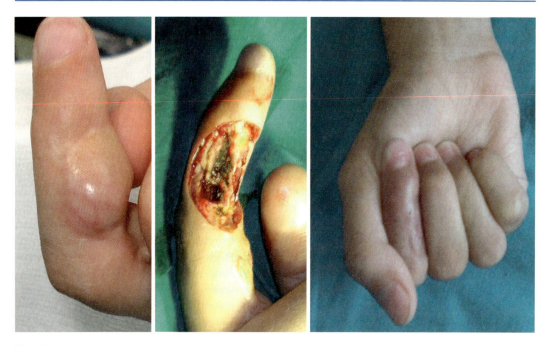

Fig. 6.3 Recurrence of retiform hemangioendothelioma needing radical excision

nodules or plaques with a size range of 1–30 cm. Although metastasis or malignancy is rare, RH is known to recur in approximately 50 % of cases.

The blood vessels are arranged in an anastomosing pattern that resembles that of the rete testis and lined with hobnail endothelial cells with focal papillary projections. The endothelial cells reveal enlarged nuclei with vesicular chromatin and rare mitosis. Some lymphocytic infiltrate is observed. Immunohistochemically, the endothelial cells are diffusely positive for factor VIII-related antigen [12].

Due to the tendency for recurrence, surgical excision must be performed under histopathologically tumor-free margins (Fig. 6.3).

Papillary Intralymphatic Angioendothelioma (PILA, Dabska Tumor)

PILA is a locally aggressive, rarely metastasizing vascular lesion characterized by lymphatic and vascular-like channels and papillary endothelial proliferation. The tumor is extremely rare and often affects the skin and subcutaneous tissues of children. The clinical appearance is variable. However, in general, it presents as a slow-growing, usually intradermal nodule that grows up to 2–3 cm in diameter. Symptoms of pain can be present. Microscopically, the cuboidal or hobnail endothelial cells lining the vascular structures are characterized by a high nuclear cytoplasmic ratio and an apically placed nucleus that produces a surface bulge, accounting for the term "hobnail." A growing number of cases described in the literature and the accumulating knowledge reveal that presence of highly specific lymphatic endothelial marker D2-40 and tumor marker vascular endothelial cell growth factor receptor type 3 (VEGFR3) suggests the tumor's lymphatic origin.

Dabska tumor and retiform hemangioendotheliomas are considered vascular neoplasms of intermediate malignancy, based on their limited capacity for lymph node metastasis, mortality from distant metastasis has been reported [12].

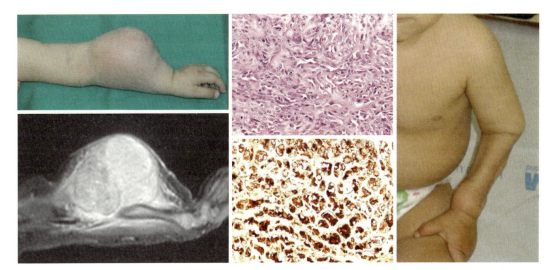

Fig. 6.4 ß-HCG-secretor angiosarcoma of the forearm

Composite Hemangioendothelioma

Composite hemangioendothelioma is the term that has been coined to name locally aggressive vascular neoplasms of low-grade malignancy showing varying combinations of benign, low-grade malignant, and high-grade malignant vascular components. The proportion of each component varies from case to case, but retiform hemangioendothelioma, epithelioid hemangioendothelioma, and spindle cell hemangioma are the predominant components in most cases [13].

Kaposi Sarcoma

Kaposi sarcoma (KS) is a low-grade vascular tumor associated with Kaposi sarcoma herpesvirus/human herpesvirus 8 (KSHV/HHV8) infection. Only 1 clinical subtype, the endemic/African subtype, commonly affects the pediatric population. Kaposi sarcoma lesions evolve from early (patch stage) macules into plaques (plaque stage) that grow into larger nodules (tumor stage). Newer histologic variants, related to different responses to recently established therapies, include anaplastic, hyperkeratotic, lymphangioma-like, bullous, telangiectatic, ecchymotic, keloidal, pyogenic granuloma-like, micronodular, intravascular, glomeruloid, and pigmented KS, as well as KS with sarcoid-like granulomas and KS with myoid nodules [14]. In a recent study strong familial incidence has been noticed. KS patients forming the clusters were indeed close relatives. One family with five affected individuals in two generations and several families with two first-degree relatives were identified.

Angiosarcoma

Angiosarcomas are rare tumors, representing approximately 2–4 % of all sarcomas, which predominantly affect adults and elderly patients. They are extremely rare in children and adolescents. The classic presentation is an enlarging, painful mass of several weeks' duration, and they are occasionally associated with acute hemorrhage, anemia, or a coagulopathy (Fig. 6.4).

Most angiosarcomas rapidly become metastatic because their vascular origin permits direct tumor dissemination into the lungs without the need for initial recruitment of new blood vessels (Fig. 6.5). The topmost upregulated genes in angiosarcomas included angiogenic regulators such as *TIE1*, *VEGFR2*, *SNRK*, *TEK*, and

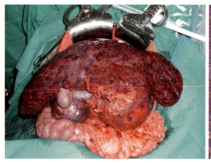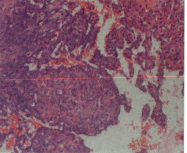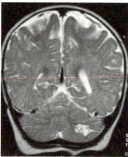

Fig. 6.5 Liver angiosarcoma. Brain metastasis 1 year after liver transplantation

VEGFR1, revealing that aberrant angiogenic signaling is a key feature of this sarcoma. MYC amplification has been also recently described as key feature of this tumor. Aberrant MYC signaling is associated with poor clinical outcomes, increased rates of metastasis, tumor recurrence, and patient mortality. Unfortunately, despite intense research efforts to inhibit MYC activity, this protein has thus far remained an elusive therapy target [15].

Epithelioid Hemangioendothelioma (EHE)

EHE is a rare vascular tumor that can arise in the soft tissue, bone, and parenchymal organs such as the liver and lung. The natural history of EHE is highly variable. EHE is characterized by a reciprocal t(1;3)(p36;q25) translocation. EHE may arise as a solitary lesion but also has a tendency to present with multifocal/metastatic involvement, especially when it arises in the liver and lung. 61 % of liver EHE develop metastasis. Disease-specific mortality has been estimated around 13–18 % for EHE arising in soft tissue, while the disease-specific mortality rate for EHE in the lung and liver is 40 and 65 %, respectively.

A novel staging system with prognostic value for EHE has been recently proposed. Pleural effusion or other signs of uncontained tumor growth, hemoptysis, and osseous involvement of more than two bones imply worse survival than do localized and discrete tumors, regardless of

the number of organs involved. No specific organ or combination of organ involvement differentially affected survival, and survival was no different between patients with multiple- vs. single-organ involvement [15].

References

1. Hoeger PH, Colmenero I (2013) Vascular tumours in infants. Part I: benign vascular tumours other than infantile haemangioma. Br J Dermatol. 2014;171(3):466–473
2. Luu M, Frieden IJ (2013) Haemangioma: clinical course, complications and management. Br J Dermatol 169(1):20–30
3. Corella F, Garcia-Navarro X, Ribe A, Alomar A, Baselga E (2008) Abortive or minimal-growth hemangiomas: immunohistochemical evidence that they represent true infantile hemangiomas. J Am Acad Dermatol 58(4):685–690
4. Glick ZR, Frieden IJ, Garzon MC, Mully TW, Drolet BA (2012) Diffuse neonatal hemangiomatosis: an evidence-based review of case reports in the literature. J Am Acad Dermatol 67(5):898–903
5. Mulliken JB, Enjolras O (2004) Congenital hemangiomas and infantile hemangioma: missing links. J Am Acad Dermatol 50(6):875–882
6. Berenguer B, Mulliken JB, Enjolras O, Boon LM, Wassef M, Josset P, Burrows PE, Perez-Atayde AR, Kozakewich HP (2003) Rapidly involuting congenital hemangioma: clinical and histopathologic features. Pediatr Dev Pathol 6(6):495–510
7. Gorincour G, Kokta V, Rypens F, Garel L, Powell J, Dubois J (2005) Imaging characteristics of two subtypes of congenital hemangiomas: rapidly involuting congenital hemangiomas and non-involuting congenital hemangiomas. Pediatr Radiol 35(12):1178–1185
8. Nasseri E, Piram M, McCuaig CC, Kokta V, Dubois J, Powell J (2014) Partially involuting congenital hemangiomas: a report of 8 cases and review of the literature.

J Am Acad Dermatol. 2014;70(1):75–79. doi:10.1016/j. jaad.2013.09.018, pii: S0190-9622(13)00969-9

9. Tlougan BE, Lee MT, Drolet BA, Frieden IJ, Adams DM, Garzon MC (2013) Medical management of tumors associated with kasabach-merritt phenomenon: an expert survey. J Pediatr Hematol Oncol 35(8):618–622

10. Croteau SE, Liang MG, Kozakewich HP, Alomari AI, Fishman SJ, Mulliken JB, Trenor CC 3rd (2013) Kaposiform hemangioendothelioma: atypical features and risks of Kasabach-Merritt phenomenon in 107 referrals. J Pediatr 162(1):142–147

11. Fernandez-Pineda I, Lopez-Gutierrez JC, Chocarro G, Bernabeu-Wittel J, Ramirez-Villar GL (2013) Long-term outcome of vincristine-aspirin-ticlopidine (VAT) therapy for vascular tumors associated with Kasabach-Merritt phenomenon. Pediatr Blood Cancer 60(9):1478–1481

12. Requena L, Kutzner H (2013) Hemangioendothelioma. Semin Diagn Pathol 30(1):29–44

13. McNab PM, Quigley BC, Glass LF, Jukic DM (2013) Composite hemangioendothelioma and its classification as a low-grade malignancy. Am J Dermatopathol 35(4):517–522

14. Ravi V, Patel S (2013) Vascular sarcomas. Curr Oncol Rep 15(4):347–355

15. Cioffi A, Reichert S, Antonescu CR, Maki RG (2013) Angiosarcomas and other sarcomas of endothelial origin. Hematol Oncol Clin North Am 27(5):975–988

Hemangiomas: Clinical Picture

7

Maria Rosa Cordisco

Infantile hemangioma (IH) is the most common tumor of infancy, affecting approximately 4 % of children [1, 2]. Lesions typically first appear at about 2 weeks of age (or less commonly are present at birth) as a blanched, blushed, or telangiectatic patch or ulcerated appearance, suggesting the possibility that hypoxemia precedes tumor growth. The area then can rapidly proliferate for several months (Fig. 7.1a, b).

The territory of the IH is delineated by the premonitory mark, yet in some cases only a part of the area proliferates [3, 4] (Fig. 7.2). They are characterized by a wide clinical heterogeneity (depth of cutaneous involvement, size).

During the last years, IH have been classified according to the level of the skin affected and into three groups: superficial, deep, and mixed hemangiomas [5, 6]. Superficial hemangiomas involve the superficial dermis and appear as bright red lesions (Fig. 7.3). These lesions may be plaque-like or more rounded papules or nodules. Deep hemangiomas involve the deep dermis and subcutis and present as bluish to skin-colored nodules (Fig. 7.4). Mixed hemangiomas have both superficial and deep components and therefore have features of both (Fig. 7.5). The skin and

subcutis appear to be most commonly affected, even factoring in more obvious presentation, whereas deep skeletal muscle is spared.

Chiller et al. proposed a new clinical classification, in which they were divided into four groups: localized, segmental, indeterminate, and multifocal hemangiomas. "Segmental hemangiomas" were those hemangiomas or clusters of hemangiomas with a configuration corresponding to known embryologic prominences, derived from the neuroectoderm. They have a geographic

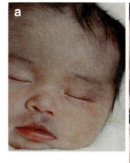
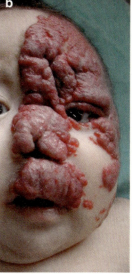

Fig. 7.1 Early hemangioma in a newborn (**a**). Hemangioma in rapid proliferative phase in the same patient, who presented with associated PHACE syndrome (**b**)

M.R. Cordisco
Department of Dermatology, Strong Memorial
Hospital/Golisano Children Hospital,
University of Rochester,
New York, USA
e-mail: mariacordisco2000@yahoo.com

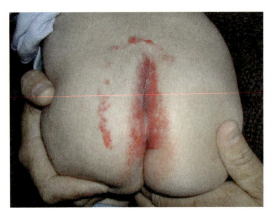

Fig. 7.2 Hemangioma with minimal or arrested growth, fine telangiectasias, and a proliferative component in the periphery in lumbosacral area. The patient has spinal dysraphism

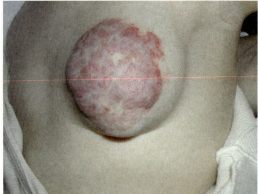

Fig. 7.5 Mixed hemangioma

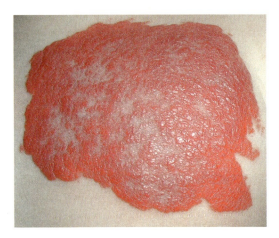

Fig. 7.3 Superficial hemangioma

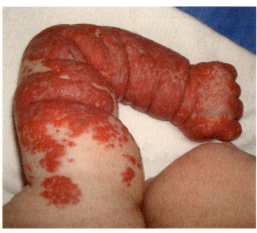

Fig. 7.6 Segmental hemangioma

shape, have large size and involve an anatomic region, and can be reticular or telangiectatic or flat cherry-red patches [6–8] (Fig. 7.6).

Four segments or patterns of involvement occur in facial area regions. Segment 1 involved the lateral forehead and temporal and lateral frontal scalp. Segments 2 and 3 correspond to the maxillary and mandibular, and Segment 4 involved the nose, philtrum, and medial frontal scalp. These segmental hemangiomas tend to be greater than 5 cm in diameter and most often span one side of the face and neck (Fig. 7.7).

"Localized hemangiomas" were defined as those hemangiomas that seem to grow from a single focal point or were localized to an area without any apparent linear or developmental configuration. They are usually oval or round.

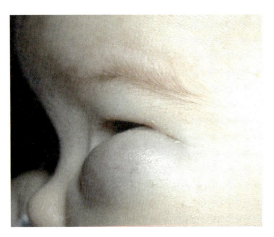

Fig. 7.4 Deep hemangiomas

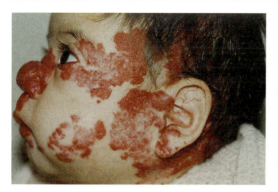

Fig. 7.7 Facial segmental hemangioma associated with PHACE syndrome (the four facial segments are partially involved)

"Indeterminate hemangiomas" were those that were not readily classified as either localized or segmental, and "multifocal hemangiomas" were defined as more than ten cutaneous hemangiomas [6].

Although approximately 60 % of hemangiomas occur on the head and neck, they can also occur in any region of the body on the trunk (25 %), extremities, and genitals (15 %) [7, 8]. Most present as solitary cutaneous and/or subcutaneous lesions (80–90 %), and a significant percentage of patients (15 %) have multiple lesions [7, 8] (Fig. 7.8).

Hemangiomas, whether small and innocuos or large and deforming but are united by a predictable biological behavior characterized by three distinct stages: a rapidly proliferating, high-flow stage (8–12 months), followed by a prolonged involuting stage (1–12 years), and finally by a variably prominent end-stage with fibrofatty residuum. [3, 5, 9–11].

However others leave only residual telangiectasias (Fig. 7.9).

Most hemangioma growth occurs in the first 5–9 months, at which point 80 % of the final size has often been reached [4].

The deep and mixed IH with segmental or indeterminate distribution differ in their growth pattern [12]. These IH sometimes appear later and continue to grow for a longer period than superficial hemangiomas (sometimes the prolonged growth has been observed until 2 years of age). Cervicofacial IH and those involving the parotid gland are a typical example of IH with this growth pattern. This group is known as

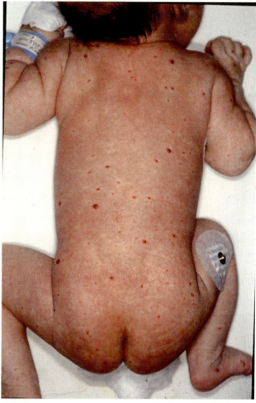

Fig. 7.8 Multifocal hemangiomas in a patient with visceral involvement

hemangiomas with prolonged growth phase [12, 13] (Fig. 7.10a, b).

Another subgroup of IH exhibits a pattern of minimal growth, and they presented a reticular or telangiectatic appearance with a proliferative component predominating in the periphery consisting of papules a few millimeters in diameter. They electively are located in the trunk and limbs and lumbosacral area [14–16] (Fig. 7.2). The beginning of involution is even more difficult to predict but usually manifested by changes in color from bright red to a paler red or gray, with a whitish discoloration that occurs always in the center of the hemangioma and extends centrifugally. Deep lesions become less blue and less warm. IH involutes over different periods of time, some in a few years, while others can take several years.

IH during the proliferative phase is composed of well-defined masses of capillaries lined by

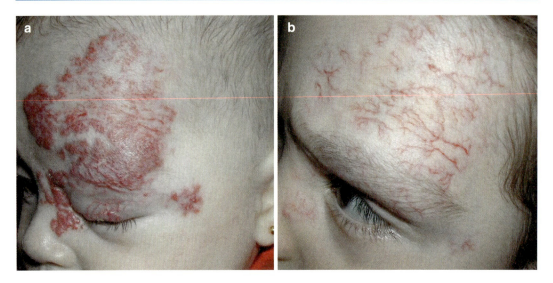

Fig. 7.9 Hemangioma in proliferative phase (**a**), post-involution telangiectasias (**b**)

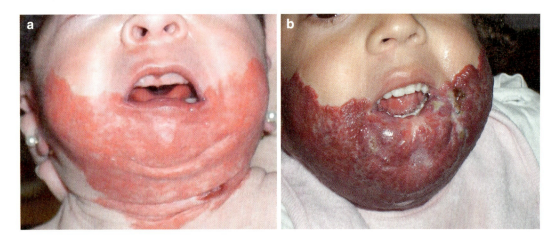

Fig. 7.10 Segmental hemangioma with "beard distribution" in proliferative phase at 2 weeks of age with associated underlying airway hemangioma (**a**) and at 22 months of age with continued growth (**b**)

plump endothelial cells. Normally configured mitotic figures may be numerous. GLUT-1 (the erythrocyte-type glucose transporter protein) is strongly expressed by endothelial cells of infantile hemangiomas at all stages of their evolution and is not expressed by other benign vascular anomalies and reactive proliferations. This appears to be an exclusive marker for IH and is an invaluable tool used to distinguish hemangiomas from other vascular lesions [17].

The diagnosis of a hemangioma is best made by clinical history and physical exam. In cases of unclear diagnosis, the best radiographic modalities to use are either a Doppler ultrasound or MRI. Biopsy should only be considered when history, physical examination, and imaging studies fail to clearly define the pathology.

Complications

The majority of infantile hemangiomas are innocuous (80 %), but a significant minority during the rapid growth phase are associated with important

Table 7.1 Hemangioma high-risk locations

Location	Complication
Eyelid	Functional impairment amblyopia
Ear	Functional impairment
Beard area	Functional impairment/airway involvement
Forehead and nasal tip	Disfigurement
Upper and lower lip	Disfigurement/ulceration
Neck/anogenital area	Ulceration
Large segmental facial and scalp area	PHACE syndrome/visceral hemangiomas
Large segmental lumbosacral area	Spinal dysraphism, anogenital/urogenital/limb abnormalities

complications such as ulceration, bleeding, risk for permanent disfigurement, compromised organ function, vision and airway obstruction, or high-output cardiac failure. In these cases, quick active and aggressive therapeutic intervention is mandatory [7, 8, 18] (Table 7.1).

Ulceration

This occurs during the proliferation phase in 15 % of IH (3–4 months of age); however it could occur in precursor lesions prior to the development of IH.

The most commonly affected areas include the anogenital area, head, and neck, particularly the lips and perioral and intertriginous areas; nevertheless IH on any site could be ulcerated (Fig. 7.11). The ulcer could persist for several weeks or months and result in pain, bleeding, infection, and sometimes permanent scarring [19]. The causes of ulceration are understood; the factors that may play a role are friction, maceration, or both. Ulceration is more frequent in mixed or superficial and larger segmental hemangiomas than in the focal subtype [18–21].

Visual Compromise

Periorbital hemangiomas most often involve the upper lid, but the lower lid and retrobulbar space are also common. We can define the anatomic location of the ocular hemangiomas as preseptal, extraconal, and intraconal [22, 23]. All the lesions that affect the visual axis may cause amblyopia, and that is the complication of most concern (Fig. 7.12a, b).

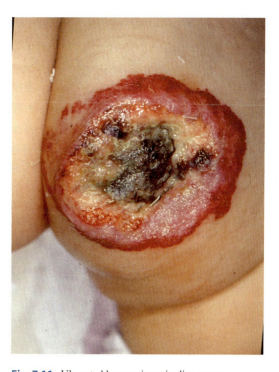

Fig. 7.11 Ulcerated hemangioma in diaper area

Amblyopia may result from different mechanisms:

1. Anisometropia (if there is a refractive difference between the eyes): In the case of hemangiomas, astigmatism is usually secondary to pressure from the tumor on the globe, which causes an irregular corneal curvature.
2. Strabismic amblyopia can occur if the hemangiomas affect the movement of extraocular muscles.
3. Deprivation amblyopia arising from partial or complete eyelid closure is particularly devastating if it occurs during the first few months of life, when it can cause profound visual impairment.

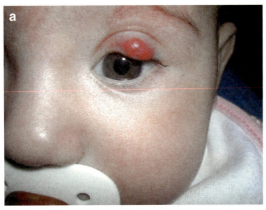
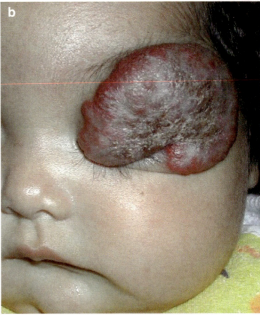

Fig. 7.12 (**a**) *Left upper* eyelid focal hemangioma causing astigmatism. (**b**) *Left upper* eyelid hemangioma The child presented with complete visual axis obstruction

Intraconal IH that involves the posterior orbit could result in proptosis, displacement of the globe, or visual axis obstruction [24, 25].

Another relatively common complication of IH is lacrimal duct obstruction because of pressure in the region of the lacrimal duct, resulting in increased tearing and recurrent conjunctivitis.

Airway Hemangiomas

Infantile hemangiomas (IH) involving the "beard area"(which encompasses the preauricular area, mandible, chin, lower lip, and anterior neck) have a high likelihood of concomitant airway hemangiomas, and this association is even more pronounced when the IH involves multiple rather than one component of the "beard area"[26] (Fig. 7.11). Of course, airway hemangiomas can occur in the absence of cutaneous IH, and some cases have been reported with localized cutaneous IH either on the face or in extra-facial locations [27, 28].

Airway hemangiomas can involve any site from the nares to the tracheobronchial tree; however they are most commonly seen in the subglottis, and laryngeal localization represents 1.5 % of congenital lesions of the larynx [29] (Fig. 7.13a, b).

Most of the subglottic hemangiomas become symptomatic during the first year of life. They are located in the posterior or lateral subglottic space, and besides hoarseness, dyspnea, and feeding difficulties, they produce a typical gradually worsening croupous stridor as the main symptom [29].

Multifocal Hemangiomas

The term diffuse neonatal hemangiomatosis (DNH) has been used to describe infants with multiple hemangiomas affecting the skin and viscera. Lesions range in size from a few millimeters to centimeters in diameter and may be present at birth but usually develop during the first week of life (Fig. 7.8).

These infants represent variable degrees of involvement ranging from only skin benign neonatal hemangiomatosis (BNH) to combined cutaneous and visceral involvement diffuse neonatal

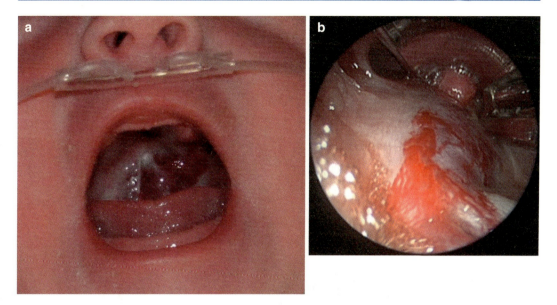

Fig. 7.13 Hemangioma in hard palate without skin involvement (**a**). Subglottic hemangioma in the same patient (**b**)

hemangiomatosis (DNH). Arbitrarily more than five cutaneous lesions have been recognized as a clue to potential visceral hemangiomas [30, 31].

Recently Glick et al. proposed replacing the old term DNH for "multifocal cutaneous hemangiomas with visceral involvement" because the significance of this disorder depends less on the number of the cutaneous hemangiomas and more on the location and potential complications of the visceral lesions [32]. All these patients should be screened for inner organ involvement. Most of these internal lesions are found on the liver but can also develop in the lungs, bowel, and brain. True IH may occur in the brain, but this has been poorly demonstrated histologically.

Large diffuse hemangiomas of the liver can also cause hypothyroidism, because IH express type 3 iodothyronine deiodinase, an enzyme that inactivates blood thyroid hormone [33].

Multifocal hemangiomas should be distinguished from other multifocal vascular lesions as multifocal pyogenic granuloma (not very common) and from multifocal lymphangioendotheliomatosis with thrombocytopenia. In the last one the cutaneous lesions are congenitally variable in number and appearance and are associated with diffuse gastrointestinal involvement. Histopathologic findings show vessels lined

by hobnail endothelial cells that are GLUT-1 negative and LYVE-1 (a lymphatic endothelial cell marker) positive [34].

Hemangiomas and Associated Structural Anomalies

Segmental hemangiomas are frequently associated with structural anomalies and/or visceral hemangiomas.

Patients with segmental hemangiomas should also undergo investigation to rule out PHACES syndrome (posterior fossa brain malformations, hemangiomas of the face, arterial cerebrovascular anomalies, cardiovascular anomalies, eye anomalies, and sternal defects or supraumbilical raphe) [35].

Which patients are at risk for PHACE? The size and distribution of IH play an important role. The risk of PHACE and associated anomalies varies with IH distribution. Children with segmental infantile hemangioma (SIH) that involved the S1 segment alone or in combination with other segments were much more likely to have PHACE and central nervous system manifestations (CNS) (Figs. 7.1 and 7.7). In contrast those patients with SIH involving S2 and S3 with spar-

Table 7.2 PHACE syndrome diagnostic criteria

Organ system	Major criteria	Minor criteria
Cerebrovascular	Anomaly of major cerebral arteries Dysplasia of the large cerebral arteries Arterial stenosis or occlusion Absence, hypoplasia, or aberrant origin or course of the large cerebral arteries, persistent trigeminal artery	Persistent embryonic artery
Structural brain	Posterior fossa abnormality: Dandy-Walker complex Cerebellar hypoplasia/atrophy Arachnoid cyst	Enhancing extra-axial lesion with features consistent with intracranial hemangioma
Cardiovascular	Aortic arch anomaly Aberrant origin of the subclavian artery	Ventricular septal defect Right aortic arch (double aortic arch)
Ocular	Posterior segment abnormality Persistent fetal vasculature Retinal vascular anomalies Morning glory disk anomaly Optic nerve hypoplasia Peripapillary staphyloma Coloboma	Anterior segment abnormality Cataract Coloboma Microphthalmia
Ventral or midline	Partial or complete agenesis of sternum Sternal cleft of pit Supraumbilical raphe Supraumbilical raphe Sternal defect	Hypopituitarism Ectopic thyroid

ing of S1 had a lower incidence of PHACE and CNS anomalies. Brain and intracranial arterial anomalies constitute the most common extracutaneous features. Persistent embryonic arteries, dysplasia, narrowing, or occlusion may lead to progressive changes and subsequent ischemia and stroke. Accordingly, neurologic and cognitive impairments are the greatest source of potential morbidity in PHACE [36].

A spectrum of congenital structural brain abnormalities has been described among patients with PHACE, of which malformations of the cerebellum and posterior fossa structures are the most commonly observed. Specific anomalies reported range from the Dandy-Walker complex to focal dysplasia and/or hypoplasia of the cerebellum. Microphthalmia is one of the more commonly reported ophthalmologic features of PHACE. Optic nerve findings reported in PHACE include peripapillary staphyloma, optic nerve hypoplasia, and the morning glory disk anomaly.

A wide variety of cardiac lesions have been described: aortic arch anomalies, atrial and ventricular septal defects, patent ductus arteriosus, persistent left superior vena cava, and, rarely, complex congenital heart disease, coarctation on the transverse aorta, right aortic arc, and aberrant origin of the brachiocephalic arteries especially the right subclavian artery [37].

Affected children are classified into two categories, definite PHACE syndrome and possible PHACE syndrome, based on the nature and number of criteria met. Definite PHACE syndrome requires the presence of a characteristic segmental hemangioma greater than 5 cm in diameter on the face (or scalp) plus one of the major criterion or two minor criteria listed in Table 7.2. Possible PHACE syndrome can be diagnosed in one of three different combinations: (a) facial hemangioma greater than 5 cm in diameter plus 1 minor criterion; (b) hemangioma of the neck or upper torso plus 1 major criterion or 2 minor criteria; or (c) no hemangioma plus 2 major criteria [38].

Although multiple cutaneous IH are known to be associated with visceral, Metry et al. observed

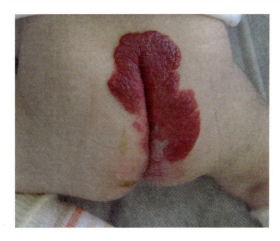

Fig. 7.14 Lumbosacral hemangioma with underlying tethered cord

segmental hemangiomas most often involving the face in association with visceral IH, and the liver was the most common visceral involvement followed by the gastrointestinal tract, brain, mediastinum, and lung [39].

The association of segmental lumbosacral hemangiomas with tethered spinal cord or genitourinary anomalies or both has been recognized for many years.

Segmental IH of the lower body and particularly those located over the lumbar or sacral spine bear their own unique risks of spinal dysraphism or genitourinary anomalies.

Recently different acronyms have been proposed: PELVIS syndrome (perineal hemangioma, external genitalia malformations, lipomyelomeningocele, vesicorenal abnormalities, imperforate anus, and skin tag), SACRAL syndrome (spinal dysraphism; anogenital, cutaneous, renal, and urologic anomalies; and hemangioma with "angioma" of lumbosacral localization), and LUMBAR syndrome (lower body hemangioma and other skin defects, urogenital abnormalities, ulceration, myelopathy, bony deformities, anorectal malformations, and arterial and renal abnormalities) [40–42].

Those patients at risk for this group of anomalies typically have segmental IH which span the midline and, in the case of spinal dysraphism, nearly always involve the lumbosacral skin. In some cases, the hemangiomas are bulky, but more often they have a flat,

telangiectatic appearance. The presence of a gluteal cleft deviation in this setting is of greatest concern for underlying spinal dysraphism (Figs. 7.2 and 7.14).

Differential Diagnosis

We should not forget that not all lesions that look like strawberry lesions are infantile hemangiomas.

Multiple tumors, both benign and malignant could masquerade as IH. It is very important to differentiate between IH and other vascular lesions and tumors such as nasal glioma, xanthogranuloma, dermoid cyst, pilomatrixoma, congenital angiofibroma, plexiform neurofibroma, hemangioendothelioma, infantile fibrosarcoma, Ewing sarcoma, rhabdomyosarcoma, metastasis of neuroblastoma, and cutaneous lesions of leukemia cutis. In all the cases based in clinical history, physical examination, and radiological findings, biopsy is mandatory to rule out the diagnosis.

References

1. Bowers RE, Graham EA, Thominson KM (1960) The natural history of the strawberry nevus. Arch Dermatol 82:667–670
2. Powell TG, West CR, Pharoah PO, Cooke RW (1987) Epidemiology of strawberry hemangioma in low birth weight infants. Br J Dermatol 116:635–641
3. Bruckner AL, Frieden IJ (2003) Hemangiomas of infancy. J Am Acad Dermatol 48:477–493
4. Chang LC, Haggstrom AN, Drolet BA, Hemangioma Investigator Group et al (2008) Growth characteristics of infantile hemangiomas: implications for management. Pediatrics 122(2):360–367
5. Drolet BA, Esterly NB, Frieden IJ (1999) Hemangiomas in children. N Engl J Med 341(3):173–181
6. Chiller KG, Passaro D, Frieden IJ (2002) Hemangiomas of infancy: clinical characteristics, morphologic subtypes, and their relationship to race, ethnicity, and sex. Arch Dermatol 138(12):1567–1576
7. Waner M, North PE, Scherer KA et al (2003) The nonrandom distribution of facial hemangiomas. Arch Dermatol 139(7):869–875
8. Haggstrom AN, Lammer EJ, Schneider RA et al (2006) Patterns of infantile hemangiomas: new clues to hemangioma pathogenesis and embryonic facial development. Pediatrics 117(3):698–703
9. Waner M, Suen JY (1999) The natural history of hemangiomas. In: Waner M, Suen JY (eds) Hemangiomas

and vascular malformations of the head and neck. A John Wiley & Sons, Inc., New York, pp 13–45

10. Martínez-Pérez D, Fein NA, Boon LM, Mulliken JB (1995) Not all hemangiomas look like strawberries. Pediatr Dermatol 12(1):1–6

11. Mulliken JB, Fishman SJ, Burrows PE (2000) Vascular anomalies. Curr Probl Surg 37:519–584

12. Brandling-Bennett HA, Metry DW, Baselga E et al (2008) Infantile hemangiomas with unusually prolonged growth phase: a case series. Arch Dermatol 144(12):1632–1637

13. Blei F, Isakoff M, Deb G (1997) The response of parotid hemangiomas to the use of systemic interferon alfa-2a or corticosteroids. Arch Otolaryngol Head Neck Surg 123(8):841–844

14. Shu K, Frieden I (2010) Infantile hemangioma with minimal or arrested growth. Arch Dermatol 146(9): 971–976

15. Mulliken JB, Marler JJ, Burrows PE, Kozakewich HP (2007) Reticular infantile hemangioma of the limb can be associated with ventral-caudal anomalies, refractory ulceration, and cardiac overload. Pediatr Dermatol 24(4):356–362

16. Corella F, Garcia-Navarro X, Ribe A, Alomar A, Baselga E (2008) Abortive or minimal growth hemangiomas. J Am Acad Dermatol 58(4):685–690

17. North PE, Waner M, Mizeracki A et al (2000) GLUT1: a newly discovered immunohistochemical marker for juvenile hemangiomas. Hum Pathol 31(1):11–22

18. Haggstrom AN, Drolet BA, Baselga E et al (2006) Prospective study of infantile hemangiomas: clinical characteristics predicting complications and treatment. Pediatrics 118(3):882–887

19. Kim HJ, Colombo M, Frieden IJ (2001) Ulcerated hemangiomas: clinical characteristics and response to therapy. J Am Acad Dermatol 44:962–972

20. Chamlin SL, Haggstrom AN, Drolet BA et al (2007) Multicenter prospective study of ulcerated hemangiomas. J Pediatr 151(6):684

21. Shin HT, Orlow SJ, Chang MW (2007) Ulcerated haemangioma of infancy: a retrospective review of 47 patients. Br J Dermatol 156(5):1050–1052

22. Bilyk JR, Adamis AP, Mulliken JB (1992) Treatment options for periorbital hemangioma of infancy. Int Ophthalmol Clin 32(3):95–109

23. Dubois J, Milot J, Jaeger B, McCuaig C, Rousseau E, Powell J (2006) Orbit and eyelid hemangiomas: is there a relationship between location and ocular problems? J Am Acad Dermatol 55:614–619

24. Millischer-Bellaiche AE, Enjolras O, Andre C, Bursztyn J, Kalifa G, Adamsbaum C (2004) Eyelid hemangiomas in infants: contribution of MRI. J Radiol 85:2019–2028

25. Ceisler EJ, Santos L, Blei F (2004) Periocular hemangiomas: what every physician should know. Pediatr Dermatol 21:1–9

26. Orlow SJ, Isakoff MS, Blei F (1997) Increased risk of symptomatic hemangiomas of the airway in association with cutaneous hemangiomas in a beard distribution. J Pediatr 131(4):643–646

27. Suh K-Y, Rosbe C, Meyer A, Frieden I (2011) Extensive airway hemangiomas in two patients without beard hemangiomas. Pediatr Dermatol 28(3):347–348

28. Sherrington CA, Sim DKY, Freezer NJ et al (1997) Subglottic hemangioma. Arch Dis Child 76:458–459

29. Rahbar R, Nicollas R, Roger G et al (2004) The biology and management of subglottic hemangioma: past, present, future. Laryngoscope 114(11):1880–1891

30. Golitz LE, Rudikoff J, O'Meara OP (1986) Diffuse neonatal hemangiomatosis. Pediatr Dermatol 3(2): 145–152

31. Holden KR, Alexander F (1970) Diffuse neonatal hemangiomatosis. Pediatr Dermatol 46:411–421

32. Glick Z, Frieden I, Garzon M, Mully T, Drolet B (2012) Diffuse neonatal hemangiomatosis: an evidence-based review of case reports in the literature. J Am Acad Dermatol 67:898–903

33. Horii KA, Drolet BA, Frieden IJ et al (2011) Prospective study of the frequency of hepatic hemangiomas in infants with multiple cutaneous infantile hemangiomas. Pediatr Dermatol 28(3):245–253

34. North PE, Kahn T, Cordisco MR, Dadras SS, Detmar M, Frieden IJ (2004) Multifocal lymphangioendotheliomatosis with thrombocytopenia: a newly recognized clinicopathological entity. Arch Dermatol 140: 599–606

35. Frieden IJ, Reese V, Cohen D (1996) PHACE syndrome. The association of posterior fossa brain malformations, hemangiomas, arterial anomalies, coarctation of the aorta and cardiac defects, and eye abnormalities. Arch Dermatol 132(3):307–311

36. Haggstrom A, Garzon M, Baselga E, Chamlin S, Frieden IJ, Holland K, Maguiness S, Mancini A, McCuaig C, Metry S, Morel K, Powell J, Perkins S, Siegel D, Drolet B (2010) Risk for PHACE syndrome in infants with large facial hemangiomas. Pediatrics 126:e418–e426

37. Bayer M, Frommelt P, Blei M, Cordisco M, Frieden I, Goddard D, Holland KE, Krol A, Maheshwar M, Metry D, Morel K, North P, Pope E, Shieh J, Southern J, Wargon O, Siegel D, Drolet B (2013) Congenital cardiac, aortic arch, and vascular bed anomalies in PHACE syndrome: The International PHACE Syndrome Registry Review. Am J Cardiol 112: 1948–52

38. Metry D, Heyer G, Hess C et al (2009) Consensus statement on diagnostic criteria for PHACE syndrome. Pediatrics 124(5):1447–1456

39. Metry D, Hawrot A, Altman C, Frieden I (2004) Association of solitary, segmental hemangiomas of the skin with visceral hemangiomatosis. Arch Dermatol 140:591–596

40. Girard C, Bigorre M, Guillot B et al (2006) PELVIS syndrome. Arch Dermatol 142(7):884–888

41. Stockman A, Boralevi F, Taieb A et al (2007) SACRAL syndrome: spinal dysraphism, anogenital, cutaneous, renal and urologic anomalies, associated with an angioma of lumbosacral localization. Dermatology 214(1): 40–45

42. Iacobas I, Burrows PE, Frieden I, Drolet B (2012) LUMBAR: association between cutaneous infantile hemangiomas of lower body and regional congenital anomalies. J Pediatr 157(5):795–801 e1–7

Diagnosis of Hemangiomas

8

Juan Carlos Lopez Gutierrez

Up to 90 % of infantile hemangiomas (IH) involving the epidermis can be easily diagnosed by their typical appearance, while in 10 % of the cases, deep location, abnormal growth pattern, or visceral involvement makes differential diagnosis necessary.

Vascular tumors and highly vascularized solid tumors can mimic one another. Mesenchymal hamartomas of the liver or intraconal rhabdomyosarcomas of the orbit usually proliferate in the first 3 months of life as hemangiomas do. Experienced and a well-trained multidisciplinary team are the key to avoid misdiagnosis with eventually fatal consequences (Fig. 8.1).

Diagnosis of hemangiomas is based first on the medical history. Two questions are of paramount importance:

Was the lesion present at birth? Did proportional or disproportional growth of the lesion after birth occur?

A careful history that includes age of onset, color, and location, along with physical examination findings, is generally sufficient in determining the pathological condition. The presence of the lesion at birth supports the diagnosis of vascular malformation or congenital hemangioma. Infantile hemangiomas are characterized by a

postnatal rapid proliferation phase in the first 6–9 months of life, followed by a slow involution phase, and in many cases complete regression. Congenital hemangiomas fully developed before birth present as erythematous warm vascular plaques or nodules with a rim of pallor and do not undergo postnatal growth. Congenital hemangiomas are divided into two categories – rapidly involuting congenital hemangiomas (RICH) and non-involuting congenital hemangiomas (NICH). As the name implies, RICH lesions begin to involute almost immediately after birth and in many cases fully involute by 1 year of age. A NICH may partially involute or soften, but full resolution does not occur (Fig. 8.2). Despite RICH involute much faster than common hemangiomas, some patients may develop significant health problems (e.g., cardiac failure or bleeding) due to arteriovenous shunting [1–3]. After physical examination hemangiomas should be classified as superficial, deep, or mixed type, according to their location in the skin and subcutaneous tissue and focal or segmental according to their extension. Superficial infantile hemangiomas may be mistaken for capillary malformations (port-wine stains). Deep infantile hemangiomas typically present as a fluctuant, compressible bluish mass and may resemble lymphatic, venous, or mixed (venous and lymphatic) malformations [4, 5]. Congenital hemangiomas may be confused with venous malformations or mixed malformations. RICH may not be distinguished from a NICH at birth and only clinical observation

8

J.C. Lopez Gutierrez, MD, PhD
Department of Pediatric Surgery,
Vascular Anomalies Center,
La Paz Children's Hospital, Madrid, Spain
e-mail: queminfantil.hulp@salud.madrid.org

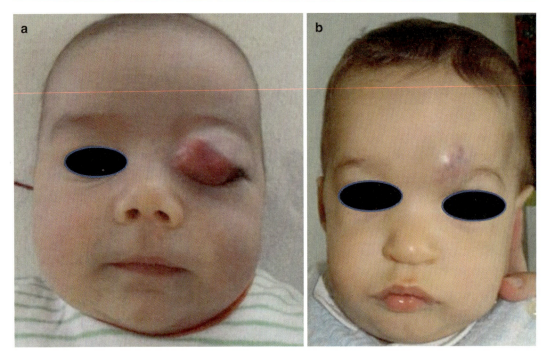

Fig. 8.1 Congenital orbital rhabdomyosarcoma (**a**) and leukemia (**b**) previously misdiagnosed as hemangiomas, received an unsuccessful course of propranolol

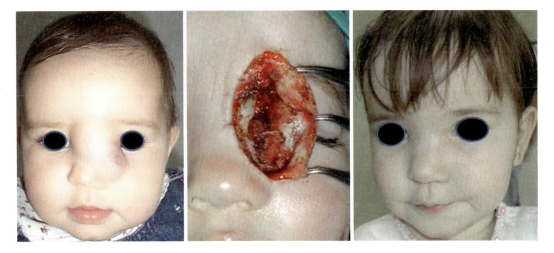

Fig. 8.2 Ultrasound and MRI findings were unable to determinate the diagnosis of glioma versus hemangioma. Excisional biopsy leads to final diagnosis of hemangioma

would allow differentiation. In the newborn, lesions may not be evident or may present as a red, white, telangiectatic, or blue patch. A peripheral rim of pallor due to vasoconstriction may be seen at this stage. As the tumor proliferates, the lesion may take on the more classic appearance, which depends on the depth of lesion and stage of evolution [6].

In cases in which clinical examination alone is inconclusive, other diagnostic modalities such as ultrasonography and magnetic resonance imaging (MRI) may be utilized. Ultrasound Doppler

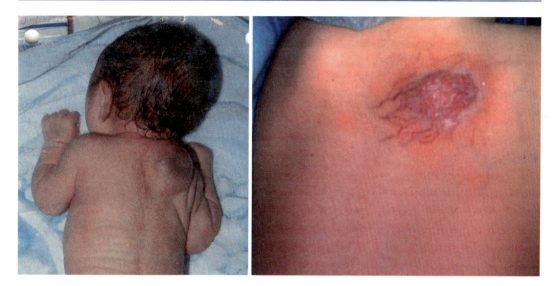

Fig. 8.3 Non-involuting or partially involuting congenital hemangioma

can assess the flow of hemangiomas, characterized by a shunt pattern with decreased arterial resistance and increased venous velocity. In deep cutaneous or visceral hemangiomas, contrast-enhanced MRI demonstrates the extent of the lesion and helps differentiation between hemangiomas and other disorders presenting with similar findings on US examination. Hemangiomas have a typical solid appearance with intermediate intensity on a T1-weighted spin-echo image, which is more intense compared with venous or lymphatic malformations. During the proliferative stage, hemangiomas show a relatively low intensity in a T2-weighted spin-echo image, while in the involution phase, they have a very low intensity. Contrast-enhanced T1-weighted MRI shows moderate intensity with prominent flow voids during the proliferative stage because of the high flow at this stage. In contrast, hemangiomas show low intensity during involution as a result of the low flow at that stage. The appropriate diagnostic tests for congenital hemangiomas are ultrasonography with Doppler (the lesions are uniformly hypoechoic, mostly confined to the subcutaneous fat and diffusely vascular, being traversed by multiple tubular vascular channels) and magnetic resonance imaging (RICH has areas of inhomogeneity and larger flow voids). Angiography is only indicated if embolization

has to be performed (large and irregular feeding arteries in disorganized patterns, arterial aneurysms, direct arteriovenous shunts, and intravascular thrombi are common features in RICH and are rarely seen in infantile hemangiomas) [7].

The type of lesion can usually be determined based on the medical history and clinical examination. Imaging is mostly useful for confirming the clinical diagnosis, estimating the extent of the lesion and determining the feasibility of surgical resection.

The differential diagnosis also includes angiosarcoma, glioma (Fig. 8.3), congenital fibrosarcoma, infantile myofibromatosis, kaposiform hemangioendothelioma, pyogenic granuloma, teratoma, tufted angioma, or rhabdomyosarcoma. Frequently, an ultrasound examination of a growing deep vascularized tumor in a 2-month-old patient concludes that the final diagnosis would probably be "hemangioma," considering "congenital fibrosarcoma" as an alternative option. In those instances, both physicians and parents consider a biopsy as necessary for a safer accurate final diagnosis [8–12].

Skin biopsy can be helpful in distinguishing unusual or atypical hemangiomas from other vascular lesions. Specimens may be evaluated by routine histological examination and immunohistochemical analysis. The histological appearance of RICH differed from NICH and common infantile hemangioma, but some overlap was noted among the three lesions. RICH is composed of small-to-large lobules of capillaries with moderately plump endothelial cells and pericytes; the lobules are surrounded by abundant fibrous tissue. One-half of the specimens have a central involuting zone characterized by lobular loss, fibrous tissue, and draining channels that are often large and abnormal.

Additionally hemangiomas have a unique vascular phenotype demonstrated by glucose transporter 1 (GLUT-1) staining marker. Since its first description by P. E. North in 2000, its use has become widely spread by clinicians and researchers in the field of vascular anomalies. Endothelial cells in RICH and other vascular tumors or malformations do not express glucose transporter-1 protein [13].

Unfortunately and despite cardinal advances in the diagnosis of hemangiomas, the use of a wrong nomenclature remains as the most frequent origin of incorrect diagnosis and inappropriate treatments.

References

1. Hand JL, Frieden IJ (2002) Vascular birthmarks of infancy: resolving nosologic confusion. Am J Med Genet 108:257–264
2. Chiller KG, Passaro D, Frieden IJ (2002) Hemangiomas of infancy: clinical characteristics, morphologic subtypes, and their relationship to race, ethnicity, and sex. Arch Dermatol 138:1567–1576
3. Boon LM, Enjolras O, Mulliken JB (1996) Congenital hemangioma: evidence of accelerated involution. J Pediatr 128:329–335
4. Haggstrom AN, Drolet BA, Baselga E, Chamlin SL, Garzon MC, Horii KA, Lucky AW, Mancini AJ, Metry DW, Newell B, Nopper AJ, Frieden IJ (2006) Prospective study of infantile hemangiomas: clinical characteristics predicting complications and treatment. Pediatrics 118(3):882–887
5. Frieden IJ, Haggstrom AN, Drolet BA, Mancini AJ, Friedlander SF, Boon L, Chamlin SL, Baselga E, Garzon MC, Nopper AJ, Siegel DH, Mathes EW, Goddard DS, Bischoff J, North PE, Esterly NB (2005) Infantile hemangiomas: current knowledge, future directions. Proceedings of a research workshop on infantile hemangiomas, April 7–9, 2005, Bethesda, Maryland, USA. Pediatr Dermatol 22(5):383–406
6. Frieden I, Enjolras O, Esterly N (2003) Vascular birthmarks and other abnormalities of blood vessels and lymphatics. In: Schachner LA, Hanse RC (eds). Pediatric Dermatology, 3rd Ed. London, Mosby, pp 833–861
7. Burrows PE (1998) Diagnostic imaging in the evaluation of vascular birthmarks. Dermatol Clin 16:455–488
8. Boon LM, Fishman SJ, Lund DP, Mulliken JB (1995) Congenital fibrosarcoma masquerading as congenital hemangioma: report of two cases. J Pediatr Surg 30(9):1378–1381
9. Mullen M, Rabban J, Frieden IJ (2013) Sacrococcygeal teratoma masquerading as congenital hemangioma. Pediatr Dermatol 30(1):112–116
10. Friedman BJ, Shah KN, Taylor JA, Rubin AI (2013) Congenital myofibroma masquerading as an ulcerated infantile hemangioma in a neonate. Pediatr Dermatol 30(6):e248–e249
11. Frieden IJ, Rogers M, Garzon MC (2009) Conditions masquerading as infantile haemangioma: part 1. Australas J Dermatol 50(2):77–97
12. Frieden IJ, Rogers M, Garzon MC (2009) Conditions masquerading as infantile haemangioma: part 2. Australas J Dermatol 50(3):153–168
13. North PE, Waner M, Mizeracki A, Mihm MC Jr (2000) GLUT1: a newly discovered immunohistochemical marker for juvenile hemangiomas. Hum Pathol 31:11–22

Diagnostics of Infantile Hemangiomas Including Visceral Hemangioma

9

Josee Dubois and Francoise Rypens

Most infantile hemangiomas (IHs) are identified according to clinical criteria. However, some cases are challenging either because of an atypical presentation (e.g., soft-tissue mass with normal overlying skin) or because of classification difficulties.

Most of the time, IHs can be found in soft tissue. Visceral hemangiomas can also be seen, associated or not, with multiple cutaneous hemangiomas (>5). The most common visceral IHs are found in the liver but can be observed anywhere.

Most liver hemangiomas are clinically silent and remain undetected. Others are discovered incidentally on prenatal ultrasound or postnatal imaging. It is hard to differentiate liver infantile hemangioma from congenital hemangioma and from hemangioendothelioma considering that most of them do not require biopsy. However, the subtype classification is helpful to make the diagnosis. The subtype classification of liver hemangiomas includes focal lesions, probably corresponding to rapidly involuting congenital hemangioma (RICH); multifocal lesions, corresponding to infantile hemangioma; and diffuse lesions [1]. Diffuse lesions are rare and present with extensive hepatic involvement, numerous small lesions in the liver leading to severe hepatomegaly, and abdominal compartment syndrome, hypothyroidism due to overproduction of type III iodothyronine deiodinase, cardiac failure, and mental retardation [2].

Imaging is needed in these clinically uncertain cases of soft-tissue mass, in PHACE syndrome, or in cases of suspicion of visceral infantile hemangioma to establish the correct diagnosis, in order to decide on the most appropriate treatment and to inform the parents of the prognosis. The imaging findings of soft-tissue infantile hemangioma are similar to visceral infantile hemangioma.

High-resolution grayscale and *Doppler ultrasound* allow for an excellent visualization of most superficial soft-tissue or visceral masses. Doppler ultrasound is the easiest mean to assess the hemodynamics of a vascular lesion and to clarify a doubtful diagnosis between an infantile hemangioma and other vascular tumor or vascular malformation. MRI is the best technique for evaluating the extent of the lesions and their relationship with adjacent structures [3–5].

On ultrasound, a variable, well-defined echogenic mass can be seen during the proliferative phase. The echogenicity is nonspecific; hyperechoic or hypoechoic lesions can be found in the proliferative phase. Sometimes, one or a few vessels are visible in the soft-tissue mass, which most often correspond to arteries. Occasionally, in the periphery

J. Dubois (✉)
Department of Medical Imaging,
CHU Sainte-Justine, Montreal, QC, Canada
e-mail: Josee-dubois@ssss.gouv.qc.ca

F. Rypens
Department of Radiology,
Radio-Oncology and Nuclear Medicine,
CHU Sainte-Justine, Montreal, QC, Canada
e-mail: francoise_rypens@ssss.gouv.qc.ca

R. Mattassi et al. (eds.), *Hemangiomas and Vascular Malformations: An Atlas of Diagnosis and Treatment*,
DOI 10.1007/978-88-470-5673-2_9, © Springer-Verlag Italia 2009, 2015

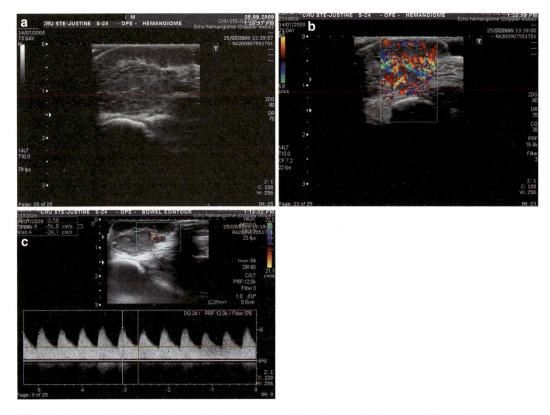

Fig. 9.1 Three-month-old girl with a soft-tissue mass. (**a**) Lesion is well limited with variable echogenicity. (**b**) Highly vascularized ≥5 vessels/cm² are observed and (**c**) High-peak systolic Doppler shifts >2 KHz with low-resistive index mean (0.61)

of the lesion, dilated veins can be seen and are related to the presence of microshunts within the hemangioma. Calcifications are never observed in soft-tissue or visceral infantile hemangioma.

Color Doppler ultrasound is used to make the diagnosis of infantile hemangioma and to differentiate it from other vascular lesions. The lesion displays an increased color flow due to numerous arteries and veins. The high-vessel density (over 5 vessels/cm²) with high Doppler shift (>2 kHz) and low-resistive index are characteristics of infantile hemangiomas. Arteriovenous shunting is visible on spectral Doppler analysis and is frequently misinterpreted as an arteriovenous malformation [6, 7] (Figs. 9.1, 9.2, and 9.3).

During the involuting phase, the lesion appears as a sonographically heterogeneous mass that becomes hyperechoic ultimately. The mass decreases in volume with a reduced number of vessels, but most of the time, the high Doppler shift persists in the remaining vessels.

On CT scan, during the proliferative phase, an infantile hemangioma shows a homogeneous mass with intense, persistent homogeneous enhancement, usually organized in a lobular pattern. During the involuting phase, *CT scan* shows a heterogeneous mass with less intense staining, as well as intralesional fibrofatty tissue.

MRI typically shows a well-defined, non-infiltrating lesion, with an intermediate signal intensity on T1-weighted sequences and increased signal intensity on T2-weighted sequences. Fast-flow vessels are identified by the presence of flow voids within and around the soft-tissue mass on spin-echo sequences and as high-signal intensity on gradient-recalled echo sequences. Perilesional edema should not be seen. The vessels with fast-flowing blood appear within and at the periphery of the mass. After

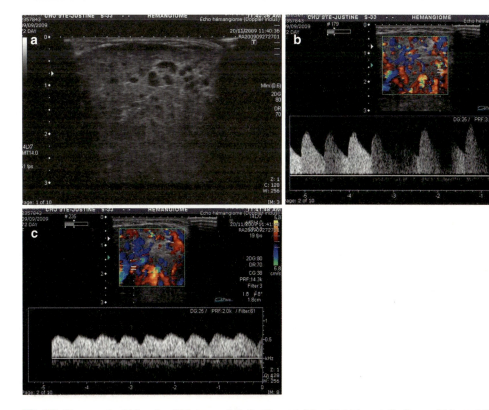

Fig. 9.2 Two-month-old female with intraparotid infantile hemangioma. (**a**) Ultrasound reveals a soft-tissue lesion with visible vessels. (**b**) Numerous arteries and veins are visible with high-systolic flow and (**c**) arterialization of the veins associated with arteriovenous fistula

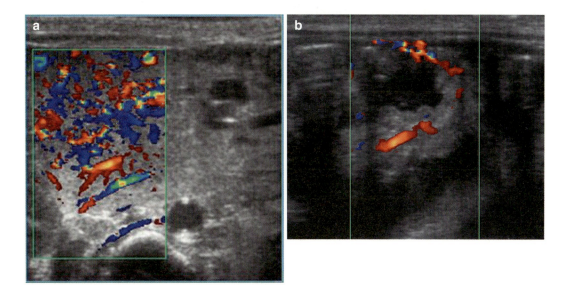

Fig. 9.3 Five-week-old female with severe intestinal bleeding required multiple transfusions. At physical exam, a segmental hemangioma of the leg was noticed. (**a**) Abdominal color ultrasound reveals a high-flow lesion in the head of pancreas and (**b**) in the small intestines. She was treated with octreotide, Cyklokapron, propanolol, and steroid with complete regression of the lesion

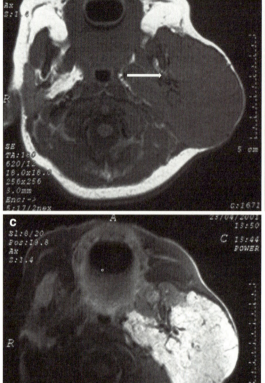

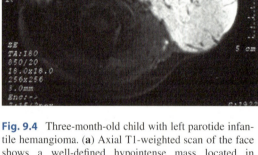

Fig. 9.4 Three-month-old child with left parotide infantile hemangioma. (**a**) Axial T1-weighted scan of the face shows a well-defined hypointense mass located in the parotid gland. Vessels are also identified by the presence of flow voids within the mass (*arrow*). (**b**) On axial T2-weighted scan with fat suppression, the mass is hyperintense. Flow void areas are still detected. No perilesional edema is visible, and (**c**) axial T1-weighted scan performed after fat suppression and gadolinium injection shows high enhancement of the lesion

gadolinium injection, high enhancement is observed. The *MRI* signal in involuting hemangiomas depends on the amount of fibrosis (hypointense on T1 and T2) and the quantity of fat (hyperintense on T1 and T2). The gadolinium enhancement decreases significantly with the involution [8–10] (Figs. 9.4, 9.5, and 9.6).

Differential Diagnostic

Congenital hemangiomas

RICH and NICH share similar imaging findings. Most of these can display the same appearance as infantile hemangioma on *US* and *CT* or *MR*. Some differences like various-sized vascular aneurysms, intravascular thrombi (calcifications), more visible vessels, and venous ectasia are observed in these congenital hemangiomas. Microarteriovenous shunting is frequently identified and sometimes arterial aneurysms are present [11, 12] (Figs. 9.7 and 9.8).

Hemangioendotheliomas

On ultrasound, hemangioendotheliomas are ill-defined, noncompressible soft-tissue masses with variable echogenicity. Calcifications and necrosis are occasionally present looking like cavities. Doppler shows a high-, moderate-, or low-vessel density, and most hemangioendotheliomas have a high Doppler shift >2 kHz with low-resistive index. Arteriovenous shunting is rarely observed [13] (Fig. 9.9).

CT scan displays a heterogeneous mass with ill-defined borders and skin thickening with subcutaneous stranding. Post-contrast *CT scan* shows inhomogeneous enhancement.

MR imaging: T1-weighted *MRI* sequences show a heterogeneous soft-tissue mass that is isointense or hypointense compared to the muscle. T2-weighted sequences show a hyperintense lesion with subcutaneous stranding. Signal voids can be seen on gradient-recalled echo and

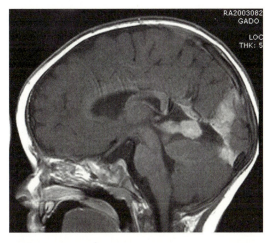

Fig. 9.5 One-month-old male with hemiface infantile hemangioma. Sagittal brain contrast T1-weighted image with fat suppression shows an enhancement of the pineal, meningeal, and tentorial areas, confirming the IH diagnosis. One year later, the MR reveals the complete regression of these lesions

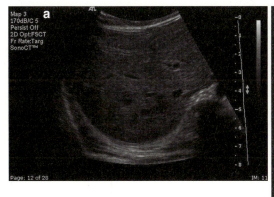
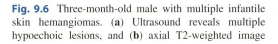
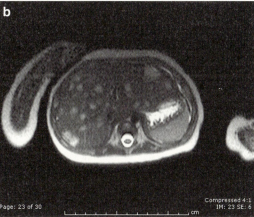

Fig. 9.6 Three-month-old male with multiple infantile skin hemangiomas. (**a**) Ultrasound reveals multiple hypoechoic lesions, and (**b**) axial T2-weighted image reveals multiple hyperintense lesions in the liver, confirming the IH diagnosis

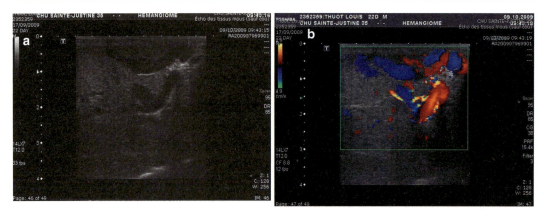

Fig. 9.7 Two-week-old child with soft-tissue lesion. (**a**) Gray-scale US shows a well-defined lesion with visible vessels, and (**b**) color Doppler reveals numerous arteries and veins. The evolution confirms the RICH diagnosis

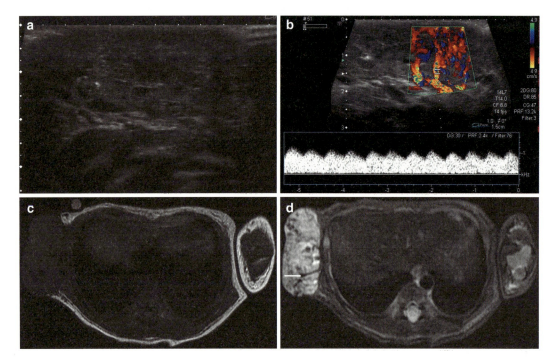

Fig. 9.8 Eighteen-month-old boy with soft-tissue mass of the thoracic wall which appeared at birth without any regression. (**a**) Ultrasound reveals a heterogeneous lesion with hypoechoic visible vessels. (**b**) Color doppler analysis reveals a high-systolic flow with low resistance with micro-fistula. (**c**) Axial T1-weighted image reveals a well-defined isodense, and (**d**) axial T2-weighted image with fat suppression shows a hyperintense lesion with flow void (*arrow*)

represent hemosiderin or other blood product. Post-gadolinium imaging displays a diffuse, heterogeneous enhancement in the soft-tissue mass.

Others Tumors

Soft-tissue sarcomas, neuroblastomas, myofibromatosis, tufted angiomas, hemangiopericytomas,

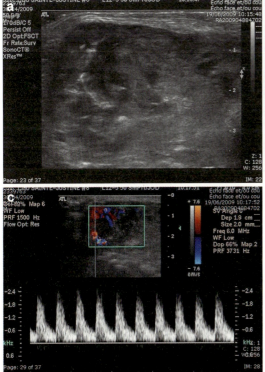

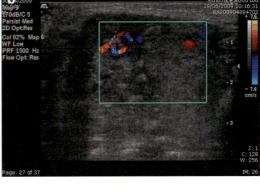

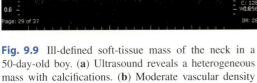

Fig. 9.9 Ill-defined soft-tissue mass of the neck in a 50-day-old boy. (**a**) Ultrasound reveals a heterogeneous mass with calcifications. (**b**) Moderate vascular density and (**c**) high-arterial resistive index. Biopsy reveals a hemangioendothelioma

infantile myofibromatosis, fibrosarcomas, rhabdomyosarcomas, metastatic neuroblastomas, or other tumors can be misdiagnosed as an infantile hemangioma.

and the imaging is not present, a biopsy has to be done.

Conclusion

The presence of a distinct mass at sonography, the high-vessel density, and the low-resistive index with Doppler are the most important diagnostic criteria of soft-tissue infantile hemangioma and visceral infantile hemangioma.

If the soft-tissue mass shows few arteries or veins, the spectral analysis shows a high-resistive index, and if you notice perilesional edema on T2 MR imaging, a malignant tumoral lesion should be suspected. If the correlation between the clinical findings

References

1. Christison-Lagay ER, Burrows PE, Alomari A, Dubois J, Kozakewich HP, Lane TS, Paltiel HJ, Klement G, Mulliken JB, Fishman SJ (2007) Hepatic hemangiomas: subtype classification and development of a clinical practice algorithm and registry. J Pediatr Surg 42:62–67; discussion 67–68
2. Huang SA, Tu HM, Harney JW, Venihaki M, Butte AJ, Kozakewich HP, Fishman SJ, Larsen PR (2000) Severe hypothyroidism caused by type 3 iodothyronine deiodinase in infantile hemangiomas. N Engl J Med 343:185–189
3. Dubois J, Garel L, Grignon A, David M, Laberge L, Filiatrault D, Powell J (1998) Imaging of hemangiomas and vascular malformations in children. Acad Radiol 5:390–400

4. Dubois J, Alison M (2010) Vascular anomalies: what a radiologist needs to know. Pediatr Radiol 40: 895–905

5. Legiehn GM, Heran MKS (2006) Classification, diagnosis, and interventional radiologic management of vascular malformations. Orthop Clin North Am 37:435–474

6. Dubois J, Patriquin HB, Garel L, Powell J, Filiatrault D, David M, Grignon A (1998) Soft-tissue hemangiomas in infants and children: diagnosis using Doppler sonography. AJR Am J Roentgenol 171:247–252

7. Paltiel HJ, Burrows PE, Kozakewich HP, Zurakowski D, Mulliken JB (2000) Soft-tissue vascular anomalies: utility of US for diagnosis. Radiology 214: 747–754

8. Konez O, Burrows PE (2002) Magnetic resonance of vascular anomalies. Magn Reson Imaging Clin N Am 10:363–388

9. Legiehn GM, Heran MK (2010) A step-by-step practical approach to imaging, diagnosis and interventional radiologic therapy in vascular malformations. Semin Intervent Radiol 27:209–231

10. Thawait SK, Puttgen K, Carrino JA, Fayad LM, Mitchell SE, Huisman TAGM, Tekes A (2013) MR imaging characteristics of soft tissue vascular anomalies in children. Eur J Pediatr 172: 591–600

11. Gorincour G, Kokta V, Rypens F, Garel L, Powell J, Dubois J (2005) Imaging characteristics of two subtypes of congenital hemangiomas: rapidly involuting congenital hemangiomas and non-involuting congenital hemangiomas. Pediatr Radiol 35:1178–1185

12. Rogers M, Lam A, Fischer G (2002) Sonographic findings in a series of rapidly involuting congenital hemangiomas (RICH). Pediatr Dermatol 9:5–11

13. Dubois J, Garel L, David M, Powell J (2002) Vascular soft-tissue tumors in infancy: distinguishing features on Doppler sonography. AJR Am J Roentgenol 178:1541–1545

Principles of Treatment of Hemangiomas

Hans-Peter Berlien and Carsten Philipp

In contrast to vascular malformations, where a spontaneous regression never occurs, in congenital vascular tumors such as infantile hemangiomas, there is a great potential for *spontaneous regression*. However, the indication for active therapy is wider and earlier in endangered regions than it is in other regions. So not the diagnosis itself gives the indication of any treatment but only a precise grading [1] based on stage, localization, biological behavior, and risk of complication. While the diagnosis is given clinically for the description of the above criterion, the color-coded duplex ultrasound is mandatory (Table 10.1).

Spontaneous Course

Because hemangiomas may involute spontaneously, waiting for spontaneous regression remains a viable therapeutic option. But the "wait-and-see" principle is always wrong (Table 10.2). If it means that treatment arrives too late, then *"see and wait"* as a control is correct, because at the first sign of progression of complication an action can be taken. Therefore, in case of small, uncomplicated infantile hemangiomas in non-problematic areas (extremities, body) without any tendency to proliferate,

especially in cutaneous hemangiomas, one can "see and wait." If delayed growth cannot be excluded, frequent controls are required. Clinical checkups alone may not be sufficient, as subcutaneous infantile hemangiomas may remain unnoticed as they grow deeply and are then only recognized after complications result. This is why a periodic duplex scan control is mandatory. For hemangiomas in the quiescent or regression phase, a "see-and-wait" attitude should normally be recommended. However, if complications are expected from ulcerations, treatment is also required for these forms. As therapy may cause adverse systemic or cutaneous side effects, particularly scarring, sometimes intervention has been reserved for patients with significant complications. Therefore, it is difficult to choose a therapy that eliminates hemangiomas before the development of complications and without systemic side effects [2]. For this reason, the following infantile hemangiomas must be considered as *"problem hemangiomas,"* for which active treatment is mandatory (Table 10.3):

- Hemangiomas of the face, particularly periorbitally, periorally, and in the areas of the ear, lips, and nose
- Hemangiomas at the mammary gland and in the anogenital area, particularly the vulva, the urethral orifice, and the anal derma
- Rapidly growing, diffuse infiltrating hemangiomas at any anatomic site
- Hemangiomatosis, either aggressive, diffuse, or visceral involvement.

H.-P. Berlien (✉) • C. Philipp
Center for Laser Medicine, Elisabeth Hospital, Berlin, Germany
e-mail: Lasermed.elisabeth@pgdiakonie.de

Table 10.1 Classification of infantile hemangioma

Stage	Clinic	CCDS
I. Prodromal phase	Red/white spot; telangiectasia	Structureless; low-echo space
	Blurred vision; swelling	No signs of pathological vessels
II. Initial phase	Loss of typical skin structure	Hyposonoric center
	Increasing thickness and induration	Hypervascularization beginning at edges
III. Proliferation phase	Bright red cutaneous infiltration; flat spreading	Increasing intratumoral hyperperfusion
	Subcutaneous growth of thickness;	Central vessel density
	Infiltration of surroundings possibly even at organ borders	Nutrition of tumor vessels
	Possible early primary central ulceration	Drainage veins with arterial flow profile
IV. Maturation phase	Pale and livid color	Declining central vessel density
	Possible central exulceration	Increasing ectatic drainage veins
	Decreasing growth	Declining arterialization of drainage veins
	Possible late ulceration over drainage veins	Central increasing hypersonoric aspect
V. Regression phase	Hypopigmentation; wrinkled skin/telangiectasis	Circumscribed hypersonoric area
	Surrounding subcutaneous drainage veins	Loss of typical tissue structure
	Subcutaneous palpable induration	Nearly no central tumor vessels
		Residuals supplying tumor arteries
		Residuals of ectatic drainage veins

Correlation of clinic and CCDS. The diagnosis itself is clinical. But for a correct definition of the stage and the involved organ structures, CCDS is mandatory

Table 10.2 Grade 1 means uncomplicated hemangioma with no risks; Grade 2a hemangiomas with low risk factors need controls; Grade 2b with risk factors needs close controls and laser therapy if any progress is observed; Grade 3 has a laser indication due to risks of complication; and Grade 4 requires additional systemic therapy

Grade	Definition	Procedure
G1	Uncritical region/organ	No treatment
No action	Signs of/or final regression	No control
G2a	Uncritical region/organ	Control; if no progress or sign of regression, follow G1
Control	No expectation of progress	If with slight progress follow G2b
G2b	Although no progress expected but critical region/organ	If with slight progress and no complication, close control
Close control		If with major progress or slight progress but with complication, follow G3a
	Uncritical region/organ but progress expected	Follow G3a
G3a	Progress, in case of further progress complication expected	If progress or no progress but remaining hemangioma causes functional impairment; start laser therapy to prevent complication
Laser treatment		
	No further progress, but critical region/organ complication expected	If regression starts, follow G2b
		If complication occurs, follow G3b
G3b	Critical region/organ complication has occurred with early regression/reduction necessary	If primary complication due to critical localization and/or biological aggressivity occurs, perform additional laser therapy systemic therapy
Add. systemic treatment		
	Monotherapy not successful	If stabilization achieved, follow G3a

Table 10.3 Therapeutic algorithm for infantile hemangiomas and congenital hemangioendotheliomas

Diagnostical pathway
Congenital vascular tumor

Legend acc. ISO 9000
Funct.: functional impairment
Progr.: progress/ regrow
Compl.: complications any kind
Coag.: coagulopathy
Crit. region: critical endangered region
Oro/anogen: perioral/anogenital

–: No
+: Yes
Criterion

Examination
+: Typical finding
–: No/untypical finding

The symbols are according to ISO 9000. The grading for infantile hemangioma is given in Table 10.2. Abbreviations: *DIC* disseminated intravascular coagulopathy, *CCDS* color-coded duplex sonography, *cHE* congenital hemangioendothelioma, *iH* infantile hemangioma, *RICH* rapid involuting congenital hemangioendothelioma, *NICH* non-involuting congenital hemangioendothelioma, *KHE* kaposiform congenital hemangioendothelioma, *Thermogr.* infrared thermography

Hemangiomas in problem zones (face, anogenital region) should be treated in their early stages to prevent complications [3]. This is the rule for hemangiomas near the eyes (threat to vision), lips (little regression tendency), and nose area (malformations of the nose – Cyrano nose). Treatment is also indicated when hemangiomas are located on the fingers (tactile problems), toes (shoe problems expected later on), breast, and cleavage area in women. Extended, highly proliferating hemangiomas or those already causing complications, as well as diffuse infiltrating hemangiomas, should be treated actively. Early treatment initiation can be decisive for the further course. In particular, as a rule, diffusely growing, infiltrating hemangiomas also require a systemic approach. Of the hemangioendotheliomas, rapidly involuting congenital hemangioendothelioma (RICH) needs only frequent ultrasound controls. For non-involuting congenital hemangioendothelioma (NICH) (Table 10.4), provided

Table 10.4 Different natural courses between infantile hemangioma and congenital hemangioendothelioma

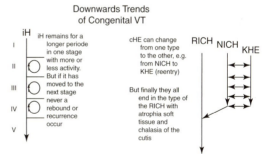

An infantile hemangioma never recurs after regression; in congenital hemangioendothelioma recurrences are possible

there is tight color-coded duplex sonography (CCDS) and thrombocyte monitoring, one may wait for a possible spontaneous regression as in RICH. If transition to a *Kaposi-like hemangioendothelioma* is suspected, however, due to an increase in inflammatory infiltrates and a

Table 10.5 Treatment options for congenital vascular tumors

Principles of Treatment of infantile Hemangioma

1. **Spontaneous course G1/2A**
   (don't forget: 80% of all hemangiomas never need any treatment)

   if not sufficient enough:

2. **Induction of regression**
   G2B/3A focal iH -> Local procedure:
   LASER *(Cryotherapy, Scarification, topical creams)*

   aggressive growth and/or endangered region or
   infiltrating-diffuse („segmental") or dissiminated iH
   additionally stop progression
   G3B -> Systemic therapy:

Antiangiogenesis	**Antiproliferating drugs**
Corticoids	Corticoids
Propranolol	*(Cytostatics)*
(Vascular growth Inhibitors)	*(Interferon)*

   to prevent the need of

3. **Surgery** *for*

Early complications	**or**	**Residuals**

thickening of interstitial septa in the sonogram, therapy should be started prior to manifestation of a Kasabach-Merritt syndrome (KMS). In addition to a local Nd:YAG laser therapy, high-dose prednisolone treatment is required. A treatment with cytostatics can thus often be avoided.

trauma, or infection, one principle used in the past for treatment was the scarification technique, compression, or ligation. However, these procedures like cryotherapy cause scars on the skin, so the reason for reporting it here is purely historical.

Induction of Regression

Due to the potential for spontaneous regression, the basic of therapy is to push this spontaneous course. Antiproliferative drugs will not induce this natural regression process but inhibit only the actual progress. This means that for focal iH, a local therapy is the first choice for *induced regression*. Only in cases where this is not sufficient enough or in disseminated or *diffuse infiltrating iH* ("segmental") an additional systemic therapy is recommended (Table 10.5).

Embolization

Comparable to ligation due to the collaterals of congenital vascular tumors, embolization is nonsensical [4]. One exceptional indication for embolization is in infantile liver hemangiomas with massive cardiac failure or massive bleeding from ulcerated hemangiomas [5]. In special cases of kaposiform hemangioendothelioma such as KMS, which cannot be treated successfully by cytostatics and laser, an embolization may be considered, but only as the last option.

Local Procedures

Mechanical Procedures

Due to the observation that hemangiomas can start involution after spontaneous ulceration,

Physical Procedures

The application of physical energy can be divided into direct tissue removal or destruction and secondary apoptosis by primary inflammation.

X-Ray Therapy

Comparable to the procedure in X-ray therapy of keloids or other inflammatory diseases, radiotherapy has also been used. But this ionizing radiation carries a high risk of mutagenicity and carcinogenicity. Furthermore, a secondary cataract is a major complication if x-ray therapy is performed near the eyes. Therefore, for infantile hemangiomas and kaposiform hemangioendothelioma, X-ray therapy is discussed here only as a historical treatment and is no longer applicable today.

Cryotherapy

Cryotherapy has no specific absorption in the tissue and works only by thermal conductivity. After application blisters and crusts occur. This causes a destruction of the overlying epithelial layer and severe frostbite with a congelatio escharotica III [6]. Complications include hypopigmentations (10–15 %) and scars or atrophies. Furthermore, there is no place for cryotherapy in treating any type of hemangioendothelioma.

Laser Therapy

Due to the high specific absorption of the correctly selected wavelength in the dermal or subcutaneous layer, *laser therapy* has been demonstrated as effective and safe for the treatment of congenital vascular tumors in children while significantly minimizing any cutaneous adverse effects. Several clinical trials have been reported positively. Through laser treatment an early and careful therapy of hemangiomas has also become possible, so that hemangiomas can be treated in early or prodromal phases to avoid enlargement [7]. However, laser treatment is required in rapidly growing hemangiomas of the head, when these lesions interfere with important functions (e.g., hands and feet) or when they endanger delicate structures because of their location (e.g., eye, anogenital region). Treatment of large hemangiomas also may be desirable.

Chemical Procedures

The basis of chemical agents for the therapy of congenital vascular tumors is comparable to the indication of physical energy: induction of inflammation.

Sclerotherapy

Sclerotherapy of varices is a safe and successful procedure. However, in infantile hemangioma or in congenital hemangioendothelioma, there is a diffuse microcirculation which does not allow a complete compression to avoid a systemic outflow. In newborns even low concentrations of the drug can cause myocarditis. For this reason the administration of sclerosing drugs is replaced by laser therapy [8]. Likewise therapy with oxidizing metals such as copper and magnesium is outdated [9]. An interstitial direct corticoid crystal injection has been reported for localized infantile hemangiomas. In the eye there is a high risk of crystal embolization of the artery resulting in permanent blindness [10, 11]. As with sclerotherapy, this procedure has been completely replaced by the different laser techniques.

Topical Pharmacotherapy

Imiquimod works by destruction and ulceration of the epithelial layer followed by a secondary inflammation in the hemangioma itself. So scars can occur. Topical corticoid creams can cause skin atrophy and systemic side effects due to uncontrolled resorption [12]. Topical propranolol has the same problem. This side effect is well known in ophthalmology for more than 50 years. Both have no effect on deep dermal or subcutaneous hemangiomas. In congenital hemangioendothelioma due to the epidermal barrier, this procedure has no effect.

Systemic Procedures

There is no specific systemic treatment for infantile hemangioma or congenital hemangioendothelioma. Two main principles are in use:

Table 10.6 Different indications of systemic therapy for infantile hemangioma and congenital hemangioendothelioma

Systemic Therapies in Congenital Vascular Tumours

IH
(aggressive and/or endangered)

Propranolol oral
1mg/kg/d for 2-3d,
increasing to 2mg/kg/d
total systemic duration: >6M
start hospitalization 1W

if med. contraindications or unsafe social situation:

Prednisolon oral
5mg/kg/d for 14d, Reduction
abs. 2,5 -5mg/w dep. on body w.
Total systemic duration: 2M
outpatient start

KHE
(e.g. Kasabach-Merrit-Symptome)

Prednisolon oral
5mg/kg/d for 14d, Reduction
abs. 2,5 -5mg/w dep. on body w.

if no stabilization of thrombocytes overlapping start with

Endoxane i.v
10mg/kg*3d every 3weeks
max 5 cycles

or
Rapamycin
(only individual indication)

antiproliferative drugs [13] and antiangiogenesis (Table 10.6).

Antiproliferative Drugs
The higher the proliferation rate, the more effective the therapy with antiproliferative drugs. However, several complications in infantile hemangiomas are caused even at a low proliferation rate due to the complicated localization. Furthermore, not all antiproliferative drugs are able to induce regression, explaining the risk of the rebound effect after systemic therapy. Therefore, systemic therapy is an adjuvant for complicated infantile hemangiomas or congenital hemangioendotheliomas and requires additional induction of regression, especially by differentiated laser therapy. In endotracheal or periorbital infantile hemangiomas, the laser-induced regression sometimes comes too late, necessitating an adjuvant systemic therapy to stop further growth. Furthermore, in kaposiform hemangioendothelioma with KMS, an immediate halt to progression is important to stop the coagulopathy [14].

Antiangiogenesis
Inhibitors of vascular growth factors have been well investigated for the therapy of malignancies. The problem in infantile hemangioma is that this tumor forms vessels as a sign of maturation and not as a sign of aggression. So in several investigations a strong relationship between vascular endothelial growth factor and the activity of the infantile hemangioma was not found. On the other hand, the long-term side effects in early childhood have not been completely investigated, so at this time antiangiogenic factors are only experimental in congenital vascular tumors [15].

Table 10.7   Treatment algorithm for infantile hemangiomas and congenital hemangioendotheliomas

Therapeutic pathway

Congenital vascular tumor

[Flow diagram with the following nodes and connections:]

- end — RICH — cHE — iH — G1 — end
- regress — CCDS Thermo — NICH — Biopsy — G2a — CCDS — n.progr/ regress
- CCDS Thermo Thrombocyt — KMS — LASER — other Tumor — specific Protocol — slight progr — CCDS — regress
- Biopsy — KHE — exc. progr — G2b — CCDS — progr
- comb LASER/ syst. therapy — comb LASER/ syst. therapy — G3b — G3a — exc. progr
- CCDS Thermo Therombocyt — CCDS — LASER
- stabil. — stabil. — exc. progr — progr — slight progr

The symbols are according to ISO 9000. The therapeutic principle is a downgrade to an uncomplicated form either of infantile hemangioma or congenital hemangioendothelioma to allow spontaneous regression

Removal

In the complete obstruction of the visual axis or in *ulcerated hemangiomas* with massive bleeding, an immediate resection of the infantile hemangioma may be *necessary*. However, an early local recurrence may be possible.

The longer the infantile hemangioma grows, the more commonly one can find huge residuals of fibrolipomatous tissue or cutis laxa after spontaneous or induced regression. Furthermore, after regression of infantile hemangiomas on a hairy head, there may be hair loss. In these cases a plastic correction after the end of the regression phase is an important option. Due to early therapy to prevent such uncontrolled growth, the number of indications is reduced. Even in late involuting congenital hemangioendotheliomas, either RICH or laser-induced NICH or KHE, a surgical

resection of the remaining tissue is sometimes necessary. However, in most cases the growth stops so early due to the early therapy that a near-complete resorption of the tumor tissue occurs (Table 10.7).

References

1. Poetke M et al (2011). In: Raulin C, Karsai S (eds) Laser therapy of infantile haemangioma and other congenital vascular tumours in infants. Springer, Berlin/Heidelberg. ISBN 978-3-642-03437-4
2. Poetke M, Berlien H-P (2005) Angeborne Gefäßanomalien. In: Pschyrembel Handbuch Therapie 3. Auflage S, De Gruyter Berlin, pp 327–329
3. AWMF-online (2012) Haemangiome im Saeuglings- und Kindesalter AWMF-Leitlinen register 006/100
4. Tonner PH, Scholz J (1994) Mögliche Lungenembolie nach Embolisation eines Hämangioms mit Fibrinkleber. Anaesthesist 43:614–617

5. Demuth RJ, Miller SH, Keller F (1984) Complications of embolization treatment for problem cavernous hemangiomas. Ann Plast Surg 13:135

6. Scholz A, Sebastian G, Baerthold W, Matthaus W, Passler L (1980) Ergebnisse der Kryochirurgie bei der Behandlung benigner vaskulärer Fehl- und Neubildungen. Arch Geschwulstforsch 50:785–793

7. Berlien HP, Cremer H, Djawari D, Grantzow R, Gubisch W (1993/1994) Leitlinien zur Behandlung angeborener Gefäßerkrankungen. Pädiatr Praxis 46:87–92

8. Winter H (1996) 20jährige Erfahrungen mit der Sklerosierungstherapie von Hämangiomen. Zbl Haut 168:7

9. Li ZP (1992) Therapeutic coagulation induced in cavernous hemangioma by use of percutaneous copper needles. Plast Reconstr Surg 89:613–622

10. Kushner BJ, Lemke BN (1993) Bilateral retinal embolization associated with intralesional corticosteroid injection for capillary hemangioma of infancy [letter; comment]. J Pediatr Ophthalmol Strabismus 30:397–399

11. Chowdri NA, Darzi MA, Fazili Z, Iqbal S (1994) Intralesional corticosteroid therapy for childhood cutaneous hemangiomas. Ann Plast Surg 33:46–51

12. Elsas FJ, Lewis AR (1994) Topical treatment of periocular capillary hemangioma. J Pediatr Ophthalmol Strabismus 31:153–156

13. Mazzuccioni MG (2007) Therapy with high-dose dexamethasone (HD-DXM) in previously untreated patients affected by idiopathic thrombocytopenic purpura: a GIMEMA experience. Blood 109:1401–1407

14. Poetke M, Jamil B, Müller U, Berlien H-P (2002) Diffuse neonatal hemangiomatosis associated with Simpson-Golabi-Behmel syndrome: a case report. Eur J Pediatr Surg 12:59–60

15. Tsang WYW, Chan JKC, Fletcher CDM (1991) Kaposi-like infantile haemangioendothelioma: a distinctive vascular neoplasm of the retroperitoneum. Am J Surg Pathol 15:982–989

Propanolol and Beta-Blockers in the Medical Treatment of Infantile Hemangiomas

Christine Léauté-Labrèze

Summary

Propranolol effectiveness on infantile hemangiomas (IHs) has been fortuitously observed. The mechanisms of action of propranolol on IHs are still poorly understood, but, since 2008, many reports have confirmed its efficacy, pooling case series and randomized studies one can say that propranolol presents a satisfactory short-term safety profile, and many teams advise oral propranolol as a first-line therapy in complicated IHs. Propranolol is indicated in case of life-threatening IHs, in case of functional consequences of the IH, or a risk of permanent disfigurement. After excluding contraindications, oral propranolol should be administered at the dose of 2–3 mg/kg/day for 6 months, about 10–15 % of infants needed to be retreated for 3–6 months more, especially if they present a large segmental IH and/or an IH with a deep component. Local beta-blockers, such as timolol, could be used for superficial IHs.

Most of the time multimodal management of complicated infantile hemangiomas (IHs) includes medical treatment in order to control the growth of the tumor. No official treatment guidelines for the treatment of IH are available; however, given the recent proven rapid efficacy and safety of beta-blockers in the therapy of IHs [1, 2], many teams advise oral propranolol as a first-line therapy.

C. Léauté-Labrèze
Unit of Pediatric Dermatology,
Reference Center for Rare Skin Diseases,
CHU Bordeaux-Pellegrin-Enfants Hospital,
Bordeaux, France
e-mail: Christine.labreze@chu-bordeaux.fr

Oral Beta-Blockers

Propranolol

Propranolol effectiveness has been fortuitously observed in an infant with an IH treated with corticosteroids and who had developed a hypertrophic cardiomyopathy with tachycardia [1]. The mechanisms of action of propranolol on IHs are still poorly understood. Propranolol is a nonselective beta-blocker commonly used in high blood pressure, tachycardia, or migraines; it is responsible for the vasoconstriction of small vessels resulting in a very rapid change in color and softening of the IH. Propranolol also lowers the rate of renin and thus has a modulating effect on angiotensin II [3]. In addition, beta-adrenergic receptors belong to the family of G-protein-coupled receptors, which, when activated by adrenergic catecholamines, can promote a series of intracellular signal transduction pathways including that of angiogenic factors such as VEGF or bFGF [4–6] and some metalloproteinases such as MMP2 and MMP9 [7]. Finally, propranolol could lead to an early apoptosis of endothelial cells that make up the majority of the tumor [8].

Propranolol has been used in a large number of case series with a good efficacy [9, 10], and two placebo-controlled studies have confirmed its effectiveness. A randomized study involving a heterogeneous population of 40 children aged 2 months to 5 years with an HI of the face treated for 6 months with propranolol or placebo showed a significant difference between the two arms in terms of volume in favor of propranolol [11], and a pilot study in infants less than 4 months treated with propranolol (3–4 mg/kg/day) showed, after only 1 month of treatment, a decrease by half in the thickness of the HI, measured by ultrasound, in children treated with propranolol, whereas in the placebo arm there was a slight increase in thickness [12]. Recently, an adaptive multicenter randomized double-blind phase II/III study of infants aged 1–5 months at baseline has compared four arms of propranolol (1 or 3 mg/kg/day for 3–6 months) versus placebo (to be published). The latter study showed that the oral suspension propranolol administered at 3 mg/kg/day for 6 months has a highly significant efficacy with a good safety profile. A recent meta-analysis of 35 studies [13] concluded that propranolol has more efficacy than other therapies in treating IHs; propranolol is more effective than steroids, vincristine, and laser in treating cutaneous IHs, periocular IHs, airway IHs, and hepatic IHs.

IH resistance to propranolol is rare; only isolated cases have been reported [14]. In more than 90 % of infants treated, 24 h after beginning treatment a change in IH color from intense red to purple is noted, associated with softening of the lesion. Symptoms such as dyspnea in airway IHs or hemodynamic abnormalities in large IHs usually resolve within 48 h [15]. In case of orbital IH with eyelid occlusion, spontaneous ocular opening could be observed within 7 days [9, 16]. After these dramatic initial responses, all symptoms of IH usually continue to improve in color and thickness. Most of the time, in 3–6 months, the IH becomes nearly flat with the single persistence of residual skin telangiectasias (Fig. 11.1). Of note, this latter aspect was usually obtained after several years of spontaneous regression. When performed, ultrasound examination may disclose objective regression in thickness associ-

Table 11.1 Oral propranolol in infantile hemangiomas for practitioners

When?
In life-threatening IH, in case of functional risks (i.e., risk of amblyopia), painful ulcerated IH, and to avoid sequels needing surgery (i.e., IH involving the nose or lips)
The earliest is the best to avoid definitive anatomical distortion and development of fibrofatty tissue
How?
After elimination of contraindications (sinus bradycardia and partial auriculoventricular block)
2–3 mg/kg/day in two or three intakes, under close monitoring for the first intake: blood pressure and heart rate for 4 h
What is the best dosage?
Begin at 1 mg/kg/day for 1 week, then increase to 2 mg/kg/day, and then 3 mg/kg/day if the tolerance is good
In case of incomplete result after 1 month, increase at 4 mg/kg/day (maximum dosage not known, but probably not useful to give more than 4 mg/kg/day)
What is the duration of treatment?
6 months of treatment
3 or 6 months more in case of relapse (lH with a deep component and/or segmental IH)
What to do to avoid expected side effects?
Minor side effects: nothing to do in case of cold hands or asymptomatic low systolic blood pressur0e. For nightmares avoid giving the treatment after 5 pm and/or reduce the dosage
Severe side effects: to avoid hypoglycemia, be sure that the infant feeds regularly; in case of poor food intake stop temporarily the propranolol; in case of wheezing, stop also temporarily the propranolol
Necessity to monitor potassium blood rate in case of very large and/or ulcerated hemangioma

ated with an increase in the resistivity parameters of IH vascularization [9]. Propranolol is effective in cutaneous IH, even in the case of ulceration [17].

In practice, after eliminating contraindications, oral propranolol is given at a progressive dosage until 2–3 mg/kg/day under medical supervision (see Table 11.1) [2]. The main contraindications are cardiologic, especially sinus bradycardia and partial auriculoventricular block, which should be excluded by cardiologic examination. Concerning PHACES syndrome with cerebrovascular involvement, recent data are reassuring; clinical series did not report side effects [18], and hemodynamic data showed no

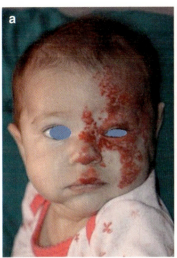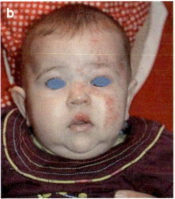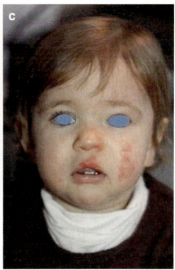

Fig. 11.1 A young girl with a segmental IH and PHACE syndrome (dysplasia of left carotid artery) treated with oral propranolol. (**a**) At 1 month of age (D_0), (**b**) after 3 months of treatment, and (**c**) at 12 months of age when stopping propranolol

difference in terms of cerebral vascularization before and after propranolol treatment [19]. Asthma is also a classic contraindication, but it is difficult to detect in young infants; predisposed babies can start wheezing during the beta-blocker treatment, especially in case of concomitant viral infection. In this situation, it is recommended to stop temporarily the propranolol or definitively in case of relapse. Parents should be strongly informed of the risk of hypoglycemia [20], and the child should be carefully monitored especially if there is a discordance in appetite, i.e., the child does not eat at regular times. Other adverse effects can be noted during the treatment including asymptomatic blood pressure drop or bradycardia, insomnia, agitation, and nightmares [2]. Some cases of hyperkalemia have been reported [21]; hyperkalemia is not due to the drug itself but is the result of tumor lysis. As a consequence, blood potassium rate should be monitored in case of a large and/or ulcerated IH treated with beta-blockers.

Propranolol intake should be maintained for 6 months. When stopping propranolol treatment, mild recoloration may be noted in ¼ of cases [2, 9, 22]; among these infants 50 % needed to be retreated 3 or 6 months more because of regrowth of the IH. Segmental IH as well as IH with a deep component is more at risk for relapse [22].

Other Beta-Blockers

Good clinical results have also been reported with other beta-blockers, but as small series or case reports; randomized comparative studies are lacking. Acebutolol [23] and atenolol [24] are both cardioselective beta-blockers; they are said to induce less bronchospasm, and they are proposed as an alternative therapy in infants predisposed to asthma. However, at high dosages the cardioselectivity is not warranted. They are also less lipophilic than propranolol and thus less responsible for nightmares. Nadolol has shown good efficacy but with the same rate of short-term side effects as propranolol [25].

Topical Beta-Blockers

For common non alarming IH, therapeutic abstention is the rule in most instances. Local treatments (corticosteroids, imiquimod, liquid nitrogen applications, etc.) have not yet provided

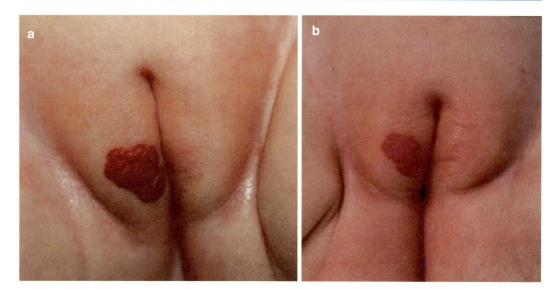

Fig. 11.2 Superficial hemangioma of the right labia majora in a young girl treated with topical timolol. (**a**) At 2 months of age (D_0) and (**b**) after 3 months of extended-release 0.5 % timolol solution applied twice daily

evidence of a good benefit/risk ratio, and their efficacy is not clearly established.

The development of local treatments based on the dramatic efficacy of beta-blockers seems logical, and some authors have published a positive experience with topical timolol. The local treatment concerns only superficial IH (Fig. 11.2); ophthalmic gels have been used first on eyelids [26] and then extended to the skin [27]. Recently, a randomized placebo-controlled study showed that topical timolol maleate 0.5 % gel with a maximum dose of 0.5 mg/day is a safe and effective option for small superficial IHs that have not ulcerated and are not on mucosal surfaces [28]. In our experience, the treatment is more efficient under occlusion [29]; however, tolerance for the dressings is a limiting factor. A homemade topical form of propranolol seems efficient [30], and a pharmaceutical gel is under development.

References

1. Léauté-Labrèze C, Dumas de la Roque E et al (2008) Propranolol for severe hemangiomas of infancy. N Engl J Med 358:2650–2651

2. Drolet BA, Frommelt PC, Chamlin SL, Haggstrom A, Bauman NM, Chiu YE, Chun RH, Garzon MC, Holland KE, Liberman L, MacLellan-Tobert S, Mancini AJ, Metry D, Puttgen KB, Seefeldt M, Sidbury R, Ward KM, Blei F, Baselga E, Cassidy L, Darrow DH, Joachim S, Kwon EK, Martin K, Perkins J, Siegel DH, Boucek RJ, Frieden IJ (2013) Initiation and use of propranolol for infantile hemangioma: report of a consensus conference. Pediatrics 131(1):128–140

3. Itinteang T, Brasch HD, Tan ST, Day DJ (2011) Expression of components of the renin-angiotensin system in proliferating infantile haemangioma may account for the propranolol-induced accelerated involution. J Plast Reconstr Aesthet Surg 64(6):759–765

4. Iaccarino G, Ciccarelli M, Soriento D et al (2005) Ischemic neoangiogenesis enhanced by beta2-adrenergic receptors overexpression: a novel role for the endothelial adrenergic system. Circ Res 97:1182–1189

5. D'Angelo G, Lee H, Weiner RI (1997) cAMP-dependant protein kinase inhibits the mitogenic action of vascular endothelial growth factor and fibroblast growth factor in capillary endothelial cells by blocking Raf activation. J Cell Biochem 67:353–366

6. Ozeki M, Fukao T, Kondo N (2011) Propranolol for intractable diffuse lymphangiomatosis. N Engl J Med 364:1380–1382

7. Annabi B, Lachambre MP, Plouffe K et al (2009) Propranolol adrenergic blockade inhibits human brain endothelial cells tubulogenesis and matrix metalloproteinase-9 secretion. Pharmacol Res 60:438–445

8. Sommers Smith SK, Smith DM (2002) Beta blockade induces apoptosis in cultured capillary endothelial cells. In Vitro Cell Dev Biol Anim 38:298–304

9. Sans V, Dumas de la Roque E, Berge J et al (2009) Propranolol for severe infantile hemangiomas: follow-up report. Pediatrics 124:e423–e431

10. Marqueling AL, Oza V, Frieden IJ, Puttgen KB (2013) Propranolol and infantile hemangiomas four years later: a systematic review. Pediatr Dermatol 30(2):182–191

11. Hogeling M, Adams S, Wargon O (2011) A randomized controlled trial of propranolol for infantile hemangiomas. Pediatrics 128(2):e259–e266

12. Léauté-Labrèze C, Dumas de la Roque E, Nacka F, Abouelfath A, Grenier N, Rebola M, Ezzedine K, Moore N (2013) Double blind randomized pilot trial evaluating the efficacy of oral propranolol on infantile hemangiomas in infants less than 4 months of age. Br J Dermatol 169(1):181–183

13. Lou Y, Peng WJ, Cao Y, Cao DS, Xie J, Li HH (2013) The effectiveness of propranolol in treating infantile hemangiomas: a meta-analysis including 35 studies. Br J Clin Pharmacol. doi:10.1111/bcp.12235

14. Caussé S, Aubert H, Saint-Jean M, Puzenat E, Bursztejn AC, Eschard C, Mahé F, Maruani A, Mazereeuw-Hautier J, Dreyfus I, Miquel J, Chiaverini C, Boccara O, Hadj-Rabia S, Stalder JF, Barbarot S, Groupe de Recherche Clinique en Dermatologie Pédiatrique (2013) Propranolol-resistant infantile haemangiomas. Br J Dermatol 169(1):125–129

15. Denoyelle F, Leboulanger N, Enjolras O et al (2009) Role of propranolol in the therapeutic strategy of infantile laryngotracheal hemangioma. Int J Pediatr Otorhinolaryngol 73:1168–1172

16. Thoumazet F, Léauté-Labrèze C, Colin J, Mortemousque B (2012) Efficacy of systemic propranolol for severe infantile haemangioma of the orbit and eyelid: a case study of eight patients. Br J Ophthalmol 96(3):370–374

17. Saint-Jean M, Léauté-Labrèze C, Mazereeuw-Hautier J, Bodak N, Hamel-Teillac D, Kupfer-Bessaguet I, Lacour JP, Naouri M, Vabres P, Hadj-Rabia S, Nguyen JM, Stalder JF, Barbarot S, on behalf of the Groupe de Recherche Clinique en Dermatologie Pédiatrique (2011) Propranolol for treatment of ulcerated infantile hemangiomas. J Am Acad Dermatol 64:827–832

18. Metry D, Frieden IJ, Hess C, Siegel D, Maheshwari M, Baselga E, Chamlin S, Garzon M, Mancini AJ, Powell J, Drolet BA (2013) Propranolol use in PHACE syndrome with cervical and intracranial arterial anomalies: collective experience in 32 infants. Pediatr Dermatol 30(1):71–89

19. Hernandez-Martin S, Lopez-Gutierrez JC, Lopez-Fernandez S, Ramírez M, Miguel M, Coya J, Marin D, Tovar JA (2012) Brain perfusion SPECT in patients with PHACES syndrome under propranolol treatment. Eur J Pediatr Surg 22(1):54–59

20. Holland KE, Frieden IJ, Frommelt PC, Mancini AJ, Wyatt D, Drolet BA (2010) Hypoglycemia in children taking propranolol for the treatment of infantile hemangioma. Arch Dermatol 146:775–778

21. Pavlakovic H, Kietz S, Lauerer P, Zutt M, Lakomek M (2010) Hyperkalemia complicating propranolol treatment of an infantile hemangioma. Pediatrics 126(6):e1589–e1593. Epub 2010 Nov 29

22. Ahogo CK, Ezzedine K, Prey S, Colona V, Diallo A, Boralevi F, Taïeb A, Léauté-Labrèze C (2013) Factors associated with the relapse of infantile hemangiomas in children treated with oral propranolol. Br J Dermatol 169:1252–1256

23. Bigorre M, Van Kien AK, Valette H (2009) Beta-blocking agent for treatment of infantile hemangioma. Plast Reconstr Surg 123:195e–196e

24. de Graaf M, Raphael MF, Breugem CC, Knol MJ, Bruijnzeel-Koomen CA, Kon M, Breur JM, Pasmans SG (2013) Treatment of infantile haemangiomas with atenolol: comparison with a historical propranolol group. J Plast Reconstr Aesthet Surg 66(12):1732–1740

25. Pope E, Chakkittakandiyil A, Lara-Corrales I, Maki E, Weinstein M (2013) Expanding the therapeutic repertoire of infantile haemangiomas: cohort-blinded study of oral nadolol compared with propranolol. Br J Dermatol 168(1):222–224

26. Guo S, Ni N (2010) Topical treatment for capillary hemangioma of the eyelid using beta-blocker solution. Arch Ophthalmol 128:255–256

27. Pope E, Chakkittakandiyil A (2010) Topical timolol gel for infantile hemangiomas: a pilot study. Arch Dermatol 146:564–565

28. Chan H, McKay C, Adams S, Wargon O (2013) RCT of timolol maleate gel for superficial infantile hemangiomas in 5- to 24-week-olds. Pediatrics 131(6): e1739–e1747

29. Moehrle M, Léauté-Labrèze C, Schmidt V, Röcken M, Poets CF, Goelz R (2013) Topical timolol for small hemangiomas of infancy. Pediatr Dermatol 30(2):245–249

30. Kunzi-Rapp K (2012) Topical propranolol therapy for infantile hemangiomas. Pediatr Dermatol 29(2): 154–159

Other Medical Treatments for Infantile Hemangioma and Congenital Vascular Tumors

Jochen Rössler

Corticosteroids

In the 1960s, the efficacy of corticosteroids was observed coincidentally when a child with IH was treated for thrombocytopenia with corticosteroids [1]. The exact explanation on how corticosteroids inhibit the growth of IH has been studied intensively; however, the biological mechanism still remains unclear. In vitro studies have shown a number of molecular effects of corticosteroids, including the induction of apoptosis by the upregulation of mitochondrial cytochrome b and clusterin/ApoJ [2]. The inhibition of angiogenesis by the downregulation of the expression of angiogenic factors has also been demonstrated [3].

Today, the administration of corticosteroid for IH is limited to situations where propranolol is not showing effect. In this extremely rare situation, corticosteroids can be used. However, dosage and duration of corticosteroid therapy are not defined based on clinical trial results. Furthermore, the choice on the type of corticosteroid administered is based on anecdotal experience and retrospective studies. Dosages of prednisone/prednisolone range from 1 to 5 mg/kg

J. Rössler
Pediatric Hematology/Oncology,
Center of Pediatrics and Adolescent Medicine,
University Medical Center Freiburg,
Freiburg, Germany
e-mail: jochen.roessler@uniklinik-freiburg.de

body weight daily, and different durations of treatment are reported in several case series. For example, a review of 24 original case series each reporting on more than five IH patients treated with systemic corticosteroids has been published [4]. In this meta-analysis, an equivalent dose of 2.9 mg/kg/day prednisone for a mean time of 1.8 months showed a response rate of 84 %. In addition, a prednisolone dose of 3 mg/kg/day was apparently more effective than 2 mg/kg/day. In a report from Israel summarizing the experiences and results of 60 children with IH treated in over 24 years, the response to corticosteroids seemed to be dose-dependent [5]. An initial dose of 5 mg/kg/day of oral prednisone for 2 weeks followed by gradual tapering off the dose for 6–8 weeks was more effective than an initial dose of 3 mg/kg/day. In our own experience, an initial prednisone dose of 2 mg/kg body weight daily for 2–4 weeks was followed by 1 mg/kg/day for another 2–4 weeks [6]. This was followed by a slow and careful tapering off over several weeks to months. This protocol was applied systematically over several years in one institution and showed an extremely high effectiveness.

Since the introduction of propranolol as an effective medical therapy for IH, we did not use this corticosteroid protocol any more. However, for congenital vascular tumors that can easily be confounded with IH not showing spontaneous regression, corticosteroids can be used as an initial therapy. In most cases, only clinical evolution or histology can help diagnose a tufted angioma

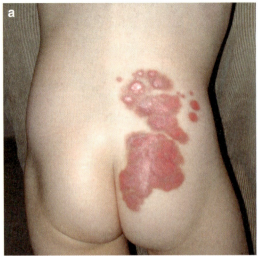

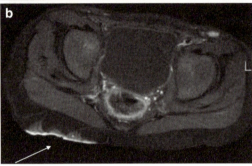

Fig. 12.1 (**a**) Kaposiform hemangioendothelioma (KHE) at the lower back in a 1.5-year-old boy. The red lesion was continuously growing during the first year of life, and biopsy was taken that confirmed KHE. (**b**) MRI with contrast enhancement of the cutaneous KHE. *Arrow* shows infiltration of the subcutis, but not the muscles or bones

or subtypes of hemangioendothelioma. Often, medical therapy has to be intensified as described below. *We present a 1.5-year-old boy with a red lesion at the lower back that showed continuous growth and was morphological not typical for IH* (Fig. 12.1). *Biopsy was taken and histology showed a kaposiform hemangioendothelioma.*

The potential side effects of corticosteroid therapy include hypertension, gastritis, and delayed growth as well as mood changes. A Cushing's syndrome with additional pituitary-adrenal axis suppression, secondary diabetes mellitus, or immunosuppression with increased susceptibility to infection is extremely rare. During corticosteroid therapy, the child should have a physical examination every 2–4 weeks

with monitoring of blood pressure, glucosuria, as well as height and weight. Prescription of oral ranitidine or a beta-blocker may be necessary. However, all side effects, especially the growth and weight retardation, are reversible [7]. Live attenuated vaccines are contraindicated during the period of corticosteroid treatment, while vaccinations with dead vaccines can be performed once the initial high dosage of steroids is reduced.

Vincristine

There are very limited reports on the use of vincristine for the treatment of proliferating, corticosteroid- and/or interferon-resistant IH [8]. However, since the introduction of propranolol, vincristine is wildly more used for function- and life-threatening congenital vascular tumors [9].

In combination with corticosteroids, vincristine can be helpful in the Kasabach-Merritt phenomenon (KMP) that often is observed in the presence of congenital vascular tumors [10]. This phenomenon is defined as thrombocytopenia and hypofibrinogenemia with elevated fibrin split products (D-dimers), suggestive of an active consumptive coagulopathy. Thrombocytes are low, ranging from 6,000 to 98,000, with fibrinogen levels less than 100 mg/dL, whereas D-dimers are elevated. Prothrombin times (PT) and activated partial thromboplastin time (PTT) can range from normal to significantly prolonged. Additionally, anemia can be present at diagnosis as a consequence of intravascular hemolysis, including red blood cell fragmentation, elevated LDH, and hyperbilirubinemia. Successful treatment of the underlying vascular tumor is critical to the correction of KMP and to the overall survival of patients. Children with KMP can die of hemorrhage or invasion/compression of vital structures by the vascular tumor. Mortality has ranged from 10 to 30 % in most series. A curative therapy of KMP can only be achieved by treatment of the underlying vascular tumor. However, supportive care to maintain hemostasis is necessary. Platelet transfusions should be reserved for active bleeding or in preparation for surgery or procedures. Aminocaproic acid and local

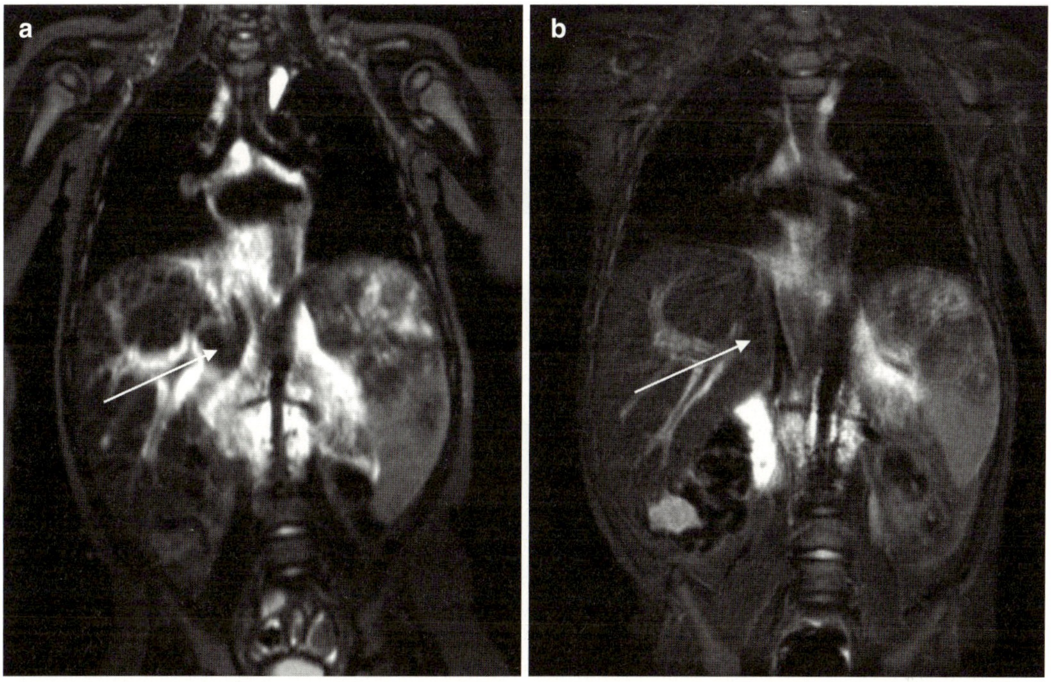

Fig. 12.2 (**a**) MRI of a 9-month-old child with a congenital vascular tumor of the retroperitoneum. (**b**) MRI 6 months after corticosteroids and vincristine therapy. *Arrows* in (**a**) and (**b**) show a diffuse lesion which has shrinked during therapy

measures may be helpful to reduce the need for platelet transfusions. Antiplatelet agents, such as acetylsalicylic acid and dipyridamole, have been used to reduce platelet aggregation within the vascular tumor. Treatment of hypofibrinogenemia with cryoprecipitate and prolonged PT or PTT with fresh frozen plasma should be a clinical decision rather than correction of a laboratory result. Symptomatic anemia should be treated with red blood cell transfusions. A retrospective study on 15 patients with different vascular lesions and KMP shows that vincristine can be a safe and effective drug not only to treat KMP but also to decrease the size of the vascular tumor [10]. A recently developed guideline on the management of KMP supports the combination of corticosteroids and vincristine as the first-line therapy for KMP [11]. *We present the MRI of a 9-months-old child with severe thrombocytopenia and anemia. Bone marrow morphology was normal and further diagnostics revealed a congenital vascular tumor at the retroperitoneum (Fig. 12.2). Therapy with corticosteroids and vincristine induced remission of KMP as well as shrinkage of the vascular tumor that could not be biopsied because of danger of bleeding.*

Vincristine is a naturally occurring vinca alkaloid isolated from the leaves of the periwinkle plant *Catharanthus roseus* [12]. It interferes with mitotic spindle microtubules by binding to tubulin, resulting in inhibition of mitosis. There is considerable experience with the use of vincristine in the treatment of malignancies in children. Vincristine is a vesicant and caution needs to be exercised if given peripherally due to the risk of extravasation. Vincristine can be administered at a dose of 1 mg/m² (or 0.05 mg/kg body weight in children <10 kg). It is generally used intravenously with weekly injections first and then tapering down by increasing the interval between injections, depending on the clinical response [13].

Neurotoxicity is the dose-limiting side effect of vincristine. A peripheral mixed sensory and motor neuropathy is common. It can also produce an autonomic neuropathy resulting in abdominal pain, constipation, and ileus. Hematologic toxicity is rarely encountered with vincristine.

Fig. 12.3 The mTOR
signaling pathway

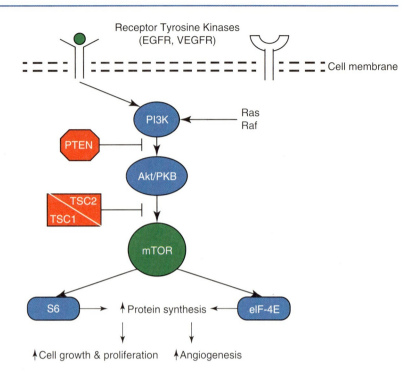

Interferon

The use of interferon alpha subcutaneously at a
dose of $1-3 \times 10^6$ million units/m² body surface
area daily has been widely reported for
corticosteroid-resistant proliferating IH in the
literature [14]. Because of its dangerous side
effects and the high effectiveness of propranolol, the use of interferon alpha for the therapy of
IH has been abandoned. Acute toxicity includes
fever, neutropenia, and anemia. Of great concern is the long-term neurotoxicity with development of spastic diplegia in up to 20 % of
treated IH [15]. Interferon alpha was initially
developed as an antiviral agent and has immu-
noregulatory, antineoplastic, and anti-angiogenic
properties [16].

In lymphangiomatosis/Gorham's disease,
where lymph vessels proliferate and destroy
involved organs such as the bones, the lungs,
soft tissue, or the spleen, interferon alpha is
administered, but only in children older than
1 year [17].

Cyclophosphamide

Some rare reports on alkylating agents used for
the treatment of congenital vascular tumors,
including cases of IH, are summarized in a review
by Hurvitz et al. [18]. Common adverse effects
include nausea, vomiting, and reversible alope-
cia. Adequate hydration and alkalization of the
urine is to be assured to prevent hemorrhagic cys-
titis and hyperuricemia. Secondary malignancies
have been reported, and, therefore, the use of
cyclophosphamide should be reserved for ultima
ratio situations.

Rapamycin

The mTOR signaling pathway seems to be activated in the endothelial cells of vascular tumors
(Fig. 12.3). Therefore, the mTOR inhibitor
rapamycin had been proposed as a potential medical treatment. Rapamycin has been administered
in an "off-label" setting for complicated vascular

anomalies, including congenital vascular tumors, such as hemangioendothelioma presenting with KMP [19]. These promising results lead to the realization of a clinical trial in the United States where rapamycin has been administered to all sorts of complicated vascular anomalies. The final results are awaited in the near future. Already today, rapamycin has been proposed as a second-line therapy for KMP if corticosteroids and vincristine are not effective [11].

Rapamycin can be administered orally, and blood levels of the drug can be measured to control a stable dosage. However, it is not yet clear which drug level should be chosen. Side effects are mucosal lesions such as aphthae as well as peripheral edema. A prophylactic administration of the antibiotic trimethoprim to prevent severe infections should be done. In times of fever, rapamycin should be stopped until recovered.

References

1. Zarem HA, Edgerton MT (1967) Induced resolution of cavernous hemangiomas following prednisolone therapy. Plast Reconstr Surg 39(1):76–83
2. Hasan Q et al (2001) Altered mitochondrial cytochrome b gene expression during the regression of hemangioma. Plast Reconstr Surg. 108(6): 1471–1476
3. Blei F et al (1993) Mechanism of action of angiostatic steroids: suppression of plasminogen activator activity via stimulation of plasminogen activator inhibitor synthesis. J Cell Physiol 155(3):568–578
4. Bennett ML et al (2001) Oral corticosteroid use is effective for cutaneous hemangiomas: an evidence-based evaluation. Arch Dermatol 137(9):1208–1213
5. Sadan N, Wolach B (1996) Treatment of hemangiomas of infants with high doses of prednisone. J Pediatr 128(1):141–146
6. Rossler J, Wehl G, Niemeyer CM (2007) Evaluating systemic prednisone therapy for proliferating haemangioma in infancy. Eur J Pediatr 167:813–815
7. Boon LM, MacDonald DM, Mulliken JB (1999) Complications of systemic corticosteroid therapy for problematic hemangioma. Plast Reconstr Surg 104(6): 1616–1623
8. Fawcett SL et al (2004) Vincristine as a treatment for a large haemangioma threatening vital functions. Br J Plast Surg 57(2):168–171
9. Perez J, Pardo J, Gomez C (2002) Vincristine – an effective treatment of corticoid-resistant life-threatening infantile hemangiomas. Acta Oncol 41(2): 197–199
10. Haisley-Royster C et al (2002) Kasabach-merritt phenomenon: a retrospective study of treatment with vincristine. J Pediatr Hematol Oncol 24(6):459–462
11. Drolet BA et al (2013) Consensus-derived practice standards plan for complicated Kaposiform hemangioendothelioma. J Pediatr 163(1):285–291
12. Gidding CE et al (1999) Vincristine revisited. Crit Rev Oncol Hematol 29(3):267–287
13. Enjolras O et al (2004) Vincristine treatment for function- and life-threatening infantile hemangioma. Arch Pediatr 11(2):99–107
14. Ezekowitz RA, Mulliken JB, Folkman J (1992) Interferon alfa-2a therapy for life-threatening hemangiomas of infancy. N Engl J Med 326(22):1456–1463
15. Barlow CF et al (1998) Spastic diplegia as a complication of interferon Alfa-2a treatment of hemangiomas of infancy. J Pediatr 132.3(Pt 1):527–530
16. Sidky YA, Borden EC (1987) Inhibition of angiogenesis by interferons: effects on tumor- and lymphocyte-induced vascular responses. Cancer Res 47(19): 5155–5161
17. Kuriyama DK et al (2010) Treatment of Gorham-Stout disease with zoledronic acid and interferon-alpha: a case report and literature review. J Pediatr Hematol Oncol 32(8):579–584
18. Hurvitz SA et al (2000) Successful treatment with cyclophosphamide of life-threatening diffuse hemangiomatosis involving the liver. J Pediatr Hematol Oncol 22(6):527–532
19. Hammill AM et al (2011) Sirolimus for the treatment of complicated vascular anomalies in children. Pediatr Blood Cancer 57(6):1018–1024

Laser Treatment of Hemangiomas

13

Hans-Peter Berlien and Margitta Poetke

Introduction

Due to the fact that especially infantile hemangiomas have a high capability of spontaneous regression and the indication for active therapy is only in cases where this spontaneous regression occurs to late or in the meantime there is an excessive growth, the aim of laser therapy is to induce this regression – except in cases where an immediate surgical intervention is needed – and not the removal of the hemangiomatous tissue. This means that any additional damage on the surrounding tissue caused by the laser therapy has to and can be avoided. The principle of laser is an inflammatory process as a result of intravascular absorption of light and vessel obstructions and generally not definitive coagulation. This means that for different forms, depths, organs, and localizations, different lasers and different laser procedures are used.

Superselective Laser Systems

The specific absorption is not only a question of the wavelength and the tissue properties; it depends also reciprocally to the exposure time [1].

This means that for superselective absorption, the lower the specific absorption, the shorter the exposure time, or the longer the exposure time, the higher the specific absorption. This results in an overlap of indications between different laser systems. Generally, the term superselective laser system is used for lasers with an exposure time of less than 100 ms (short pulsed lasers) [2].

Flashlamp-Pumped Pulsed Dye Laser ("FPDL Laser")

FPDL nowadays is generally accepted as the treatment of choice for macular port-wine stains. Also patients with diffuse telangiectases as a component of the Rothmund-Thomson syndrome or the Louis-Bar syndrome demonstrate dramatic clearing following treatment with the pulsed dye laser.

But the use of FPDL with a wavelength of 585 or 595 nm and a pulse duration of 300 μs to 2 ms is only indicated in the very early stages of infantile hemangiomas not thicker than 2 mm, provided there is no subcutaneous part [3]. Treatment is simple and quick. When the faces of newborn and small children have to be treated, anesthesia is required, while in areas other than the face, local anesthesia (e.g., with EMLA) suffices. Side effects are extremely rare. Occasionally, blisters and scabs are observed, requiring cooling and stabilization of the epidermis by a fluid cooling cuvette. The obligatory

H.-P. Berlien (✉) • M. Poetke
Center for Laser Medicine, Elisabeth Hospital,
Berlin, Germany
e-mail: Lasermed.elisabeth@pgdiakonie.de

R. Mattassi et al. (eds.), *Hemangiomas and Vascular Malformations: An Atlas of Diagnosis and Treatment*,
DOI 10.1007/978-88-470-5673-2_13, © Springer-Verlag Italia 2009, 2015

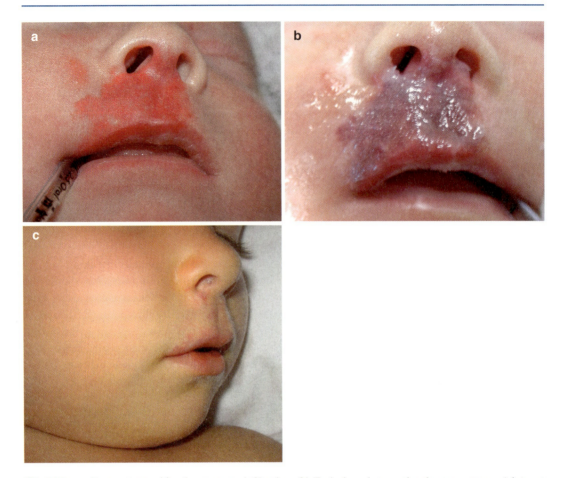

Fig. 13.1 (**a**) Hemangioma with sole cutaneous infiltration. (**b**) Typical postinterventional mauve purpura (ointment applied). (**c**) After one treatment only faint residuals left for further spontaneous regression

bluish-black coloring disappears within 14 days (Fig. 13.1a–c). Scars appear in <1 % of all cases. Particularly in the anogenital area, there is a danger of ulceration with secondary infection. An early FPDL therapy of all infantile hemangiomas and their precursor lesions brought no essential advantages compared to an untreated control group [4], but the authors of this study did not differentiate the hemangiomas according to their depth nor their various stages of development (Fig. 13.2a–d). Tuberous hemangiomas are not an indication for FPDL, and it also fails in subcutaneous and endophytically growing hemangiomas [5]. Telangiectatic changes, primary or as residues of mature infantile hemangiomas, also are not suited for FPDL (Table 13.1). This is an indication for the KTP laser.

Frequency-Doubled Nd:YAG Laser ("KTP")

This type of laser must not be mixed up with the pulsed Nd:YAG laser or even with the continuous wave Nd:YAG laser [6]. Here, the infrared light of the Nd:YAG laser passes through a potassium titanyl phosphate crystal, which produces from the near infrared (NIR) of 1,064 nm by frequency doubling half the wavelength of 532 nm. Thus the biological effect is comparable to that of an argon laser [4]. The advantage of this type of laser is that the KTP due to its better efficacy, especially when pumped with diodes, does not need water cooling unlike the argon laser. This makes it easier to handle.

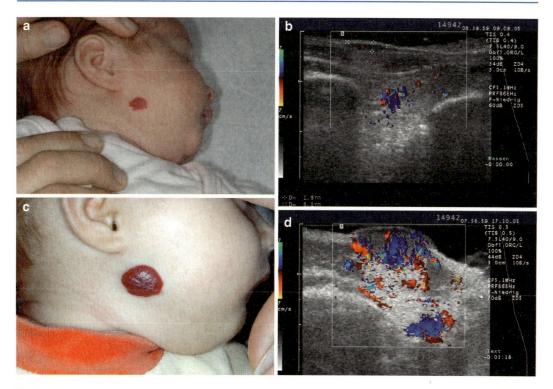

Fig. 13.2 (**a**) Hemangioma assumed to be only superficial. (**b**) In CCDS hyposonic swelling of the skin, notice the faint hypersonic modification of the subcutaneous region with some small color-coded vessels: indication of deeper infiltration. (**c**) Rapid growth despite FPDL laser therapy. (**d**) Now CCDS shows the preexisting subcutaneous infiltration more clearly

Table 13.1 Vessel size limits the effect of the flashlamp-pumped pulsed dye laser

Pressure and temperature distribution

Pulsed laser irradiation

Surface

◯ = Heat

╱ = Pressure

The shorter the pulse length, the smaller the affected volume. This explains why the pulsed dye laser is not suitable for larger telangiectatic vessels

Due to the experience with other telangiectases, such as angioma serpiginosum, small tuberous hemangiomas and residual telangiectasias after regression are being directly treated under glass spatula compression dot to dot (Fig. 13.3a, b). By short pulse durations of a maximum of 100 ms and avoidance of double exposure or overlapping, absorption only takes place in the hemoglobin of the vessels, so that no thermal side effects are to be expected in the surrounding tissue.

Pulsed Nd:YAG Laser

Unlike the KTP laser, NIR radiation is applied directly. The difference to the standard cw-Nd:YAG laser is its short pulse rate of 2–10 ms, albeit with high pulse peaks. While the biophysical penetration is the same as that of the cw-Nd:YAG laser, the actual penetration depth is limited due to the short pulse duration (Fig. 13.4a–c). For this reason, this laser is suited in anatomically endangered regions or larger vein ectasias and tuberous lesions [7]. To avoid secondary damage by scattered radiation or heat conduction, at least one

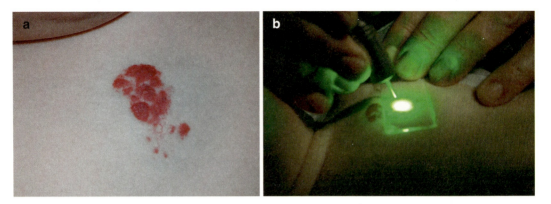

Fig. 13.3 (**a**) The cutaneous part of this combined hemangioma shows vascular ectasias and tuberous infiltrations. (**b**) KTP treatment under quartz glass compression

intermittent cooling system by cold air or ice cubes is required, unless the beam is led through the fluid cooling cuvette or the ice cube as with the cw-Nd:YAG laser.

Continuous Wave (cw-Nd:YAG) Lasers

With longer exposure times than 100 ms, thermal conductivity by the laser-heated tissue is the main effect. This means that for the primary reaction, a specific absorption is important, but the whole tissue interaction is also triggered by the exposure time (Table 13.2). Lasers with high water absorption like erbium or CO_2 lasers have in all tissue the same primary effect; the real tissue interaction depends only on the exposure time. Besides argon laser, the cw-Nd:YAG laser is the laser type that has been used for the longest time in the treatment of congenital vascular anomalies. It is the same laser which is used for endoscopic surgery. In addition to the possibility of directing the laser beam via thin glass fibers, the immense biophysical variability has made this laser the "workhorse" in the treatment of congenital vascular anomalies. The biophysically determined penetration (drop in photon density to 1/e2) is 8 mm for most tissues. But this means that with continuous wave mode at high performance, an effective photon density can still be attained in depths of 20 and 30 mm. On the other hand, the photon density and thus the effective

depth can be limited to less than 1–4 mm by short pulse durations. Suitable cooling procedures protect the penetrated surface enough despite surface absorption to allow no tissue reactions there but only deeper down. Moreover, different absorption coefficients are responsible for the selective effect. Blood and organs rich in blood absorb this near-infrared radiation considerably better than connective or fatty tissue. The tissue reaction to NIR also differs from tissue to tissue. Collagen shows considerable shrinkage and the endothelium already reacts with a serious vasculitis to power densities which do not yet trigger a reaction in other tissue. High power densities quickly lead to carbonization, which then fully absorbs the following laser radiation. Thus, vaporization sets in with two consequences: if one wants to ablate or cut, this process must occur very quickly to avoid unwanted thermal effects in the vicinity. If coagulation is intended especially in the deep regions, this process must be avoided, as no radiation gets deep down enough. The direction of these processes determines the wide usage of cw-Nd:YAG laser [8].

Transcutaneous Direct Application

In the same way such in the case of patients with Osler syndrome, small tuberous lesions and telangiectasias may also be treated with cw-Nd:YAG laser analogous to pulsed Nd:YAG laser and KTP laser. To avoid thermal damage, short

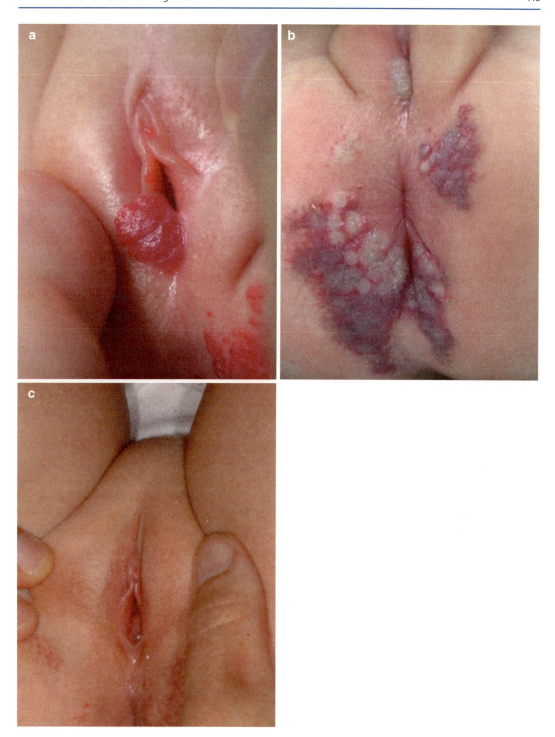

Fig. 13.4 (**a**) Markedly elevated cutaneous infiltration in the sensitive anogenital region. (**b**) Circumscribed spotted superficial coagulations after pulsed Nd:YAG laser exposition. (**c**) Only minor hemangioma residuals after healing without any scar

Table 13.2 Principle application modes of the cw-Nd:YAG laser

Types of Nd:YAG-Laser applications

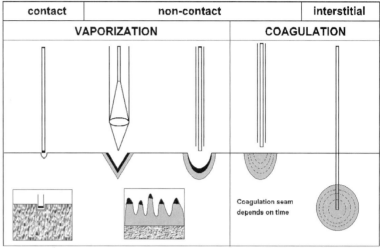

With the different procedure of surface cooling the variety of tissue interactions increases

pulse rates of a maximum of 100 ms, an output of 25 W, and a small spot diameter of up to 0.5 mm are required by using a focusing handpiece. Besides, intermittent and post cooling with ice cubes have to take place to avoid thermal damage by heat blockage.

Transcutaneous Application with Fluid Cooling Cuvette

If intermittent cooling is not sufficient, continuous cooling is required. The heat capacity of spray or cold air cooling is not sufficient for the heat blockage caused by the cw-Nd: YAG laser. Various contact cooling systems are on the market or are offered. Cooled sapphire plates are easy to handle but have a series of disadvantages. The metal frame of the cooling Peltier element may lead to frostbite in case of direct skin contact. The biggest disadvantage, however, is that their plane surface cannot adapt to the anatomic situation, especially in children's faces, so they either do not have full contact to the surface or are too heavily compressed at the edges, causing not only frostbite but also change in the microcirculation. Thus, they can actually be used only for large plane areas. The fluid cooling cuvette with

a 40 % refrigerated glycol solution has a (side of the patient) highly flexible, highly transparent latex membrane which, through changes in the outlet valve, can adapt even to difficult anatomic silhouettes (Table 13.3). An additional advantage is that this prestressing makes it possible to adjust the compression pressure and the blood flow to vary tissue absorption [9]. With maximum compression, the overlying tissue can be made transparent for the Nd:YAG laser radiation. With negative pressure (suction), the tiniest capillary vessels can be expanded, boosting specific absorption. The cooling capacity has been calculated to have a reaction in the center of the laser beam given the necessary absorption while adverse events by scattering and thermal conduction are avoided in the surrounding areas. In case of vein ectasias, this procedure is better suited than the KTP.

Transcutaneous Application with Continuous Ice Cube Cooling

If subcutaneous lesions are to be treated transcutaneously, a continuous Nd:YAG laser application would create so much heat that none of the abovementioned cooling systems would be able

Table 13.3 Cooling chamber, principle of the fluid cooling cuvette

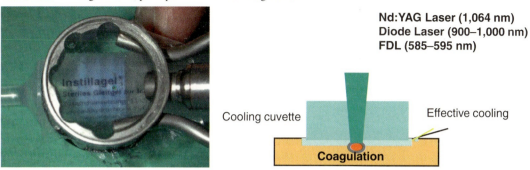

The high transparent flexible latex membrane allows a continuous control of the laser process and follows any anatomical structure without uncontrolled compression. However, the heat capacity is limited for pulsed applications

to completely protect the transient tissue from unwanted coagulation [10]. Deep freezing systems such as liquid nitrogen or deep temperature Peltier elements cannot be directed sufficiently, so frostbite would result. Here, radiation through a transparent, ice cube without air bubbles seems to be the solution. The melting of ice to water is one of the most energy-consuming processes. This high heat capacity is capable of completely rerouting the heat that builds up in the transient tissue by basic absorption, so there are no reactions on the surface. On the other hand, natural law prevents the temperature from dropping below 0 °C, avoiding frostbite. Since meltwater always guarantees good tissue contact, contact gels moreover are superfluous. This cooling effect is limited to 2 mm due to the thermal conductivity properties of the tissue, so that laser radiation can treat subcutaneous lesions thanks to its greater penetration, without causing any defects on the surface. Prerequisites are the use of a focusing handpiece with a focus diameter of 0.5–1 mm. This focus has to be positioned to the tissue surface through an ice cube, as otherwise no sufficient penetration will be attained because of diffraction scattering. As the ice cube has its own absorption for this laser radiation, a prolonged exposition would drill a hole into the ice cube ("chimney effect"), letting radiation get directly to the tissue surface. Therefore, the 6 ice cube has to be moved above the hemangioma under laser exposition, the ray itself moving in small spiral motions with a radius of about 5 mm to avoid

too high a load for a single spot. If only the laser beam would be moved above the ice cube, but not the ice cube as well, the chimney effect could be avoided, but the developing heat on the surface of the hemangioma would melt the ice cube so much that there would be no more direct tissue contact between the ice cube and hemangioma ("igloo effect"). By compression especially in large hemangiomas with the ice cube, the depth of penetration can be increased, and by pressure on the surface, the absorption decreased, boosting the protection (Table 13.4). This procedure is only recommended under anesthesia because of the associated pain. Besides, this is also necessary because of laser safety, because most hemangiomas are located in the face near the eyes. For the exact positioning of the laser parameters, an intraoperative CCDS is required, as this alone enables determination of activity and exact stage, dimension, and where applicable involvement of various layers (Fig. 13.5a–d). To choose the laser output, the following rules apply: The more active and aggressive the growth and the earlier the stage, the smaller the output to avoid an overreaction. The more vessels are visible already, the higher the output to attain involution. Moreover, the stronger the intracutaneous lesion, the smaller the output, but in exclusive subcutaneous lesions, more output. However, in exclusive subcutaneous lesions, the output is higher. Treatment next to the eyes necessitates protection from forward-scattered radiation. For this purpose, metal spatulas ("eye spatulas") are suited that float on

Table 13.4 Transcutaneous Nd:YAG laser treatment with ice cube cooling

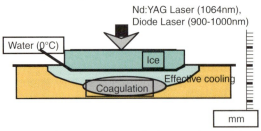

For continuous laser application, a greater heat capacity is required to save the overlying skin. Irradiation through a clear ice cube allows a deep laser reaction without any damage to the overlying skin. The protection is so perfect that in eyelid treatment it is possible to carry out a transpalpebral coagulation without notice. Therefore, the cornea in this case must be protected with a metal spatula

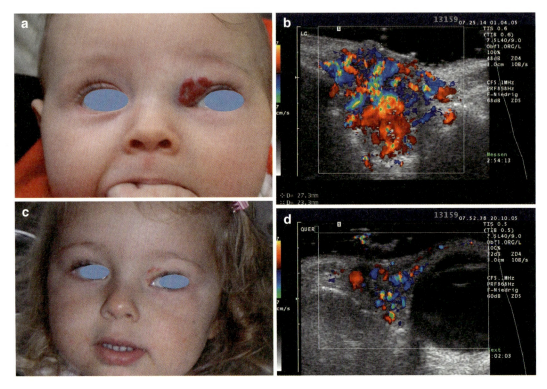

Fig. 13.5 (**a**) Besides a cutaneous infiltration the subcutaneous volume hinders eyelid motility. (**b**) CCDS detects the deep infiltration medial of the bulb. (**c**) After four transcutaneous treatments there is advanced regression in both components. (**d**) Even close to the bulb only marginal residuals

a kanamycin-ointment bed in such a way that the backside never touches the cornea. For this reason, the laser beam should always be turned away from the eyeball. At the columella, attention should be paid to the cartilage structure of the nose. In case of hemangiomas on the lips, the laser also has to be turned away from the gingiva to avoid destruction of the dental germ.

A hemangioma of the gingiva itself can then be treated with the FPDL laser. The aim is not a definite coagulation of the infantile hemangioma but the induction of a vasculitis. A visible blanching or even an involution during laser treatment should be avoided as this would be equivalent to overdosing. The optimal total dose has been reached when the hemangioma during laser

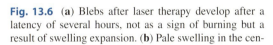
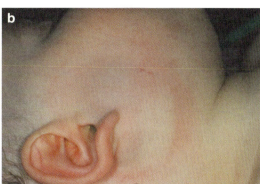

Fig. 13.6 (a) Blebs after laser therapy develop after a latency of several hours, not as a sign of burning but a result of swelling expansion. (b) Pale swelling in the cen-ter of the treatment region with surrounding reddish rim: suspect of a beginning infection

treatment starts to show a swelling and is bulging and the surrounding area turns red, which lasts up to 12 h. Occasionally, 6–24 h postoperatively, subcutaneous blue indurations develop as an expression of the vasculitis with a vessel break-down. This reaction is common in very active infantile hemangiomas in the early proliferation phase. As the overlaying epidermis is easily dam-aged, postoperatively, enough ointment should be applied, and the area should be protected against scratches with suitable measures such as the wearing of gloves. A bandage is rarely necessary, except in case of heavy mechanical abrasions. Although this treatment does not cause injuries on the surface of the skin, about 2 % of the chil-dren, 12–48 h after the operation, develop erysip-elas with a beginning lymphangitis (Fig. 13.6a, b). This is seen frequently in the face. Erysipelas does not develop in the hemangioma itself or around it, but occasionally a few centimeters away draining into the lymph. This inflammation can be differentiated from the direct postopera-tively laser-induced inflammation as this region is sensitive to touch and hardened. In already exulcerated or even secondarily infected heman-giomas, this reaction has never been noted, nor in interstitial treatment when puncturing. It thus is not a nosocomial infection. An immediate treat-ment with oral antibiotics with a broad-spectrum cephalosporin will cause the clinical symptoms to subside within a few hours. Fever and symp-toms do not exist at any time then, but the infil-trate may persist for a few days.

As regression in hemangioendotheliomas can-not be attained as easily as in infantile hemangio-mas, clearly more output up to 60 W is required as normally is used only for the treatment of vas-cular malformations. As with the treatment of vascular malformations, the incidence of side effects from Nd:YAG laser treatment of heman-giomas is quite small.

In contrast to the interstitial puncture tech-nique, uniform coagulation can be achieved, so that fibrosis will not be as pronounced after heal-ing is completed.

Impression Technique

Unlike in interstitial puncturing, the fiber in the impression technique is being put on the surface and pressed into the hemangioma. This way, a shift of the laser's effect below the surface is also attained without triggering coagulation on the surface of the hemangioma (except for the fiber contact area). Therefore, this technique should be used for the skin only in limited cases, as it may cause small scars. But it is an ideal technique for hemangiomas reachable from the mucosa includ-ing the conjunctiva (Fig. 13.7a, b), as it leads to a "restitutio ad integrum" even in the contact area. With a laser output of a maximum of 5 W, the in-depth effect can be adjusted by length of exposi-tion. This way, laser application becomes possible even near critical structures. In hemangiomas on the upper as well as the lower eyelid, a curved

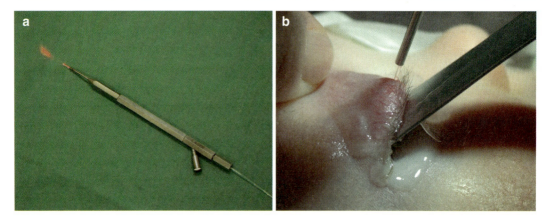

Fig. 13.7 (**a**) Fastener for bare fiber application. (**b**) Bare fiber impression technique in the sensitive region of the upper lid ridge; even without scattering protection of the eye is mandatory

fiber holder is used for laser application from the conjunctiva to the outside (Fig. 13.8a–e). The skin temperature above the hemangioma is constantly being controlled with a finger; the position of the fiber point can be controlled with the CCDS. In lip hemangiomas, likewise, the laser can be applied from enoral. The impression technique closes the gap between direct application, even with the pulsed Nd:YAG laser which operates only on the surface, and the transcutaneous ice cube application which reaches large volumes.

Interstitial Puncture Technique

In very large, deep, and particularly purely subcutaneous hemangiomas, neither the impression technique nor the transcutaneous ice cube method can totally avoid thermal damage to the surface. In these cases, the hemangioma is being punctured with a Teflon vein catheter and a fiber is being inserted (Fig. 13.9a–c). Output should be between 4 and 5 W, as with higher output, there are immediate carbonizations at the fiber tip which for one thing would burn the tissue and for another would prevent a uniform distribution of the laser radiation. Intraoperative CCDS control is obligatory [11] to avoid erroneous puncturing and to monitor adequate laser reaction via the color bruit. Skin temperature above the laser area must be monitored continually with a finger just as in the impression technique when the distance

from the fiber tip to the surface is less than 10 mm. Thermal damage of the surface thus can safely be avoided, but when nerves are being directly aimed for, for instance, with the fiber tip, they may be damaged. This can be excluded by the transcutaneous ice cube technique. By optimizing the laser parameters and the ice cube quality, the indication for the interstitial technique for infantile hemangiomas therefore has clearly dropped. Even vast parotid hemangiomas only rarely are treated this way. For large hemangioendotheliomas, be it the Kaposi-like (KHE) or the non-involuting congenital hemangioendothelioma (NICH), this technique represents an expansion of the transcutaneous ice cube technique (Fig. 13.10a–d), as by direct application subcutaneously an immediate coagulation of the hemangioendotheliomas can be achieved. In patients with a Kasabach-Merritt syndrome along with a coagulopathy, however, the bleeding risk through puncturing has to be avoided. In such cases, small coagulations of the dermis should be accepted and the ice cube technique with a high output of 60 W applied.

Endoscopy

In infantile hemangiomas, there is an indication for endoscopic treatment, primarily in subglottal and tracheal infantile hemangiomas [12] as well as in the urethra and the anal canal. While an

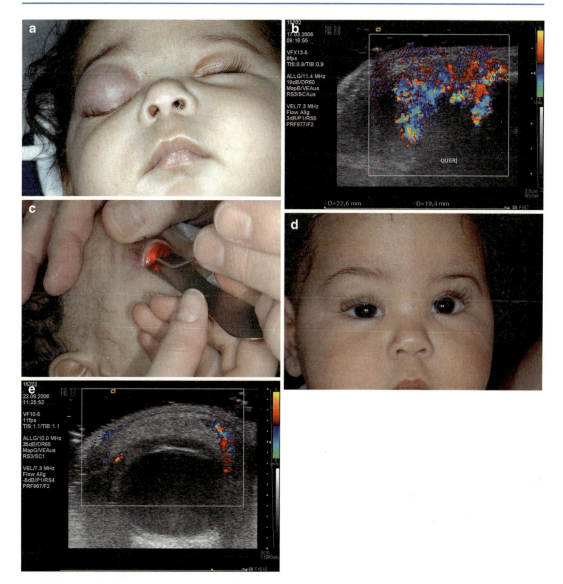

Fig. 13.8 (**a**) Purely subcutaneous hemangioma. (**b**) Infiltration depth >20 mm above the bulb. (**c**) Directional impression technique transconjunctival allows high-energy input without risk of scars. (**d**) Perfect reduction of the volume. (**e**) Five months later barely smallest residuals are left

involvement of the male urethra by an infantile hemangioma is rare and by differential diagnosis a vascular malformation should be considered, in girls, especially vulvar and perineal infantile hemangiomas are clearly more common. To exclude further lesions at the bladder neck, which also is rather affected by a vascular malformation, a cystourethroscopy should always be performed. The endoscope is entered through the working canal with the fiber and in flat disseminated hemangiomas a punctual coagulation achieved by noncontact of the fiber tip with the tissue with an output of 10 W, pulsed, and exposures lasting a maximum of 100 ms. Confluent coagulation definitely has to be avoided. In case of pad-like hemangiomas, the impression technique is performed over the endoscope as described above with a maximum output of only 5 W. Especially in subglottal and tracheal hemangiomas, the hemangioma must not be coagulated

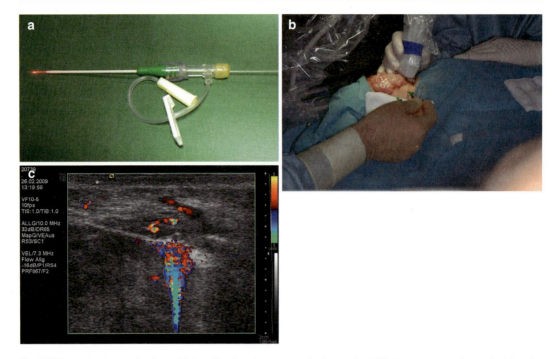

Fig. 13.9 (**a**) Equipment for interstitial application: bare fiber within a standard Teflon intravenous cannula. (**b**) Puncture, positioning of the bare fiber, and online laser monitoring under CCDS control. (**c**) The typical intralesional color bruit during laser exposition

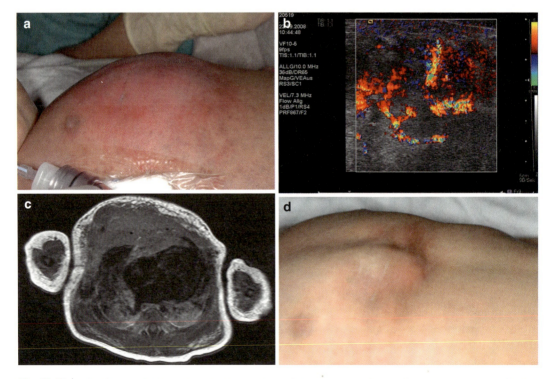

Fig. 13.10 (**a**) Widespread KHE in the right thorax. (**b**) Large infiltrating vessels in the chest wall. (**c**) MRI shows the infiltration of the pleural space and mediastinum. (**d**) Status after multimodal treatment sessions, including interstitial laser therapy

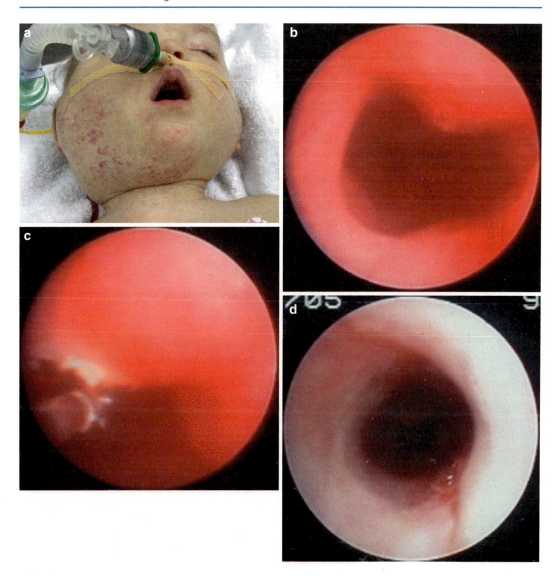

Fig. 13.11 (**a**) Extensive hemangioma in the face and neck frequently involve the subglottic trachea as well. (**b**) Hemangioma of the right anterior tracheal wall. (**c**) During Nd:YAG laser bare fiber contact coagulation. (**d**) Almost no residuals in control after only one treatment

completely, as scarred strictures may remain [13]. Circular applications should be avoided as well (Fig. 13.11a–d). In infantile hemangiomas one has to be particularly careful of the vocal cords themselves. Only short, single punctual applications are permissible to avoid fibrosis and thus limited function of the vocal cords. In no case should it be attempted to remove the hemangioma in one session. For this procedure, a postoperative intubation for safety reasons is usually not necessary. In infantile hemangiomas of the larynx and trachea, a simultaneous short-interval high-dose prednisone therapy is essential. With this regimen we were able to avoid primary tracheotomy for more than 20 years in patients with infantile hemangiomas [14].

In children who underwent tracheotomy in emergency situations elsewhere and who then came to us, the tracheostoma could be closed after a maximum of two sessions.

References

1. Anderson RR, Parish JA (1981) The optics of human skin. J Invest Dermatol 77:9–13
2. Tong AKF, Tan OT, Boll J, Parrish JA, Murphy GF (1987) Ultrastructure: effects of melanin pigment on target specificity using a pulsed dye laser (577 nm). J Invest Dermatol 88:747–752
3. Poetke M, Philipp C, Berlien HP (2000) Flashlamp-pumped pulsed dye laser for hemangiomas in infancy. Arch Dermatol 136:628–632
4. Achauer BM, Vander Kam VM (1989) Capillary hemangiomas (Strawberry Mark) of infancy: comparison of argon and Nd: YAG laser treatment. Plast Reconstr Surg 84(1):60–69
5. Ashinoff R, Geronemus RG (1993) Failure of the flashlamp-pumped pulsed dye laser to prevent progression to deep hemangioma. Pediatr Dermatol 10: 77–80
6. Poetke M, Urban P, Philipp C, Berlien HP (2004) Laserbehandlung bei Hämangiomen- Technische Grundlagen und Möglichkeiten. Monatsschr Kinderheilkunde 152:7–15
7. AWMF online (2007) Empfehlungen zur Behandlung mit Laser und hochenergetischen Blitzlampen (HBL) in der Dermatologie, Empfehlungen der Deutschen Dermatologischen Gesellschaft. AWMF-Leitlinien-Register Nr. 006/100; Hämangiome im Säuglings- und Kleinkindesalter
8. Berlien HP, Waldschmidt J, Müller G (1988) Laser treatment of cutaneous and deep vessel anomalies. In: Waidelich W (ed) Laser optoelectronics in medicine. Springer, Berlin/Heidelberg/New York, pp 526–528
9. Poetke M, Philipp C, Berlien HP (1997) Ten years of laser treatment of hemangiomas and vascular malformations: techniques and results. In: Berlien HP, Schmittenbecher PP (eds) Laser surgery in children. Springer, Berlin, pp 82–91
10. Raulin C, Karsai S (2011) Laser therapy of infantile haemangioma and other congenital vascular tumours in infants. Springer, Berlin/Heidelberg. ISBN 978-3-642-03437-4
11. Urban P, Philipp CM, Poetke M, Berlien HP (2005) Value of colour coded duplex sonography in the assessment of haemangiomas and vascular malformations. Med Laser Appl 20(4):267–278
12. Cholewa D, Waldschmidt J (1998) Laser treatment of hemangiomas of the larynx and trachea. Lasers Surg Med 23:221–232
13. Apfelberg DB, Maser MF, Lash H, White DN (1985) Benefits of CO2 laser in oral hemangioma excision. Plast Reconstr Surg 75:46
14. Berlien HP, Müller GJ (2003) Applied laser medicine. Springer, Berlin/Heidelberg, p 69

Surgery of Hemangiomas

14

Gianni Vercellio and Vittoria Baraldini

Summary

The surgical management of infantile hemangiomas (IH) usually consists of late correction of contour deformities after completed spontaneous involution with excision of remaining fibrofatty tissue and exuberant skin.

The range of indications for surgical excision of IH has been modified since 2008, after the revolution of treatments gold standard for IH, in the propranolol era [1, 2].

However, the introduction of particular techniques adopted in order to minimize intraoperative bleeding and optimize scarring made early surgical excision of IH during the proliferating phase or after partial involution feasible in case of unsuccessful treatment with propranolol.

On the basis of our experience, early surgical excision can be considered in the following situations: rapidly growing IH with expectance of relevant fibrofatty remnants after involution, voluminous tuberous IH anatomically located in scarcely exposed areas where scars would be easy to hide, pedunculated IH with a narrow implantation base, non-involutive congenital IH (NICH type), palpebral IH with secondary functional impairment of palpebral motility nonresponsive to propranolol/corticosteroids and/or laser treatment, ulcerated and bleeding IH nonresponsive to propranolol/corticosteroids and/or laser treatment, and IH of the nose producing secondary cartilage deformity.

Introduction

Among the different therapeutic options for a common IH, a marginal role was traditionally reserved to surgery. This is due to multiple reasons: IH's natural tendency toward spontaneous involution, IH's good response to medical and laser treatment, and the high incidence of worse cosmetic results after surgical excision with hypertrophic surgical scars compared to persistent fibrofatty remnants after completed spontaneous involution [3, 4].

Furthermore, when approaching a large IH in the proliferating phase, intraoperative bleeding control is the main challenge for the surgeon: a few specific techniques have been developed in order to reduce bleeding during the operation.

Although parents are normally reluctant to surgery, since it requires general anesthesia and occasionally blood transfusions, often they ask for an early excision of the mass, particularly when it affects exposed anatomical areas.

Similarly to what happens for other vascular anomalies, the assessment of indications for early surgical excision of IH requires an evaluation of different parameters: anatomical areas involved,

G. Vercellio (✉) • V. Baraldini
Vascular Malformations Centre – "V.Buzzi"
Children's Hospital, Milan, Italy
e-mail: gianni.vercellio@alice.it;
Vittoria.baraldini@icp.mi.it

R. Mattassi et al. (eds.), *Hemangiomas and Vascular Malformations: An Atlas of Diagnosis and Treatment*,
DOI 10.1007/978-88-470-5673-2_14, © Springer-Verlag Italia 2009, 2015

IH type and size, past complications, IH life cycle phase, functional implications, and level of response to alternative treatments [5].

Indications and Timing for Surgical Treatment

Indications and timing for surgical treatment are strictly related each other.

There is a general agreement about the choice to postpone surgical treatment of IH in the expectation of a complete spontaneous involution. Therefore, indications for surgery are normally restricted to the treatment of fibrofatty remnants with different techniques:

(a) Excision of exuberant fibrofatty tissue (liposuction can be employed)

(b) Correction of contour deformities [3–5]

The indications for early surgical excision of IH in the proliferative phase are more controversial [6], and they are listed as follows:

1. Rapidly growing IH with expectance of relevant fibrofatty residuum after involution
2. Voluminous tuberous IH affecting anatomical sites where scars would be easy to hide (i.e., neck, scalp)
3. Pedicled tuberous IH with a narrow implantation base (excisable using the "round-block" technique)
4. Non-involutive congenital IH (NICH type – Fig. 14.1)
5. Palpebral IH with secondary functional impairment of palpebral motility scarcely or nonresponsive to medical and/or laser treatment [7, 8]
6. IH of the nose producing secondary cartilage deformity
7. Large IH in the lip producing facial disfigurement, speech impairment, and feeding difficulties [9]
8. Ulcerated and bleeding IH nonresponsive to medical and/or laser treatment

Thanks to the introduction of medical treatment with propranolol for critical IH, nowadays the bleeding control during surgery for early IH excision has been much easier. Surgery for

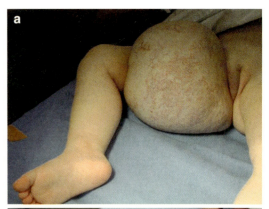

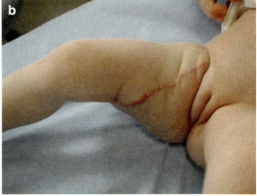

Fig. 14.1 Giant non-involuting congenital hemangioma in the thigh with functional gait impairment. Excision by lenticular incision and linear closure technique (**a**). Postoperative results (**b**)

excision of exuberant fibrofatty tissue and correction of contour deformities can now be performed during early infancy after the 6 month of medical treatment with propranolol, optimizing the cosmetic final result and minimizing the psychological side effects of stigmatization.

Techniques

The main purpose of surgery for the removal of IH, regardless of their life cycle phase (proliferative or involutive), is to optimize the final cosmetic result [10]. When approaching large hemangiomas in the proliferating phase, intraoperative bleeding control is the main challenge for the surgeon: a few surgical tricks can be employed in order to minimize intraoperative bleeding.

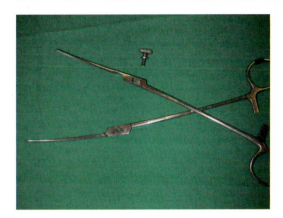

Fig. 14.2 A homemade special clamp that can be disassembled in two parts by removing a screw that acts as a hinge

Two different surgical techniques for partial or total excision of a critical hemangioma which meet this challenge can be used:

(a) The *lenticular-shaped incision and linear closure* technique
(b) The *circular excision and purse-string closure* technique, which had been previously reported as a "round-block technique" [11–14]

The first one is the traditional method used for the removal of skin masses with a *lenticular-shaped incision and linear closure*: this technique is proposed for lesions larger than 3.0 cm in diameter at the base. The skin incision must be oriented with the axis of the relaxed skin tension lines and must be drawn along the border between affected tissue and normal skin [15, 16].

Intraoperative blood losses can be conspicuous for patient's age and weight.

In order to minimize bleeding by reducing the lesion vascular supply, a technique of hemostatic "squeezing" at the tumor's base can be employed for removal of the most voluminous tumors.

A special clamp was designed. This was manufactured in such a way that it can be disassembled into two parts by removing a screw which acts as a hinge (Fig. 14.2). Reinsertion of the screw enables reassembly of the two parts as a clamp. The two parts of this disassembled clamp are blindly inserted under the skin through a small skin incision adjacent to the hemangioma and passed in the subcutaneous tissue on opposite

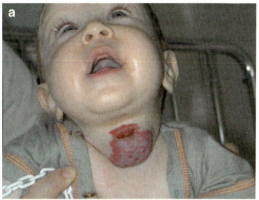

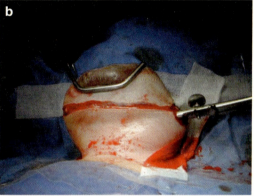

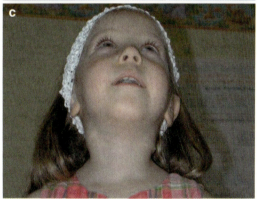

Fig. 14.3 Lenticular incision and linear closure technique for excision of a large cervical hemangioma in a 9-month-old girl (**a**). An original clamp with de-joined branches is blindly inserted under the skin for hemostatic squeezing at the base of the vascular tumor (**b**). Follow-up control 6 months after surgery (**c**)

sides of the mass. The two parts are then reassembled after insertion of the screw, and the clamp is closed underneath the hemangioma base thus compressing its blood supply (Fig. 14.3).

In order to make the clamp's blind insertion easier and reduce vascularity, a variable volume of epinephrine solution in normal saline (0.1 % dilution) is injected within the subcutaneous tissue underlying the hemangioma and circumferentially around the lesion [5].

Detachment of the vascular tumor from the deep plans and the surrounding tissues is then obtained using monopolar diathermy. After resection, the clamp is released and complete bleeding control is accomplished using bipolar diathermy on the residual afferent vessels which normally present a radial distribution.

Linear closure by side to side approximation of the wound edges is finally obtained: intradermal absorbable running suture is tailored to close the skin. Sometimes it is necessary to lengthen the skin incision along its main axis up to 1/3 of its original size from each end in order to avoid "dog ears" at the wound extremities.

The "round-block technique," described by Mulliken et al. [17] and more recently adopted by the authors, is indicated for excision of smaller lesions, sized less than 30 mm in diameter.

The advantages of using *the purse-string closure technique* for removal of localized hemangiomas consist of minimizing the subsequent scar length (up to 50 % shorter compared with results obtained from the traditional linear closure technique) and minimizing the adjacent structure distortion, since tension is equally applied along multiple radial lines with a symmetrical concentric distribution pattern rather than along a main axis perpendicular to the linear wound.

In our experience preliminary hydrostatic undermining by saline injection is always useful before performing a circular skin incision in order to detach the vascular tumor from the deep plans and the surrounding tissues and to encourage a symmetrical distortion of adjacent structures by concentric distribution of tension lines.

When conspicuous blood losses are expected, a running polypropylene or nylon 2/0 nontraumatic suture is temporarily placed around the lesion base. This suture is fixed on a silicon tourniquet (Vessel loop ®); in this way either hemostatic squeezing of the IH or radial recruiting of surrounding healthy skin is achieved at the same time [5].

After having completed the IH removal and accurate hemostasis using bipolar diathermy, the temporary hemostatic running nylon suture is removed. The circular defect is then closed with a double purse-string suture: 3/0 Vicryl running circular suture within the subcutis and 3/0 running absorbable monofilament for skin intradermal suture. If a small opening remains, one or two percutaneous additional sutures can be placed to approximate the wound edges [5].

After circular excision of a giant IH in selected cases, the large circular skin defect can be closed using a combined linear closure technique centrally with purse-string closure at the wound extremities in order to reduce the scar length.

No drain is normally needed.

Postoperative Care

An occlusive dressing with an iodopovidone gauze is left unchanged for 48 h to prevent postoperative bacterial wound contamination after both techniques. Further subsequent medication is planned after 10 days. The running absorbable sutures are left in situ until they dissolve.

Infection, delayed wound healing, and scar widening occur with a relevant incidence after IH excision with the round-block technique (20 %).

Parents need to be very well prepared and informed about the possible moderate scar widening: the eventual need of a second surgical operation a few months later to correct the scar if it is not cosmetically acceptable should be always discussed before the first operation.

Conclusions

On the basis of the authors' experience, the range of indications for the surgical removal

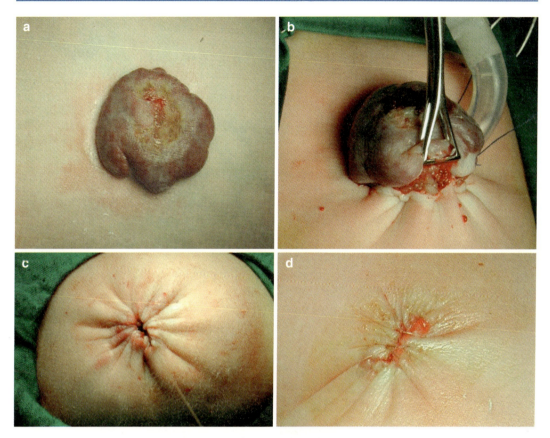

Fig. 14.4 "Round-block" technique in a tuberous hemangioma (**a**). After temporary positioning of a hemostatic circular suture at the lesion base, a round-block excision is performed with circular skin incision (**b**). Concentric purse-string sutures in the subcutaneous and intradermic layers are then tailored (**c**). Tightening the subcutaneous purse-string suture first and then the intradermal one apposes the wound margin. This procedure produces multiple radial gathered ridges which usually flatten in a few weeks (**d**)

of IH can be expanded to the proliferative phase using particular surgical techniques in order to achieve a good bleeding control and to optimize the final cosmetic result.

Early excision might prevent psychological stigmatization of affected children and parents [18, 19].

However, even for the largest tumors, early surgical removal of IH should be always evaluated by the surgeon as a treatment option after having considered the chance to obtain a rapid improvement with less invasive treatments such as propranolol administration and/or laser photocoagulation techniques.

Bleeding control is greatly ameliorated if surgery is performed during or soon after 6 months of propranolol administration.

Selected cases require a multimodal treatment strategy combining medical treatment by early administration of propranolol, surface laser photocoagulation of the affected skin, and surgical excision of fibrofatty residuum (Figs. 14.4 and 14.5).

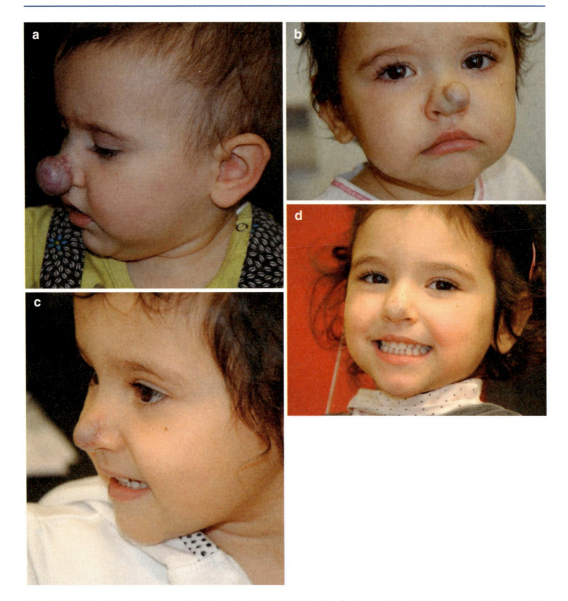

Fig. 14.5 IH "en Cirano" of the nose in a 9-month-old child (**a**). Results after 1 year of medical treatment with propranolol: partial involution and fibrofatty tuberous remnants (**b**). Results after surgical correction at 3 years of age (**c**, **d**)

References

1. Léauté-Labrèze C, Dumas de la Roque E, Hubiche T, Boralevi F, Thambo JB, Taïeb A (2008) Propranolol for severe hemangiomas of infancy. N Engl J Med 358(24):2649–2651
2. Malik MA, Menon P, Rao KL, Samujh R (2013) Effect of propranolol vs prednisolone vs propranolol with prednisolone in the management of infantile hemangioma: a randomized controlled study. J Pediatr Surg 48(12):2453–2459
3. Margileth AM, Museles M (1965) Cutaneous hemangiomas in children: diagnosis and conservative management. JAMA 194(5):523–526
4. Enjolras O, Mulliken JB (1993) The current management of vascular birthmarks. Pediatr Dermatol 10(4):311–313
5. Baraldini V, Coletti M, Cigognetti F, Vercellio G (2007) Haemostatic squeezing and purse-string sutures: optimising surgical techniques for early excision of critical infantile haemangiomas. J Pediatr Surg 42:381–385
6. Luu M, Frieden IJ (2013) Haemangioma: clinical course, complications and management. Br J Dermatol 169(1):20–30

7. Mawn LA (2013) Infantile hemangioma: treatment with surgery or steroids. Am Orthopt J 63:6–13

8. Krema H (2013) Primary surgical excision for pediatric orbital capillary hemangioma. Semin Ophthalmol 00:1–4

9. Hynes S, Narasimhan K, Courtemanche DJ, Arneja JS (2013) Complicated infantile hemangioma of the lip: outcomes of early versus late resection. Plast Reconstr Surg 131(3):373e–379e

10. Demiri EC, Pelissier P, Genin-Etcheberry T et al (2001) Treatment of facial haemangiomas: the present status of surgery. Br J Plast Surg 54(8):665–674

11. Peled IJ, Zagher U, Wexler MR (1985) Purse-string suture for reduction and closure of skin defects. Ann Plast Surg 14:465

12. Tremolada C, Blandini D, Beretta M et al (1997) The "round block" purse-string suture: a simple method to close skin defects with minimal scarring. Plast Reconstr Surg 100(1):126–131

13. Patel KK, Telfer MR, Southee R (2003) A "round block" purse-string suture in facial reconstruction after operations for skin cancer surgery. Br J Oral Maxillofac Surg 41(3):151–156

14. Weisberg NK, Greenbaum SS (2003) Revisiting the purse-string closure: some new methods and modifications. Dermatol Surg 29(6):672–676

15. Gillespie PH, Banwell PE, Hormbrey EL et al (2000) A new model for assessment in plastic surgery: knowledge of relaxed skin tension lines. Br J Plast Surg 53(3):243–244

16. Gibson T, Kenedi RM (1967) Biomechanical properties of the skin. Surg Clin North Am 47:279

17. Mulliken JB, Rogers GF, Marler JJ (2002) Circular excision of hemangioma and purse-string closure: the smallest possible scar. Plast Recontr Surg 109(5):1544–1554

18. Dieterich-Miler CA, Cohen BA, Ligget J (1992) Behaviour adjustment and self-concept of young children with haemangiomas. Pediatr Dermatol 9:241

19. Tanner JL, Dechert MP, Frieden IJ (1998) Growing up with a facial hemangioma: parent and child coping and adaptation. Pediatrics 101(3):446–452

Treatment of Hemangiomas by Embolization

15

Patricia E. Burrows and David J.E. Lord

Hemangiomas, both infantile and congenital forms, are high-flow lesions and thus are amenable to transarterial embolization. Embolization for bleeding and high-output cardiac failure can be lifesaving. Preoperative devascularization to reduce bleeding at time of resection is also useful in selected situations. Today, embolization of hemangioma is infrequently performed in pediatric institutions with multidisciplinary vascular anomalies programs, because of increased effectiveness of pharmacotherapy for both infantile hemangioma and kaposiform hemangioendothelioma as well as recognition that many congenital hemangiomas will involute rapidly without treatment.

Published literature regarding the use of embolization to treat pediatric hemangiomas consists mainly of case reports and very small series and is confusing because most reports did not distinguish between infantile and rapidly involuting congenital hemangiomas. Transcatheter embolization of a small number of hepatic hemangiomas was reported in the 1980s and 1990s [1–6]. There was definitely a discrepancy between excellent results in some patients, with onset of regression of the mass within days of embolization, and failure or death in other patients. In retrospect, review of the illustrations in these publications reveals that the lesions responding dramatically well were focal hemangiomas, almost certainly rapidly involuting congenital hemangiomas. Patients with multifocal hepatic hemangiomas, which are infantile hemangiomas, often failed embolization, and some deaths related to hepatic failure were reported [2, 3, 6, 7]. Studies investigating the vascularity of hepatic hemangiomas showed two distinct forms. The focal hemangiomas, now known to be RICH, frequently have arteriovenous, arterioportal, and porto-venous fistulas [8]. Partial embolization of a hepatic RICH is typically followed by a rapid improvement in congestive heart failure and regression of the tumor [9–11]. Multifocal hepatic hemangiomas, which are infantile hemangiomas, can also cause cardiac volume overload, but these respond less well to embolization and are more likely to develop complications. Vascular anatomy can be quite complex, with extensive arterial supply from hepatic and extra hepatic arteries often combined with large porto-venous fistulas. Extensive hepatic artery embolization can result in hepatic necrosis because there is poor hepatic perfusion from the portal veins, due to porto-venous shunting [2, 3, 10]. Fortunately, these patients often respond rapidly to treatment with beta-blockers and embolization is rarely needed.

P.E. Burrows, MD (✉)
Department of Radiology,
Children's Hospital of Wisconsin,
Medical College of Wisconsin, Milwaukee, WI, USA
e-mail: pburrows@chw.org

D.J.E. Lord
Department of Radiology,
Children's Hospital at Westmead,
The University of Sydney,
Westmead, Sydney, NSW, Australia
e-mail: David.Lord@health.nsw.gov.au

Embolization of cutaneous hemangiomas and hemangioendotheliomas associated with Kasabach-Merritt phenomenon is performed infrequently. Case reports usually describe rapid improvement in platelet counts. However, thrombocytopenia usually recurs in a few weeks, so additional embolization or pharmacotherapy is needed [12–14]. Drug treatment is preferable, reserving embolization for lesions with active bleeding and the feasibility of resection after embolization.

Disadvantages of Therapeutic Embolization in Infancy

Embolization of infantile or congenital hemangioma is usually a complex procedure, requiring significant technical skills and knowledge specific to these lesions [15]. The arterial supply of an infantile hemangioma is usually through a large number of small arterial branches. Supraselective embolization requires catheterization of numerous vessels, a process requiring administration of significant doses of fluid, contrast medium, and radiation. Nontarget embolization can occur, causing damage to healthy tissue. Congenital hepatic hemangiomas can have direct arteriovenous fistulae. Choice of the wrong embolic agent may result in pulmonary embolization. Persistent fetal circulation including patent foramen ovale can also lead to systemic migration of embolic material potentially occluding coronary, cerebral, or other vital arteries. Femoral artery thrombosis following angiography and embolization [risk is greater than 10 % of neonates] can lead to tissue damage, leg length discrepancy, and claudication. In addition to these possible complications, the benefits of embolization may be transient, if the lesion continues to proliferate.

Current Indications for Embolization of Hemangiomas and Other Vascular Tumors in Infancy

High-output cardiac failure requiring mechanical ventilation and pressor therapy. If the patient fails or cannot tolerate medical treatment, embolization should be carried out urgently.
Severe bleeding from superficial hemangiomas; embolization may also facilitate resection.
Severe thrombocytopenia secondary to Kasabach-Merritt phenomenon, not responsive to pharmacotherapy and associated with bleeding.

Embolization Techniques

Arterial Access. If possible, the umbilical artery should be used for arterial access in neonates, to minimize trauma to the femoral artery. Axillary arterial access is preferred for lesions in the abdomen and lower extremities. If the femoral artery is to be used, arterial access should be obtained with ultrasound guidance, in order to minimize trauma during cannulation [15]. To further decrease the risk of femoral artery thrombosis, the patient should be heparinized after femoral artery access and kept warm before and after the procedure. A four French sheath and guide catheter is used. Global angiography is carried out through the guide catheter [e.g., aortography for hepatic hemangiomas]. A microcatheter is then used to select the individual feeding arteries. The choice of embolic material will depend upon the anatomy and angio-architecture. For infantile hemangiomas without direct arteriovenous shunting, particles are frequently used. In congenital hemangiomas with arteriovenous shunts, coils, tissue adhesive, or Onyx are more appropriate. These agents also require less fluid and contrast medium than particles. The goal of embolization for cardiac overload is to decrease shunting. Complete occlusion of arterial supply is usually not necessary (Fig. 15.1).

Summary

Embolization is generally not a first-line treatment for infantile and congenital hemangiomas, as well as kaposiform hemangioendotheliomas, but can be effective and even lifesaving in selected situations.

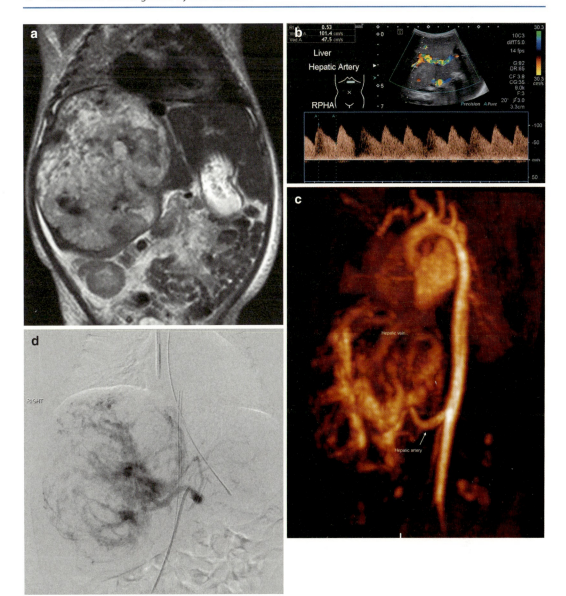

Fig. 15.1 Term neonate requiring mechanical ventilation and pressors with cardiac volume overload and respiratory insufficiency due to massive hepatic RICH. Hepatic arterial supply was partially embolized using large particles and Gelfoam, resulting in rapid clinical improvement. The infant was extubated and feeding normally within 2 days of the procedure and continues to do well. (a) T2-weighted coronal MRI shows a large spherical heterogeneous mass in the right hepatic lobe. (b) Color Doppler ultrasound image of the liver shows dilated hepatic vessels with a low-resistance Doppler waveform consistent with arteriovenous shunting. (c) MR angiography shows the extreme vascularity of the mass. (d, e) Hepatic arteriogram confirms the high-flow nature of the focal lesion, without direct arteriovenous fistulae. (f) Segmental angiogram prior to embolization. (g, h) Hepatic angiogram carried out after embolization shows subtotal occlusion of the tumor vascularity. If the patient did not improve, further embolization could be carried out in a second stage. *RPHA*, right posterior hepatic artery

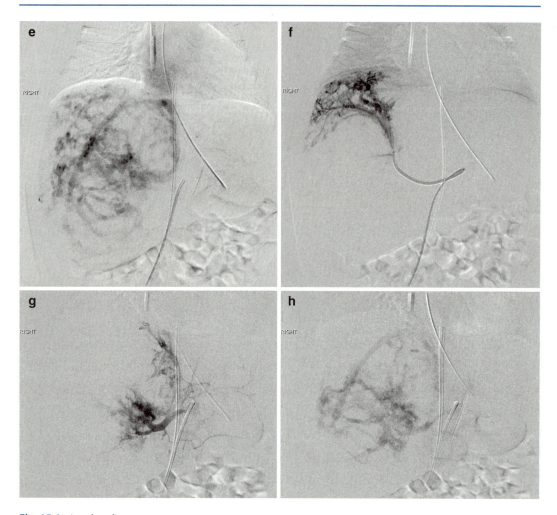

Fig. 15.1 (continued)

References

1. Stanley P, Grinnell VS, Stanton RE, Williams KO, Shore NA (1983) Therapeutic embolization of infantile hepatic hemangioma with polyvinyl alcohol. AJR Am J Roentgenol 141(5):1047–1051
2. Burrows PE, Rosenberg HC, Chuang HS (1985) Diffuse hepatic hemangiomas: percutaneous transcatheter embolization with detachable silicone balloons. Radiology 156(1):85–88
3. Burke DR, Verstandig A, Edwards O, Meranze SG, McLean GK, Stein EJ (1986) Infantile hemangioendothelioma: angiographic features and factors determining efficacy of hepatic artery embolization. Cardiovasc Intervent Radiol 9(3):154–157
4. Stanley P, Geer GD, Miller JH, Gilsanz V, Landing BH, Boechat IM (1989) Infantile hepatic hemangiomas. Clinical features, radiologic investigations, and treatment of 20 patients. Cancer 64(4):936–949
5. Fellows KE, Hoffer FA, Markowitz RI, O'Neill JA Jr (1991) Multiple collaterals to hepatic infantile hemangioendotheliomas and arteriovenous malformations: effect on embolization. Radiology 181(3):813–818
6. McHugh K, Burrows PE (1992) Infantile hepatic hemangioendotheliomas: significance of portal venous and systemic collateral arterial supply. J Vasc Interv Radiol 3(2):337–344
7. Byard RW, Burrows PE, Izakawa T, Silver MM (1991) Diffuse infantile haemangiomatosis: clinicopathological features and management problems in five fatal cases. Eur J Pediatr 150(4):224–227
8. Kassarjian A, Dubois J, Burrows PE (2002) Angiographic classification of hepatic hemangiomas in infants. Radiology 222(3):693–698
9. Kassarjian A, Zurakowski D, Dubois J, Paltiel HJ, Fishman SJ, Burrows PE (2004) Infantile hepatic hemangiomas: clinical and imaging findings and their correlation with therapy. AJR Am J Roentgenol 182(3):785–795

10. Burrows PE, Dubois J, Kassarjian A (2001) Pediatric hepatic vascular anomalies. Pediatr Radiol 31(8): 533–545
11. Roebuck D, Sebire N, Lehmann E, Barnacle A (2012) Rapidly involuting congenital haemangioma (RICH) of the liver. Pediatr Radiol 42(3): 308–314
12. Stanley P, Gomperts E, Woolley MM (1986) Kasabach-Merritt syndrome treated by therapeutic embolization with polyvinyl alcohol. Am J Pediatr Hematol Oncol 8(4):308–311
13. Burrows PE, Lasjaunias PL, Ter Brugge KG, Flodmark O (1987) Urgent and emergent embolization of lesions of the head and neck in children: indications and results. Pediatrics 80(3):386–394
14. Enomoto Y, Yoshimura S, Egashira Y, Iwama T (2011) Transarterial embolization for cervical hemangioma associated with Kasabach-merritt syndrome. Neurol Med Chir 51(5):375–378
15. Lord DJ, Chennapragada SM (2011) Embolization in neonates and infants. Tech Vasc Interv Radiol 14(1):32–41

Treatment of Infantile Hemangiomas of the Head and Neck

16

Milton Waner and Teresa O

The location of a hemangioma is not random [1]. Both focal and segmental hemangiomas are found at sites of predilection. Their anatomical location and extent are thus predictable. When confronted with a patient with a hemangioma, the following decisions should be addressed:

Should we treat?

How should we treat?

When should we treat?

The decision *should* we treat is based on a number of simple variables:

1. Lesions that are clearly exposed warrant treatment (at least 60 % of hemangiomas are central facial lesions).
2. Lesions that are unlikely to involute completely and where treatment will result in a better outcome (50 % of lesions do not involute completely [2]; after the age of 4 years, further involution in any given hemangioma is unlikely).
3. Complications such as ulceration, functional impairment, cardiac failure, and disfigurement.

4. Airway hemangiomas and periocular/orbital hemangiomas.

The decision "*how* to treat" should be made by a multidisciplinary team. The tendency to use one modality for all lesions should be avoided. The following are important considerations:

1. The type of lesion (focal or segmental)
2. The depth of the lesion
3. The stage of the lesion (proliferating, quiescent, or involuting)

In general, propranolol has replaced corticosteroids as a first line of therapy [3]. All early lesions should be given a trial of propranolol (or timolol if superficial) unless there is a contraindication or some other objection to its use. It should be kept in mind that propranolol does cross the blood-brain barrier and that short-term memory loss is a known side effect in the elderly. For this reason, nadolol, which does not cross the blood-brain barrier and appears to be as effective, is advocated by some. Topical propranolol in one or other form has also become popular for very superficial lesions, and unfortunately, some have used it for deeper lesions [4]. Its efficacy for deeper lesions is in doubt, and the degree of absorption has not yet been determined. One should therefore be cautious when dosing a patient.

A very high percentage of patients respond to propranolol, but it appears that focal lesions do not respond as well. If treated very early, a lesion may shrink and "disappear" or simply stop

M. Waner, MB, BCh (Wits), FCS (SA), MD (✉)
Teresa O, MD, M.Arch
Department of Otolaryngology, Center for Vascular Birthmarks, Vascular Birthmark Institute, New York Head and Neck Institute, Lenox Hill Hospital and Manhattan Eye, Ear, and Throat Hospital,
New York, NY, USA
e-mail: Mwmd01@gmail.com; to@vbiny.org

growing. At present, the proportion and the type of lesion that falls into each of these groups have not yet been determined. Our euphoria with this drug is still prevalent. Realistically, the response to systemic propranolol may be one of the following:

1. The response may be excellent (almost complete or complete shrinkage of the lesion).
2. The lesion may only partially respond (50 % or less). This is more often seen with focal lesions.
3. The lesion may fail to respond. This is seen with some fully grown lesions.

In a small series, 50 % of patients treated with propranolol needed treatment with some other modality (laser or surgery) in order to achieve a satisfactory response. Our belief is that early treatment with propranolol is most beneficial. Lesions will either respond and shrink or simply stop growing. If the lesion being treated was small at the time of commencement, then either of these responses is acceptable. However, when faced with a large lesion, a failure to progress without appreciable shrinkage is not acceptable. In these cases, surgery should be considered. In addition to this, residual cutaneous involvement can and should be treated with a laser [5].

We therefore only surgically intervene when the lesion warrants treatment, has failed to respond, or inadequately responds to propranolol; in some focal ulcerated hemangiomas in whom surgery will ultimately be needed; and in lesions that are obstructing the airway or visual axis where resolution is urgent. Our surgical approach is determined by the depth of the lesion and its anatomical location. The following examples demonstrate our approach.

Paranasal Hemangiomas

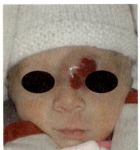 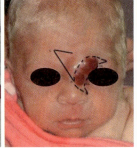 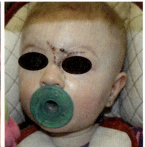 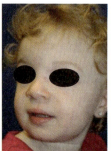

Fig. 16.1 A child with a compound (superficial and deep components) left glabellar/paranasal IH. During surgery an elliptical incision was used to remove the IH. A local rotation flap was used, and the standing cone was corrected 3 weeks later. The patient has undergone scar revision and multiple laser treatments. These procedures were done prior to the discovery of propranolol. Since we do see partial or nonresponders to propranolol, the technique of treatment described above is still relevant

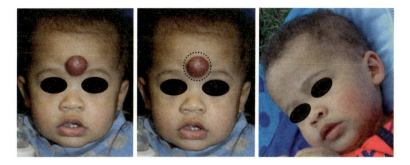

Fig. 16.2 A child with a midline forehead hemangioma. This was a pedunculated lesion, and after much discussion, the parents elected to proceed with surgery. The lesion was resected through a vertical midline ellipse (the *dotted line* represents the incision lines). Since this was a pedunculated lesion, there was sufficient skin left to prevent significant medial movement of the brows

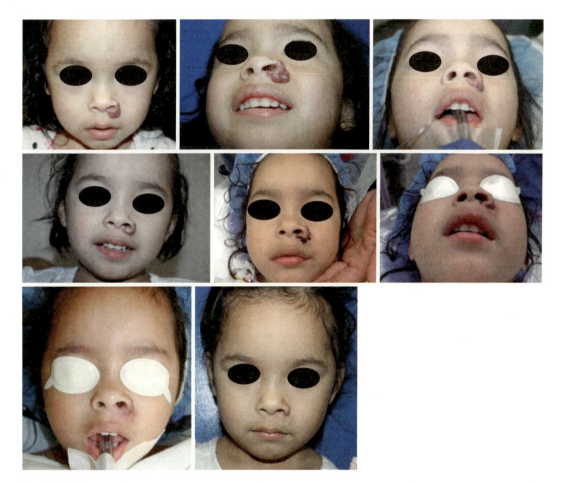

Fig. 16.3 This child is a twin who presented with a hemangioma that involved her left nostril, upper lip, and nasolabial area. The area around the nostril was resected initially. This was followed with laser treatment and a perialar flap which was used to reconstruct her nasal sill. The standing cone that resulted from this was corrected 3 weeks later. This is a difficult area to correct and should be approached in a staged manner

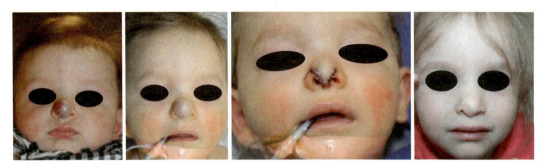

Fig. 16.4 An infant with a focal nasal tip hemangioma. This was treated with propranolol and pulsed dye laser until 10 months of age. The patient then underwent surgical resection to correct the Cyrano nasal deformity. In these cases, the hemangioma originates in the midline, between the lower lateral nasal cartilages. As it proliferates, it displaces the cartilages laterally and rotates them outward. A modified subunit approach [6] allows resection of redundant skin and approximation of the lower lateral cartilages. Even if the hemangioma was left untreated and allowed to involute spontaneously, the distortion of the lower lateral cartilages will leave a permanent nasal tip deformity

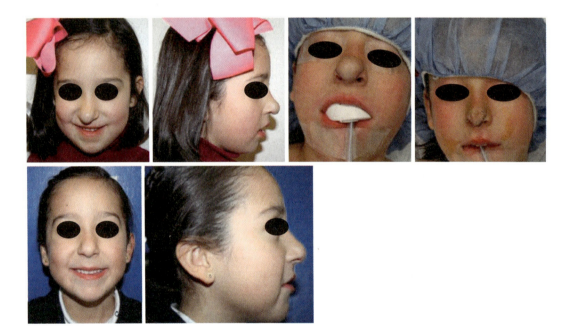

Fig. 16.5 A child in whom spontaneous involution resulted in residual fibrofatty tissue and a Cyrano nasal deformity. A modified subunit approach allowed resection of redundant skin and correction of the position of the lower lateral cartilages. The patient is seen several years postoperatively. Normal nasal development has occurred

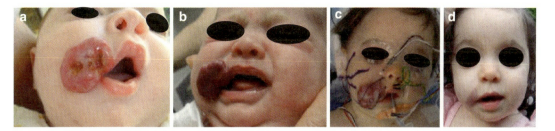

Fig. 16.6 An infant with an ulcerated nasolabial hemangioma (**a**). The child was treated with corticosteroids to treat the ulceration (pre-propranolol era) (**b**). The hemangioma was then excised using an ellipse (**c**). Excision of all of the involved skin would have everted the lateral third of the upper lip. A small ellipse of IH skin was left, but the underlying hemangioma was excised. Facial nerve monitoring was used [7], and all the nerve branches as well as the muscle were preserved. The wound was closed, and several laser treatments including pulsed dye and fractional CO_2 were used in the final stages (**d**)

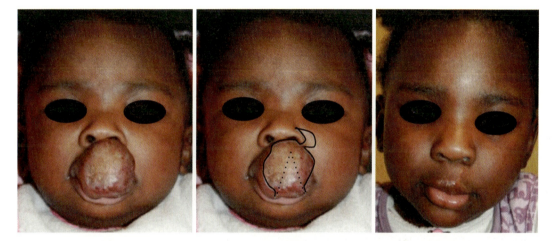

Fig. 16.7 An infant with an upper lip hemangioma. This child had not been previously treated. Surgical excision was undertaken to correct the horizontal and vertical lengthening of the upper lip [8]. A horizontal wedge resection was used to correct the horizontal dimension (the *dotted line* represents the mucosal incisions). Once this was corrected, a second stage was undertaken to develop a vermillion with a cupid's bow. Unfortunately, the patient's scar was not optimal. Concerning lesions of the upper lip, the lip is usually too long in the vertical or the horizontal dimension. The above case demonstrates a lip too long in the horizontal dimension. A lesion that causes lengthening of the vertical dimension is corrected through an incision along the vermilliocutaneous junction. The appropriate height of tissue is removed, and the junction is then reconstituted

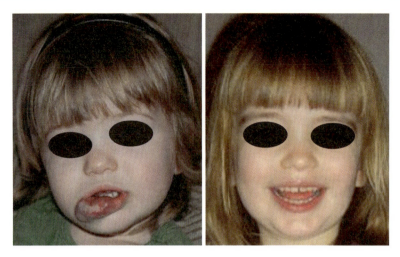

Fig. 16.8 A hemangioma of the lower lip is usually corrected through a wedge resection. In the above case, about 40 % of the lower lip was removed. As the hemangioma proliferates, it almost always stretches the lower lip making removal of a significant length of lower lip without producing a microstomia. The surgeon should use his/her judgment in these cases, but we have removed up to 50 % of the lower lip without causing microstomia

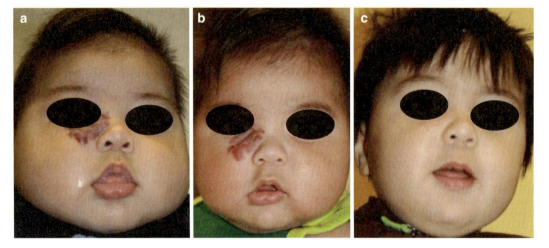

Fig. 16.9 An infant with a right paranasal hemangioma (**a**). The child was treated with propranolol for several months. The lesion shrunk but not completely (**b**). A pulsed dye laser and fractional CO_2 laser completed the treatment (**c**)

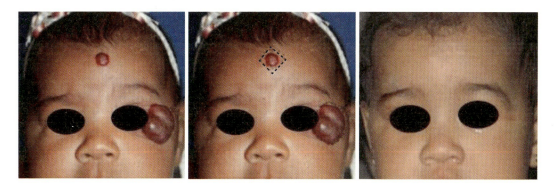

Fig. 16.10 An infant with a lesion involving her left lower eyelid and her forehead. The lower eyelid lesion was pedunculated, and this allowed excision using an ellipse with the long axis following the subciliary line and extending past the lateral canthus to the brow. There was enough skin to allow primary closure without an ectropion (the *dotted line* represents the incision lines). The forehead lesion was excised using an ellipse with its long axis, parallel to the relaxed tension lines of the brow. The most common complication following a lower eyelid excision is an ectropion. This results from insufficient skin for primary closure. In most cases, preoperative planning can prevent this. The child is seen here several months post excision

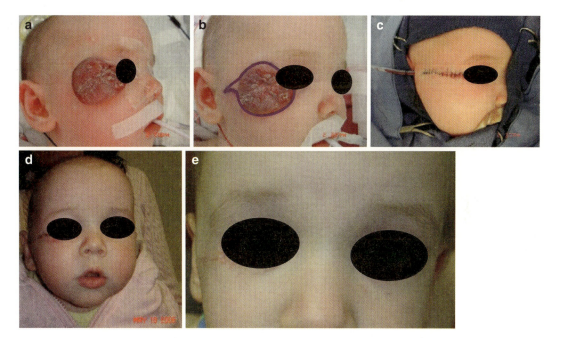

Fig. 16.11 An infant with a right lower eyelid and periorbital ulcerated hemangioma (**a**). The lesion was excised using an ellipse (**b**). Due to the extent of the lesion, primary closure was a challenge. The child is seen immediately post surgery (**c**) and a week later (**d**). Since there was insufficient skin, the child was left with an ectropion which persisted (**e**) 1 year later. This can be repaired with a small skin graft

References

1. Waner M, North PE, Scherer KA, Frieden IJ, Waner A, Mihm MC Jr (2003) The nonrandom distribution of facial hemangiomas. Arch Dermatol 139(7):869–875. Epub 2003/07/23
2. Buckmiller LM, Munson PD, Dyamenahalli U, Dai Y, Richter GT (2010) Propranolol for infantile hemangiomas: early experience at a tertiary vascular anomalies center. Laryngoscope 120(4):676–681. Epub 2010/01/30
3. Leaute-Labreze C, DumasdelaRoque E, Hubiche T, Boralevi F, Thambo JB, Taieb A (2008) Propranolol for severe hemangiomas of infancy. N Engl J Med 358(24):2649–2651. Epub 2008/06/14
4. McMahon P, Oza V, Frieden IJ (2012) Topical timolol for infantile hemangiomas: putting a note of caution in "cautiously optimistic". Pediatr Dermatol 29(1): 127–130. Epub 2012/01/20
5. Sherwood KA, Tan OT (1990) Treatment of a capillary hemangioma with the flashlamp pumped-dye laser. J Am Acad Dermatol 22(1):136–137. Epub 1990/01/01
6. Waner M, Kastenbaum J, Scherer K (2008) Hemangiomas of the nose: surgical management using a modified subunit approach. Arch Facial Plast Surg 10(5):329–334. Epub 2008/09/17
7. Ulkatan S, Waner M, Arranz-Arranz B, Weiss I, O TM, Saral M et al (2014) New methodology for facial nerve monitoring in extracranial surgeries of vascular malformations. Clin Neurophysiol 125(4):849–855. Epub 2013/10/22
8. O TM, Scheuermann-Poley C, Tan M, Waner M (2013) Distribution, clinical characteristics, and surgical treatment of lip infantile hemangiomas. JAMA Facial Plast Surg 15(4):292–304. Epub 2013/06/12

Treatment of Visceral Hemangiomas

Juan Carlos Lopez Gutierrez

IHs rarely involve thoracic or abdominal viscera. Visceral IH can be focal or segmental, localized or diffuse, immunostaining positively against GLUT-1 marker at all phases. Their clinical course depends on factors such as size, location, and proliferation rate. Ulceration and bleeding occur mainly at intestinal location. Occasionally they can develop in association with cutaneous hemangiomas.

Thoracic Hemangiomas

1. *Mediastinum*: Vascular anomalies, including hemangiomas and vascular malformations, comprise 3–6 % of mediastinal masses in childhood. Correct diagnosis almost always can be established by history, radiographic studies, and bronchoscopy if necessary. Compression of airway and great vessels by a large hemangioma is not frequent, but preventive treatment with propranolol is recommended if aggressive proliferation is noticed in an asymptomatic patient [1].
2. *Lung*: Pulmonary hemangiomas are rare. They may involve the airway or the parenchyma and may be localized or multifocal. If asymptomatic, pharmacological or surgical treatment is not indicated.
3. *Pleura*: Hemangiomatosis involving the pleura is a rare cause of bloody pleural effusion in the neonate.
4. *Heart*: Vascular tumors of the heart are also rare in children, of which congenital hemangiomas and infantile hemangiomas represent the most frequent subgroups.

It is important that the physician understand the difference between these two groups to better provide appropriate prognostic and therapeutic advice to the parents of children with these anomalies as beta-blockers will not improve the newborn with a congenital hemangioma clinical course.

The presence of hemangiomas in heart valves is an exceptional finding. Transesophageal echocardiography is used to establish a diagnosis of cardiac tumor, though careful interpretation is needed to avoid diagnostic errors such as of a prolapsing left atrial myxoma.

Abdominal Hemangiomas

1. *Stomach*: As in the esophagus, a wide variety of gastric vascular anomalies are incorrectly referred to as "hemangiomas" in the medical literature. Significant differences must be taken into consideration before deciding any surgical approach on hemangiomas and venous malformations of the stomach. Although

J.C. Lopez Gutierrez, MD, PhD
Department of Pediatric Surgery,
Vascular Anomalies Center,
La Paz Children's Hospital, Madrid, Spain
e-mail: queminfantil.hulp@salud.madrid.org

R. Mattassi et al. (eds.), *Hemangiomas and Vascular Malformations: An Atlas of Diagnosis and Treatment*, 145
DOI 10.1007/978-88-470-5673-2_17, © Springer-Verlag Italia 2009, 2015

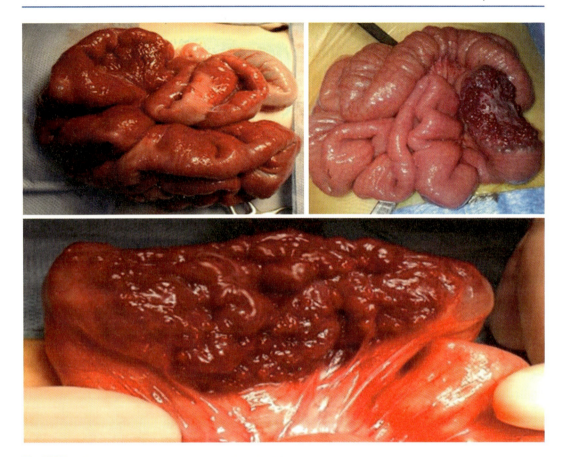

Fig. 17.1 Different macroscopic appearance of intestinal hemangiomas

bleeding is the most common symptom of both gastric hemangiomas and venous malformations, treatment differs. Pharmacological angiogenesis inhibition with propranolol is the mainstay of hemangioma therapy.

2. *Intestine*: Hemangiomas of the small bowel are rare tumors (Fig. 17.1). Once again a proper application of nomenclature is crucial to prevent the institution of improper therapies. Hemangiomas have a pathognomonic appearance on endoscopy. In case of doubt, Glut-1 immunohistochemistry on a biopsy specimen will be of help for a correct diagnosis. Capsule endoscopy can be performed safely in pediatric patients after ingestion or endoscopic placement of the capsule to diagnose bleeding vascular tumors after negative results of gastroscopy and colonoscopy.

Although intussusception caused by a hemangioma of the small bowel is a rare

condition (commonly founded in blue rubber bleb nevus syndrome), it should be taken into consideration in the differential diagnosis of abdominal pain of doubtful origin.

Only 1 % of patients with minor rectal bleeding examined by sigmoidoscopy have hemangiomas.

Hemangiomas of the greater or lesser omentum are not exceptional and very often asymptomatic in the context of diffuse neonatal hemangiomatosis.

Unfortunately many patients still undergo emergency laparotomies and intestinal resections in the context of gastrointestinal bleeding without having the option of systemic propranolol therapy.

3. *Liver*: Hemangiomas are the most common benign liver tumors in children. They can be difficult to diagnose and complex to treat. Differential diagnosis must be accurate in any

patient with atypical presentation of liver hemangioma [2]. An important differentiating factor in the evaluation of pediatric hepatic masses is the age of the patient. Hepatoblastomas, mesenchymal hamartomas, and metastatic disease from Wilms tumor or neuroblastoma are usually seen in the first 3 years of life, whereas hepatocellular carcinoma, focal nodular hyperplasia, hepatic adenoma, and metastases from lymphoma are more common in older children.

Several current studies attempt to determine how common liver hemangiomas are in children with infantile hemangiomas by comparing liver ultrasound results in patients with one to four cutaneous hemangiomas, five or more cutaneous hemangiomas, or at least one large hemangioma versus ultrasound results in children without hemangiomas identifying at the same time specific risk factors in patients who have liver hemangiomas.

Vascular anomaly specialists must be able to distinguish hemangiomas from various vascular malformations as well as appreciate their dynamic course with time. Several attempts made to classify pediatric liver vascular tumors led to an unhelpful plethora of confusing terminology. Immunohistochemistry has been used in the study of hemangiomas and supports a new classification of these tumors based on the expression of GLUT-1 as a substitution of the old and confusing term of hepatic infantile hemangioendothelioma:

1. GLUT-1-positive expression is usually demonstrated in multifocal and diffuse hepatic infantile hemangioma, which shares clinical and morphological features with cutaneous infantile hemangioma (Fig. 17.2). Diffuse neonatal hemangiomatosis is a frequently fatal disorder characterized by multiple cutaneous and visceral hemangiomas. Complications include high-output cardiac failure, hemorrhage, hepatic failure, and consumption coagulopathy. The diagnosis of consumptive hypothyroidism as a result of increased type 3 iodothyronine deiodinase activity in the hemangiomas has to be done in every patient with multifocal or diffuse lesions. Myocardial depression secondary to hypothyroidism in children with hepatic hemangioma has been reported. Coincident with the involution of the hemangiomas, the child's hypothyroidism improves.

2. GLUT-1-negative vascular liver tumors occur in neonates with unique clinical, imaging, and pathological features. They differ from diffuse hemangioma in terms of earlier presentation as solitary masses with central necrosis, rapid involution, and pathologic features showing a notable, often prolific, lymphatic compliment immunoreacting positively with the monoclonal antibody D2-40.

Following the parallelism with cutaneous anomalies, the term hepatic congenital hemangioma has been suggested comparing their behavior with rapid involuting congenital hemangiomas (RICH) described in skin and subcutaneous locations (Fig. 17.3).

To sum up, hepatic hemangiomas represent three different categories of lesions: focal, multifocal, and diffuse [3].

The natural history for focal hemangiomas is spontaneous regression in the first year of life; however, shunt embolization or complete surgical excision is required in case of cardiac failure.

In the last 30 years, a significant number of children underwent orthotopic liver transplantation (OLT) or died in the context of cardiac failure due to diffuse infantile hepatic hemangiomas (IHH). Over this period of time, steroids, vincristine, or interferon has represented the standard therapy without uniform successful response.

Reported experience in IHH management found that diffuse hemangiomas (Glut-1 positive) had a higher mortality rate than solitary ones (Glut-1 negative) [4].

Propranolol was first used at our institution for the treatment of IHH in 2008 with nine consecutive patients, showing remarkable response to the therapy in the following years. Since then, no patient with IHH underwent OLT or died. This experience has been supported by data from other centers' experience, ratifying that a new era in the management of IHH has been opened with the use of beta-blockers in the management of this potentially fatal disease [5–8].

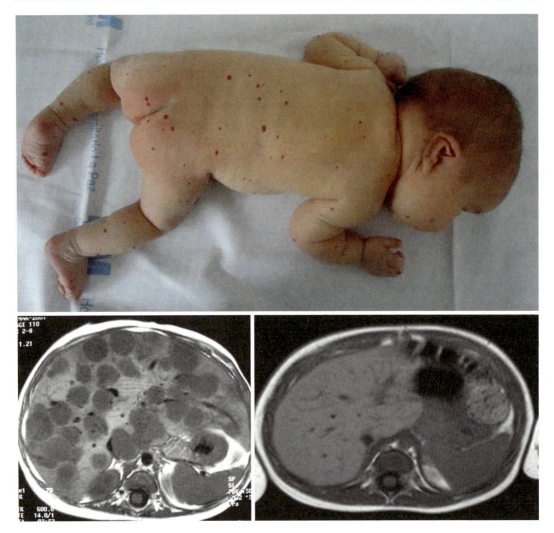

Fig. 17.2 Neonatal hemangiomatosis with multifocal liver hemangioma. Response to a 6-month course of propranolol

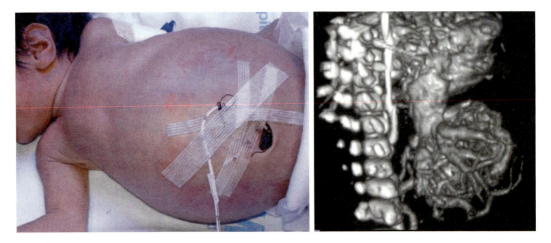

Fig. 17.3 Hepatic congenital hemangioma (RICH). Angioarchitecture on CT

In Spain, the National Transplant Organization reported no candidates for liver transplantation with IHH in the last 5 years.

In Japan, among 19 symptomatic children needing treatment for IHH (National Center for Child Health published data), 4 died after receiving steroids, vincristine, or interferon. No deaths were reported in patients being treated with propranolol [9].

In the last 5 years, propranolol has dramatically changed the scope of the newborn with IHH. Prognosis is currently considered as favorable, and those previously considered as unfortunate patients are not anymore candidates for OLT.

In patients with severe acquired hypothyroidism resulting from both increased activity of type 3 iodothyronine deiodinase and increased production of TSH-like hormone from hepatic hemangiomas, L-thyroxin replacement should be considered till the age of 3 years. Propranolol treatment for this condition has been recently reported [10].

4. *Spleen*: Hemangiomas involving the spleen are rare and seldom symptomatic; they are not to be misdiagnosed with littoral cell angioma (LCA), a different benign vascular tumor of the spleen which most commonly presents in adults as an enlarged spleen containing multiple nodules with constitutional symptoms (low-grade fever and fatigue) and signs of hypersplenism (anemia and thrombocytopenia). Hemangiomatosis of the spleen and omentum is also a finding in patients with diffuse neonatal hemangiomatosis. Response to propranolol is uniformly good, avoiding the need for splenectomy.

5. *Pancreas*: The pancreas is an unusual site for a hemangioma in an infant. Hemangioma should be considered in a younger than 6-month-old patients presenting with a history of jaundice, pale stools, and dark urine. Abdominal ultrasound scan and magnetic resonance imaging will show an enhancing mass in the pancreas. Propranolol is the first-line treatment. If there is no response to beta-blocker, biliary diversion with a Roux-en-y hepaticojejunostomy is the procedure of choice in case of obstructive jaundice.

In summary current approach to visceral IH treatment is pharmacological without consideration to their location. Response to beta-blocker treatment is similar and uniformly good in cutaneous and visceral IH with a less than 1 % reported failure rate.

In fact the rapid response of IH to propranolol can be helpful in the management of radiologically undiagnosed vascularized tumors located in difficult anatomic areas where a biopsy can entail significant morbidity. Since IH is the most frequent tumor with increased blood supply in this age group and it responds dramatically to propranolol, an oral beta-blocker test can be useful in order to reduce the need for biopsies, when ultrasound and MRI cannot ascertain the diagnosis of hemangioma or sarcoma among others. Propranolol is administrated at 3 mg/kg/day for 3 weeks. The criteria for positive response are reduction of volume and blood flow, measured by weekly ultrasound examination. Sarcomas, mesenchymal hamartomas, or metastatic diseases do not respond to propranolol and continue to progress, while IH always shows decreased perfusion and size avoiding the need for biopsies in difficult areas as the liver, heart, and orbit.

References

1. Tsang FH, Lun KS, Cheng LC (2011) Hemangioma of the diaphragm presenting with cardiac tamponade. J Card Surg 26(6):620–623
2. Maruani A, Piram M, Sirinelli D, Herbreteau D, Saliba E, Machet MC, Lorette G (2012) Visceral and mucosal involvement in neonatal haemangiomatosis. J Eur Acad Dermatol Venereol 26(10):1285–1290
3. Kulungowski AM, Alomari AI, Chawla A, Christison-Lagay ER, Fishman SJ (2012) Lessons from a liver hemangioma registry: subtype classification. J Pediatr Surg 47(1):165–170
4. Hernandez F, Navarro M, Encinas JL, Lopez Gutierrez JC (2005) The role of GLUT1 immunostaining in the diagnosis and classification of liver vascular tumors in children. J Pediatr Surg 40(5):801–804
5. Kochin IN, Miloh TA, Arnon R, Iyer KR, Suchy FJ, Kerkar N (2011) Benign liver masses and lesions in children: 53 cases over 12 years. Isr Med Assoc J 13(9):542–547
6. Avagyan S, Klein M, Kerkar N, Demattia A, Blei F, Lee S, Rosenberg HK, Arnon R (2013) Propranolol as a first-line treatment for diffuse infantile hepatic

hemangioendothelioma. J Pediatr Gastroenterol Nutr 56(3):17–20

7. Vanlander A, Decaluwe W, Vandelanotte M, Van Geet C, Cornette L (2010) Propranolol as a novel treatment for congenital visceral haemangioma. Neonatology 98(3):229–231

8. Mhanna A, Franklin WH, Mancini AJ (2011) Hepatic infantile hemangiomas treated with oral propranolol–a case series. Pediatr Dermatol 28(1): 39–45

9. Kuroda T, Kumagai M, Nosaka S, Nakazawa A, Takimoto T, Hoshino K (2011) Critical infantile hepatic hemangioma: results of a nationwide survey by the Japanese Infantile Hepatic Hemangioma Study Group. J Pediatr Surg 46(12):2239–2243

10. Vergine G, Marsciani A, Pedini A, Brocchi S, Marsciani M, Desiderio E, Bertelli S, Vecchi V (2012) Efficacy of propranolol treatment in thyroid dysfunction associated with severe infantile hepatic hemangioma. Horm Res Paediatr 78(4):256–260

Treatment of Genital Infantile Hemangiomas

Rainer Grantzow

Diagnosis

Hemangiomas in the *anogenital region* are rare and comprise about 1 % of all hemangiomas. They are seen at the perineum, the labia, and the scrotum (Figs. 18.1 and 18.2). Due to their localization, there are no optical or aesthetical problems as found with facial localization. Anogenital hemangiomas show the same development as other hemangiomas including the well-known phases of proliferation and regression. They can be classified into intracutaneous, subcutaneous, and combined types.

The diagnosis is visual except in the case of the subcutaneous type. In these cases, duplex *sonography* must be carried out to verify the diagnosis and thereby exclude other soft tissue tumors, in particular malignant tumors such as rhabdomyosarcomas.

Sometimes, it can be difficult to distinguish a hemangioma from a nevus flammeus or another form of vascular malformation. Occasionally, the appearance of labial venous malformations can imitate subcutaneous hemangioma, but duplex sonography will usually lead to the correct diagnosis. Magnetic resonance imaging (MRI) investigations are not necessary to evaluate anogenital hemangiomas; however,

MRI is mandatory to detect further pelvic venous malformation.

Perineal hemangiomas can be associated with defects such as anorectal, neurologic, renal or urinary tract, and genital malformations. Acronyms like SACRAL syndrome [1] or PELVIS syndrome [2] are proposed in such rare cases.

Complications

The major problem of perineal hemangiomas is their tendency to ulcerate. Normally, *ulceration* occurs in the phase of strong proliferation and is seen only in the first 4–5 months of life; ulceration is uncommon after this stage. Reasons for this complication are numerous. Despite the

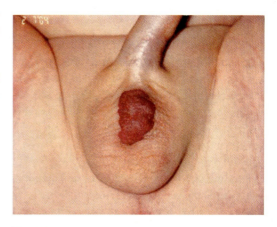

Fig. 18.1 Flat scrotal hemangioma

R. Grantzow
Department of Pediatric Surgery,
Ludwig-Maximilians-Universität, Munich, Germany
e-mail: rainer.grantzow@med.uni-muenchen.de

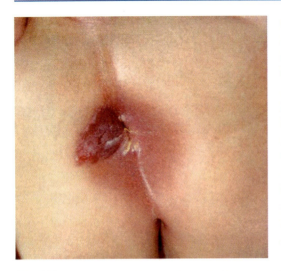

Fig. 18.2 Perianal hemangioma with a small ulceration

hyperperfusion of a hemangioma, the skin can be underperfused due to micro AV fistulas in the center of the hemangioma that have a steal effect at the surface and can lead to skin necrosis. Secondly, the moisture under a nappy can macerate and damage the skin and reduce its function as a barrier against bacterial invasion. These two mechanisms in combination result in ulceration with secondary bacterial infection. Unfortunately, these ulcerations require a long time to heal because of the negative influence of stool and urine. Furthermore, they are very painful and present a challenge in wound management.

Prevention and Therapy

The avoidance of ulceration should be a main aim, and the target of all interventions is to minimize extrinsic factors such as moisture and extended contact with urine and stool. In this situation, it is very important to advise the parents of the necessity to change nappies frequently. Additionally, the hemangioma should be covered with a barrier cream like zinc oxide paste.

In principle, the possibilities of hemangioma treatment in the anogenital region are the same as in other regions. According to size, volume, and shape of the lesion dye, Nd-YAG laser or surgical interventions can be performed. In contrast to

facial hemangiomas, aesthetical problems are irrelevant and therefore indications to active treatment are rare. Furthermore, the main problem in the therapy of perianal and genital hemangiomas is that such therapy can initiate ulceration (Fig. 18.3a) and result in deterioration [3]. In particular, swelling and thermic damage of the skin after *laser therapy* (dye and Nd-YAG laser) can trigger ulceration of the vulnerable skin, the avoidance of which is the main aim of all therapy. In addition, deeper parts of the hemangioma can grow despite dye laser treatment, because the depth of dye laser effect is only 0.8 mm [4]. This dilemma should be considered seriously before any laser application. Due to these complications, the traditional procedure of "wait and see" has many advantages for hemangiomas at this localization. The relative merits of the dye laser versus "wait-and-see" approach are discussed in the only existing randomized and controlled study [5].

Since 2008 with the introduction of the *ß-blocker propranolol* as a possibility to treat hemangiomas [6], a new tool is available, also for anogenital hemangiomas. The above described negative influence of a laser application on the skin surface does not exist in the therapy with ß-blockers, so that only systemic side effects have to be considered. Due to these advantages, it is not astonishing that within short time, the propranolol therapy became a standard despite its "off-label use" in the moment.

In case of ulceration, different aspects of therapy have to be noted. A crucial point is the dressing of the wound, which should protect against stool and urine, accelerating wound healing and making the painless change of wound dressings possible. *Hydrocolloids* are standard, if localization enables their application (Fig. 18.3b, c). Changing of the dressing should be painless and is necessary only twice weekly. If this is not possible (beneath the anus or female genitalia), Vaseline-impregnated gauze can be used but must be changed more frequently than hydrocolloids. Small defects can be treated with barrier creams like *zinc oxide* paste. Additionally, topical antibiotics can be applied, but the effects of such a treatment are uncertain. However, gentle

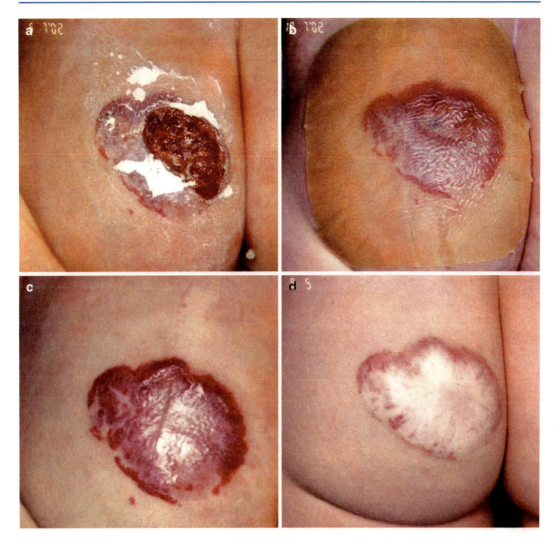

Fig. 18.3 (**a**) Ulcerated gluteal hemangioma after cryotherapy (wrong indication). (**b**) Twelve days later with hydrocolloid dressing and reduction of the wound size. (**c**) Closed wound after 6 weeks wound management with hydrocolloid dressing. (**d**) Residuals 2 years later with typical flat scar and hypopigmented skin

cleaning of the wound (shower, bath) or application of painless antiseptic liquids (Octenisept®) is the basic treatment in secondary *wound healing*. Systemic therapy with antibiotics can be necessary, if signs of infection like fever or leukocytosis are present. Impairment of wound healing after dye laser application in ulcerated hemangiomas has been reported [7, 8], but there are no controlled and randomized studies about the effect of dye laser treatment on wound healing. Unfortunately, the report of David et al. [7] concerns only 4.4 % of cases treated ($n=7$) with

an anogenital localization, while that of Kim et al. [8] concerns 14 of 22 cases.

Systemic *steroid therapy* is a further option to treat hemangiomas, but its serious side effects have to be weighed in view of the low efficacy of this kind of treatment. Furthermore, the immunosuppressive effect of steroids may have a negative influence in cases of infected ulcers. Furthermore, steroids can inhibit wound healing and prolong the time to wound healing. In summary, the cortisone therapy of hemangiomas cannot be recommended.

The last option in the treatment of anogenital hemangiomas is the *surgical excision*. This procedure is possible for small hemangiomas only, if primary closure of the wound is possible. However, these hemangiomas are usually harmless and do not need any therapy.

After healing and remission of ulcerated hemangiomas, a flat *scar* with typical *hypopigmentation* will appear (Fig. 18.3d). This scar is robust without danger of further ulceration.

References

1. Stockman A, Boralevi F, Taieb A, Léauté-Labrèze C (2007) SACRAL syndrome: spinal dysraphism, anogenital, cutaneous, renal and urologic anomalies, associated with an angioma of lumbosacral localisation. Dermatology 214:40–45

2. Girard C, Bigorre M, Guillot B, Bessis D (2006) PELVIS syndrome. Arch Dermatol 142:884–888

3. Witman PM, Wagner AM, Scherer K, Waner M (2006) Complications following pulsed dye laser treatment of superficial hemangiomas. Lasers Surg Med 38:116–123

4. Poetke M, Philipp C, Berlien HP (2000) Flashlamp pulsed dye laser for hemangiomas in infancy. Arch Dermatol 136:628–632

5. Batta K, Goodyear HM, Moss C, Williams HC, Hiller L, Waters R (2002) Randomised controlled study of early pulsed dye laser treatment of uncomplicated childhood haemangiomas: results of 1-year analysis. Lancet 360:521–527

6. Léauté-Labrèze C, Dumas de la Roque E, Hubiche T, Boralevi F et al (2008) Propranolol for severe hemangiomas of infancy. N Engl J Med 358:2649–2651

7. David LR, Malek MM, Argenta LC (2003) Efficacy of pulse dye laser therapy for the treatment of ulcerated hemangiomas: a review of 78 patients. Br J Plast Surg 56:317–327

8. Kim HJ, Colombo M, Friede IJ (2001) Ulcerated hemangiomas: clinical characteristics and response to therapy. J Am Acad Dermatol 44:962–972

Management of Syndromes Related to Infantile Hemangiomas

19

Carlo Mario Gelmetti, Riccardo Cavalli,
and Marco Rovaris

Introduction

While it is commonly accepted that infantile hemangiomas (IHs) are usually located, more or less superficially, into the skin, they have been described also elsewhere. Sites of extracutaneous hemangiomas include the following: the central nervous system, larynx, thymus, mediastine, lung, adrenal glands, liver, gallbladder, gastrointestinal tract, pancreas, spleen, lymph nodes, and urinary bladder. However, it should be noted that, in many cases, the diagnosis of extracutaneous hemangiomas is only hypothetic as well as their position in the present classification of vascular anomalies. While localized IHs are often benign, except when they are located near a noble structure such as the airways or the orbital area, segmental IHs may be associated with birth defects. These cases should be very carefully studied for life-threatening conditions (heart failure, respiratory distress), functional risks (amblyopia, swallowing disorders, digestive and renal alterations, etc.), aesthetic risks (especially IHs of the face), and painful ulcerations.

In the twentieth century, clinical and laboratory studies enable to separate vascular anomalies into two categories: vascular malformations and vascular tumors. The so-called Mulliken's classification [1] was substantially adopted by the International Society for the Study of Vascular Anomalies (ISSVA) in 1996 and is still in use and accepted by the experts in this field. Unexpectedly this classification was upset in the same year, when Frieden at al. published the first paper dealing with PHACE syndrome [2]. PHACE[1] is an acronym indicating a disorder characterized by the association of posterior fossa malformations, hemangiomas, arterial anomalies, coarctation of the aorta and other cardiac defects, and eye abnormalities [3]. Indeed the association of vascular and nonvascular intracranial malformations with IHs was published in 1978 [4] by a Spanish neuroradiologist, Pascual-Castroviejo, but his paper was overlooked by the vast majority of clinicians.

C.M. Gelmetti (✉) • M. Rovaris
Department of Pathophysiology and Transplantation (CMG), University of Milan, Milan, Italy

Clinica Dermatologica – IRCCS Fondazione Ca' Granda "Ospedale Maggiore Policlinico" di Milano (RC), Milan, Italy
e-mail: carlo.gelmetti@unimi.it

R. Cavalli
Foundation Ca' Granda "Ospedale Maggiore Policlinico", Via Pace 9, 20122 Milano, Italy

[1] Of note: Some authors call this entity PHACES syndrome (OMIM 606519), adding a final S for sternal clefting or supraumbilical raphe (i.e., midline raphe or ventral wall defects).

That's why this disease, at present, is also known as Pascual-Castroviejo type II syndrome [5][2].

Indeed the ISSVA's classification separates clearly vascular tumors (the group that includes IHs) from vascular malformations indicating, at the same time, that errors in angiogenesis or vasculogenesis that occur in embryonic phase may lead to stable lesions (i.e., vascular malformations) but, quite obviously, not to proliferative lesions (i.e., IHs). From this starting point, it was conceptually clear that vascular tumors and vascular malformations could not be present in the same individual, unless by chance[3]. However, despite the fact that the etiopathogenesis of both vascular tumors and vascular malformations is still unknown, the description of many cases of PHACE syndrome (and, in parallel, the description of LUMBAR/PELVIS/SACRAL syndrome[4] in other patients) makes likely that a pathogenic *noxa* can provoke either vascular tumors and vascular malformations in the same individual.

Generally, in the past, an infant with cutaneous vascular malformations was logically screened for other extracutaneous vascular/nonvascular malformations, while an infant with cutaneous hemangiomas was just investigated according to the localization of the lesion (with the exception of diffuse neonatal hemangiomatosis in which visceral hemangiomas, typically hepatic hemangiomas, are found contemporaneously). This attitude, after the observation of PHACE and LUMBAR/PELVIS/SACRAL

syndromes, is no more valid. Indeed, these syndromes seem to represent a transition between vascular tumors and vascular malformations [6]. By consequence, all large, plaque-like or segmental IH occurring in the head or in the pelvis should be evaluated in a multidisciplinary context in which all medical specialties are involved, depending on the site of the lesions and individual symptoms. Correlation to the anatomic location of the IH is not mandatory (hemangioma distribution does not predict the presence of cardiovascular anomalies overall) [7], but it appears to be helpful in determining which abnormalities might be present. The possible coexistence of hidden vascular tumors or malformations should also change the attitude towards a treatment. In the past, the knowledge that IH has a spontaneous regression led many doctors, namely, pediatricians, to advise a "wait and see" philosophy. Today, the sentence "Leave it alone-it will go away" is no longer an acceptable advice for IH. In contrast, especially when associated malformations are suspected, the treatment should be given as soon as possible to avoid *sequelae* [8]. The therapy, when possible, will be started after the clinical and instrumental evaluation of the patient is concluded. Due to the complexity of all those cases, the need of a case manager is particularly felt.

PHACE Syndrome

PHACE syndrome (Figs. 19.1, 19.2, and 19.3) is the association of a large IH usually on the face or neck, in combination with one or more other abnormalities (see Table 19.1 for a complete list). The fact that PHACE affects girls nine times more often than boys makes this syndrome even more enigmatic. Regardless of theoretical speculations, it is recommended that any infant with a large facial IH be evaluated by a physician who is familiar with vascular anomalies. If PHACE syndrome is suspected, special radiology tests including an MRI or MRA (magnetic resonance angiography) of the head, neck, and chest and an echocardiogram are needed. If the tests are abnormal, the patient should be

---

[2] Pascual-Castroviejo type I syndrome has nothing to do within the field of vascular anomalies and it is characterized by cerebrofaciothoracic dysplasia associated with corpus callosum hypogenesis.

[3] For example, in this case, two distinct *noxae*, pathogenetically different, affecting the vasculogenesis would have been active in different times: the first in the embryonic period (the cause of vascular malformation) and the second in the postnatal period (the cause of IH).

[4] For the spelling of the acronyms, see PELVIS (perineal hemangioma, external genitalia malformations, lipomyelomeningocele, vesicorenal abnormalities, imperforate anus, and skin tag); SACRAL (spinal dysraphism, anogenital, cutaneous, renal, and urologic anomalies, associated with an angioma of lumbosacral localization); and LUMBAR (lower body hemangioma/lipoma or other cutaneous anomalies, urogenital anomalies, myelopathy, bony deformities, anorectal/arterial anomalies, and renal anomalies).

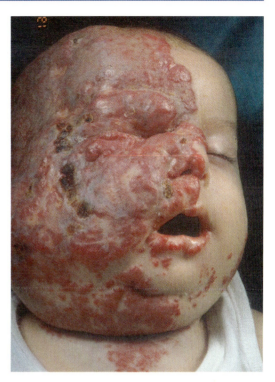

Fig 19.1 PHACE syndrome in a young girl. A large, plaque-like hemangioma is affecting the central part of the face and it was particularly aggressive on the nose. Unfortunately this patient had also lissencephaly that caused major neurodevelopmental problems

Fig 19.3 This case summarizes some of the possible findings in PHACE syndrome: a large plaque-like hemangioma involves the right half of the face (closing the *visus* of the right eye) and, bilaterally, the "beard" area (with a possible involvement of the airways)

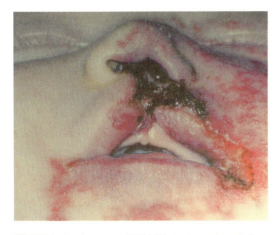

Fig 19.2 Another case of PHACE syndrome in an infant. This picture illustrates dramatically the involvement of the nose and the upper lip with significant loss of tissue in both. These complications will require a future reconstructive approach

referred to a tertiary-level hospital and seen by a multidisciplinary vascular anomaly team. The physicians who may be needed to study and treat these infants are ideally all pediatric specialists; however, dermatologists, hematologists/oncologists, ophthalmologists, radiologists, neurologists and neuroradiologists, geneticists, cardiologists, and otolaryngologists should be consulted. Given the fact that airway hemangiomas (Fig. 19.3) can be rapidly fatal, otolaryngologists should be involved first. Soon after, neurologists and neuroradiologists together with ophthalmologists, radiologists, cardiologists, and cardiothoracic surgeons should be called. When the patient is out of danger, hematologists/oncologists and geneticists can be helpful. However, it should not be forgotten that patients with PHACE syndrome may be at risk for other neurological problems even after the IH has gotten better. These problems may include migraine, headaches, seizures, developmental delays, speech delays, and, very rarely, ischemic strokes. These symptoms may be the result of structural defects or cerebrovascular events from the arterial defects; thus a strict

Table 19.1 Medical findings associated with PHACE syndrome

Posterior fossa anomalies-brain structure
  Dandy-Walker complex
  Cerebellar hypoplasia
  Unilateral cerebellar hypoplasia
  Subependymal or arachnoid cysts
  Dilated lateral ventricles
  Hypoplasia of cerebrum
  Hypoplasia of corpus callosum
  Hypoplasia of septum pellucidum
  Hypoplasia of vermis
  Absent foramen lacerum
  Polymicrogyria
  Microcephaly
  Heterotopia
  Absent pituitary or partially empty sella turcica
Arterial lesions-cerebrovascular
  Dysplasia of the large cerebral arteries[a]
  Stenosis, occlusion, absence or moderate to severe hypoplasia of the large cerebral arteries[a]
  Aberrant origin or course of the large cerebral arteries[a]
  Saccular aneurysms
  Persistent embryonic arteries
  Cerebral sinus malformations
  Sinus pericranii
  Dural arteriovenous malformations
  Moyamoya vasculopathy
  Acute arterial stroke
Cardiac/aortic coarctation/cardiovascular
  Coarctation or interrupted aortic arch
  Aneurysms of aortic arch
  Right aortic arch
  Double aortic arch
  Congenital valvular aortic stenosis
  Aberrant origin of a subclavian with or without a vascular ring
  Subclavian steal syndrome
  Anomalous coronary arteries
  Patent ductus arteriosus
  Anomalous pulmonary veins
  Patent foramen ovale
  Cor triatriatum
  Tricuspid atresia/stenosis
  Dextrocardia
  Persistent left superior vena cava
  Ventral and atrial septal defects
  Pulmonary stenosis
  Tetralogy of Fallot

Table 19.1 (continued)

  Ectopia cordis or Cantrell's syndrome
  Arteriovenous shunting
Eye abnormalities
  Posterior segment abnormalities
  Retinal vascular abnormality
  Persistent fetal retinal vessels
  Iris vessel hypertrophy
  "Morning-glory" disk
  Peripapillary staphyloma
  Optic nerve hypoplasia
  Anterior segment abnormalities
  Microphthalmos
  Coloboma
  Congenital cataracts.
  Sclerocornea
  Iris hypoplasia
  Exophthalmos
  Congenital third nerve palsy
  Horner syndrome
Other associated anomalies
Ventral developmental
  Partial or complete agenesis of sternum
  Sternal cleft or pit
  Sternal papule
  Lingual ectopic thyroid
  Supraumbilical raphe
  Omphalocele
Miscellaneous
  Pituitary insufficiency
  Micrognathia
  Auricular hypoplasia or agenesis/"low-set" ears
  Orofacial clefting
  Airway hemangioma
  Carcinoid endobronchial tumor
  Spina bifida occulta
  Esophageal diverticulum
  Cervical cyst
  Ipsilateral sensorineural hearing loss
  Congenital scrotal/hemiscrotal agenesis
  Hemangioma of the liver

Modified from Ref. [3]
[a]Internal carotid artery, middle cerebral artery, anterior cerebral artery, posterior cerebral artery, or vertebrobasilar system

collaboration between the various experts is crucial to design the optimal treatment. A formal therapeutic guideline cannot be given, because the patients are not identical; therefore it should be remembered that every infant diagnosed with PHACE syndrome has different medical needs. What is sure is that propranolol is helpful also in PHACE syndrome. However, this beta-blocking drug could be theoretically responsible for an eventually increased risk of ischemic stroke due to the underlying cerebral vascular disease. Clinical [9] and investigational [10] studies have ruled out this possibility, so propranolol should be considered a first-choice treatment also in the case of PHACE syndrome.

LUMBAR/PELVIS/SACRAL Syndrome

In 2006, 10 years after the description of PHACE syndrome, the association of a pelvic hemangioma and malformations in the pelvic region was described as PELVIS syndrome [11]. One year after, always by analogy with PHACE syndrome, the term SACRAL syndrome was proposed [12]. Subsequent collaboration and unification of the features have led to a more comprehensive acronym, LUMBAR, that will be used in this context [13] (Figs. 19.4 and 19.5a, b). In short, by analogy with PHACE syndrome, LUMBAR

syndrome describe the association of segmented hemangioma of the lower extremities associated with other trunk or lower-body malformations. As

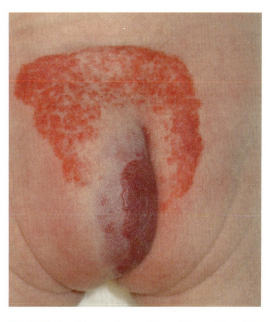

Fig 19.4 In this newborn girl, a big nodular deep hemangioma is accompanied by a plaque-like superficial hemangioma; in addition, a deviation of the gluteal fold is also present

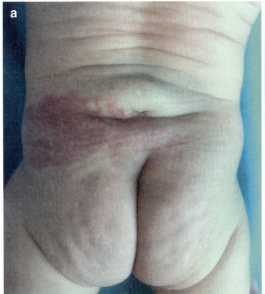

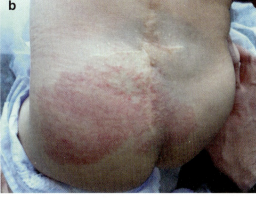

Fig 19.5 (**a**) In this infant, the lumbar region is intersected by a plaque-like hemangioma accompanied with a capillary malformation, a subcutaneous mass in the lower part of the spine, an important skin depression, and a clear deviation of the gluteal fold. The patient presented also angiolipomatosis and dysraphism. (**b**) The same patient after neurosurgery

it is the case for PHACE syndrome, LUMBAR syndrome is often incomplete, but a complete list of all possible defects is theoretically endless given the individual variations of the underlying malformations [14]. Therefore, the list of the recommended diagnostic test for LUMBAR syndrome, as it happens for PHACE syndrome, could be very long. In this case, however, the biggest difference is the usefulness of ultrasound and Doppler examination for LUMBAR syndrome. Indeed, for patients younger than 3–4 months, ultrasound and Doppler examination of the spine, abdomen, and pelvis can give significant data. For older patients, any lumbar hemangioma or hemangioma in either the sacral area and/or on the perineum/genitals in a patient with suspected myelopathy, an MRI of the spine, abdomen, and pelvis is recommended (an MRI of only the abdomen and pelvis is appropriate for patients without myelopathy). When segmental IHs affect the lower extremities, a magnetic resonance angiography/magnetic resonance venography of the abdomen, pelvis, and the affected limb should be performed along with standard radiographs of the lower extremities [15]. By analogy with PHACE syndrome, LUMBAR syndrome should be managed according to different medical needs. Together with medical treatment with propranolol, neurologists, radiologists, and neuroradiologists should be consulted first. While airway hemangiomas and cerebrovascular problems are not expected, the presence of imperforate anus is an emergency requiring a prompt surgical correction. Neurosurgeons (Figs. 19.5a, b), urologists, gynecologists (in females), nephrologists, general and vascular surgeons, gastroenterologists, and geneticists can join the team if needed.

Diffuse Neonatal Hemangiomatosis

Diffuse neonatal hemangiomatosis presents with multiple, progressive, rapidly growing cutaneous hemangiomas associated with widespread visceral hemangiomas in the liver, lungs, gastrointestinal tract, brain, and meninges [16]. It is a rare condition, characterized by the presence, at birth or in the following weeks, of tens or hundreds of IHs over the entire skin and internal organs, with symptoms linked to the constant development of new elements and to their locations, resulting in the most various complications such as intestinal bleeding, heart failure, and impairment of respiratory and nervous systems. There is also a benign form (benign neonatal hemangiomatosis) with only cutaneous and hepatic lesions or even only cutaneous ones. An evidence-based review of case reports in the literature has shown that many cases reported in the literature as diffuse neonatal hemangiomatosis represent newly described multifocal vascular anomalies such as multifocal lymphangioendotheliomatosis with thrombocytopenia, which has a strikingly higher mortality than common IHs. Therefore, the term "multifocal infantile hemangioma – with or without extracutaneous disease" instead of "diffuse neonatal hemangiomatosis" for multiple cutaneous IHs has been proposed [17]. More recently, a case of diffuse neonatal hemangiomatosis associated also with an isolated cerebellar arteriovenous malformation has been described, raising the question whether diffuse neonatal hemangiomatosis and PHACE and LUMBAR syndromes are related [18]. It is, however, of note that propranolol coupled with supportive treatment in case of congestive heart failure can be used also for diffuse neonatal hemangiomatosis [19]. Propranolol seems useful for cutaneous as well for visceral lesions [20].

Conclusion

Lacking a clear biologic definition of IH, the description of syndrome related to IH, and consequently their management, is questionable. In ISSVA classification, there is still a grey area in which all these forms (e.g., PHACE syndrome, LUMBAR syndrome, etc.) should be collocated. Thus, if in the past a multidisciplinary approach for IH was advisable, today it seems mandatory with the only exception, perhaps, of small, isolated, non-segmental, non-ulcerated IHs which are not located in critical areas.

References

1. Mulliken JB, Young AE (1988) Vascular birthmarks; hemangiomas and malformations. WB Saunders, Philadelphia
2. Frieden IJ, Reese V, Cohen D (1996) PHACE syndrome. The association of posterior fossa brain malformations, hemangiomas, arterial anomalies, coarctation of the aorta and cardiac defects, and eye abnormalities. Arch Dermatol 132(3):307–311
3. www.chw.org/display/PPF/DocID/.../router.asp. Updated in Dec 2013
4. Pascual-Castroviejo I (1978) Vascular and nonvascular intracranial malformation associated with external capillary hemangiomas. Neuroradiology 16:82–84
5. Pascual-Castroviejo I, Alvarez-Linera J, Coya J, Viaño J, Pascual-Pascual SI, Velázquez-Fragua R, López-Gutiérrez JC (2011) Pascual-Castroviejo type II syndrome (P-CIIS). Importance of the presence of persistent embryonic arteries. Childs Nerv Syst 27(4):617–625
6. Höger PH (2012) Hemangioma. New aspects of pathogenesis, differential diagnosis and therapy. Hautarzt 63(2):112–120
7. Bayer ML, Frommelt PC, Blei F, Breur JM, Cordisco MR, Frieden IJ, Goddard DS, Holland KE, Krol AL, Maheshwari M, Metry DW, Morel KD, North PE, Pope E, Shieh JT, Southern JF, Wargon O, Siegel DH, Drolet BA (2013) Congenital cardiac, aortic arch, and vascular bed anomalies in PHACE syndrome (from the International PHACE Syndrome Registry). Am J Cardiol 112(12):1948–1952
8. Kaushik SB, Kwatra SG, McLean TW, Powers A, Atala AJ, Yosipovitch G (2013) Segmental ulcerated perineal hemangioma of infancy: a complex case of PELVIS syndrome successfully treated using a multidisciplinary approach. Pediatr Dermatol 30(6):e257–e258
9. Mohanan S, Besra L, Chandrashekar L, Thappa DM (2012) Excellent response of infantile hemangioma associated with PHACES syndrome to propranolol. Indian J Dermatol Venereol Leprol 78(1):114–115
10. Hernandez-Martin S, Lopez-Gutierrez JC, Lopez-Fernandez S, Ramírez M, Miguel M, Coya J, Marin D, Tovar JA (2012) Brain perfusion SPECT in patients with PHACES syndrome under propranolol treatment. Eur J Pediatr Surg 22(1):54–59
11. Girard C, Bigorre M, Guillot B, Bessis D (2006) PELVIS syndrome. Arch Dermatol 142(7):884–888
12. Stockman A, Boralevi F, Taïeb A, Léauté-Labrèze C (2007) SACRAL syndrome: spinal dysraphism, anogenital, cutaneous, renal and urologic anomalies, associated with an angioma of lumbosacral localization. Dermatology 214(1):40–45
13. Frade F, Kadlub N, Soupre V, Cassier S, Audry G, Vazquez MP, Picard A (2012) PELVIS or LUMBAR syndrome: the same entity. Two case reports. Arch Pediatr 19(1):55–58
14. Yadav DK, Panda SS, Teckchandani N, Bagga D (2013) SACRAL syndrome. BMJ Case Rep 31:2013
15. Tlougan BE, Gonzalez ME, Orlow SJ (2011) Abortive segmental perineal hemangioma. Dermatol Online J 17(10):8
16. Patiroglu T, Sarici D, Unal E, Yikilmaz A, Tucer B, Karakukcu M, Ozdemir MA, Canoz O, Akcakus M (2012) Cerebellar hemangioblastoma associated with diffuse neonatal hemangiomatosis in an infant. Childs Nerv Syst 28(10):1801–1805
17. Glick ZR, Frieden IJ, Garzon MC, Mully TW, Drolet BA (2012) Diffuse neonatal hemangiomatosis: an evidence-based review of case reports in the literature. J Am Acad Dermatol 67(5):898–903
18. Ferrandiz L, Toledo-Pastrana T, Moreno-Ramirez D, Bardallo-Cruzado L, Perez-Bertolez S, Luna-Lagares S, Rios-Martin JJ (2013) Diffuse neonatal hemangiomatosis with partial response to propranolol. Int J Dermatol 8
19. Dotan M, Lorber A (2013) Congestive heart failure with diffuse neonatal hemangiomatosis, case report and literature review. Acta Paediatr 102(5):e232–e238
20. Mazereeuw-Hautier J, Hoeger PH, Benlahrech S, Ammour A, Broue P, Vial J, Ohanessian G, Léauté-Labrèze C, Labenne M, Vabres P, Rössler J, Bodemer C (2010) Efficacy of propranolol in hepatic infantile hemangiomas with diffuse neonatal hemangiomatosis. J Pediatr 157(2):340–342

Part III

Vascular Malformations

Epidemiology of Vascular Malformations

20

Byung-Boong Lee, James Laredo, Richard F. Neville, Young-Wook Kim, and Young-Soo Do

Incidence and Prevalence

Congenital vascular malformation (CVM) has been a symbol of confusion among various vascular disorders through decades, and naturally its epidemiological data as well were based on much confusing definition and classification of the CVMs [1–3].

Despite a new era of the CVMs based on the contemporary concept of the Hamburg Classification [4–6] that has taken over the old era of "angiodysplasia" with mostly name-based eponyms/classifications through the last three decades, a substantial confusion remained misguiding clinical interpretation of the CVMs including their epidemiologic data as well.

For example, the term "hemangioma" is still mistakenly used for the extratruncular type of venous malformation (VM) despite a genuine hemangioma that is *NOT* a vascular malformation but a vascular tumor [7–9]. Hence, many of the VMs were misrepresented as a hemangioma and classified erroneously in hospital records, publications, etc. Besides, the majority of "mixed" conditions of various CVMs were recorded separately from other CVMs as one of numerous syndrome-based vascular disorders.

Therefore, the epidemiologic data available in the literatures in the mid of this confusing era often misguide true incidence and prevalence of the CVMs altogether with the confusing definition of new and old terminology, and the overall dependability of the data for its incidence and prevalence is quite limited.

Nevertheless, Stevenson AC et al. reported an overall frequency of major and minor malformations of 12.7 % in single births and 4.6 % in multiple births in a large-scale study sponsored by the World Health Organization in 1977 based on the survey of 426,932 live and stillborn births [10].

Similarly, Myrianthopoulos NC [11] reported the epidemiological characteristics of CVM occurring in 53,394 consecutive single births and in 1,197 twin births in a prospective Collaborative Perinatal Project based on the information recorded according to preestablished uniform guidelines; at the end of the first year of life, malformations were detected in 15.6 % of singletons. Multiple malformations were diagnosed in 2.6 % of the single offspring; the highest frequency was associated with the cardiovascular system (74.4 %).

B.B. Lee, MD, PhD, FACS (✉) • J. Laredo
R.F. Neville
Division of Vascular Surgery, Department of Surgery,
George Washington University Medical Center,
Washington, DC, USA
e-mail: bblee@mfa.gwu.edu; bblee38@comcast.net;
jlaredo@mfa.gwu.edu; rneville@mfa.gwu.edu

Y.W. Kim, MD, PhD
Division of Vascular Surgery, Cardiac and Vascular
Center, Samsung Medical Center, Sungkyunkwan
University School of Medicine, Seoul, Korea

Y.S. Do, MD, PhD
Department of Radiology, SamSung Medical Center,
Sungkyunkwan University School of Medicine,
Seoul, Republic of Korea

R. Mattassi et al. (eds.), *Hemangiomas and Vascular Malformations: An Atlas of Diagnosis and Treatment*,
DOI 10.1007/978-88-470-5673-2_20, © Springer-Verlag Italia 2009, 2015

Kennedy WP et al. also reported the overall incidence of CVM as 1.08 % ranging from 0.83 to 4.5 % based on comprehensive review of 238 studies on the world literature reporting more than 20 million births [12]. These overall incidences of CVM were obtained from hospital records, birth certificates, and also retrospective questionnaires from intensive examinations of children. However, this study highlighted the variability in reporting methods due to differences in terminology and inconsistent diagnostic criteria.

These landmark studies, however, represent the era of marked misconceptions on the CVMs with confusing nomenclature before great advances were made in the understanding of the pathophysiology, classification, nomenclature, and treatment of all vascular lesions through the past three decades.

A new concept is now established for the CVMs (e.g., Hamburg Classification) with appropriate differentiation with often confusing vascular tumor represented by the hemangioma (e.g., ISSVA Classification). The CVMs solely represent the group of various birth defects affecting the vascular system(s); over 90 % present at birth with a male–female ratio of 1:1 [13–15].

Depending upon the vascular system(s) affected and also the embryological stage when the developmental arrest has occurred, the CVMs present strikingly different characteristics from each other with a much different clinical condition morphologically, pathophysiologically, and also hemodynamically (e.g., extratruncular and truncular lesions) [16–18].

Within this boundary of new concept, further reliable epidemiological data became available through the last decade; Tasnadi G et al. (1993) reported overall incidence of the CVM in 1.2 % (43 out of 3,573) based on a study carried on 3,573 3-year-old children: infiltrating or localized venous malformation (VM) and/or arteriovenous malformation (AVM) in 16 cases (37 %), capillary malformation (CM)/port-wine stain in 15 cases (35 %), lymphatic malformation (LM)/primary lymphedema in 5 cases (12 %), phlebectasia with nevus and limb length discrepancy in 5 cases (12 %), and phlebectasia in 2 cases (4 %) [19].

Eifert S and Villavicencio JL et al. also reported (2000) the prevalence of deep venous anomalies among the VMs, diagnosed with modern technology: duplex scanning, plethysmography, computerized tomography, magnetic resonance imaging, and angiography. Among 392 patients with various CVMs, 257 (65.5 %) were confirmed as VM of deep venous anomalies in various conditions of phlebectasia, aplasia or hypoplasia of venous trunks, aneurysms, and avalvulia [20]. Phlebectasia was the most frequent (36 %), followed by aplasia or hypoplasia of the deep venous trunks (8 %) and venous aneurysms (8 %). At least one deep venous anomaly was present in 47 % of the patients with predominantly VMs.

Although most of the published data on the CVMs by referral centers suggest that the VM is the most common CVMs, they are estimated to occur in 1 in 5,000–10,000 childbirths [21].

But, the CM with clinical manifestation as port-wine stain of the skin and mucosa is still much more common than the VM, occurring in 0.3 % of childbirths [22].

Besides, the VMs [23–25] are certainly the most frequent type of the CVMs to need a medical attention since the AVMs [26–28] are relatively rare, and much less visible LMs [29–31], especially the truncular type known as a primary lymphedema, are often neglected as one of the CVMs.

Lee BB et al. reported that the LMs are as common as the VMs among a total of 797 CVM cases (315/797) (1995–2001: 446 females and 351 males; mean age 22.1 years in the range of 14 days to 81 years), when both extratruncular LM/lymphangioma and truncular LM/primary lymphedema are counted together: LM 315 (39.5 %), VM 294 (36.9 %), AVM 76 (9.5 %), and combined CVMs/hemolymphatic malformation (HLM) 66 (8.3 %), although unclassified CVMs – 40 (5.0 %) – that are mostly VM to be confirmed later were not counted [32].

Lee BB et al. made further extended review on the predilection site of the CVMs among a total of 1,203 patients (1994–2003), which revealed the lower extremity as the most prevalent site: 464 (38.6 %) patients with LM 224, VM 144, AVM 32, combined 27, and unclassified 37, followed by the head and neck (275–22.9 %) with

VM 114, LM 63, AVM 38, combined 29, CM[1] 4, AM[2] 1, and unclassified 26. However, among 1,203 patients, 237 patients were confirmed for the CVM scattered throughout multiple sites, which consist of VM 110, LM 49, AVM 19, combined forms 39, CM 2, and unclassified 18. Besides, the upper extremity is also affected by the CVM in a significant degree (138, 11.5 %), and the torso/thorax (53–4.4 %) also became a unique site for various CVM lesions together with the abdominopelvic-genitalia regions (35–2.1 %).

Among the VMs, the lower extremity was the most common site (144), followed by the head and neck (114); multiple site involvement was also common (110). The LMs were also most prevalent in the lower extremity (224) followed by the head and neck (63) and also as one of multiple sites (49). Interestingly, the combined CVMs were found most common as a part of multiple site involvement (39), followed by the head and neck (29) and lower extremity (26). The AVMs, however, showed a different pattern with even distribution among the head and neck (38), upper extremity (35), and lower extremity (32), and multiple site involvement was relatively rare (19).

In view of entirely different clinical behavior and prognosis by two subtypes of LM – extratruncular lesion/lymphangioma and truncular lesion/primary lymphedema – Lee et al. made an additional review on the subtypes of the LM separately among 1,203 CVM patients. Predominant LM existing as an independent lesion consists of 271 truncular LM and 122 extratruncular LM lesions. Of the 122 patients with predominantly extratruncular LM, 89 had the macrocystic type with a predilection for the head, neck, and thorax (63/122). Of the 271 patients with truncular LM, 247 had an aplastic and/or obstructing type with a predilection for the extremities (253), mostly of the lower extremity (224). Of the 1,203 CVM patients, 108 had LM lesion which was combined/coexisting with VM as HLM [33].

Lee BB et al. made a further analysis of expanded group (1994–2004) of 1,475 CVM patients to show a very similar distribution of the main CVM groups in comparison to the earlier version reported previously based on 1,203 patients [18] except VM was more prevalent than LM: VM 569 (38.6 %), LM 445 (30.2 %), AVM 177 (12.0 %), HLM 136 (9.2 %), and unclassified 148 (10.0 %). The majority of the "unclassified" belongs to the VM clinically but not confirmed yet with appropriate tests deferred till needed for the treatment.

Therefore, we consider that the extratruncular VMs are the most frequent malformations of all as an independent CVM lesion and present in either diffuse or localized forms [34]. The estimated incidence of predominantly VMs is approximately 0.8–1 % in the general population [19].

But when both extratruncular and truncular LMs are combined, its overall incidence is close to those of the VM, if not higher [33].

The peripheral AVMs are the least common CVMs representing approximately 10–15 % in the range of 5–10 % to 15–20 % [19, 35] of all clinically significant CVM lesions, while the VMs comprise approximately 2/3 of all CVMs [36, 37]. And the "extratruncular" AVM (formerly angiomatous AVM) lesion comprises the majority of AVM cases [15]. However, most of the current data available regarding the incidence and prevalence of AVMs are based on cerebrospinal AVMs: approximately 250,000 people in the USA with equal or female >male (2:1) ratio in [38, 39].

Although the majority of CVMs are either independent VMs [16, 40] or LMs [30, 33], a significant number of the CVMs are also known to remain mixed in various extents, and these complex forms classified to HLM can include arterial, capillary, venous, or lymphatic elements as well (e.g., Klippel–Trenaunay Syndrome, Parkes Weber Syndrome).

Lately, Yamaki T et al. reported the prevalence of the VM component among the Klippel–Trenaunay Syndrome based on 61 patients examined with duplex ultrasound and magnetic resonance imaging: Extratruncular VMs were

---

[1] CM – isolated/independent capillary malformation as a sole CVM lesion

[2] AM – arterial malformation: truncular

detected in 47 patients (77 %), while truncular VMs were found in 50 patients (82 %). Among these, embryonic lateral marginal vein showed the highest occurrence: 53 % (32 patients). Deep vein hypoplasia was found in seven patients (12 %), while five patients (8 %) had deep vein aplasia [41].

To date, no racial, demographic, or environmental risk factors for CVMs have been identified.

References

1. Lee BB, Laredo J, Lee TS, Huh S, Neville R (2007) Terminology and classification of congenital vascular malformations. Phlebology 22(6):249–252
2. Lee BB, Bergan J, Gloviczki P, Laredo J, Loose DA, Mattassi R et al (2009) Diagnosis and treatment of venous malformations – consensus document of the International Union of Phlebology (IUP)-2009. Int Angiol 28(6):434–451
3. Lee BB, Villavicencio L (2010) Chapter 68. General considerations. Congenital vascular malformations. Section 9. Arteriovenous anomalies. In: Cronenwett JL, Johnston KW (eds) Rutherford's vascular surgery, 7th edn. Saunders Elsevier, Philadelphia. pp1046–1064
4. Belov S (1989) Classification, terminology, and nosology of congenital vascular defects. In: Belov S, Loose DA, Weber J (eds) Vascular malformations. Einhorn-Presse, Reinbek, pp 25–30
5. Lee BB, Laredo J (2012) Classification of congenital vascular malformations: the last challenge for congenital vascular malformations. Phlebology 27(6): 267–269
6. Rutherford RB (1995) Classification of peripheral congenital vascular malformations. In: Ernst C, Stanley J (eds) Current therapy in vascular surgery, 3rd edn. Mosby, St. Louis, pp 834–838
7. Lee BB, Laredo J (2012) Hemangioma and venous/vascular malformation are different as an apple and orange! Editorial. Acta Phlebol 13:1–3
8. Lee BB (2012) Venous malformation is NOT a hemangioma. Editorial. Flebologia Y Linfologia – Lecturas Vasculares 7(17):1021–1023.
9. Lee BB (2013) Venous malformation and haemangioma: differential diagnosis, diagnosis, natural history and consequences. Phlebology 28(Suppl 1): 176–187
10. Stevenson AC, Johnston HA, Stewart MIP, Golding DR (1966) Congenital malformations. A report of a study of series of consecutive births in 24 centres. Bull WHO 34(Suppl):9, and 100–102 (Extracts)
11. Myrianthopoulos NC, Chung CS (1974) Congenital malformations in singletons. Epidemiologic survey. Reports from the Collaborative Perinatal project. Birth Defects Orig Artic Ser 10(11):1–58
12. Kennedy WP (1977) Epidemiologic aspects of the problem of congenital malformations. In: Persaud TNV (ed) Problems of birth defects. University Park Press, Baltimore, pp 35–52
13. Enjolras O, Wassef M, Chapot R (2007) Introduction: ISSVA classification. In: Color atlas of vascular tumors and vascular malformations. Cambridge University Press, New York, pp 1–11
14. Gloviczki P, Duncan AA, Kalra M, Oderich GS, Ricotta JJ, Bower TC et al (2009) Vascular malformations: an update. Perspect Vasc Surg Endovasc Ther 21(2):133–148
15. Lee BB, Baumgartner I, Berlien HP, Bianchini G, Burrows P, Do YS, Ivancev K, Kool LS, Laredo J, Loose DA, Lopez-Gutierrez JC, Mattassi R, Parsi K, Rimon U, Rosenblatt M, Shortell C, Simkin R, Stillo F, Villavicencio L, Yakes W (2013) Consensus document of the International Union of Angiology (IUA)-2013. Current concept on the management of arterio-venous management. Int Angiol 32(1):9–36
16. Lee BB (2010) Not all venous malformations needed therapy because they are not arteriovenous malformations. Dermatol Surg 36(3):347, Comments on Dermatol Surg. 2010;36(3):340–346
17. Lee BB, Lardeo J, Neville R (2009) Arterio-venous malformation: how much do we know? Phlebology 24:193–200
18. Lee BB (2008) Changing concept on vascular malformation: no longer enigma. Ann Vasc Dis 1(1):11–19
19. Tasnadi G (1993) Epidemiology and etiology of congenital vascular malformations. Semin Vasc Surg 6: 200–203
20. Eifert S, Villavicencio JL, Kao TC et al (2000) Prevalence of deep venous anomalies in congenital vascular malformations of venous predominance. J Vasc Surg 31:462–471
21. Vikkula M, Boon LM, Mullikan JB (2001) Molecular genetics of vascular malformations. Matrix Biol 20: 327–335
22. Eerola I, Boon LM, Mulliken JB et al (2003) Capillary malformation – arteriovenous malformation, a new clinical and genetic disorder caused by RASA1 mutations. Am J Hum Genet 73:1240–1249
23. Lee BB, Kim DI, Huh S, Kim HH, Choo IW, Byun HS, Do YS (2001) New experiences with absolute ethanol sclerotherapy in the management of a complex form of congenital venous malformation. J Vasc Surg 33(4):764–772
24. Lee BB, Do YS, Byun HS, Choo IW, Kim DI, Huh SH (2003) Advanced management of venous malformation (VM) with ethanol sclerotherapy: mid-term results. J Vasc Surg 37(3):533–538
25. Lee BB (2003) Current concept of venous malformation (VM). Phlebolymphology 43:197–203
26. Lee BB, Do YS, Yakes W, Kim DI, Mattassi R, Hyun WS, Byun HS (2004) Management of arterial-venous shunting malformations (AVM) by surgery and

embolosclerotherapy. A multidisciplinary approach. J Vasc Surg 3:596–600

27. Kim JY, Kim DI, Do YS, Kim YW, Lee BB (2006) Surgical treatment for congenital arteriovenous malformation: 10 years' experience. Eur J Vasc Endovasc Surg 32(1):101–106. Epub 2006 Feb

28. Lee BB, Laredo J, Deaton DH, Neville RF (2009) Chapter 53. Arteriovenous malformations: evaluation and treatment. In: Gloviczki P (ed) Handbook of venous disorders: guidelines of the American Venous Forum, 3rd edn. A Hodder Arnold, London, pp 583–593

29. Lee BB, Andrade M, Bergan J, Boccardo F, Campisi C, Damstra R, Flour M, Gloviczki P, Laredo J, Piller N, Michelini S, Mortimer P, Villavicencio JL (2010) Diagnosis and treatment of primary lymphedema – consensus document of the International Union of Phlebology (IUP)-2009. Int Angiol 29(5):454–470

30. Lee BB, Villavicencio JL (2010) Primary lymphedema and lymphatic malformation: are they the two sides of the same coin? Eur J Vasc Endovasc Surg 39:646–653

31. Lee BB (2005) Lymphedema-angiodysplasia syndrome: a prodigal form of lymphatic malformation (LM). Phlebolymphology 47:324–332

32. Do YS, Yakes W, Shin SW, Lee BB (2005) Ethanol embolization of arteriovenous malformations: interim results. Radiology 235:674–682

33. Lee BB, Laredo J, Seo JM, Neville R (2009) Chapter 29. Treatment of lymphatic malformations. In: Mattassi R, Loose DA, Vaghi M (eds) Hemangiomas and vascular malformations. Springer, Milan, pp 231–250

34. Lee BB, Baumgartner I, Berlien P, Bianchini G, Burrows P, Gloviczki P et al (2014). Diagnosis and treatment of venous malformations – consensus document of the International Union of Phlebology (IUP)-2013. Int Angiol. [Epub ahead of print]

35. Cho SK, Do YS, Shin SW, Choo SW, Choo IW et al (2006) Arteriovenous malformations of the body and extremities: analysis of therapeutic outcomes and approaches according to a modified angiographic classification. J Endovasc Ther 13(4):527–538

36. Villavicencio JL, Scultetus A, Lee BB (2002) Congenital vascular malformations: when and how to treat them. Semin Vasc Surg 15(1):65–71

37. Young AE (1988) Pathogenesis of vascular malformations. In: Mulliken JB, Young AE (eds) Vascular birthmarks: hemangiomas and malformations. W.B. Saunders Co, Philadelphia, pp 107–113

38. Jackson JE, Mansfield AO, Allison DJ (1996) Treatment of high-flow vascular malformations by venous embolization aided by flow occlusion techniques. Cardiovasc Intervent Radiol 19(5):323–328

39. Al-Shahi R, Warlow C (2001) A systematic review of the frequency and prognosis of arteriovenous malformations of the brain in adults. Brain 124(10):1900–1926

40. Lee BB, Laredo J, Neville R (2010) Embryological background of truncular venous malformation in the extracranial venous pathways as the cause of chronic cerebrospinal venous insufficiency. Int Angiol 29(2):95–108

41. Yamaki T, Konoeda H, Fujisawa D, Ogino K, Osada A et al (2013) Prevalence of various congenital vascular malformations in patients with Klippel-Trenaunay syndrome. J Vasc Surgery Venous Lymphat Disord 1(2):187–193

Histology of Vascular Malformations

21

Paula E. North

Introduction

Vascular anomalies as a broad group are usefully divided into the vascular tumors, which are intrinsically proliferative lesions such as infantile hemangioma (IH), and the vascular malformations, which represent congenital errors in vascular morphogenesis and grow more commensurately with the growth of the child. This division into tumors and malformations is compliant with the classification scheme endorsed by the multidisciplinary International Society for the Study of Vascular Anomalies (ISSVA), originally derived from that proposed in 1992 by Mulliken and Glowacki, in which vascular anomalies were divided into tumors (e.g., the "angiomas") and malformations, based on presence or absence of endothelial mitotic activity [1]. Accumulated experience has proved that presence of endothelial mitotic activity alone is not sufficient as a single factor to separate tumors from malformations, since there are secondary effects such as ischemia and turbulence that may stimulate mitotic activity. When combined with correlations with other histological features and clinical behavior, however,

consideration of endothelial mitotic activity was a rational starting point that has enlightened our approach to these perplexing lesions.

Although now broadly accepted, this distinction between "angiomas" and malformations represents a significant departure from the traditional diagnostic approach of pathologists, in which the term *hemangioma* has been applied without regard to etiology or clinical behavior and at best has been modified by morphological descriptors such as *capillary* or *cavernous*. Many experienced pathologists still refer to *venous malformations*, which consist of mitotically quiescent collections of developmentally abnormal veins, as *cavernous hemangiomas*. Similarly, developmental abnormalities of the lymphatic vasculature (*lymphatic malformations* by the new classification scheme) have previously been referred to as *lymphangiomas*, and *arteriovenous malformations* have been termed *arteriovenous hemangiomas*. Continued use of this poor traditional nosology encourages past misconceptions despite new etiological clarity. Refinements and additions to the ISSVA-sanctioned scheme will be necessary, as entities that defy classification based on simple criteria are clarified and discoveries in vascular developmental biology progress. Nevertheless, this approach has already proven itself in international practice to be a useful starting point in a biology-based system of histopathological diagnosis in which the various types of vascular malformations, as true errors of vasculogenesis, can

P.E. North, MD, PhD
Department of Pathology, Medical College of Wisconsin, Milwaukee, WI, USA

Department of Pathology and Laboratory Medicine, Children's Hospital of Wisconsin, Milwaukee, WI, USA
e-mail: pnorth@mcw.edu

be recognized and appropriately classified based upon their characteristic clinical, histological, immunophenotypical, and imaging findings, supplemented when possible by pathognomonic molecular diagnostic test results.

Histology

Vascular malformations may contain venous, capillary, lymphatic, or arterial components in any combination and have been associated with various dysmorphic syndromes [2, 3]. Both blood vascular and lymphatic vascular malformations represent developmental errors of the embryonic vasculature, grow slowly with the child, and persist throughout life. Histopathological distinction between vascular malformations and vascular tumors can be difficult, not only due to lack of clinical history but also because the gross and microscopic appearances of developmental vascular malformations tend to evolve during postnatal life and may include areas of vascular proliferation. Factors causing this evolution include progressive or intermittent vascular ectasia, recruitment of collateral vessels, organizing thrombosis, hormonal modulation, and reactive neovascularization in response to abnormal intralesional hemodynamics. It is also possible that the intrinsic genetic defects that cause abnormal in utero vascular development, and thus vascular malformations, may sometimes continue in postnatal life and cause increased mitotic potential or aberrant responses to angiogenic factors. To complicate things further, rare macrocystic lymphatic malformations may appear to regress if scarring prevents filling of the cystic vessels. Despite these uncertainties, vascular malformations can usually be recognized by their presence at birth, slow proportionate growth, lack of regressive behavior, and relative mitotic quiescence. Some malformations that are presumed to be congenital may be temporarily hidden because of their deep location, which complicates preoperative diagnosis. The histopathologist's task is to confirm or dispute the clinical impression and to subclassify malformations based on the constituent vessels and (for blood vascular malformations) presence or absence of histological

evidence of arteriovenous shunting. Correlation with clinical and radiological information is often essential. Summarized below are the key clinical features and current histopathological diagnostic criteria for each of the major categories of vascular malformations, beginning with those arising from the blood vasculature. It is useful to remember that the endothelial cells of all vascular malformations, both lymphatic and blood vascular, are immunonegative for markers that are specific for IH, such as GLUT1 [4–9].

Cutaneous Capillary/Venulocapillary Malformations (Port-Wine Stains)

Clinical

Abnormalities of the superficial cutaneous vascular plexus are heterogeneous in etiology and presentation. They include both capillary/venulocapillary malformations and telangiectasias. Some of these are multifocal and associated with syndromes linked to known genetic mutations. These inherited disorders are rarely encountered by pathologists and are reviewed in Chap. 37. The section below focuses upon a well-recognized sporadic cutaneous clinicopathological entity referred to by clinicians as *port-wine stain* (PWS). PWSs affecting the ophthalmic branch of the trigeminal nerve are often associated with venulocapillary abnormalities of the ipsilateral leptomeninges and eye, producing the neurocutaneous disorder known as Sturge-Weber syndrome (SWS). The strongly segmental pattern of PWS and Sturge-Weber syndrome has long suggested the possibility of mosaicism due to somatic mutation of otherwise lethal genes. Very recently, the causative somatic mutation of most, and possibly all, cases of Sturge-Weber syndrome and nonsyndromic PWSs of the head and neck was discovered – an activating mutation in the GNAQ gene [10].

Microscopic Features

PWS biopsies from infants and young children may not reveal the characteristic vessel ectasia

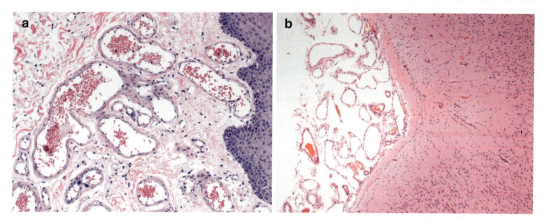

Fig. 21.1 (**a**) Cutaneous venulocapillary malformation (port-wine stain). (**b**) Leptomeningeal venulocapillary malformation, Sturge-Weber Syndrome

that generally becomes prominent in histological sections after the patient is about 10 years of age, despite clinically evident red discoloration of the skin at birth. Over time, dermal vessels of venulocapillary size become progressively dilated and filled with erythrocytes (Fig. 21.1). These vessels are rounded in contour and lined by thin, elongated endothelial cells associated with peripheral pericytes, neither cell population showing evidence of mitotic activity. Histologically similar vessels comprise the leptomeningeal malformation in PWS patients with SWS (Fig. 21.1b). PWS vessel walls become more thickened and fibrous with time. Beyond this fibrous wall thickening, vessels in areas demonstrating generalized soft tissue hypertrophy may develop plump coats of loosely organized, well-differentiated smooth muscle fibers [11]. The "cobblestoning" clinically noted in many mature PWSs reflects protrusion of dermis containing dilated vessels between adnexal anchors. Gross nodule formation reflects focally exaggerated vascular ectasia and/or late development of complex epithelial, mesenchymal, and neural hamartomatous changes [12].

Venous Malformations

Clinical

Terms used in the past to refer to lesions now recognized as venous malformations (VM) include *cavernous hemangioma* and *venous hemangi-*

oma. Use of these outdated terms as diagnostic labels for lesions that are biologically consistent with VM is confusing to clinicians (and inaccurate) and should be abandoned. It is of interest that so-called cavernous hemangiomas or cavernomas of the brain, terms still firmly entrenched among neurosurgeons, are localized collections of massively dilated capillaries or venules, rather than veins.

Venous malformations are typically singular lesions, either localized or segmental, with no associated abnormalities, although some occur as part of complex syndromes. Superficial lesions appear blue in color and enlarge under conditions that increase venous pressure (e.g., dependency or exertion). Extensive lesions may be complicated by chronic, low-grade consumptive coagulopathy, and phleboliths are common.

Multiple venous malformations occur as a familial mucocutaneous disorder and also in the poorly understood dysmorphic syndrome known as *blue rubber bleb nevus syndrome*, first described in 1958 by Bean [13]. Blue rubber bleb nevus syndrome comprises an association between multiple venous malformations of the skin and the gastrointestinal tract, complicated by gastrointestinal bleeding. Venous malformations have also been described in patients with Turner's syndrome [14]. *Multiple mucocutaneous venous malformations* inherited as an autosomal dominant trait have been linked to a locus (*VMCM1*) on chromosome 9p21 and are associated with activating missense mutations in the endothelial

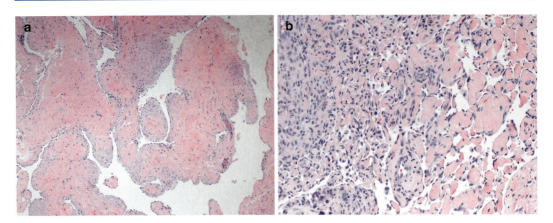

Fig. 21.2 (**a**) Venous malformation. (**b**) Venous malformation, intravascular papillary endothelial hyperplasia

cell-specific TIE-2 tyrosine kinase gene [15, 16, 17]. Recent studies have also identified somatic TIE-2 mutations in a large percentage of sporadic venous malformations [17, 18]. Multiple VM also occur without recognized etiology in Maffucci syndrome, a rare congenital disorder also characterized by dyschondroplasia, multiple enchondromas, and spindle cell hemangiomas. Similarly, multiple gastrocutaneous VM seen in blue rubber bleb nevus syndrome are associated with gastrointestinal bleeding and anemia; some cases are sporadic, and others autosomal dominant, all without known etiology.

Microscopic Features

Venous malformations are characterized by abnormal collections of veins that are superficial or deep, diffuse or localized, and solitary or multiple. They have flat, mitotically inactive endothelial cells (Fig. 21.2a). The venous nature of these malformations is implied by the presence of a variable amount of well-differentiated smooth muscle in the vessel walls (usually scant relative to luminal diameter), the absence of an internal elastic membrane, and erythrocyte-filled lumina. Vessels of capillary or venular proportions may also be present within the lesion. Component veins vary with regard to luminal size and wall thickness both between and within individual lesions. Those excised from some patients, particularly with Klippel-Trénaunay syndrome, may

show extreme disorganization of component smooth muscle fibers. Lining endothelial cells are positive for CD31, vWF, and CD34 and are negative for GLUT1 and other IH-associated markers [5].

Luminal thrombi in various stages of organization are common in venous malformations, reflective of stasis in these low-flow lesions. Recanalizing thrombi may demonstrate *intravascular papillary endothelial hyperplasia* (Fig. 21.2b). Although the latter may appear concerning for possible malignancy, this histological pattern represents an exuberant response of endothelial cells to organizing thrombus. It was first described by Masson in 1923 in hemorrhoidal veins and has been referred to as Masson's tumor or Masson's pseudoangiosarcoma. Early stages of this organizing process show growth of endothelial cells into fibrinous thrombus material, which divides it into papillary fronds lined by a single layer of plump endothelial cells without significant cytologic atypia. In later stages, the fibrin cores of the papillae become collagenized and hyalinized, and the endothelial lining becomes attenuated. Fusion of the lesional papillae may form an anastomosing meshwork of vessels separated by connective tissue stroma reminiscent of angiosarcoma; the pleomorphism, necrosis, and relatively high mitotic rate of angiosarcoma are lacking. This type of lesion can also present as a mass within an apparently normal vein, most commonly in adults, and rarely as an organizing extravascular hematoma. Foci of intravascular papillary endothelial hyperplasia are common in VM and help distinguish these low-flow lesions from high-flow arteriovenous malformations.

Glomuvenous Malformations

Lesions characterized by presence of benign glomus cells have been subclassified historically into categories such as diffuse type, solitary type, multiple type, solid type, adult type, and pediatric type. Current evidence supports division of these lesions into two major categories: (1) the glomus tumor proper, a cellular neoplasm that tends to be well circumscribed, solitary, and subungual, and (2) the so-called glomangioma, a frequently multifocal lesion, more properly termed *glomuvenous malformation*, that presents in infants or children and histologically resembles a venous malformation in which lesional vessels are surrounded by layers of glomus cells. The following discussion is restricted to this second category, which accounts for 10–20 % of all glomus cell lesions.

Clinical

Glomuvenous malformations (GVMs) are superficial lesions becoming evident in childhood or adolescence and generally covering a large area of skin and/or subcutis. They appear either as multiple, widely distributed to confluent, soft, red-to-blue nodules, or as pink to deep blue multifocal plaques. Although clinically resembling venous malformations, GVMs differ in a number of ways. They tend to be more nodular or cobblestone-like in appearance, appear bluer and less compressible, and do not swell with exercise or dependency [19].

GVM is less painful than the glomus tumor proper but may be tender to palpation, and attacks of pain may occur during menstruation and pregnancy. All reported cases have behaved in a benign fashion. Due to their more expansive, multifocal nature, GVM is less amenable to surgery than common adult-type glomus tumors and may recur locally following subtotal resections and may progress locally [20]. Sclerotherapy is less effec-

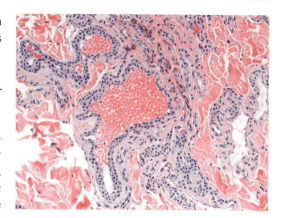

Fig. 21.3 Glomuvenous malformation

tive for GVMs than for venous malformations [20, 21]. Most GVM is sporadic; some rare familial cases have demonstrated an autosomal dominant pattern of inheritance [22, 23]. Based on linkage disequilibrium studies with these families, a locus for glomangiomas (termed *VMGLOM*) has been mapped to chromosome 1p21-p22 and codes for a protein of still uncertain function termed glomulin [24–26]. Sporadic glomangiomas likely result from somatic mutations at this locus.

Microscopic Features

GVM consists of dilated, thin-walled veins in the dermis and subcutis, often distributed as separate nodules. They are histologically similar to those comprising venous malformations but are surrounded by one or more layers of cuboidal glomus cells (Fig. 21.3). The glomus cell component can be quite variable from region to region and vessel to vessel, making adequate sampling important. Like venous malformations without glomus cells, many GVMs contain organizing thrombi or phleboliths.

Arteriovenous Malformations

Clinical

Like all vascular malformations, arteriovenous malformations (AVMs) are the result of errors in vascular morphogenesis and are not neoplastic in

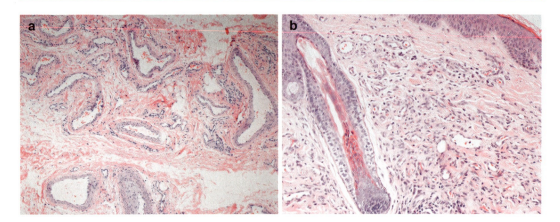

Fig. 21.4 (**a**) Arteriovenous malformation. (**b**) Arteriovenous malformation, cutaneous

origin. Use of the outdated term "arteriovenous hemangioma" is thus inappropriate. AVM is usually evident at birth and associated with an often clinically significant degree of arteriovenous shunting. Those with superficial extension may produce a palpable thrill or pulsation. Clinically significant hemorrhage and local tissue ischemia due to arterial steal are relatively common. Deep lesions may not become apparent until later in childhood or even adolescence or adulthood if shunting is low grade. AVMs tend to progress over time as collateral arterial flow is recruited into the low-resistance vascular bed. For the same reason, they often recur with a vengeance if incompletely excised or inadequately embolized. Unlike AV fistulas, which are often acquired lesions and are characterized by one or a few large AV shunts, AVMs are more complex developmental anomalies with a myriad, perhaps millions, of small abnormal AV connections that bypass a normally controlled, high-resistance vascular bed.

The vast majority of AVMs are sporadically occurring single lesions of unknown etiology. AV shunts are seen less commonly in familial disorders such as hereditary hemorrhagic telangiectasia (HHT) and the capillary malformation-arteriovenous malformation disorder (CMAVM). CMAVM, characterized by multiple atypical cutaneous capillary stains and increased incidence of arteriovenous malformations, is caused by inactivating mutations in *RASA1* [27]. HHT, also known as Osler-Rendu-Weber syndrome, is an autosomal dominant disorder characterized by multisystemic

angiodysplasia leading to frequent epistaxis, telangiectasias, GI bleeding, and arteriovenous shunts in the liver, brain, and lung. It has been linked to mutations in two genes and has therefore been designated HHT type 1 (HHT1; gene, *endoglin*; chromosome 9q34.1) and HHT type 2 (HHT2; gene, *ALK-1*, chromosome 12q11-q14) [28, 29]. HHT in association with juvenile polyposis has been linked to mutations in *SMAD4* [30].

Microscopic Features

The histological appearance of AVMs often varies considerably from one area to another, and the actual arteriovenous shunts are difficult to find without extensive sectioning or special techniques. Most histological sections show beds of arterioles, capillaries, and venules within a densely fibrous or fibromyxomatous background, intermixed with numerous larger caliber arteries and thick-walled veins (Fig. 21.4a). The arteries are often tortuous, and the veins typically show adventitial fibrosis and irregular intimal fibrosis. There is no evidence of thrombosis or intravascular papillary endothelial hyperplasia, consistent with the abnormally high venous flow. Involved skin often contains a prominent "pseudoangiosarcomatous" proliferation of small vessels, creating a ragged, cellular appearance that lacks the delicate lobularity of IH (Fig. 21.4b). Isolated foci of mitotically active small vessel proliferation reminiscent of a vascular tumor such as infantile hemangioma or pyogenic granuloma can also be seen in more deeply seated regions of many AVM, admixed with the large vessel component. This proliferative component may dominate the histological picture in deep intramuscular AVMs, particularly those involving the tongue, potentially leading to a misdiagnosis of hemangioma. These unusually cellular AVMs, like the more typical forms of AVM, are negative for GLUT1 and other infantile hemangioma-associated antigens [5, 31]. Clinical and radiological correlation with histology is essential in the diagnosis of AVM.

Arterial embolization using polyvinyl alcohol or other foreign materials precedes most surgical resections of AVMs, in order to reduce intraoperative bleeding. This elicits a variable acute inflammatory response within the involved tissues. Tissue necrosis is a rare complication.

Lymphatic Malformations

Clinical

Lymphatic malformations (LM) have traditionally been referred to as "lymphangiomas," despite general absence of significant endothelial mitotic activity. Just as blood vascular malformations are presumed to be developmental errors in morphogenesis of the blood vasculature, LM are thought to be errors in morphogenesis of the lymphatic vascular system. Relatively superficial LM are usually evident at birth or within the first year or two of life. In addition to the more common presentations in skin and subcutis, LM may also involve deeper soft tissues, bone, or viscera and may not become evident until older childhood or later. They can be localized or regional and may diffusely involve many tissue planes or organ systems.

In current practice, it has been found to be useful to subclassify LM as either macrocystic, microcystic, or combined. Macrocystic LMs, defined arbitrarily by a cyst diameter of at least 0.5 cm, have traditionally been termed "cystic hydromas." Microcystic LMs are more common and may develop anywhere. Macrocystic LM most commonly occurs in the loose connective tissue of the neck, axilla, chest wall, or groin and often changes in size due to progressive distention of the lymphatic spaces by lymph fluid. LM often enlarges with systemic or local infection. Surgical excision of macrocystic LM has significant morbidity, and a mainstay of therapy has become sclerotherapy with irritants such as killed bacteria (OK-432) or doxycycline [32, 33]. Combined microcystic and macrocystic LMs are common and perhaps even the norm. Treatment of microcystic and combined microcystic-macrocystic LM is problematic; sclerotherapy for these is generally ineffective.

LM is often associated with significant soft tissue (particularly fat) and bony overgrowth. LM involving the superficial skin or mucosae typically forms fragile, clear surface vesicles that often ulcerate or bleed and become dark. Many dermal or mucosal lymphatic malformations are associated with more deeply seated lesions composed of larger vessels, explaining the frequent recurrence of resected dermal lesions. Upper airway obstruction is a significant risk in LM involving the tongue or oropharynx. Chylous ascites/intestinal lymphangiectasia or pleural or pericardial effusions may complicate abdominal and thoracic LM.

Generalized lymphatic anomaly (GLA), often called "lymphangiomatosis," is an extensive LM involving viscera and/or bone, often with coincident involvement of skin or soft tissues. Spleen, liver, lung, and intestine are commonly involved viscera. Clinical morbidity is high due to the lung involvement, effusions, and bone erosion and fracture.

Microscopic Features

Microcystic LMs are comprised by dilated small vessels with angular-to-rounded contours lined by a single layer of flattened-to-slightly hobnailed endothelial cells, rimmed by rare pericytes and little or no smooth muscle (Fig. 21.5a). These are filled with clear fluid and sometimes a few lymphocytes and/or macrophages. Traumatized lymphatic vessels may contain abundant erythrocytes.

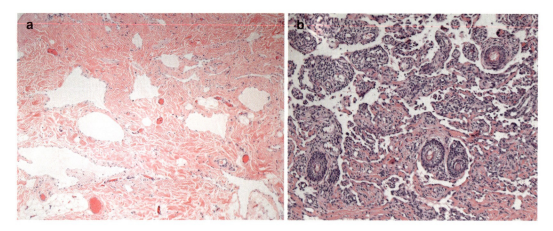

Fig. 21.5 (**a**) Lymphatic malformation. (**b**) Lymphatic malformation, infiltrative pattern

In microcystic LMs involving skin or mucosa, the dilated lymphatic vessels often protrude into superficial vascular papillae, causing bleb formation and epidermal/mucosal hyperplasia. Overlying epidermis may appear hyperkeratotic and verrucous, and the surrounding stroma may be fibrotic and chronically inflamed. The vessels of diffusely infiltrative microcystic LMs often wrap extensively around tissue structures, producing the appearance of free-floating tissue elements and a complex anastomosing vasculature reminiscent of lymphangiosarcoma (Fig. 21.5b). Focal lymphoendothelial spindling and hyperplasia may be evident in some of the lesional vessels of these diffuse LM. A low but appreciable level of proliferative activity indicated by cell cycle markers such as Ki-67 may be present.

Macrocystic LM vessels have thicker, irregular coats of smooth muscle and/or fibrous tissue and may have valves. Vessel lumens usually contain proteinaceous material and a few lymphocytes and/or macrophages. In many LM, the enlarged lumina contain abundant blood or organizing myxoid thrombus material resulting from vessel wall injury or communication with the venous system. This makes it difficult to distinguish veins from lymphatics and may suggest a venous or mixed venous-lymphatic malformation. This distinction can usually be made by immunoreaction for antigens such as podoplanin (with the D2-40 antibody) that are expressed by lymphatic endothelial, but not blood vascular endothelial cells (Fig. 21.6). The surrounding

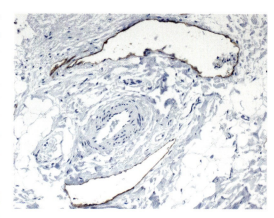

Fig. 21.6 Lymphatic malformation, podoplanin immunostain

stroma often shows a lymphocytic infiltrate varying from a few scattered cells to striking, organoid aggregates containing lymphoid follicles.

Gorham-Stout disease, aka "disappearing bone disease," is a form of GLA characterized by prominent, typically multifocal intraosseous LM. The affected bones undergo cystic cortical osteolysis due to progressively dilated intraosseous lymphatic spaces, resulting in "disappearance" of bones in imaging studies, particularly plain film. Histologically, dilated, extremely thin-walled lymphatic vessels that may be extremely difficult to appreciate in routine sections expand the marrow space, compressing and eventually thinning the cortical bone, sometimes to the point of pathological fracture. Immunohistochemistry for the pan-endothelial marker CD31 is useful to identify the endothelial lining of the cystically dilated spaces, and immunohistochemistry for podoplanin confirms lymphatic differentiation. In many patients with multifocal bony involvement by LM, viscera (especially spleen) are also affected by LM. Periosseous soft tissue extension into soft tissue is common. Rare cases of osteolysis with similar but localized clinical and radiological presentation may be associated with VM or AV fistula instead of LM.

Some spontaneously aborted fetuses with posterior cervical swellings traditionally referred to as "cystic hydroma" have been shown to have increased cutaneous lymphatics (e.g., trisomies 13 and 21), whereas those with monosomy X (Turner's syndrome) do not show increased or dilated lymphatics [34].

Combined Venous-Lymphatic Malformations

The close relationship between the lymphatic and venous systems during embryonic development may explain why some low-flow malformations include both lymphatic and venous and/or capillary components. Lesions from patients with Klippel-Trénaunay syndrome (KTS) and related disorders most consistently exemplify this phenomenon, but solitary mixed malformations of lymphatic, venous, and capillary vessels are also commonly observed in nonsyndromic patients. KTS envelops a spectrum of complex, segmental congenital disorders characterized by a variable combination of lymphatic and capillary-venous malformations associated with skeletal and adipose tissue overgrowth in the involved segment [2, 3].

Microscopic Features

The histology of KTS is generally typical of VM and LM, with variably distributed components of each. Overlying areas of cutaneous involvement compounded by reaction to expansion of dermal papillae by ectatic capillaries or lymphatics create a PWS-like surface stain (although distinct from PWS histologically) punctuated by angiokeratoma-like lesions. Eccrine glands are often notably enlarged and surrounded by myxoid stroma. Veins may demonstrate striking mural smooth muscle disarray. The malformations are largely cutaneous and subcutaneous but may also infiltrate deep skeletal muscle. Subcutaneous fat is increased.

References

1. Mulliken JB, Glowacki J (1982) Hemangiomas and vascular malformations in infants and children: a classification based on endothelial characteristics. Plast Reconstr Surg 69:412–422
2. Easterly NB (1995) Cutaneous hemangiomas, vascular stains and malformations, and associated syndromes [Review]. Curr Probl Dermatol 7:67–108
3. Mulliken JB, Fishman SJ, Burrows PE (2000) Vascular anomalies. Curr Probl Surg 37:519–584
4. North PE, Waner M, Mizeracki A et al (2000) GLUT1: a newly discovered immunohistochemical marker for juvenile hemangiomas. Hum Pathol 31:11–22
5. North PE, Waner M, Mizeracki A et al (2001) A unique microvascular phenotype shared by juvenile hemangiomas and human placenta. Arch Dermatol 137:559–570
6. North PE, Waner M, Buckmiller L, James CA, Mihm MC (2006) Vascular tumors of infancy and childhood: beyond capillary hemangioma. Cardiovasc Pathol 15:303–317
7. North PE (2008) Vascular tumors and malformations of infancy and childhood. Pathol Case Rev 13(6):213–235
8. North PE, Mihm MC Jr (2001) Histopathological diagnosis of infantile hemangiomas and vascular malformations. In: Hochman M (ed) Vascular lesions. Facial Plast Surg Clin North Am 9:505–524
9. North PE (2010) Vascular tumors and malformations, in surgical pathology clinics, vol 3(3). Elsevier Saunders, Philadelphia, pp 455–494
10. Shirley MD, Tang H, Gallione CJ, Baugher JD, Frelin LP, Cohen B, North PE, Marchuk DA, Comi AM, Pevsner J (2013) Sturge-Weber syndrome and port-wine stains caused by somatic mutation in GNAQ. N Engl J Med 368(21):1971–1979
11. North PE, Sanchez-Carpintero I, Mizeracki A, Waner M, Mihm MC (2003) The distinctive histology of lip enlargement in port-wine stains: a clinicopathological study. Lab Invest 83(1):96A
12. Sanchez-Carpintero I, Mihm MC, Waner M, Mizeracki A, North PE (2004) Epithelial and mesenchymal hamartomatous changes in mature port-wine stains: morphological evidence for a multiple germ layer field defect. J Am Acad Dermatol 50(4):606–612
13. Bean WB (1958) Anomalous vascular spiders and related lesions of the skin. Charles C. Thomas, Springfield

14. Weiss SW (1988) Pedal hemangioma (venous malformation) occurring in Turner's syndrome: an additional manifestation of the syndrome. Hum Pathol 19:1015–1018

15. Calvert JT, Riney TJ, Kontos CD et al (1999) Allelic and locus heterogeneity in inherited venous malformations. Hum Mol Genet 8:1279–1289

16. Vikkula M, Boon LM, Carraway KL 3rd et al (1996) Vascular dysmorphogenesis caused by an activating mutation in the receptor tyrosine kinase TIE2. [see comments]. Cell 87:1181–1190

17. Suri C, Jones PF, Patan S et al (1996) Requisite role of anigopoietin-1, a ligand for the TIE2 receptor, during embryonic angiogenesis. Cell 87:1171–1180

18. Soblet J, Limaye N, Uebelhoer M, Boon LM, Vikkula M (2013) Variable somatic TIE2 mutations in half of sporadic venous malformations. Mol Syndromol 4: 179–183

19. Mounaycr C, Wassef M, Enjolras O et al (2001) Facial 'glomangiomas': large facial venous malformations with glomus cells. J Am Acad Dermatol 45:239–245

20. Gould EW, Manivel JC, Albores-Saavedra J et al (1990) Locally infiltrative glomus tumors and glomangiosarcomas. A clinical, ultrastructural, and immunohistochemical study. Cancer 65:310–318

21. Yang JS, Ko JW, Suh KS et al (1999) Congenital multiple plaque-like glomangiomyoma. Am J Dermatopathol 21:454–457

22. Rycroft RJ, Menter MA, Sharvill DE et al (1975) Hereditary multiple glomus tumours. Report of four families and a review of literature. Trans St Johns Hosp Dermatol Soc 61:70–81

23. Wood WS, Dimmick JE (1977) Multiple infiltrating glomus tumors in children. Cancer 40:1680–1685

24. Irrthum A, Brouillard P, Enjolras O et al (2001) Linkage disequilibrium narrows locus for venous malformation with glomus cells (VMGLOM) to a single 1.48 Mbp YAC. Eur J Hum Genet 9:34–38

25. Brouillard P, Olsen BR, Vikkula M (2000) High-resolution physical and transcript map of the locus for venous malformations with glomus cells (VMGLOM) on chromosome 1p21-p22. Genomics 67:96–101

26. Brouillard P, Boon LM, Vikkula M (2002) Mutations in a novel factor, glomulin, are responsible for glomuvenous malformations ("glomangiomas"). Am J Hum Genet 70:866–874

27. Eerola I, Boon LM, Mulliken JB et al (2003) Capillary malformation-arteriovenous malformation, a heretofore undescribed clinical and genetic entity, is caused by RASA1 mutations. Am J Hum Genet 73:1240–1249

28. McAllister KA, Grogg KM, Johnson DW et al (1994) Endoglin, a TGF-beta binding protein of endothelial cells, is the gene for hereditary haemorrhagic telangiectasia type 1. Nat Genet 8:345–351

29. Johnson DW, Berg JN, Baldwin MA et al (1996) Mutations in the activin receptor-like kinase 1 gcnc in hereditary haemorrhagic telangiectasia type 2. Nat Genet 13:189–195

30. Gallione CJ, Repetto GM, Legius E et al (2004) A combined syndrome of juvenile polyposis and hereditary haemorrhagic telangiectasia associated with mutations in MADH4 (SMAD4). Lancet 363:852–859

31. North PE, Mizeracki A, Thomas JR et al (2000) Intramuscular "hemangiomas" are vascular malformations immunodistinct from juvenile hemangiomas. Lab Invest 80:14A

32. Brewis C, Pracy JP, Albert DM (2000) Treatment of lymphangiomas of the head and neck in children by intralesional injection of OK-432 (Picibanil). Clin Otolaryngol 25:130–135

33. Molitch HI, Unger EC, White EL et al (1995) Percutaneous sclerotherapy of lymphangiomas. Radiology 194:343–347

34. Chitayat D, Kalousek DK, Bamforth JS et al (1989) Lymphatic abnormalities in fetuses with posterior cervical cystic hydroma. Am J Med Genet 33:352–356

Classification of Vascular Malformations

22

Raul Mattassi and Dirk A. Loose

Because of their great variability, congenital vascular malformations (CVM) were difficult to understand. Evolution of classification and terminology reflected that main problem which exists even today.

Classification

In the past centuries, several classifications were based on description. Early reports were effective to understand some clinical pictures, like the accurate description of John Bell of arteriovenous malformations [1].

At this time and till much later, the difference between hemangioma and CVM was not clear, and many descriptions include one or the other disease or both in the same series.

In 1863 Rudolf Virchow, the father of cellular pathology, called all vascular anomalous masses "angioma." They divided them in *angioma simplex*, *angioma cavernosum*, and *angioma racemosum* [2]. The difference was based on the type of vessels of the defect: the angioma simplex was composed of capillaries, angioma cavernosum by large vascular channels, and angioma racemosum by a large number of dilated vessels that may connect. The classification of Virchow was for a long time the most accepted internationally.

Further attempts to classify the unclear group of "vascular tumors" were centered on the effort to differentiate tumors of malformative origin from true neoplasm.

In 1928, Cushing and Bailey, working on the tumors of the central nervous system, made a difference between *hamartomas*, anomalous agglomerations of vessels present at birth with or without a proliferative tendency but not malign, and *angiomas*, neoplasms that have a late onset. They introduced also the term "hemangioblastoma," a tumor of the central nervous system that originates from the vessels [3].

In 1930 Costa, based on a review of the literature, divided vascular neoformations in *hamartomas*, of a neoformative origin (divided in capillary, simple, cavernous, and arteriovenous), and *angioblastomas* with a proliferative tendency. The last group was divided in benign forms, as hypertrophic angioma, hemangioendothelioma, and hemangiopericytoma, and true tumors [4].

In 1942 Thomas divided vascular tumors in benign and malign angiomas: in the second group he included hemangioendothelioma and angiosarcoma [5].

Masson (1953) divided angiomas in *dysgenetic* (capillary angioma, cavernoma, venous angioma, and arteriovenous angioma), *hyperplastic*

R. Mattassi (✉)
Center for Vascular Malformations "Stefan Belov",
Department of Vascular Surgery,
Clinical Institute Humanitas "Mater Domini",
Castellanza (Varese), Italy
e-mail: raulmattassi@gmail.com

D.A. Loose
Section Vascular Surgery and Angiology,
Facharztklinik Hamburg, Hamburg, Germany
e-mail: info@prof-loose.de

R. Mattassi et al. (eds.), *Hemangiomas and Vascular Malformations: An Atlas of Diagnosis and Treatment*,
DOI 10.1007/978-88-470-5673-2_22, © Springer-Verlag Italia 2009, 2015

(hypertrophic and hyperplastic angioma, pyogenic granuloma, hemangioendothelioma, hemangiopericytoma, and plexiform angioma), and *neoplastic hemangiomas* (angiosarcoma and angioplastic sarcoma) [6].

Landing and Farber in 1956 expressed the opinion, in accordance with several authors including Masson, that simple angiomas are congenital and originate from embryonic seizures of the mesodermal tissue [7].

In 1967, Stout and Lattes propose a new classification that presented in a simple form of the topic. They called all the defects "hemangiomatosis" and distinguished *angiomatosis* (capillary, venous and arteriovenous hemangioma, and all synonyms), *lymphangiomatosis* (all lymphatic dysplasia), and *angiosarcomatosis* (malignant vascular tumors, like hemangioendothelioma and hemangiopericytoma) [8].

The main progress in the understanding and classification of CVM was the publication of Malan and Puglionisi in 1964 [9]. Based on his extensive practical work, he proposed a classification centered on *anatomo-clinical pictures*. "We find it far more desirable to differentiate the vascular malformations into a number of anatomo-clinical pictures, each with a precise definition of the pathogenetic role of the vascular abnormality, of its evolution and of the therapeutic possibilities," the authors wrote [10]. He introduced the concept of the "predominant type of involved vessel," as he noticed that malformations rarely affect one type of vessel alone but often polyangiopathies are in question. His classification of CVM (or "angiodysplasias," as he suggested to call them), widely accepted for a long time in the international literature (even today in some groups), distinguished between venous, arterial, and associated arterial and venous defects. In the last group he included arteriovenous malformations. Capillary malformations were not included [9] (Table 22.1).

In this classification for the first time, they clearly made a difference between defects of the main vessels (like congenital aneurysms, abnormal course, and aplasia) and direct communication between the main artery and vein (arteriovenous fistulas), which he called "troncular" (derived from the embryological term used by several embryologists at the beginning of the century) [11, 12] and

Table 22.1 Classification of Malan and Puglionisi [9]

Venous angiodysplasias
Phlebectatic dysplasias
Phlebangiomas
Phlebangiomatosis
Combinations
Arterial angiodysplasias
Associated arterial and venous angiodysplasias
True phlebarteriectasia
Angiodysplasia with arteriovenous shunt
Mixed angiodysplasias

"angioma" indicating areas of fistulous tissue or areas of dysplastic veins infiltrating tissues.

He considered that the difference between both groups was due to a different embryological phase in which the vessel development is affected by a pathological process: in the early phase, remnants of the primitive vascular network remain in tissues, while in the late phase anomalies of the main vessels may develop.

Stefan Belov, a Bulgarian pioneer in the treatment of CVM, proposed a classification which was influenced by the publications of Malan and was also based on *morphology* which he considered crucial to understand CVM. He took over the distinction of Malan between defects of the main vessels and peripheral malformations. However, in a much more clearer and organic classification, he distinguished the *defects of the main vessels* that referred separately to arteries, veins, and lymphatics, including direct arteriovenous fistulas, in the "troncular" group. *Peripheral defects* were divided into limited and infiltrating forms of the single types (venous, arteriovenous, or lymphatic) and called "extratruncular," to differentiate them from the first group [13–15] (Table 22.2). As Malan, he accepted the concept that the truncular and extratruncular forms are the result of a defect in the embryological development of vessels. The new data about genetics may confirm that concepts (see chap. 2). The distinction between the truncular and extratruncular forms, not clearly pointed out by other classifications, proved effective also in the practical approach. This classification was called "Hamburg Classification" because she was discussed and approved during a workshop held in Hamburg (Germany) in 1988 by the working group of vascular anomalies which later became ISSVA (International Society for the

Table 22.2 Hamburg classification (1989)

Types	Forms	
	Truncular	Extratruncular
Predominantly arterial defects	Aplasia or obstruction	Infiltrating
	Dilatation	Limited
Predominantly venous defects	Aplasia or obstruction	Infiltrating
	Dilatation	Limited
Predominantly AV shunting defects	Deep	Infiltrating
	Superficial	Limited
Combined/mixed defects	Arterial and venous without shunt	Infiltrating hemolymphatic
	Hemolymphatic with or without shunt	Limited hemolymphatic

Table 22.3 ISSVA classification (1996)

Tumors	Malformations	
	Simple	Combined
Hemangioma	Capillary (C)	AVF, AVM, CVM
	Lymphatic (L)	LVM, CAVM, CLAVM
Others	Venous (V)	

Table 22.4 Classification of Mulliken and Glowacki [17]

Slow flow
Capillary (CM)
Lymphatic (LM)
Venous (VM)
Fast flow
Arterial (AM): aneurysm, coarctation, ectasias
Arteriovenous fistulas (AVF)
Arteriovenous (AVM)
Complex combined (often associated with skeletal overgrowth)
Regional syndromes

Table 22.5 Modified Hamburg classification (2007)

Primary classification
Arterial malformations
Venous malformations
Arteriovenous malformations
Lymphatic malformations
Capillary malformation
Combined vascular malformations
Morphological/embryological subclassification
Extratruncular forms
Diffuse, infiltrating
Limited, localized
Truncular forms
Obstruction or narrowing
Aplasia, hypoplasia, hyperplasia
Obstruction due to atresia or membranous occlusion
Stenosis due to coarctation, spur, or membrane
Dilatation
Localized (aneurysm)
Diffuse (ectasias)

Study of Vascular Anomalies (see Chap. 3), as a guidance to diagnosis.

The original Hamburg classification was later modified by adding the capillary malformations, which was missing in the original form and was one of the critics moved to it [16] (Table 22.3).

The difference between hemangiomas and vascular malformations remains unclear until the studies of Judah Volkmann in Boston who demonstrated that hemangiomas are lesions that have a hyperplasia of the endothelium, while malformations have a normal endothelial turnover.

The publication of Mulliken and Glowacki in 1982, which reported the studies of Volkmann, definitively distinguished hemangiomas from vascular malformations as two different entities, based on cellular kinetics, physical examination, and natural history. They proposed a classification which they called "biological classification," underlining the specific difference between hemangiomas and CVM [17–19].

Their classification of CVM was based on *hemodynamics*, dividing CVM in high-flow and low-flow lesions, adding syndromes of complex cases in a group of combined complex defects. This classification proved to be an excellent guide to understand the hemodynamics of CVM and is today widely accepted (Table 22.4).

In 1994, during the international workshop in Budapest, ISSVA nominated a commission of two experts, Dirk Loose from Germany and Odile Enjolras from France, in order to propose a common classification. The result of their work was presented during the workshop in Rome, in 1996,

Table 22.6 ISSVA classification of vascular anomalies (updated 2014)

Vascular anomalies				
Vascular tumors			Vascular malformations	
	Simple	Combined	Of major named vessels	Associated with other anomalies
Benign	Capillary (CM)	CVM, CLM	Arteries, veins, lymphatics	Include 11 types
Locally aggressive or borderline	Lymphatic (LM) Venous (VM)	LVM, CLVM	Anomalies of origin, course, Anomalies of origin, course, CLAVM	
Malignant	Arteriovenous (AVM)			
	Artreriovenous fistulas (AVF)			

and was accepted officially by ISSVA (Table 22.5). Several updates and changes of this classification were published independently by several authors in the latter years. The classification is accepted and extensively used internationally [20–22].

The Hamburg classification is also widely accepted today, including two main international consensus, one about management of venous malformations and one about arteriovenous and in some main textbooks of vascular surgery [23–25].

In the international workshop of ISSVA held in Melbourne in 2014, an updated ISSVA classification was presented and accepted. The new, updated version, a result of the tremendous work of Michel Vassef from Paris, will distinguish capillary, lymphatic, venous, and arteriovenous malformations and arteriovenous fistulas. Also defects of the main named vessels (called also "truncal": the same as the "truncular" defects of the Hamburg classification), combined forms, and association with other defects are considered (Table 22.6). Several subgroups will be included in order to include all new discoveries, like the genetic-related clinical pictures and others. The whole classification, aiming to include all subgroups of vascular defects, the recently known genetic data and also the unclassified defects, is very complex, including several tables. This new proposal includes the principal points of the Hamburg classification and may bring to a general accordance about classification.

Some other classifications has been proposed for specific topics in CVM, like the one proposed by Schobinger, based on the clinical picture of the patient, which is widely used today (Table 22.7).

Capillary malformations of the skin, called also port-wine stains (PWS), can be classified

Table 22.7 Clinical classification of Schobinger

Stage I – Quiescence: pink-bluish stain, warmth, and arteriovenous shunting are revealed by Doppler scanning. The arteriovenous malformation mimics a capillary malformation or involuting hemangioma

Stage II – Expansion: stage I plus enlargement, pulsations, thrill, bruit, and tortuous/tense veins

Stage III – Destruction: stage II plus dystrophic skin changes, ulceration, bleeding, tissue necrosis. Bony lytic lesions may occur

Stage IV – Decompensation: stage III plus congestive cardiac failure with increased cardiac output and left ventricle hypertrophy

Table 22.8 Wagner grading system of capillary malformations

Grade	Description
1	Light pink macules, vessel diameter <80 μm
2	Dark pink macules, vessel diameter 80–120 μm
3	Red macules, vessel diameter 120–150 μm
4	Purple macules and papules, vessel diameter >150 μm

according to the Wagner grading system [26] Table 22.8.

Angiographic pictures of venous and of AV malformations have contributed to the development of specific classifications, mainly related to treatment. More details are discussed in Chaps. 29 and 33.

Terminology

Few diseases have generated a large number of different names as CVM. Old terms of only historical significance, like nevus angiectoides, varice aneurysm, cirsoid aneurysm, red angioma telangiectaticum, hamartoma, racemose aneu-rysm, nevus anemicus, and many others, can be found in the literature.

However, even today there is still a diffuse, incorrect use of terminology regarding CVM which is the cause of confusion and difficult comprehension of the diseases.

The term "angioma." In order to reduce confusion with infantile hemangioma, in a session dedicated to terminology and classification during the workshop of vascular malformations, held in Hamburg, Germany, in 1988, it has been recommended to avoid using that term.

"Hemangioma," a term that should be well known in its meaning, is even today used in incorrect forms. In a review of the literature, "hemangioma" has been incorrectly used in 71.3 % of publications [27].

"Cavernous hemangioma" is even more extensively used to describe vascular malformations (mainly venous) all over the body: a literature control of the term is demonstrated in over 7,000 papers, which includes the term "posttraumatic cavernous hemangioma."

Another confusing terminology is that related to some clinical pictures of CVM, described in literature with the definition of syndromes. The best known is the paper of Klippel-Trenaunay, which referred about cases of CVM of the lower limbs with a clinical "triad" of cutaneous nevus, dilated veins, and limb elongation [28]; Parkes Weber described similar cases with also clinical signs of arteriovenous shunt [29]. Today, the terminology of "Klippel-Trenaunay syndrome" (KTS) or Parkes Weber syndrome (PWS) should be used only after a specific diagnosis in order to recognize the vascular defects in a complex situation. However, KTS has become a way to express an easy diagnosis, often by inexperienced people. It is common to find a diagnosis of KTS or (less common) PWS, given without any instrumental examination, based simply on a clinical observation of the patient. Those diagnoses have also been given to locations outside the limbs, as, for example, "KT of the ear" for an AV malformation of the ear lobe! It is also common to meet the diagnosis of "Klippel-Trenaunay-Weber syndrome," a compromise between forms with and without AV malformations which is nonsense. Those superficial diagnoses, often incorrect, may have severe psychological consequences for the patient and parents. The main recommendation should be to strictly avoid the KTS and PWS diagnosis which should be reserved to experienced physicians, dedicated to CVM. The use of a much simpler and less challenging term of "probable vascular malformation" will be by far better accepted by the patients.

References

1. Bell J (1815) The principles of surgery. Longman, Hurst and Rees, London, pp 456–489
2. Virchof R (1863) Angiome. In: Die Krankhaften Geschwülste. Hischwald, Berlin
3. Cushing HW, Bailey P (1928) Tumors arising from the blood vessels of the brain; angiomatous malformations and hemangioblastomas. I Thomas, Springfield, p 195
4. Costa A (1930) Sulla classificazione e la dottrina degli emangiomi e delle malformazioni capillari. Policlinico Chir 37:57
5. Thomas A (1942) Vascular tumors of bone. A pathological and clinical study of twenty seven cases. Surg Gynecol Obstet 74:777–795
6. Masson F (1953) Tumeurs humaines. Librerie Maloine, Paris
7. Landing BH, Farber S (1956) Tumors of the cardiovascular system, Atlas of tumor pathology. Armed Forces Institute of Pathology, Washington, D.C
8. Stout AP, Lattes R (1967) Tumors of the soft tissues, Atlas of tumor pathology. Second series, Fascicle I. Armed Forces Institute of Pathology, Washington, D.C, pp 67–83
9. Malan E, Puglionisi A (1964) Congenital angiodysplasias of the extremities. Note I: Generalitires and classification; venous dysplasias. J Cardiovasc Surg 5:87–130
10. Malan E (1974) Vascular malformations (angiodysplasias). Carlo Erba Foundation, Milan, 17
11. Woolard HH (1922) (Woolard) The development of the principal arteries stem in the forelimb of the pig. Contrib Embryol Carnegie Inst 4:141–154
12. Reinhoff WF (1924) Congenital arteriovenous fistula, an embryological study with the report of a case. Bull Johns Hopkins Hosp 35:271–284
13. Belov S, Loose DA, Weber J (1989) Vascular malformations. Einhorn Presse, Reinbeck, p 29, Editor's comment: classification
14. Belov S (1990) Classification of congenital vascular defects. Int Angiol 9(3):141–146
15. Belov S (1993) Anatomopathological classification of congenital vascular defects. Semin Vasc Surg 6(4): 219–224

16. Lee BB, Laredo J, Lee TS et al (2007) Terminology and classification of congenital vascular malformations. Phlebology 22:249–252
17. Mulliken JB, Glowacki J (1982) Hemangiomas and vascular malformations in infants and children: a classification based on endothelial characteristics. Plast Reconstr Surg 69:412–420
18. Mulliken J (1993) Cutaneous vascular anomalies. Semin Vasc Surg 6(4):204–218
19. Mulliken JB (1988) Classification of vascular birthmarks. In: Grainger RG, Allison DJ (eds) Vascular birthmarks, haemangiomas, and malformations. WB Saunders, Philadelphia, pp 24–37
20. Mulliken JB, Burrows PE, Fishman SJ (2013) Vascular anomalies. Hemangiomas and malformations. Oxford University Press, New York
21. Enjolras O, Wassef W, Chapot R (2007) Color atlas of vascular tumors and vascular malformations. Cambridge University Press, New York
22. Nozaki T, Matusako M, Mimura H et al (2013) Imaging of vascular tumors with an emphasis on ISSVA classification. Jpn J Radiol 31(12):775–85
23. Lee BB,, Baumgartner I, Berlien P, Bianchini G, Burrow P, Gloviczki P, Huang, Y, Laredo J, Loose DA, Markovic J, Mattassi R, Parsi K, Rabe E, Rosenblatt M, Shortell C, Stillo F, Villavicencio L, Zamboni P; (2014). Diagnosis and treatment of venous malformations. Consensus document of the International Union of Phlebology (IUP) updated 2013. Int Angiol, June (Epub ahead of print)
24. Lee BB, Baumgartner I, Burrows P, Do YS, Ivancev K, Kool LS, Laredo J, Loose DA, Lopez-Gutierrez JC, Mattassi R, Rimon U, Shortell C, Simkin R, Stillo F, Villavicencio L, Parsi K, Yakes W (2013) Consensus document of the International Union of Angiology (IUA)-2013. Current concepts on the management of arterio-venous malformations. Int Angiol 32(1):9–36
25. Lee BB, Villavicencio L (2010) Congenital vascular malformations. General considerations. In: Cronenwett G, Johnston KW (eds) Rutherford's vascular surgery. Saunders, Philadelphia
26. Waner M, Suen JY (eds) (1999) Hemangiomas and vascular malformations of the head and neck. Wiley-Liss, New York
27. Hassanein AH, Mulliken JB, Fishman SJ, Green AK (2011) Evaluation of terminology for vascular anomalies in current literature. Plast Reconstr Surg 127(1):347–351
28. Klippel M, Trenaunay P (1900) Du noevus variqueux et osteohypertrophique. Arch Gen Med 3:641–672
29. Weber PF (1918) Haemangiectatic hypertrophy of limbs-congenital phlebarteriectasia and so-called congenital varicose veins. Br J Child Dis 15:13–17

Principles of Diagnostics

23

Raul Mattassi, Dirk A. Loose, and Massimo Vaghi

Introduction

Congenital vascular malformations (CVM) are extremely variable in type, site, extension, and secondary effects.

For these reasons, the diagnostic process may be difficult and often incomplete if there is not a guideline that helps to follow specific steps toward a complete comprehension of the single defect.

To proceed with diagnostics, some specific points should be cleared:

- Type of the defect
- Morphology
- Site
- Hemodynamic characteristics
- Secondary effects on structures and organs

According to the data to be recorded, the diagnostic process can be divided in three steps:

R. Mattassi (✉)
Center for Vascular Malformations "Stefan Belov",
Department of Vascular Surgery,
Clinical Institute Humanitas "Mater Domini",
Castellanza (Varese), Italy
e-mail: raulmattassi@gmail.com

D.A. Loose
Section Vascular Surgery and Angiology,
Facharztklinik Hamburg, Hamburg, Germany
e-mail: info@prof-loose.de

M. Vaghi
Department of Vascular Surgery, A.O.G. Salvini
Hospital, Garbagnate Milanese, Italy
e-mail: vaghim@yahoo.it

Step 1: Recognition or exclusion of a CVM. Hemodynamic study is crucial.

Step 2: Establishing anatomical localization, morphology, extension, and involvement of structures as well as secondary effects of the defect (bone growth anomalies, cardiac overloading).

Step 3: Definitive classification of the VM.

Diagnostic process should progress along the line that goes from clinical examination to noninvasive then less invasive up to invasive tests.

The first diagnostic tool after clinical evaluation is *duplex ultrasonography examination*, B mode for morphologic study and spectral, color, and power Doppler to find out flow characteristics [1]. This exam is effective and recommended in almost all cases of CVM. However, knowledge and experience on CVM of the physician/technician who performs the examination are required; otherwise, results will be incomplete. Duplex ultrasonography will be discussed in detail in Chap. 26.

The second examinations are *MR and CT without or with contrast*. These exams allow a better morphologic study and also hemodynamic data. Selection criteria between both will be discussed in Chap. 27.

The third group of examinations includes different tests performed mainly after the former two, according to the data obtained. It includes *lymphoscintigraphy*, *whole blood pool scintigraphy*, *transarterial lung perfusion scintigraphy*, *bone scanogram*, and others. Nuclear medicine test will be discussed in Chap. 28.

R. Mattassi et al. (eds.), *Hemangiomas and Vascular Malformations: An Atlas of Diagnosis and Treatment*,
DOI 10.1007/978-88-470-5673-2_23, © Springer-Verlag Italia 2009, 2015

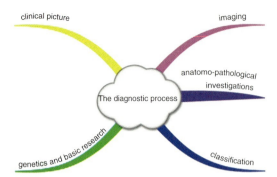

Fig. 23.1 Components of a complete diagnostic approach to a vascular malformation

The fourth group is the invasive tests group, including *catheter angiography* (mainly used during an intention-to-treat session, rather than as a pure diagnostic test), *phlebography* (performed only in selected cases and with specific skills), and *lymphography* (very rarely used today).

The final goal of the diagnostic process should be the precise definition, according to a classification, of the single case (see Chap. 22). Single diagnostic tools will be discussed in detail in the following chapters (Figs. 23.1) [2–4].

References

1. Laroche JP, Becker F, Khau-Van-Kien A, Baudoin P, Brisot D, Buffler A, Coupé M, Jurus C, Mestre S, Miserey G, Soulier-Sotto V, Tissot A, Viard A, Vignes S, Quéré I, Société française de médecine vasculaire (2013) Quality standards for ultrasonographic assessment of peripheral vascular malformations and vascular tumors. Report of the French Society for Vascular Medicine. J Mal Vasc 38(1):29–42
2. Lee BB, Baumgartner I, Berlien HP, Bianchini G, Burrows P, Do YS, Ivancev K, Kool LS, Laredo J, Loose DA, Lopez-Gutierrez JC, Mattassi R, Parsi K, Rimon U, Rosenblatt M, Shortell C, Simkin R, Stillo F, Villavicencio L, Yakes W (2013) Consensus document of the International Union of Angiology (IUA)-2013. Current concept on the management of arterio-venous. Int Angiol 32(1):9–36
3. Lee BB, Baumgartner I, Berlien P, Bianchini G, Burrows P, Gloviczki P, Huang Y, Laredo J, Loose DA, Markovic J, Mattassi R, Parsi K, Rabe E, Rosenblatt M, Shortell C, Stillo F, Vaghi M, Villavicencio L, Zamboni P (2014) Diagnosis and treatment of venous malformations consensus document of the International Union of Phlebology (IUP): updated 2013. Int Angiol. [Epub ahead of print]
4. Legiehn GM, Heran MK (2010) A step-by-step practical approach to imaging diagnosis and interventional radiologic therapy in vascular malformations. Semin Intervent Radiol 27(2):209–231

Clinical Aspects in Vascular Malformations

24

Byung-Boong Lee, James Laredo,
and Richard F. Neville

General Overview

Since the turn of the last century, relentless efforts were made on the congenital vascular malformation (CVM) for better understanding. But, the CVM still remains as an enigma in modern medicine with such wide range of clinical presentation, unpredictable clinical course, and erratic response to the treatment with high recurrence: the most difficult and confusing diagnostic as well as therapeutic challenge among various vascular disorders [1–3].

To make the condition worse, the old terminology and classification, based solely on the limited clinical knowledge, added more confusion on its definition and management till lately [4–6]. The most serious mistake old terminology caused to CVM was to have it mixed up with genuine hemangioma by misunderstanding and calling it hemangioma as well.

(Neonatal/infantile) hemangioma is *NOT* a vascular malformation. Hemangioma is a postnatal vascular tumor with a distinctive pattern of initial proliferative phase of explosive growth followed by involutional phase of spontaneous

regression. Hemangioma would therefore need "wait and see" watching for its natural regression first till proven otherwise. But, the CVM as the outcome of defective development of vascular structure would never go away but steadily grow throughout life. They need the treatment and not the conservation [7–9] (Fig. 24.1).

In other words, both CVM and hemangioma are two entirely different conditions with different management and prognosis. The CVMs are "self-perpetuating" slowly progressing embryonic tissue remnant as a birth defect. On the contrary, the hemangioma is a "self-limited" vascular (Fig. 24.1) tumor starting in early neonatal period as a rapid growing lesion in its majority but soon followed by steady regression before reaching to the age of 7. Therefore, the differentiation between the CVM and (infantile/neonatal) hemangioma will be the first most important step for the proper diagnosis of the CVMs for correct management [10–12].

The second most important aspect of the CVM is that "CVM is NOT a single vascular disorder;" it represents a group of various vascular defects with much different characteristics and clinical behaviors. The CVM is the outcome of developmental arrest during various stages of the embryogenesis, depending upon the circulation systems affected by this inborn error – artery, vein, lymphatic, and capillary – and also the embryonic stages, early or late, when it developed; the CVM will become a venous, arterial, lymphatic, as well as capillary malformation

B.-B. Lee, MD, PhD, FACS (✉) • J. Laredo
R.F. Neville
Division of Vascular Surgery, Department of Surgery,
George Washington University Medical Center,
Washington, DC, USA
e-mail: bblee@mfa.gwu.edu; bblee38@comcast.net;
jlaredo@mfa.gwu.edu; rneville@mfa.gwu.edu

R. Mattassi et al. (eds.), *Hemangiomas and Vascular Malformations: An Atlas of Diagnosis and Treatment*,   189
DOI 10.1007/978-88-470-5673-2_24, © Springer-Verlag Italia 2009, 2015

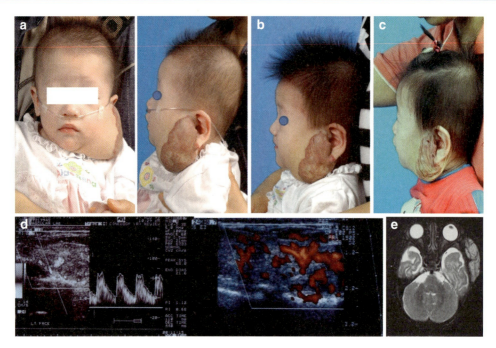

Fig. 24.1 (**a–e**) (Infantile) Hemangioma for differential diagnosis with vascular malformation (**a**) depicts a typical clinical finding of (infantile) hemangioma along the left cheek, appeared suddenly as a small lump month after the birth; soon the tumor started to grow exponentially reaching to the size shown in (**b**) within a few months. Following initial explosive growth through proliferative stage, the lesion shown in (**a**) started to regress within first year of age to reach remarkably shrunken condition shown in (**b**) as unique characteristic of the hemangioma. Before reaching to the age of 4 years, the lesion was almost completely regressed as shown in (**c**). In such situation, careful history and physical examination are more than enough for correct diagnosis as a hemangioma. However, occasionally simple tests like Duplex ultrasonography or further additional MRI might be needed to confirm the clinical impression for differential diagnosis between vascular malformation and hemangioma; as shown in (**d**), hemangioma in proliferative stage depicts hypervascular condition, compatible to the findings shown in MRI (**e**)

either as an "extratruncular" or "truncular" form with entirely different clinical significance and prognosis [13–15] (Fig. 24.2).

Therefore, proper differentiation among various CVMs is extremely important following the differentiation with the hemangioma. Although the CVM is often called AV malformation (AVM), the AVM is only one of the CVMs, and AVM should not represent the entire group of the CVMs [16–18].

The CVM, especially of the venous nature, named the venous malformation (VM) is often called the cystic/cavernous hemangioma. But again, this is the wrong term based on the old concept/classification misguiding the clinicians, and its misuse should be stopped [19–21].

The name-based eponyms (e.g., Klippel-Trenaunay syndrome, Parkes Weber syndrome), which have been used for a century, should also be used with proper discretion. In the past era when the clinical findings were the only criteria for the diagnosis, the CVMs had to be classified only with these clinical findings and named after the physicians who first described it. Such old classifications are not able to provide the mandatory information on the etiology, anatomy, embryology, and pathophysiology including the hemodynamic status for the contemporary concept of the CVMs [22–24] (Fig. 24.3 and 24.4).

Hamburg classification, named after the consensus workshop held in Hamburg in 1988, is capable to clear all these confusions caused by old nomenclatures/classifications and became a new guideline for the contemporary management of the CVMs [25–27] (Table 23.1A and B).

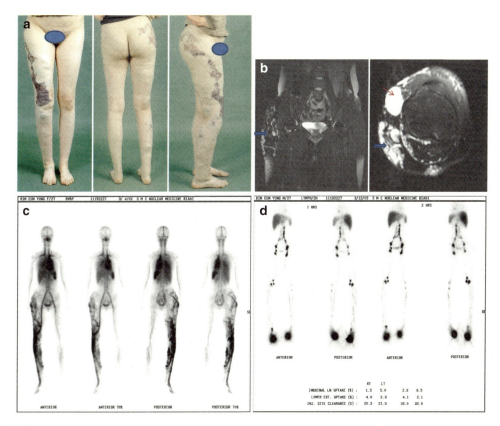

Fig. 24.2 (**a–d**) Combined form of vascular malformation: (**a**) represents a clinical condition of diffusely swollen right lower extremity by combined condition of three different vascular malformations: venous, lymphatic and capillary malformations (CM). (**b**) shows the MRI findings to confirm two different types of venous malformation: extratruncular (*thick blue arrow*) and truncular (*thin red arrow*) venous malformation (VM) lesions while (**c**) confirms abnormal blood pool by two different types of the VM lesions altogether throughout right lower extremity, detected by Whole Body Blood Pool Scintigraphy (WBBPS). (**d**) illustrates overall lymphatic transport condition of both lower extremities assessed with radionuclide lymphoscintigraphy (LSG); right lower extremity shows reduced isotope uptake at the proximal/inguinal lymph nodes together with delayed clearance with mild dermal backflow as well as collateral routes suggesting substantial lymphatic dysfunction by truncular lymphatic malformation (LM) known as 'primary' lymphedema [28]

Much advanced technology through the century is now able to provide accurate diagnosis of such complicated CVM condition; often non- to minimally invasive tests are more than adequate for the diagnosis per se in its majority, and further invasive tests can be reserved as a road map for the group later when the treatment is indicated [28–30].

NOT every CVM would need the treatment; only the CVM lesions with appropriate indications should be selected as a candidate for the treatment. Decision on whether the treatment is indicated or not should be based on the consensus among the multidisciplinary team members;

proper evaluation on the benefit versus the risk is essential since the majority of the conventional treatment accompanies high morbidity [31–33].

The VM [34–36] and LM (lymphatic malformation) [37–39] are generally not a life- or limb-threatening condition in its majority on the contrary to the AVMs [40–42]; AVM, VM, and LM are therefore mandated for different treatment principles since their clinical behavior and the prognosis are so different. Identical treatment principle cannot be implemented indiscriminately to all these different types of the CVMs; the treatment principle/strategy for the VM and LM should be different from those for the AVM [43–45].

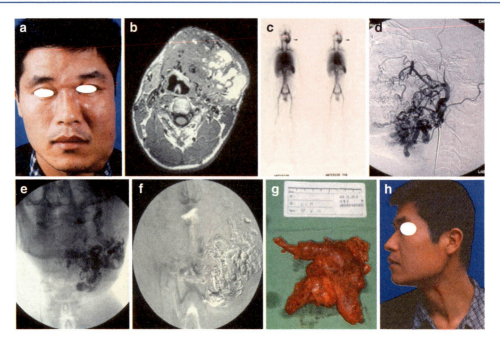

Fig. 24.3 (**a–h**) AV malformation (**a**) portrays rapidly expanding swelling along entire left face following minor blunt trauma, which was further extended to the left upper neck across the chin line and also to reach to periorbital region within a year. As shown in MRI (**b**), the lesion was confirmed as AV malformation (AVM) in infiltrating nature, compatible to Duplex ultrasonographic finding as a high flow lesion. As shown in (**c**), the lesion was confined only left face and neck and no other lesions were depicted on WBBPS to make it manageable by surgical excision. (**d**) represents arteriographic finding of the AVM as infiltrating extratruncular lesion, and the lesion was filled with n-BCA glue done preoperatively as shown in (**e**); this glue filled lesion depicted in (**f**) became a road map for subsequent surgical excision to allow minimal risk of bleeding and collateral tissue damage. Whole lesions were safely resected in total, shown in surgical specimen (**g**), and follow up clinical finding in 5 years was excellent shown in (**h**). Such contemporary approach of surgical and endovascular therapy combined can provide much improved outcome of the management in comparison to two procedures done separately [32]

Selection of the treatment modalities in addition to the basic conservative treatment regimen such as surgical or nonsurgical (e.g., sclerotherapy) should be made by a multidisciplinary team [46–48].

Accurate and thorough hemodynamic assessment of the deep venous system of the lower extremity is absolutely required for the safe management of the CVMs located in the lower extremity, especially for the hemolymphatic malformation (HLM) consisted of the LM and VM combined [49–51]. Priority for treatment among multiple lesion types should be based on the relative degree, extent, and severity of the specific lesion.

Every treatment strategy should be set accordingly based on the multidisciplinary approach with full integration of open surgery and endovascular surgery to improve the treatment outcome.

The endovascular surgery with various modalities of embolotherapy and sclerotherapy should be considered with priority as an independent therapy to the "surgically inaccessible/difficult" lesion. Even the "surgically accessible" lesion should be treated by the combined approach of preoperative endovascular therapy and subsequent open excisional surgery whenever possible to reduce the complication and morbidity [52–54] (Fig. 24.3).

Active incorporation of the pre- and/or postoperative endovascular therapy with embolotherapy/sclerotherapy allows substantial expansion of the traditional role of surgical therapy especially for the "infiltrating extratruncular" form of CVM while maintaining acceptable range of surgical risk. Such perioperative, especially preoperative, therapy could reduce surgical morbidity

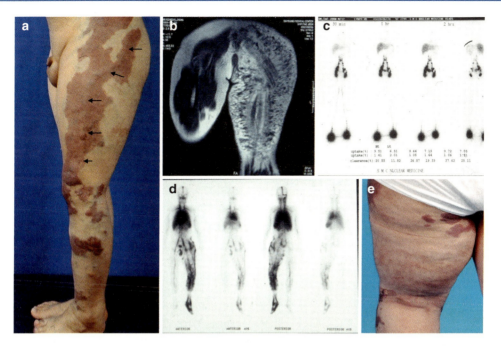

Fig. 24.4 (**a–e**) Hemolymphatic Malformation (**a**) renders typical limb swelling involved to complicated condition of hemolymphatic malformation consisted of VM, LM, and CM, also known as Klippel Trenaunay Syndrome. This photo (4A) was taken soon after the marginal vein (MV) was resected -see the outline of surgical incision by black arrows- due to the lymphatic leakage from upper buttock. Preoperative MRI finding, shown in (**b**), was lymphedematous soft tissue swelling by truncular LM; further assessment of lymph transporting function with LSG shown in (**c**) confirmed reduced isotope uptake at inguinal lymph nodes as well as delayed clearance, which is compatible with clinical findings as primary lymphedema but there was no clear evidence for extratruncular LM/ lymphangioma was involved. Based on the WBBPS findings (**d**) to confirm extratruncular VM and truncular VM both as the major cause of deteriorating venous symptoms (e.g. venous stasis ulcer), surgical excision of a truncular VM confirmed as MV in this patient was performed with priority. But within 2 weeks following MV resection, the lymph started to leak from posterior aspect of left buttock shown in (**e**) precipitating the local as well as general sepsis to require intense antibiotic therapy, etc. It took more than 6 months to be relieved from recurrent bouts of massive leakage

as well as complications drastically so that such benefit can exceed beyond the boundary for the traditional surgical approach [55–57] (Fig. 24.3).

Such approach with fully integrated endovascular therapy and the traditional open surgical therapy can achieve acceptable goal for the contemporary management of the CVMs as a new strategy. And the treatment strategy should be reviewed periodically based on the response to the initial and subsequent therapy by the multidisciplinary team and should be readjusted accordingly [52–57].

However, not every CVM lesion is amenable to the treatment. Furthermore, not every CVM lesion should be treated. Its mere presence often makes the practitioner feel obligated to treat. The only lesion assessed by the multidisciplinary team with justified indications such as severe symptoms or complications of the lesion (e.g., leakage, sepsis) should be considered for treatment. Although extratruncular CVM lesions are more serious than truncular lesions with much poorer long-term outcome, an overzealous approach sometimes does more harm than good [40, 58, 59].

"Cure" with devastating complication and morbidity is NOT better than limited "control" with less complication and morbidity even for the AVM. Observation sometimes remains the best approach yet until figuring out the exact condition of the lesion; "not to intervene" is sometimes a wiser choice than to casually intervene without a full understanding of the biology and natural history of the CVM lesion.

Table 24.1 (A & B)

A. Hamburg classification[a] of congenital vascular malformations (CVMs) – species

    Arterial malformation

    Venous malformation

    Arterio-venous malformation

    Lymphatic malformation

    Capillary malformation

    Combined vascular malformation

B. Hamburg classification of CVMs[b]: forms – embryological subtypes

    1. Extratruncular forms

        Infiltrating, diffuse

        Limited, localized

    2. Truncular forms

        Obstruction or stenosis

        Aplasia; hypoplasia; hyperplasia

        Stenosis; membrane; congenital spur

        Dilatation

        Localized (aneurysm)

        Diffuse (ectasia)

[a]Original classification was based on the consensus on the CVM through the international workshop held in Hamburg, Germany, 1988, and subsequently modified based on the predominant lesion

[b]Represents the developmental arrest at the different stages of embryonic life: Earlier stage – Extratruncular form; Later stage – Truncular form

[c]Both forms (truncular and extratruncular) may exist together; may be combined with other various malformations (e.g. capillary, arterial, AV shunting, venous, hemo-lymphatic and/or lymphatic); and/or may exist with hemangioma)

A "controlled" aggressive approach is therefore favored especially for the less vicious CVM lesion like LM, where every effort is made to minimize collateral damage during treatment. The decision to initiate treatment should be based on the accepted indications.

When the benefit of treatment outweighs the risk of complications and morbidity, less risky treatment options (e.g., foam/liquid sclerotherapy) should be the first-line therapy. "No treatment is the best option if feasible." In contrast to the treatment of AVMs, all the VM and LM lesions can be treated using a less aggressive approach.

The traditional conservative approach to the young pediatric patient with a VM and LM is still valid, especially for the common CVMs as far as there is NO evidence of bony involvement (e.g., leg length discrepancy). It is usually safe to delay treatment until the child reaches to the age of 2 or more years before beginning diagnostic procedures and treatment.

Nevertheless, CVM lesions producing the vascular-bone syndrome (e.g., angio-osteohypotrophy/hypertrophy) are best treated early in order to prevent long bone growth discrepancy [60–62].

Also, for the VM or LM lesion at a life- or limb-threatening anatomic location, an earlier treatment approach is preferred over a more conservative one (e.g., surgical decompression); for the lesion complicated with a life- or limb-threatening condition (e.g., hemorrhage, sepsis, pulmonary embolism), the treatment should be started expeditiously despite the risk of the associated morbidity [63–65].

Another important aspect of the CVM management is to refer complicated case to an experienced center where the patient can be treated effectively by well-organized team in early childhood and not having to wait until after reaching adolescence.

Special Consideration- Combined Form of CVMs

The majority of the CVMs exist as an independent lesion affecting one circulation system in general (e.g., VM, LM) except AVM. But substantial numbers of the CVMs exist together and classified separately as a combined form: Hamburg classification named this group as "hemolymphatic malformation (HLM)" to represent the majority of combined CVMs [66–68].

Because HLM is NOT a simple condition of numerical adding of various CVMs, they are much more difficult to manage due to unpredictable interaction between various CVM components and often negatively. Do anticipate with proper preparation on potential impact of one CVM component therapy to another remaining component (e.g., increased lymph leak with sepsis by ill-planned marginal vein resection).

In general, however, the AVMs and VMs are clinically more virulent vascular malformations compared with LMs so that the AVM should get the priority followed by the VMs in principle. Treatment of the LM should be addressed after successful management of the VM and/or AVM when present.

But the management of the LM belonging to the HLM is different from those of (independent) LM alone due to the interrelationship with other vascular malformations: truncular and/or extra-truncular VM and/or AVM. When a LM coexists with another CVM such as a VM, for example, the decision to treat is usually based on the severity of symptoms associated with the concomitant CVM [69–71].

In other words, when both extratruncular and truncular LMs and also extratruncular and truncular VMs exist together, which is infrequent among Klippel-Trenaunay syndrome (KTS) patients, the treatment of this complex HLM should be based on the treatment of the VM component (either truncular or extratruncular forms) with a priority. And also the extratruncular VM lesion should be treated initially by, for example, excision and/or sclerotherapy unless otherwise indicated (e.g., massive pulmonary embolism by the marginal vein as coexisitng VM component) (Fig. 24.3 and 24.4).

But the treatment of the concomitant VM often results in a transient worsening of the lymphatic dysfunction due to the interrelated venous and lymphatic systems. This often occurs following surgical resection of a marginal/lateral embryonic vein (e.g., increased lymphatic leakage and/or sepsis of lymphatic origin) (Fig. 24.4). When the deep venous system is involved in VM, such as in deep vein hypoplasia, further care/support of an already compromised lymphatic system is essential to prevent associated complications, such as recurrent cellulitis [72–74].

Besides, HLM lesions can have both truncular and extratruncular LM components among KTS, which make clinical management more complicated. When extratruncular and truncular LM lesions should occur together where surgical excision is required, extreme care should be taken not to risk further damage to the lymph-transporting system that is already jeopardized by the truncular LM lesion causing the chronic lymphedema; a staged approach should be taken. This approach should minimize its impact on an already poorly functioning lymphatic system. Aggressive MLD (manual lymphatic drainage)-based decongestive lymphatic therapy should prevent further deterioration of lymphatic function.

References

1. Lee BB, Kim HH, Mattassi R, Yakes W, Loose D, Tasnadi G (2003) A new approach to the congenital vascular malformation with new concept – Seoul Consensus. Int J Angiol 12:248–251
2. Lee BB, Mattassi R, Loose D, Yakes W, Tasnadi G, Kim HH (2004) Consensus on controversial issues in contemporary diagnosis and management of congenital vascular malformation – Seoul communication. Int J Angiol 13(4):182–192
3. Lee BB (2008) Changing concept on vascular malformation: no longer enigma. Ann Vasc Dis 1(1):11–19
4. Malan E, Puglionisi A (1965) Congenital angiodysplasias of the extremities, note II: arterial, arterial and venous, and hemolymphatic dysplasias. J Cardiovasc Surg (Torino) 6:255–345
5. Malan E (1974) History and nosography. In: Malan E (ed) Vascular malformations (angiodysplasias). Carlo Erba Foundation, Milan, pp 15–19
6. Villavicencio JL (2007) Congenital vascular malformations: historical background. Special issue. Phlebology 22:247–248
7. Mulliken JB (1988) Treatment of hemangiomas. In: Mulliken JB, Young AE (eds) Vascular birthmarks, hemangiomas and malformations. WB Saunders, Philadelphia, pp 88–90
8. Mulliken JB, Glowacki J (1982) Hemangiomas and vascular malformations in infants and children: a classification based on endothelial characteristics. Plast Reconstr Surg 69:412–422
9. Mulliken JB (1988) Classification of vascular birthmarks. In: Grainger RG, Allison DJ (eds) Vascular birthmarks, haemangiomas, and malformations. WB Saunders, Philadelphia, pp 24–37
10. Lee BB (2002) Advanced management of congenital vascular malformation (CVM). Int Angiol 21(3):209–213
11. Lee BB (2004) Critical issues on the management of congenital vascular malformation. Ann Vasc Surg 18(3):380–392
12. Lee BB, Laredo J (2012) Hemangioma and venous/vascular malformation are different as an apple and orange! Editorial. Acta Phlebol 13:1–3
13. Lee BB, Laredo J, Lee TS, Huh S, Neville R (2007) Terminology and classification of congenital vascular malformations. Phlebology 22(6):249–252
14. Bastide G, Lefebvre D (1989) Anatomy and organogenesis and vascular malformations. In: Belov S, Loose DA, Weber J (eds) Vascular malformations. Einhorn-Presse Verlag GmbH, Reinbek, pp 20–22
15. Woolard HH (1922) The development of the principal arterial stems in the forelimb of the pig. Contrib Embryol 14:139–154
16. Lee BB (2013) Venous malformation and haemangioma: differential diagnosis, diagnosis, natural history and consequences. Phlebology 28(Suppl 1):176–187

17. Lee BB, Lardeo J, Neville R (2009) Arterio-venous malformation: how much do we know? Phlebology 24:193–200

18. Lee BB, Laredo J (2012) Classification of congenital vascular malformations: the last challenge for congenital vascular malformations. Phlebology 27(6):267–269

19. Lee BB (2012) Venous embryology: the key to understanding anomalous venous conditions. Phlebolymphology 19(4):170–181

20. Lee BB (2012) Venous malformation is NOT a hemangioma. Editorial. Flebologia Y Linfologia – Lecturas Vasculares 7(17):1021–1023

21. Lee BB, Laredo J (2013) Venous malformation: treatment needs a bird's eye view. Phlebology 28:62–63

22. Lee BB (2012) Klippel-Trenaunay syndrome: is this term still worthy to use? Acta Phlebol 13:1–2

23. Klippel M, Trenaunay J (1900) Du noevus variqueux et osteohypertrophique. Arch Gén Méd 3:641–672

24. Gloviczki P, Driscoll DJ (2007) Klippel–Trenaunay syndrome: current management. Phlebology 22:291–298

25. Belov S (1990) Classification of congenital vascular defects. Int Angiol 9:141–146

26. Belov S (1993) Anatomopathological classification of congenital vascular defects. Semin Vasc Surg 6:219–224

27. Belov S (1989) Classification, terminology, and nosology of congenital vascular defects. In: Belov S, Loose DA, Weber J (eds) Vascular malformations. Einhorn-Presse, Reinbek, pp 25–30

28. Lee BB, Laredo J, Lee SJ, Huh SH, Joe JH, Neville R (2007) Congenital vascular malformations: general diagnostic principles. Phlebology 22(6):253–257

29. Lee BB, Bergan J, Gloviczki P, Laredo J, Loose DA, Mattassi R, Parsi K, Villavicencio JL, Zamboni P (2009) Diagnosis and treatment of venous malformations - consensus document of the International Union of Phlebology (IUP)-2009. Int Angiol 28(6):434–451

30. Lee BB, Choe YH, Ahn JM, Do YS, Kim DI, Huh SH, Byun HS (2004) The new role of MRI (magnetic resonance imaging) in the contemporary diagnosis of venous malformation: can it replace angiography? J Am Coll Surg 198(4):549–558

31. Lee BB. Not all venous malformations needed therapy because they are not arteriovenous malformations. Comments on Dermatol Surg. 2010;36(3):340–346. Dermatol Surg. 2010;36(3):347

32. Lee BB, Bergan JJ (2002) Advanced management of congenital vascular malformations: a multidisciplinary approach. J Cardiovasc Surg 10(6):523–533

33. Lee BB, Do YS, Yakes W, Kim DI, Mattassi R, Hyun WS, Byun HS (2004) Management of arterial-venous shunting malformations (AVM) by surgery and embolosclerotherapy. A multidisciplinary approach. J Vasc Surg 3:596–600

34. Lee BB (2003) Current concept of venous malformation (VM). Phlebolymphology 43:197–203

35. Lee BB, Do YS, Byun HS, Choo IW, Kim DI, Huh SH (2003) Advanced management of venous malformation (VM) with ethanol sclerotherapy: mid-term results. J Vasc Surg 37(3):533–538

36. Lee BB, Bergan J (2008) Chapter 12. Transition from alcohol to foam sclerotherapy for localized venous malformation with high risk. In: Bergan J, Cheng VL (eds) A textbook- foam sclerotherapy. The Royal Society of Medicine Press Ltd, London, pp 129–139

37. Lee BB, Villavicencio JL (2010) Primary lymphedema and lymphatic malformation: are they the two sides of the same coin? Eur J Vasc Endovasc Surg 39:646–653

38. Lee BB, Andrade M, Bergan J, Boccardo F, Campisi C, Damstra R, Flour M, Gloviczki P, Laredo J, Piller N, Michelini S, Mortimer P, Villavicencio JL (2010) Diagnosis and treatment of primary lymphedema – consensus document of the International Union of Phlebology (IUP)-2009. Int Angiol 29(5):454–470

39. Lee BB, Kim YW, Seo JM, Hwang JH, Do YS, Kim DI, Byun HS, Lee SK, Huh SH, Hyun WS (2005) Current concepts in lymphatic malformation (LM). Vasc Endovasc Surg 39(1):67–81

40. Kim JY, Kim DI, Do YS, Kim YW, Lee BB (2006) Surgical treatment for congenital arteriovenous malformation: 10 years' experience. Eur J Vasc Endovasc Surg 32(1):101–106, Epub 2006 Feb

41. Lee BB, Laredo J, Deaton DH, Neville RF (2009) Chapter 53. Arteriovenous malformations: evaluation and treatment. In: Gloviczki P, Hodder Arnold A, Gloviczki P (eds) Handbook of venous disorders: guidelines of the American Venous Forum, 3rd edn. A Hodder Arnold, London, pp 583–593

42. Lee BB (2006) Chapter 76. Mastery of vascular and endovascular surgery. In: Zelenock GB, Huber TS, Messina LM, Lumsden AB, Moneta GL (eds) Arteriovenous malformation. Lippincott, Williams and Wilkins, Philadelphia, pp 597–607

43. Lee BB (2005) New approaches to the treatment of congenital vascular malformations (CVMs) – single center experiences – (editorial review). Eur J Vasc Endovasc Surg 30(2):184–197

44. Lee BB, Laredo J, Kim YW, Neville R (2007) Congenital vascular malformations: general treatment principles. Phlebology 22(6):258–263

45. Lee BB, Laredo J, Seo JM, Neville R (2009) Chapter 29. Treatment of lymphatic malformations. In: Mattassi R, Loose DA, Vaghi M (eds) Hemangiomas and vascular malformations. Springer Italia, Milan, pp 231–250

46. Villavicencio JL, Scultetus A, Lee BB (2002) Congenital vascular malformation: when and how to treat them. Semin Vasc Surg 15(1):65–71

47. Kim KH, Kim HH, Lee SK, Seo JM, Lee BB, Chang WY (2001) OK-432 intralesional therapy for lymphangioma in children. J Korean Assoc Pediatr Surg 7(2):142–146

48. Lee BB, Baumgartner I, Berlien HP, Bianchini G, Burrows P, Do YS, Ivancev K, Kool LS, Laredo J, Loose DA, Lopez-Gutierrez JC, Mattassi R, Parsi K, Rimon U, Rosenblatt M, Shortell C, Simkin R, Stillo F, Villavicencio L, Yakes W (2013) Consensus document of the International Union of Angiology (IUA)-

2013. Current concept on the management of arterio-venous management. Int Angiol 32(1):9–36

49. Lee BB, Mattassi R, Choe YH et al (2005) Critical role of duplex ultrasonography for the advanced management of a venous malformation (VM). Phlebology 20:28–37

50. Lee BB (2013) Marginal vein is not a simple varicose vein: it is a silent killer! Review. Damar Cer Derg 22(1):4–14

51. Lee BB, Laredo J, Neville R, Mattassi R (2011) Chapter 52. Primary lymphedema and Klippel-Trenaunay syndrome. Section 11 – lymphedema and congenital vascular malformation. In: Byung-Boong L, Bergan J, Rockson SG (eds) Lymphedema: a concise compendium of theory and practice, 1st edn. Springer, London, pp 427–436

52. Loose DA, Weber J (1991) Indications and tactics for a combined treatment of congenital vascular malformations. In: Balas P (ed) Progress in angiology. Chapt Miscellanea. Minerva Medica, Torino, pp 379–482

53. Loose DA (2009) Combined treatment of arteriovenous malformations. In: Mattassi R, Loose DA, Vaghi M (eds) Hemangiomas and vascular malformations. Springer, Milan, pp 195–204

54. Yakes WF, Parker SH, Gibson MD, Haas DK, Pevsner PH, Carter TE (1989) Alcohol embolotherapy of vascular malformations. Semin Intervent Radiol 6:146–161

55. Cromwell LD, Kerber CW (1979) Modification of cyano-acrylate for therapeutic embolization: preliminary experience. Am J Roentgenol 132:799

56. Weber JH (1993) Vaso-occlusive angiotherapy (VAT) in congenital vascular malformations. Semin Vasc Surg 6:279–296

57. Natali J, Merland JJ (1976) Superselective arteriography and therapeutic embolization for vascular malformations (angiodysplasias). J Cardiovasc Surg 17:465–472

58. Lee BB (1999) Congenital venous malformation: changing concept on the current diagnosis and management. Asian J Surg 22(2):152–154

59. Lee BB, Kim DI, Huh S, Kim HH, Choo IW, Byun HS, Do YS (2001) New experiences with absolute ethanol sclerotherapy in the management of a complex form of congenital venous malformation. J Vasc Surg 33(4):764–772

60. Mattassi R (1993) Differential diagnosis in congenital vascular-bone syndromes. Semin Vasc Surg 6:233–244

61. Kim YW, Do YS, Lee SH, Lee BB (2006) Risk factors for leg length discrepancy in patients with congenital vascular malformation. J Vasc Surg 44:545–553

62. Mattassi R, Vaghi M (2007) Vascular bone syndrome-angi-osteodystrophy: current concept. Phlebology 22:287–290

63. Mattassi R, Vaghi M (2007) Management of the marginal vein: current issues. Phlebology 22:283–286

64. Aggarwal K, Jain VK, Gupta S, Aggarwal HK, Sen J, Goyal V (2003) Klippel-Trenaunay syndrome with a life-threatening thromboembolic event. J Dermatol 30(3):236–240

65. Walder B, Kapelanski DP, Auger WR, Fedullo PF (2000) Successful pulmonary thromboendarterectomy in a patient with Klippel-Trenaunay syndrome. Chest 117(5):1520–1522

66. Villavicencio JL, Conaway CW, Pikoulis E, Gannon MX (1997) Congenital vascular malformations of venous predominance. The Klippel Trenaunay syndrome. In: Raju S, Villavicencio JL (eds) Surgical management of venous disease. Williams and Wilkins, Media, pp 445–467

67. Jacob AG, Driscoll DJ, Shaughnessy WJ, Stanson AW, Clay RP, Gloviczki P (1998) Klippel-Trenaunay syndrome: spectrum and management. Mayo Clin Proc 73(1):28–36

68. Gloviczki P, Stanson AW, Stickler GB, Johnson CM, Toomey BJ, Meland NB, Rooke TW, Cherry KJ Jr (1991) Klippel-Trenaunay syndrome: the risks and benefits of vascular interventions. Surgery 110(3):469–479

69. Lee BB, Kim DI, Kim HH, Choi JY, Do YS, Choo SW, Kim BT (2000) Hidden risk of the deterioration of the lymphatic function following the management of venous component of the hemolymphatic malformation (HLM). Abstract, 13th International Society for the Study of Vascular Anomalies, Montreal, May 10–13, 2000

70. al-Salman MM (1997) Klippel-Trenaunay syndrome: clinical features, complications, and management. Surg Today 27(8):735–740

71. Servelle M, Babillot J (1980) Deep vein malformations in the Klippel-Trenaunay syndrome. Phlebologie 33(1):31–36

72. Kim YW, Lee BB, Cho JH, Do YS, Kim DI, Kim ES (2007) Haemodynamic and clinical assessment of lateral marginal vein excision in patients with a predominantly venous malformation of the lower extremity. Eur J Vasc Endovasc Surg 33(1):122–127

73. Eifert S, Villavicencio JL, Kao TC et al (2000) Prevalence of deep venous anomalies in congenital vascular malformations of venous predominance. J Vasc Surg 31:462–471

74. Telander RL, Kaufman BH, Gloviczki P, Stickler GB, Hollier LH (1984) Prognosis and management of lesions of the trunk in children with Klippel-Trenaunay syndrome. J Pediatr Surg 19(4):417–422

Dermatological Manifestations of Vascular Malformations

25

Kurosh Parsi

Introduction

Patients with congenital vascular malformations (CVM) present with a variety of dermatological manifestations. These can range from common manifestations of venous hypertension seen in truncular venous malformations (VM), secondary skin changes associated with lymphedema commonly found in truncular lymphatic malformations (LM), and specific conditions such as acroangiodermatitis pointing to an underlying arteriovenous malformation (AVM). In addition, capillary malformations (CM) in combination with other vascular anomalies present with typical clinical signs. In this chapter, we briefly examine the dermatological manifestations of CVM.

Arteriovenous Malformations (AVM)

General Morphology

AVMs are always present at birth, but the clinical signs may be quite subtle in neonates, infants, and young children. The lesions enlarge in time proportionate to the child's growth, and hence the physical signs evolve over time.

K. Parsi
Department of Dermatology,
St. Vincent's Hospital, Sydney, Australia
e-mail: Kurosh.Parsi@svha.org.au

Dermal AVMs may appear as a faint pink patch in neonates but enlarge to form cutaneous lesions. An important clinical sign of a subdermal or subcutaneous AVM may be pallor of the overlying skin due to a cutaneous "steal" where arterial blood is shunted away into the draining veins, bypassing the cutaneous capillary network (Fig. 25.1a). The resulting pallor has geographical borders following a multi-angulated "stellate" pattern that correlates with the cutaneous arteriolar supply (Fig. 25.1b) [1, 2].

A mature subcutaneous AVM may manifest as a warm, enlarged pulsating mass. The mass effect is due to enlargement of the anomalous vessels as well as an associated soft tissue hypertrophy and fibrosis. Lesions in deeper tissues may not always be clinically recognizable and hemorrhage can be a presenting sign of an occult AVM.

Associated Findings

AVMs often cause soft tissue and bony hypertrophy. The soft tissue hypertrophy results in asymmetry and in time can cause disfigurement. Soft tissue and bony hypertrophy can result in enlargement of the affected limb in length and circumference. This can lead to a secondary scoliosis. When there is an associated venous or lymphatic malformation (Parkes Weber syndrome), typical signs of chronic venous hypertension or lymphedema may be present.

Fig. 25.1 Cutaneous steal presenting as pallor in the skin overlying arteriovenous malformations (AVM). (**a**) Pallor surrounding fine telangiectasias overlying a dermal AVM. (**b**) Pallor surrounding a combined venous, microcystic lymphatic malformation overlying a subcutaneous AVM

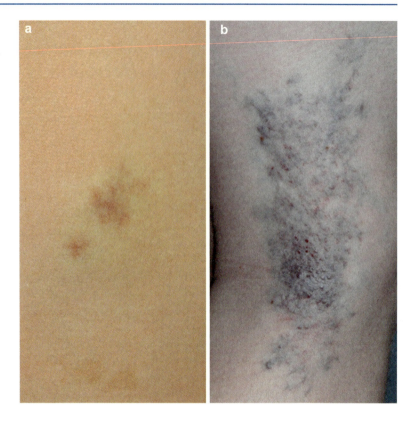

Stewart-Bluefarb Syndrome

Stewart-Bluefarb syndrome (SBS) refers to acroangiodermatitis secondary to an underlying AVM [3]. First described by Bluefarb and Adams and later by Stewart in 1967, the term Stewart-Bluefarb syndrome was conceived by Earhart in 1974 [4].

Acroangiodermatitis is an angioproliferative skin eruption that represents a reactive endothelial hyperplasia [5]. It is possibly driven by an angiogenic response to high perfusion rates and the associated increase in venous and capillary pressures. Clinically, it presents with violaceous brown macules, papules, and nodules that may become confluent to form large plaques. Lesions may eventually ulcerate. Acroangiodermatitis has a predilection for extensor surfaces and in particular the dorsal aspect of the foot and the first three toes (Fig. 25.2a) [6].

Histologically, acroangiodermatitis is characterized by profuse thin-walled capillaries lined by a single layer of endothelial cells and a perivascular proliferation of dermal fibroblasts. Secondary changes include extensive extravasation of erythrocytes and hemosiderin deposition in the dermis. There may be an associated inflammatory mononuclear infiltrate (Fig. 25.2b).

Clinically, acroangiodermatitis resembles Kaposi's sarcoma (KS) and is often referred to as "Pseudo-KS." Acroangiodermatitis lacks the typical histological features of KS such as the vascular slit pattern, the diverse inflammatory infiltrate, and a positive human herpes virus type 8 (HHV-8), factor VIII-associated antigen, and CD34+ antigen in endothelial cells.

Acroangiodermatitis is not always secondary to an AVM and may have an acquired etiology. The acquired form is referred to as

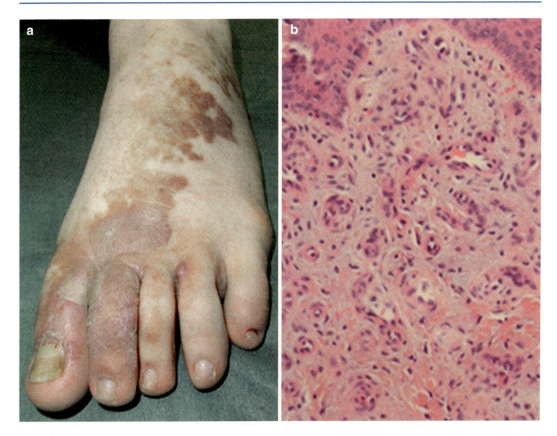

Fig. 25.2 (**a**) Acroangiodermatitis involving the dorsum of the foot. (**b**) Histology of acroangiodermatitis comprised of multiple capillaries lined by a single layer of endothelial vessels surrounded by fibroblasts

"acroangiodermatitis of Mali" and is seen in the presence of severe venous hypertension at later stages of chronic venous insufficiency (CVI) or secondary to an iatrogenic AV fistula. While SBS is usually unilateral, acroangiodermatitis of Mali may be bilateral. Unlike SBS, histological changes in acroangiodermatitis of Mali are limited to the superficial dermis.

> **Clinical Pearl**
> A distinct violaceous pigmentation involving the dorsum of the toes and the feet should trigger a biopsy to diagnose acroangiodermatitis and a search for an underlying AVM.

Venous Malformations (VM)

Truncular Venous Malformations

Truncular VMs present as structural abnormalities such as aplasia, hypoplasia, obstruction, dilation, duplication, aneurysm, and valvular agenesis of the affected vessels. The clinical presentation is quite variable and correlates with the anatomical abnormality. Truncular VMs involving the lower limb veins can cause venous hypertension and present with typical dermatological signs of CVI. These include venous eczema, hyperpigmentation, depigmentation, atrophie blanche, lipodermatosclerosis, and ulceration. In severe cases, subcutaneous calcification and ossification can occur.

Fig. 25.3
Klippel-Trenaunay
syndrome (KTS)

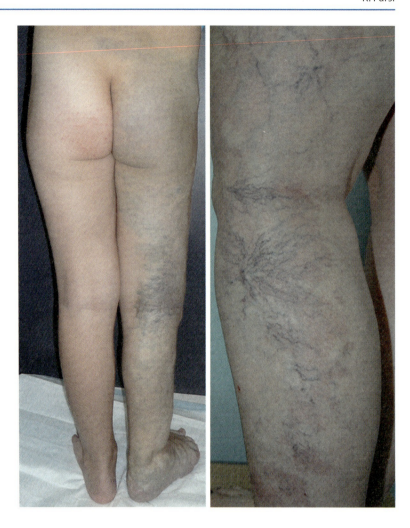

CVI secondary to an incompetent embryonic lateral marginal vein of the thigh will present with skin changes involving the lateral distal calf and ankle. Combined malformations such as the Klippel-Trenaunay syndrome (KTS) can present with typical signs of venous hypertension as well as signs of the associated anomalies. While KTS presents with hypertrophy of the affected limb (Fig. 25.3), Servelle-Martorell syndrome presents with bony hypotrophy and limb shortening.

Extratruncular Venous Malformations

Extratruncular VMs present as lesions. Intradermal lesions may present as blanchable dermal telangiectasias and venulectasias that can cover large surface areas (Fig. 25.4). Subcutaneous and intramuscular VMs may present as partially or fully compressible masses. The enlargement may be positional as lesions may fill up and enlarge in dependent positions.

Particular subtypes of extratruncular VMs include glomovenous malformations (GVM) and the blue rubber bleb syndrome (BRB). Both conditions present as intradermal or subdermal blue lesions. GVMs are in general darker than BRB lesions. These lesions are blanchable on light pressure unless thrombosed. Thrombosed VMs on the lips can be confused with a melanoma due to the dark color. Occult lesions can be located using infrared-based vein illumination devices (Fig. 25.5).

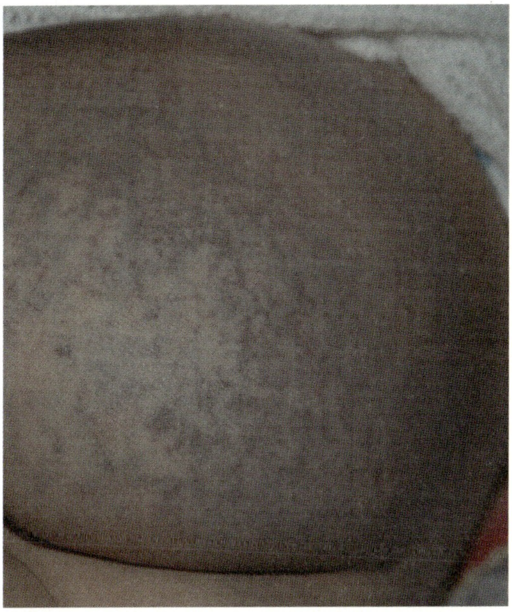

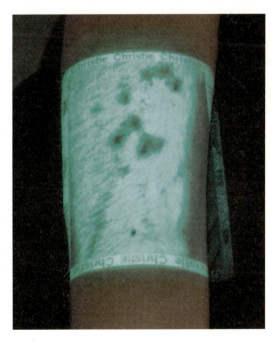

Fig. 25.4 Dermal venous malformation

Lymphatic Malformations (LM)

Truncular Lymphatic Malformations

Patients with truncular LMs can present with advanced signs of lymphedema at a very young age. These include cutaneous changes such as erythema, induration, verrucous change, and hyperkeratosis. Lymphedema can be complicated by secondary dermatophyte or bacterial infections and present with cellulitis or lymphangitis.

Patients with primary lymphedema should have a complete dermatological examination that should include examination of skin, hair, nails, and eyelashes. In lymphedema-distichiasis syndrome (FOXC2 mutation), lymphedema is associated with the growth of extra eyelashes in the inner lining of the eyelid. In the yellow nail syndrome, lymphedema (secondary to lymphatic hypoplasia) is associated with yellow dystrophic nails, bronchiectasis, and chronic sinusitis.

Extratruncular Lymphatic Malformations

Extratruncular LMs can infiltrate other tissues in a localized or generalized distribution. They present with cystic lesions that may be macrocystic or microcystic. Macrocystic lesions present as a mass, whereas microcystic lesions present as multiple vesicles which may appear verrucous. The vesicles normally contain clear fluid but bleeding from the fragile cystic walls can result in a blood-stained appearance (Fig. 25.6a, b).

Lymphangiectasia

Lymphangiectasias are saccular dilations of the superficial lymphatics. These present as translucent vesicles that can enlarge to form small bullae and nodules. Some lesions may be pedunculated and develop a hyperkeratotic verrucous surface.

Lymphangiectasias develop secondary to increased intralymphatic pressure that results from lymph accumulation in the superficial vessels. An accompanying lymphedema is seen in most

Fig. 25.5 Glomovenous malformations. Occult lesions located with infrared illumination

Other Findings

Both extratruncular and truncular VMs can present with thrombophlebitis.

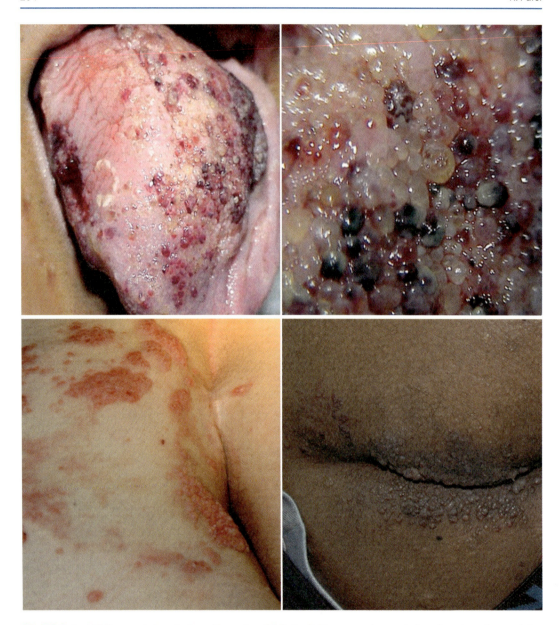

Fig. 25.6 (**a**, **b**) Microcystic lymphatic malformation (LM). (**c**, **d**) Verrucous changes in lymphangiectasias overlying macrocystic LM

patients who present with lymphangiectasias. *Lymphangioma circumscriptum* refers to lymphangiectasias involving the skin and the subcutaneous tissues secondary to an underlying LM (Fig. 25.6c, d).

Stewart-Treves Syndrome

Stewart-Treves syndrome is the development of a cutaneous angiosarcoma in long-standing chronic lymphedema. This syndrome has been reported in patients with primary lymphedema secondary

to a truncular LM but is more likely to occur in secondary lymphedemas.

Capillary Malformations and Angiokeratomas

Capillary Malformations (CM)

These lesions typically present as a light-pink to deep-red macule or patch in a geographical or dermatomal pattern. The color deepens to a darker red, and the lesion thickens with time and becomes more nodular. CM can accompany other vascular tumors or malformations and are found in KTS and Parkes Weber syndrome. A facial CM in a V1 and V2 distribution may be a manifestation of Sturge-Weber syndrome.

Capillary-Lymphatic Malformations (Angiokeratomas)

Capillary-lymphatic malformations (CLM) are combined anomalies of the capillary and lymphatic vessels. CLMs present as demarcated papules or nodules. The lesions are referred to as angiokeratomas when the surface is hyperkeratotic and verrucous. The most common form is the *angiokeratoma of Fordyce* which is found on the genitals.

Other Conditions

Cutis Marmorata Telangiectatica Congenita (CMTC)

Cutis marmorata telangiectatica congenita (CMTC), or van Lohuizen's syndrome, is a complex congenital malformation composed predominantly of capillary and venous vessels. CMTC is characterized by a partly blanchable, branched pattern of livedo racemosa. The rings are incomplete and present with central pallor. The involved skin may become atrophic and ulcerate. Ulceration is more likely in skin overlying elbows and knees. The subcutaneous fat may show signs of atrophy and induration, and the involved limb itself may be hypoplastic. The cutaneous eruption is initially more prominent and accompanied by telangiectatic vessels but tends to fade with time.

CMTC should be differentiated from cutis marmorata, a physiological response to cold seen in newborns presenting with a fully blanchable, symmetrical, and diffuse mottled pattern of livedo reticularis. In neonates, the lesions of CMTC may appear very similar to cutis marmorata. In contradistinction to cutis marmorata, the cutaneous presentation of CMTC is branched (hence *racemosa*), asymmetrical, localized, and segmental and will not resolve completely with warming of the skin. This distinction is very important as CMTC is associated with a number of associated abnormalities such as glaucoma, neurological, and psychomotor disorders.

Phakomatosis Pigmentovascularis

This condition is an association of a widespread vascular nevus (usually a CM) with an extensive pigmentary nevus including dermal melanocytosis (Mongolian spot), nevus spilus, and nevus of Ota.

References

1. Parsi K, Partsch H, Rabe E et al (2011) Reticulate eruptions. Part 1: vascular networks and physiology. Australas J Dermatol 52:159–166
2. Parsi K, Partsch H, Rabe E et al (2011) Reticulate eruptions: part 2. Historical perspectives, morphology, terminology and classification. Australas J Dermatol 52:237–244
3. Parsi K, O'Connor A, Bester L. Stewart-Bluefarb syndrome: Report of five cases and a review of literature. Phlebology. 2014 Aug 13. pii: 0268355514548090
4. Earhart RN, Aeling JA, Nuss DD et al (1974) Pseudo-Kaposi sarcoma. A patient with arteriovenous malformation and skin lesions simulating Kaposi sarcoma. Arch Dermatol 110:907–910
5. Requena L, Fariña MC, Renedo G et al (1999) Intravascular and diffuse dermal reactive angioendotheliomatosis secondary to iatrogenic arteriovenous fistulas. J Cutan Pathol 26:159–164
6. Amon RB (1975) Arteriovenous malformation resembling Kaposi sarcoma. Arch Dermatol 111: 1656–1657

Ultrasound Diagnostics

26

Massimo Vaghi

Introduction

Ultrasound examination is the ideal completion of clinical examination. It represents the extension of the examining hand in order to discover the characteristics of the underlying tissues, involved vessels, and blood flow properties. The merge of these characteristics in conjunction with clinical history and clinical examination allows to get morphological and hemodynamic characteristics of the malformation and to classify it.

The main advantages of ultrasound are the low cost and the physiologic acquisition of images in real time. Main disadvantages are the time lasting examination, the spatial limit of the scan probe, and the most important condition that the test should be performed by a person experienced in vascular malformations.

Steps of the Examination

An ultrasound examination of a CVM is more complex than the study of venous insufficiency or arterial occlusive disease. It can be divided in four steps (Fig. 26.1):

M. Vaghi, MD
Department of Vascular Surgery, A.O.G. Salvini
Hospital, Garbagnate Milanese, Italy
e-mail: vaghim@yahoo.it

1. Search and recognition of a vascular anomaly, its site, and involved vessels.
2. Definition of the main morphology, finding out if it is a truncular or an extratruncular defect or even a combination, according to the Hamburg classification.
3. Definition of the borders, including easily to detect anatomical landmarks, size, and in- and outflow vessels. Calcifications, thrombosis, and infiltration of organs and tissues should be recognized. At the end of the examination, it should be possible to classify the malformation according to the Hamburg classification.
4. Fourth level is the ultrasound examination to plan and to guide treatment (surgical, percutaneous, or interventional therapy) (Fig. 26.1) [1–6].

Technique

Study should be performed according to guidelines for the examination of abdomen, neck, and limbs. At the limbs, a bilateral study is recommended to recognize other eventually existing unknown malformations and also to compare the malformed anatomy with the normal limb.

Subcutaneous and soft tissues with a contralateral comparison are necessary to recognize and measure tissue hypertrophy or atrophy

Examination of the limbs should be performed in both upright and lying position, as some venous malformations may not be visible in lying

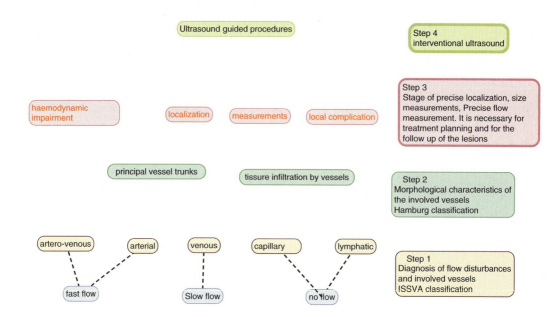

Fig. 26.1 Diagnostic steps in ultrasound diagnosis of vascular anomalies

position due to a collapse of low-flow structures. All flow evocative tests should be undertaken in order to clarify as much as possible the hemodynamic map of the limb [7].

Examination should include all axial principal vessels (arteries and veins) and their flow characteristics. After that, the attention should be addressed to the vascular anomalies which are external to the axial vessels (extratruncular anomalies) [1].

Hemodynamic Patterns

Three types of flow pattern are recognizable in CVM:

Slow-flow pattern: Typical of venous malformations. Flow may be spontaneous or only evocated by provocation maneuvers. The physiologic direction of flow should be unidirectional (to the heart). The presence of a reflux component longer than 0.5 may be a sign of incompetence of the underlying vein (Fig. 26.2).

This component may be analyzed in order to highlight the reflux time and the reflux volume.

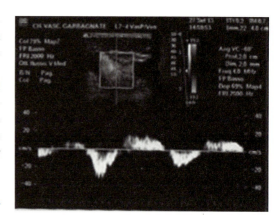

Fig. 26.2 Reflux in truncular malformed veins

In presence of a reflux, the origin and the pattern should be defined. A continuous venous flow without influence of the respiratory activity to the proximal veins is sign of a possible venous stenosis.

Fast-flow pattern: Typical pulsatile arterial pattern which includes monophasic and triphasic waves. Monophasic waves are typical of low-resistance vessels that perfuse kidneys and brain. This pattern is also typical of AV shunts associated with pulsatile flow in the outflow

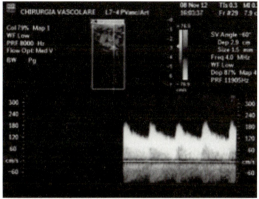

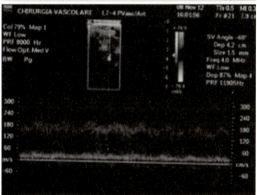

Fig. 26.3 Flow characteristics in AV shunt. (**a**) Arterial component with high diastolic velocity. (**b**) Venous component with pulsatile flow

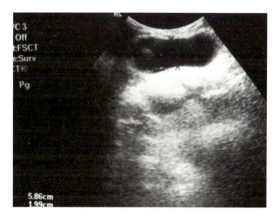

Fig. 26.4 Lymphatic superficial macrocyst

Morphology

Truncular anomalies are characterized by the presence of aplasia/obstruction, hypoplasia, or dilatation of the involved vessels (see Chap. 22). Persistence of embryonic structures like sciatic artery, sciatic vein, and embryonal vein is also possible and may be combined with the other truncular defects or with areas of dysplastic vessels in the tissues (extratruncular forms). Course of all vessels should be investigated in order to find out/exclude anomalies of number, position, and morphology.

More complex is the examination of extratruncular malformations. The tissue echogenicity may be very different in relation to the ratio vessels/tissue and to the existing edema [8].

Thrombosis can be recognized by tissue compression and flow analysis. *Flow absence* is a normal result after malformation sclerosis: in a partially occluded malformation, areas with flow may coexist with others without flow. *Quantitative evaluation* of morphology is possible by size measure of the defect. Malformations can increase their size because of normal development of the pathology, as a result of vessel thrombosis or as the early reaction to sclerosis with ethanol or other fluids (inflammation and edema).

In lymphatic extratruncular malformations, macro- and microcystic forms can be differentiated by ultrasound measure of cyst diameter (micro less than 2 cm, macro over 2 cm). Sometimes, difference between extreme low-flow venous malformations and lymphatic defects

veins. Distal to the shunt, we observe a slowing and dampening of the arterial velocity profile which may be responsible of peripheral ischemia. Contemporary on the venous side, we can record pulsatile flow proximal to the shunt and blood stasis distally (Fig. 26.3) [6].

No-flow pattern: Typical of capillary and pure lymphatic malformations. No flow data can be found also in thrombosed venous malformations (Fig. 26.4) [2–5].

Hemodynamic parameters obtained from the study should be recorded in order to allow a quantifiable follow-up of the malformation. Most useful data are flow rate, resistivity index, pulsatility index in AV shunts, and reflux time and reflux volume in venous malformations. Additional important hemodynamic data are segmental pressure measurement in arterial and arteriovenous malformations and dynamic venous measurement in venous malformations (by an invasive method).

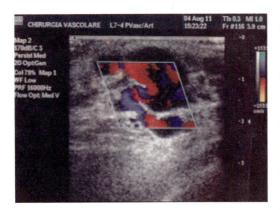

Fig. 26.5 Ultrasonographic morphological study of an AV shunt: note the presence of an artery to an enlarged vein

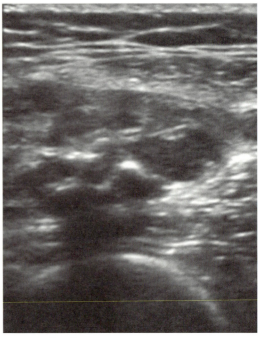

may be difficult [9]. Ultrasound is also useful in the prenatal diagnosis of vascular malformations particularly the diagnosis of lymphatic cystic malformations of the neck which are potentially dangerous during delivery [10, 11].

In lymphedema, the study of the thickness of subcutaneous tissue and morphology of lymph nodes is possible (Fig. 26.4).

Ultrasound is useful to guide treatment, percutaneous or intraoperative. The site and morphology of venous malformations and characteristics of outflow vessels can be determined; probability of success in ethanol injection can be predicted [12–14]. In AV shunts, the morphology and the number of outflow veins are recognizable (Fig. 26.5) [13, 14]. Intraoperative, a portable Doppler is effective to find out the site of an AV nidus inside tissues.

According to the site of the malformation, some specific test can be performed:

CVM in muscles: Muscle involvement is common. Involved muscular fibers show often edema. Muscular fibers may have a normal function or may have lost their contractibility. Muscle function can be tested by ultrasound study of muscle contraction (Fig. 26.6).

CVM in nerves: Nerve involvement is not infrequent and may explain origin of some atypical pain. Direct nerve infiltration or compression by the malformation itself or, sometimes, painful compression by phleboliths is possible. Careful ultrasound examination of main

Fig. 26.6 Structural muscular distortion secondary to extratruncular venous malformation (Taken from the previous edition)

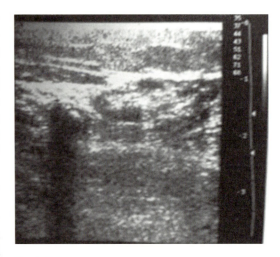

Fig. 26.7 Phlebolith in soft tissue (note the acoustic shadowing)

nerves in case of pain is recommended (Fig. 26.7).

CVM in bones: AVM inside the bone is well known. Bone high-flow vessels, entering and exiting the bone, may be detected using transcranial setting (Fig. 26.8).

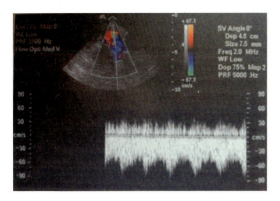

Fig. 26.8 Demonstration of AV shunt in a tibial bone

CVM in joints: Joint involvement may also be detected by careful ultrasound investigation.

Visceral venous malformations: Ultrasound investigation may be helpful in the diagnosis of visceral vein pathologies, like the nutcracker and Budd-Chiari syndrome.

Ultrasound investigation is the key for diagnosis and follow-up of CVM [15]. If a better spatial data for treatment planning is required, other examinations are required. They will be discussed in Chaps. 27, 28, and 29.

References

1. Laroche JP, Becker F, Khau-Van-Kien A, Baudoin P, Brisot D, Buffler A, Coupé M, Jurus C, Mestre S, Miserey G, Soulier-Sotto V, Tissot A, Viard A, Vignes S, Quéré I (2013) Société française de médecine vasculaire. Quality standards for ultrasonographic assessment of peripheral vascular malformations and vascular tumors. Report of the French Society for Vascular Medicine. J Mal Vasc 38(1):29–42

2. Bataille AC, Boon LM (2006) Aspects cliniques des malformations capillaires. Ann Chir Plast Esthet 51:335–347

3. Dubois J, Alison M (2010) Vascular anomalies: what a radiologist needs to know. Pediatr Radiol 40:895–905

4. McCafferty IJ, Jones RG (2011) Imaging and management of vascular malformations. Clin Radiol 66:1208–1218

5. Laurian C, Enjolras O, Bisdorff A, Franceschi C, Marteau V (2010) Hémangiomes et malformations vasculaires. EMC Angéiol 2010:19–17306

6. González SB, Busquets JC, Figueiras RG, Martín CV, Pose CS, de Alegría AM et al (2009) Imaging arteriovenous fistulas. Am J Roentgenol 193:1425–1433

7. Paltiel HJ, Burrows PE, Kozakewich HP, Zurakowski D, Mulliken JB (2000) Soft-tissue vascular anomalies: utility of US for diagnosis. Radiology 214:747–754

8. Eivazi B, Fasunla AJ, Hundt W, Wiegand S, Teymoortash A (2011) Low flow vascular malformations of the head and neck: a study on brightness mode, color coded duplex and spectral Doppler sonography. Eur Arch Otorhinolaryngol 268:1505–1511

9. Lee BB, Laredo J, Lee SJ, Huh SH, Joe JH, Neville R (2007) Congenital vascular malformations: general diagnostic principles. Phlebology 22(6):253–257

10. Connell F, Homfray T, Thilaganathan B, Bhide A, Jeffrey I, Hutt R, Mortimer P, Mansour S (2008) Congenital vascular malformations: a series of five prenatally diagnosed cases. Am J Med Genet A 146A(20):2673–2680

11. Yagel S, Kivilevitch Z, Cohend SM, Valsky V, Messing B, Shen O, Achiron R (2010) The fetal venous system, part I: normal embryology, anatomy, hemodynamics, ultrasound evaluation and Doppler investigation. Ultrasound Obstet Gynecol 35:741–750

12. Puig S, Casati B, Staudenherz A, Paya K (2005) Vascular low flow malformations in children: current concepts for classification, diagnosis and therapy. Eur J Radiol 53(1):35–45

13. Bo Park K, Soo Do Y, Kim DI, Wook Kim Y, Seop Shin B, Suk Park H, Wook Shin S, Ki Cho S, Wook Choo S, Gyu Song Y, Choo IW, Lee BB (2012) Predictive factors or response of peripheral arteriovenous malformations to embolization therapy: analysis of clinical data and imaging findings. J Vasc Interv Radiol 23(11):1478–1486

14. Cho SK, Do YS, Kim DI, Kim YW, Shin SW, Park KB, Ko JS, Lee AR, Choo SW, Choo IW (2008) Peripheral arteriovenous malformations with a dominant outflow vein: results of ethanol embolization. Korean J Radiol 9(3):258–267

15. Blei F (2008) Congenital lymphatic malformations. Ann N Y Acad Sci 1131:185–194

Role of MR and CT in Diagnostics

27

Josee Dubois and Gilles Soulez

MRI

MRI is the best method to evaluate the extension of the malformation and its relationship with adjacent structures [1]. The MR exam evaluates the extension; the size of the malformation; the infiltration of muscles, bones, tendons, and articulations; and the location of nerves, vessels, arteries, veins, and lymphatics included in the vascular malformations. MRI is also helpful in evaluating responses to treatment [2].

Routine sequences should include T1-weighted spin-echo or fast SE sequences, T2-weighted fat-suppressed fast SE acquisitions, and T1-weighted post-contrast fat-suppressed sequences. Depending on the clinical context and the result of Doppler US imaging, specific sequences are recommended depending whether we are investigating a slow- or fast-flow malformation.

Regarding slow-flow malformations, T1-weighted spin-echo sequences and T2-weighted fat suppression with short TI (inversion time) inversion recovery (STIR) are useful to determine the extent of the venous or lymphatic malformations. A T1-weighted spin-echo acquisition with fat suppression after gadolinium injection is required to document the enhancement of the malformation and differentiate venous malformation that will enhance from lymphatic malformation displaying minimal enhancement on the septa. 3D ultrafast spoiled gradient-echo acquisitions are also useful to evaluate the enhancement of the malformation after gadolinium injection. They can be repeated at different time frame to document the pattern of enhancement [3].

3D gadolinium-enhanced fat gradient-echo acquisition is helpful to evaluate the vascularization of the malformation [4]. To evaluate the dynamic circulation of the vascular anomalies, time-resolved MR angiography sequences are used and allow to differentiate the arterial inflow and venous drainage [5, 6].

CT Scan

Computed tomography plays a limited role for the evaluation of vascular anomalies given the inherent lack of soft tissue details and the advance of MR imaging. However, CT scan is useful for the evaluation of bone erosion and phleboliths, although last generation of multidetector CT can be used to obtain a three-dimensional reformation of vessels and to plan the embolization in cases of complex vascular anomalies. They are also useful to document aneurysm formation in high-flow malformations.

J. Dubois (✉)
Department of Medical Imaging,
CHU Sainte-Justine, Montreal, QC, Canada
e-mail: josee-dubois@ssss.gouv.qc.ca

G. Soulez
Department of Radiology,
CHUM Notre-Dame (University of Montreal),
Montreal, QC, Canada
e-mail: gilles.soulez.chum@ssss.gouv.qc.ca

R. Mattassi et al. (eds.), *Hemangiomas and Vascular Malformations: An Atlas of Diagnosis and Treatment*, DOI 10.1007/978-88-470-5673-2_27, © Springer-Verlag Italia 2009, 2015

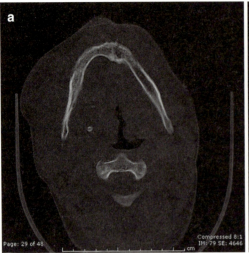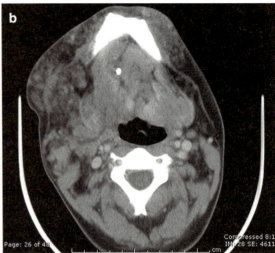

Fig. 27.1 Fourteen-year-old boy with venous malformation. (**a**, **b**) CT scan with contrast shows an extensive heterogeneous lesion of the face with infiltration of the masseter, buccal floor, tongue, parapharyngeal region, and mandibular bone. Phlebolith was seen

Venous Malformations

Different patterns of venous malformations (VMs) can be observed. The most common is a cavitary lesion with a delayed enhancement with or without abnormal draining vein. The second pattern is the presence of dysplastic veins that can be localized or diffuse in particular in upper or lower limbs. These patterns are better differentiated with percutaneous phlebography of the lesion before sclerotherapy.

Also, VMs can be a component of many syndromes, such as Klippel-Trénaunay, blue rubber bleb nevus, Maffucci's, Proteus, Cloves, or Bannayan-Riley-Ruvalcaba syndromes.

On *CT scan*, venous malformation shows a hypodense or heterogeneous lesion before contrast which enhances peripherally and slowly after injection of contrast. Phleboliths, bone erosion, or bony overgrowth is more clearly depicted on CT scan images (Fig. 27.1).

MRI – The first acquisition has to be done with a wide field of view to assess the extent of the lesion. VM can be seen on every part of the body. On T1-weighted images, VM is hypointense or isointense compared to the muscle. They may present with a heterogeneous or intermediate signal secondary to thrombosis or hemorrhage.

Absence of flow void is mandatory for the diagnosis of VM. On fat-sat T2-weighted sequences, high-signal intensity is observed. Sometimes, low-signal intensity is related to thrombosis or phleboliths. Fat suppression with short TI (inversion time) inversion recovery (STIR) T2-weighted sequence with a 512 matrix is well suited for this purpose. T2-weighted gradient-echo sequences can also be used to demonstrate calcifications or hemosiderin. On gradient-echo sequences, the absence of signal in the blood vessel in the vicinity of the malformation suggests a slow-flow malformation. Fluid-fluid level can be seen in regions of low or no flow.

FSE T1-weighted sequences with fat suppression should be performed after gadolinium injection to evaluate the perfusion of the malformation. Heterogeneous enhancement is seen after injection of gadolinium. MRI may also demonstrate soft tissue changes related to the VM, such as fatty replacement, atrophy of the adjacent musculature, or hypertrophy of the subcutaneous fat compared with the contralateral side [7].

To evaluate the dynamics of the VM, we perform a dynamic perfusion study 1, 2, 5, and 10 min after contrast infusion using a 3D ultrafast spoiled gradient-echo acquisition (volumetric interpolated breath-hold examination (VIBE)

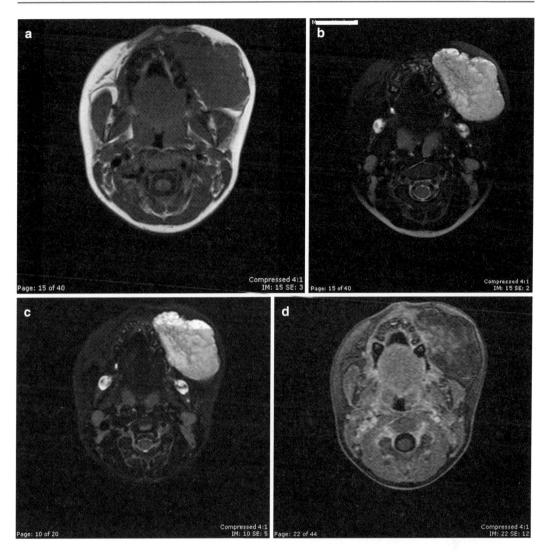

Fig. 27.2 Five-year-old girl with cheek venous malformation. (**a**) Axial T1-weighted image shows an isodense lesion of the left cheek. (**b**) Axial fast SE T2-weighted fat-suppressed image demonstrates a well-defined hyperintense lesion without perilesional edema. (**c**) STIR sequence). These contrast-enhanced 3D acquisitions images show hyperintense lesion with small signal voids (phleboliths). (**d**) Dynamic VIBE acquisition was performed. At 10 min, heterogeneous filling of the malformation by gadolinium was seen

sequence). These contrast-enhanced 3D acquisitions are also useful to appreciate the drainage of the malformation in the venous system [1, 8].

On 3D contrast-enhanced MRA, the lesions and their drainage into the systemic venous system can be mapped and should be documented on the report. The absence of deep venous system can be a contraindication for sclerosing treatment in some complex cases (Figs. 27.2, 27.3, and 27.4).

Arteriovenous Malformations

Arteriovenous malformations (AVMs) are isolated anomalies or are part of a syndrome, such as Parkes Weber or Rendu-Osler-Weber.

On *CT scan*, AVMs appear as highly enhancing lesions with numerous feeding and draining vessels, without persistent tissue staining (Fig. 27.5).

MRI shows arteries and veins with low-signal intensity due to the flow void phenomenon

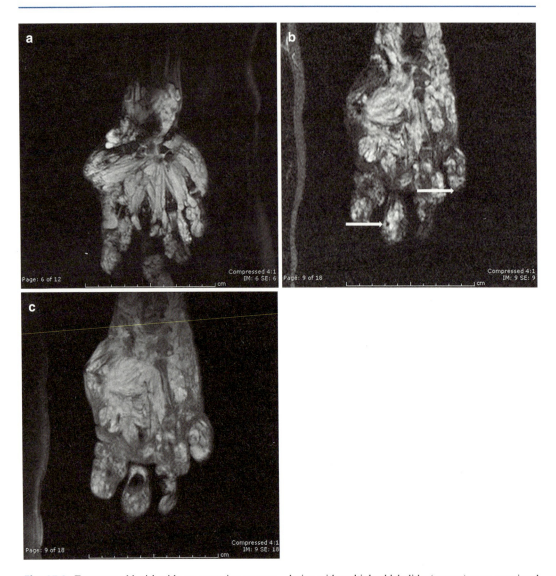

Fig. 27.3 Four-year-old girl with an extensive venous malformation of the hand. (**a**) Coronal axial T2 fat-suppressed image reveals a hyperintense signal of a significant infiltrative lesion of the muscle tendon of the hand. (**b**) STIR image shows the presence of hyperintense lesion with multiple phleboliths (*arrows*), seen as a signal void in the lesion. (**c**) Delayed contrast-enhanced fat-suppressed VIBE T1-weighted image shows diffuse enhancement of the venous malformation

of rapid and/or turbulent blood flow on both T1- and T2-weighted spin-echo sequences. Except for the presence of fat occasionally, no soft tissue mass is visible. A hypersignal is observed on gradient-echo and angiographic sequences. Occasionally, there are numerous interspersed small punctuated areas of high-signal intensity caused by hemorrhage and thrombosis. Gadolinium-enhanced MR angiography is helpful to evaluate feeding arteries and draining veins. The presence of an early venous filling is typically seen in AVMs. Using time-resolved MR angiography sequences, it is now possible to evaluate the dynamic opacification of AVM

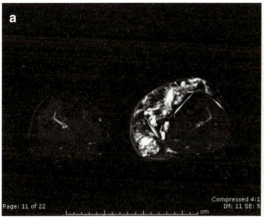
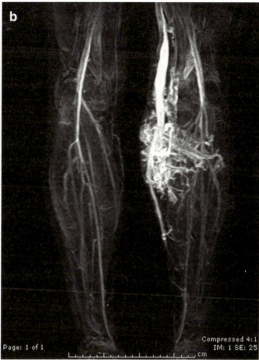

Fig. 27.4 Eighteen-year-old female with Klippel-Trénaunay syndrome. (**a**) Axial T2-weighted image demonstrates numerous hyperintense vessels in the subcutaneous fat. (**b**) Coronal contrast VIBE sub mip image shows numerous abnormal veins draining in a medial marginal vein. The deep venous system is normal

with the arterial feeders, nidus, and draining veins [6, 9, 10]. Since these sequences have a high temporal resolution, there is a compromise on spatial resolution which is lower than conventional 3D MR angiography using parallel imaging techniques (Fig. 27.6). In this setting, it can be useful to perform a 3D gradient-echo acquisition at high resolution during the steady-state phase of contrast enhancement to have a good delineation of the extension of the malformation.

Capillary Malformations

Capillary malformations are superficial vascular malformations. The only indication for MR imaging is to rule out an underlying AVM or associated complex anomalies such as Sturge-Weber, Klippel-Trénaunay, Parkes Weber, Cobb, or Proteus syndromes.

MRI – Capillary malformations are hyperintense on fluid-sensitive sequences and hypointense on T1-weighted images and display enhancement after contrast administration.

Lymphatic Malformations

Lymphatic malformations are divided into two types: macrocystic or microcystic. We will not discuss the lymphedema or complex syndrome associated with lymphatic malformations (Fig. 27.7).

CT scan of macrocystic lymphatic malformations shows a low-attenuation mass with enhancement of the septa after contrast injection [11].

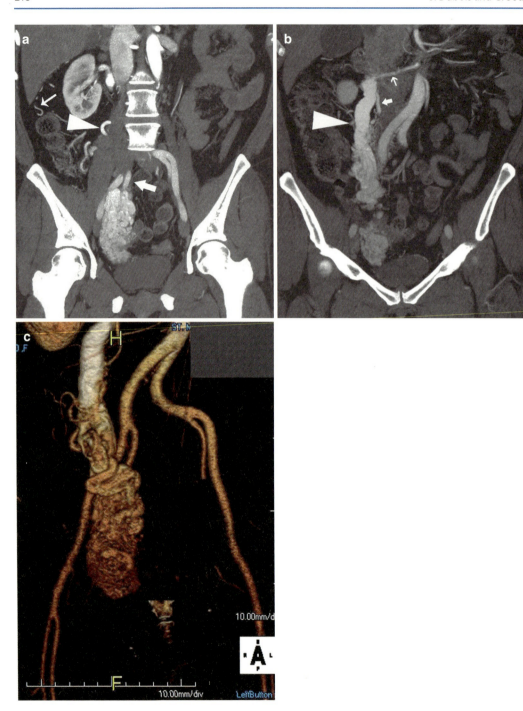

Fig. 27.5 Patient presenting a pelvic AVM involving the right ovary and parameter. (**a**) Coronal reformation of a CTA in arterial phase showing the large AVM and the contribution of the right internal iliac artery (*large arrow*). Contributions of an enlarged right ovarian artery (*arrowhead*) and renal capsular arteries (*small arrow*) can be seen. (**b**) A large ovarian vein (*arrowhead*) draining the AVM is observed on a posterior coronal reformation. The proximal portion of the enlarged ovarian artery (*large arrow*) arising from an accessory renal artery (*small arrow*) is also demonstrated. (**c**) The extension and 3D anatomy of the AVM are well seen on this volume rendering reformation

A pure microcystic lymphangioma is ill defined with fat infiltration and no enhancement after contrast injection is observed.

MRI shows a septated mass with low-signal intensity on T1 and high-signal intensity on T2. Because of varying amounts of protein or hemorrhage within the lesion, lymphatic malformations occasionally present with variable-signal intensity on T1 and T2 sequences. Sometimes, a high signal on T1 sequence or a fluid level can be observed in cases of cyst with a high content

of protein or a hemorrhagic content [3]. No gadolinium enhancement is visible, except in the septa. Pure microcystic lymphatic malformations are isointense on T1 and display a heterogeneous signal on T2, with or without a slight heterogeneous enhancement on T1 post gadolinium. Stranding of the adjacent subcutaneous fat may be present.

Bone lesions can be seen on T2-weighted sequences secondary to osteolysis, as seen in Gorham-Stout syndrome, also known as disappearing bone disease [12].

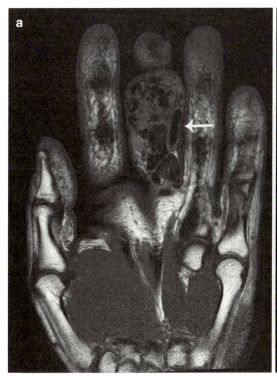 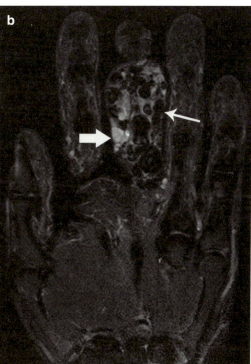

Fig. 27.6 Patient presenting an AVM of the third finger with worsening symptoms of venous congestion. (**a**) T1-weighted spin-echo acquisition showing the high-flow AVM with multiple vascular channels displaying flow void signals (*arrow*). (**b**) T2-weighted short tau inversion recovery (STIR) acquisition showing high-flow vessels with flow void on the arterial and venous side (*small arrow*) and several congestive veins with a low-flow paradoxical enhancement (*large arrow*). (**c**) Time-resolved acquisition (4D track) after gadolinium injec-

tion in the arterial phase showing both digital arteries feeding the AVM and the nidus. (**d**) On the venous phase (4D track), the dilated veins and the venous drainage are well demonstrated. (**e**) High-resolution 3D T1-weighted fast-field echo (FFE) with fat suppression in the coronal. It is not possible on these acquisitions to differentiate arterial feeders from draining veins. Small thrombi can be seen on the venous side, probably related to the venous congestion (*arrows*)

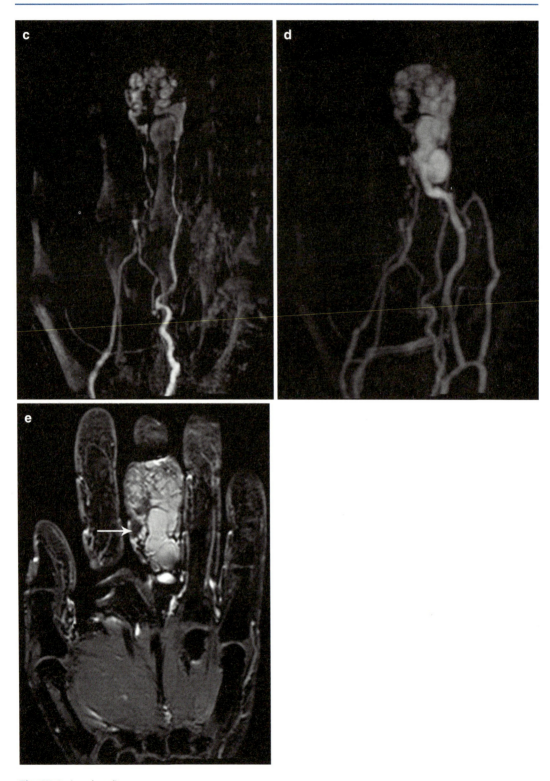

Fig. 27.6 (continued)

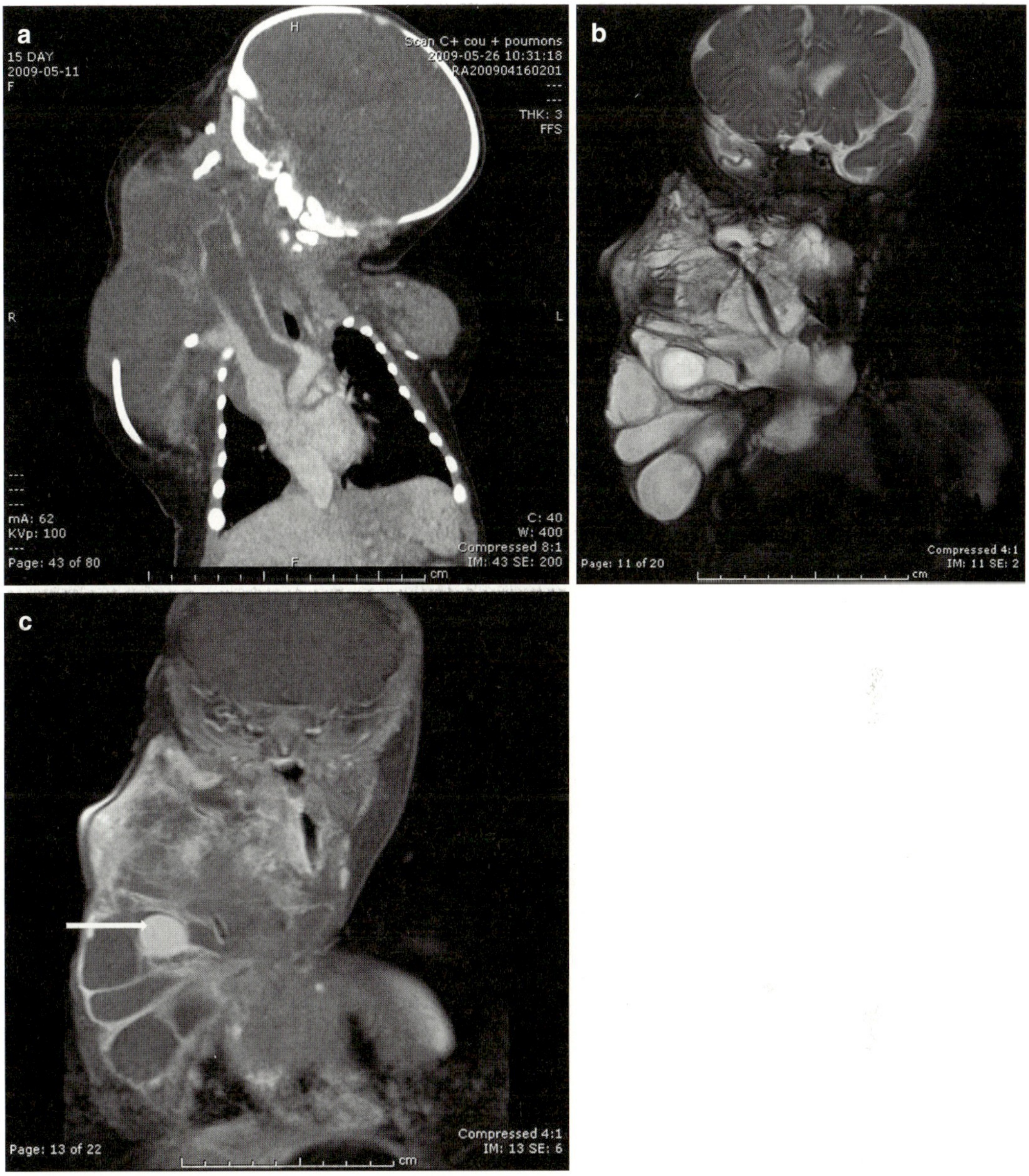

Fig. 27.7 Fifteen-day-old female child with a huge right cervico-mediastinal lesion, confirming a lymphatic malformation diagnosis. (**a**) CT scan shows a hypodense lesion with discrete enhancement of septa and significant displacement of the neck vessels. (**b**) Coronal T2-weighted image demonstrates a hyperintense macrocystic lesion. (**c**) Coronal T1-weighted contrast image shows an enhancement of the septa. The hypersignal in one of the cysts represents hemorrhage (*arrow*)

References

1. Dubois J, Soulez G, Oliva VL, Berthiaume MJ, Lapierre C, Therasse E (2001) Soft-tissue venous malformations in adult patients: imaging and therapeutic issues. Radiographics 21:1519–1531

2. Thawait SK, Puttgen K, Carrino JA, Fayad LM, Mitchell SE, Huisman TAGM, Tekes A (2013) MR imaging characteristics of soft tissue vascular anomalies in children. Eur J Pediatr 172:591–600

3. Caty V, Kauffmann C, Dubois J, Mansour A, Giroux MF, Oliva V, Piché N, Therasse E, Soulez G (2014) Clinical validation of semi-automated software for volumetric and dynamic contrast enhancement analysis of soft tissue venous malformations on magnetic resonance imaging examination. Eur Radiol 24(2): 542–551

4. Dobson MJ, Hartley RW, Ashleigh R, Watson Y, Hawnaur JM (1997) MR angiography and MR imaging of symptomatic vascular malformations. Clin Radiol 52:595–602

5. Ohgiya Y, Hashimoto T, Gokan T et al (2005) Dynamic MRI for distinguishing high-flow from low-flow peripheral vascular malformations. AJR Am J Roentgenol 185:1131–1137

6. Taschner CA, Gieseke J, Le Thuc V et al (2008) Intracranial arteriovenous malformation: time-resolved contrast-enhanced MR angiography with combination of parallel imaging, keyhole acquisition, and k-space sampling techniques at 1.5 T. Radiology 246:871–879

7. Rak KM, Yakes WF, Ray RL et al (1992) MR imaging of symptomatic peripheral vascular malformations. AJR Am J Roentgenol 159:107–112

8. Li W, David V, Kaplan R, Edelman RR (1998) Three-dimensional low dose gadolinium-enhanced peripheral MR venography. J Magn Reson Imaging 8:630–633

9. Reinacher PC, Stracke P, Reinges MH, Hans FJ, Krings T (2007) Contrast-enhanced time-resolved 3-D MRA: applications in neurosurgery and interventional neuroradiology. Neuroradiology 49(Suppl 1):S3–S13

10. Ziyeh S, Strecker R, Berlis A, Weber J, Klisch J, Mader I (2005) Dynamic 3D MR angiography of intra- and extracranial vascular malformations at 3 T: a technical note. AJNR Am J Neuroradiol 26:630–634

11. Dubois J, Alison M (2010) Vascular anomalies: what a radiologist needs to know. Pediatr Radiol 40:895–905

12. Konez O, Vyas PK, Goyal M (2000) Disseminated lymphangiomatosis presenting with massive chylothorax. Pediatr Radiol 30:35–37

Nuclear Medicine Diagnostics

28

Roberto Dentici and Raul Mattassi

Introduction

Nuclear imaging technique may have a more important role in the evaluation of angiodysplastic malformations, where tissue structure subversion, unpredictability of the morphological picture, frequent multifocality, and, in a few cases, the remarkable extent of the corporeal districts cannot be unequivocally answered with the use of more traditional methods.

The frequent lack of a recognized anatomic and structural consideration and the difficult distinction between masses generically defined as "liquid" may result in ambiguous nuclear magnetic resonance (NMR) patterns, while the presence of an anomalous escape course, segregated vascular districts, low recirculation speed, or the pathological mixture typical of lymphovenous abnormalities represents an impasse for angiographic interpretation.

In this corner of "diagnostic half-light," nuclear investigations make a useful contribution, albeit with the intrinsic limitations of a discipline that

found its methodology more on functional than on morphological aspects [1].

While there are some procedures that have been made obsolete by the technical and diagnostic refining of radiological studies, the nuclear methods that have resisted represent a real complementary diagnostic tool for the evaluation of angiodysplasia, thanks to their procedural simplicity, lack of invasiveness, high tolerability, and low biological cost from a dosimetric point of view [2].

Whole-Body Blood Pool Scintigraphy (WBBPS)

WBBPS (Fig. 28.1) is valuable for the initial screening of malformations and as an intermediate evaluation parameter for partial corrective procedures (post-interventional and/or post-embolization control). On the other hand, therapeutic or conservative treatments must be attempted several times in the instrumental follow-up of suspicious recidivism. WBBPS, a simple procedure from a technical point of view, makes red blood cells visible through the use of physiological contrast medium. This allows the vascular tree to be visualized in its entirety, as if a radiological contrast medium had been used. In this way, areas of high and/or altered "hematic" signal indicate the presence of the vascular malformation (Fig. 28.2).

As an example, in the truncular forms of vascular malformation, it is possible to distinguish anomalies of both arterial and venous course,

R. Dentici
Nuclear Medicine Service, Hospital "Caduti Bollatesi",
Bollate (Milan), Italy

R. Mattassi (✉)
Center for Vascular Malformations "Stefan Belov",
Department of Vascular Surgery,
Clinical Institute Humanitas "Mater Domini",
Castellanza (Varese), Italy
e-mail: raulmattassi@gmail.com

R. Mattassi et al. (eds.), *Hemangiomas and Vascular Malformations: An Atlas of Diagnosis and Treatment*,   223
DOI 10.1007/978-88-470-5673-2_28, © Springer-Verlag Italia 2009, 2015

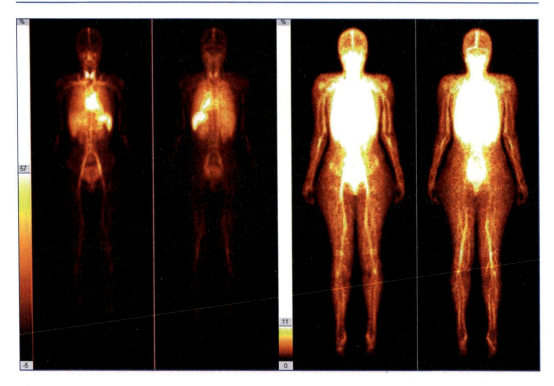

Fig. 28.1 Red blood cell angioscintigraphy: normal whole-body scan

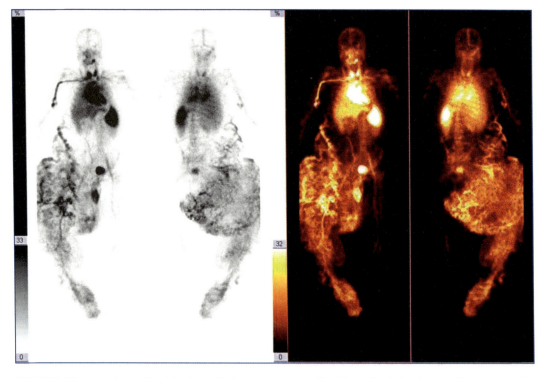

Fig. 28.2 Young patient with right lower limb over-growth. The labelled RBC study demonstrates a total sub-version of the vascular tree of the right leg. The dysplastic mass is spreading to the abdominal wall, partially surrounding the splanchnic tissues. The tomographic three-dimensional reconstruction emphasizes the chaotic structural complexity of this malformation

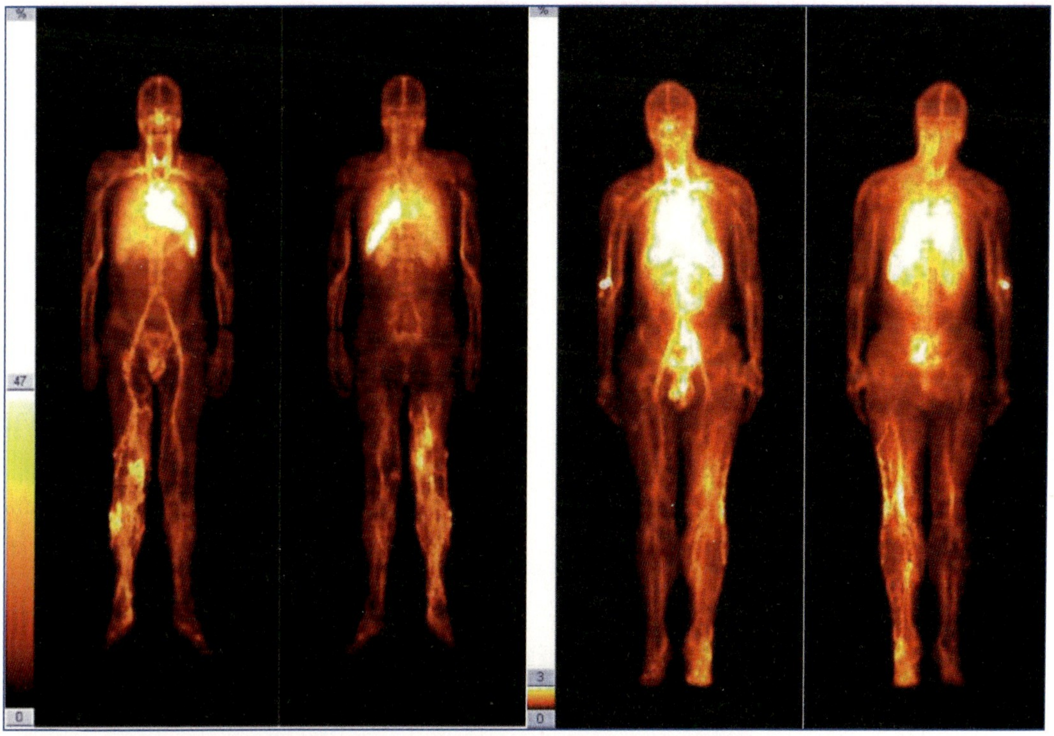

Fig. 28.3 Two cases of marginal vein of the inferior limb. Deep venous trunks are faintly visualized

stenotic occlusions, and expansions of the vessels. The poor or absent evidence of an artery or vein section, such as the slowing down or the absence of downstream flow, demonstrates hypoplasia or aplasia of the vessel, respectively (Fig. 28.3). Aneurysms are also recognizable with a typical and irregular increase in caliber.

In the extratruncular forms of vascular malformation, the tracer "accumulates" in pathological areas, providing a clear vision of the extent of the dysplasia. With images acquired in mutually orthogonal projections and especially with the three-dimensional tomographic reconstruction, it is also possible to better define and locate the lesion.

Of great interest is the possibility of identifying vascular malformations that, because of their liquid or mucinous aspect, can deceive sophisticated methods such as computer tomography (CT) and NMR: areas already catalogued as "angiomatous" but that are "cold" (not vascularized) according to scintigraphy should be carefully reexamined. Finally, in some cases, whole-body acquisition can reveal hidden abnormalities.

Furthermore, the study can be extended to the following day: this is possible because the biological contrast medium, represented by radiolabelled erythrocytes, remains active throughout its radioisotope decay. This is particularly suitable for the evaluation of lymphovenous abnormalities in which the slow recirculation time and mixture among the two pathological circuits do not allow an immediate evaluation using the most traditional radiological techniques, which are limited by the rapid elimination of contrast medium (Fig. 28.4).

It is possible to view the "discharge" or the "effusion" of the autologous cells from the intravascular compartment to the lymphatic one, achieving results of absolute diagnostic value. The main limitation of this method is the poorly detailed image, which does not allow discrimination between venous and arterial structures.

It is possible to differentiate between high-flow malformations (arteriovenous malformations [AVM]) and low-flow masses (prevailing venous component) by the comparative analysis of the transit time of the tracer in the pathological

Fig. 28.4 Lymphovenous shunt, detected by angioscintigraphy. At the second-day scan, a progressive subdermal hematic spillage is observed (*arrows*) (Reproduced from Dentici et al. [3])

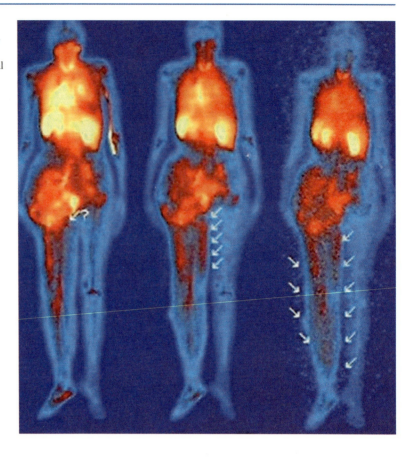

and corresponding healthy districts: the presence of an AVM is almost always revealed by activity-time curves obtained by the acquired dynamic sequence during the intravenous administering of radiotracer. The estimation of intralesional hemodynamics is essential in determining the appropriate treatment: surgical resection, arterial embolization, or sclerotherapy (Fig. 28.5).

Flow study (with the analysis of transit time or with direct puncture into the intravascular space of the lesion) provides a quantitative indicator of intralesional hemodynamics in low-flow lesions, in addition to accurate distinction between high-flow and low-flow lesions. For the percutaneous injection of sclerosing agents, the estimation of the flow characteristics of soft tissue vascular anomalies is essential for determining appropriate patient management. The last promising methodological aspect of great interest is represented by whole-body tomographic study, which can be extended to any corporeal district.

The tomographic approach in nuclear medicine has been used for the study of cerebral and myocardial perfusion (with ad hoc radiolabelled tracers) and for the evaluation of vascular malformations (prevalently hepatic), thanks to the possibility of revealing the "vascular nature" of lesions, not seen with methods such as echography, CT angiogram, and NMR.

The most recent generation of nuclear equipment and the availability of iterative rebuilding algorithms allow images of higher definition and total body images in three-dimensional rotation to be obtained; these can help to better define the highlighted lesions and their topographical relationships.

The availability of updated image-fusion software allows exams acquired with radiological methods to be imported and nuclear medicine imaging (NMI), CT, and NMR images to be melted, obtaining an iconography of high diagnostic content, in which structural and functional

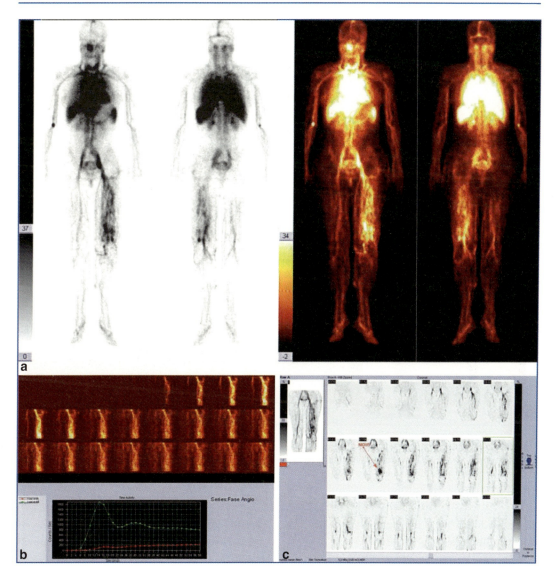

Fig. 28.5 (**a**) In this patient, the whole-body scan demonstrates a complex intra- and extratruncular malformation. (**b**) Study of the tracer's transit time is barely suggestive of an arteriovenous shunt. (**c**) At tomographic reconstruction, the AVM nidus is visible above the knee joint and in front of femoral artery

aspects of primary importance are merged in areas not accessible for clinical or sonographic exams, for instance, angiomatous intracranial or facial malformations (Fig. 28.6).

Recently, WBBPS was evaluated in 137 patients suspected to have venous or lymphatic malformations as a whole-body screening and diagnostic tool. WBBPS successfully detected abnormal blood pooling lesions in 96.8 % (120/124) of the patients with venous malformations, while no

tracer entered in lymphatic defects, demonstrating a good differential diagnosis possibility. In addition, WBBPS discovered 41 other lesions not recognized by clinical evaluation. WWBP was considered a valuable initial diagnostic tool with an accuracy of 97.1 % [4].

For postoperative evaluation of results of treatment, WBBPS was successfully used; a positive result after alcohol treatment was considered the reduction of the 50 % decrease in

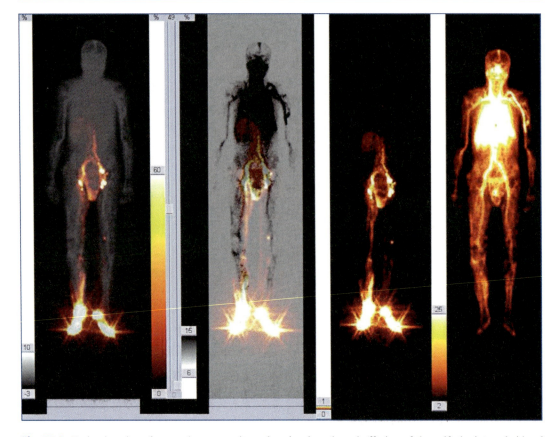

Fig. 28.6 Fusion imaging of a complex composite malformation involving the right inferior limb and the pelvis. The venous dysplasia mainly includes the calf and the lateral side of the knee and thigh. The lymphatic defect involves dermal effusion of the calf, the internal side of the thigh, the scrotum, and the peritoneal space, configuring a picture of probable lymphocele complicated by abdominal spillage. No evidence of lymphovenous shunt

abnormal blood pool ratio compared with pretreatment images [5].

This new gold standard is today within the reach of nuclear equipment supplemented with a single "hybrid" diagnostic position, a multihead gamma camera, and a multislice CT.

The integration of NMI and NMR is anticipated in the near future.

Lymphoscintigraphy

Historically, the instrumental approach to the alterations of the lymphatic system was carried out by radiological lymphangiography with a contrast medium. This method represents the gold standard for the study of a series of alterations and compromises of the lymphatic system, from the simple lymphedema to the staging of neoplasia involving the pelvis and the abdominal area [6].

While this method is able to reveal every detail of the lymphatic grid, escape routes, the presence of morphological alterations, and the caliber of vessels, it does have some drawbacks, which relegate it as an historical instrument of the radiologist rather than as one of the active tools of diagnostic practice.

Radiological lymphangiography is technically very difficult, requiring a microsurgical approach to the interdigital lymphatic capillaries; it also employs an oily contrast medium that remains in circulation and which may cause local complications at the injection point (up to skin necrosis), may be the cause of lymphangitis (in some cases worsening the clinical picture and

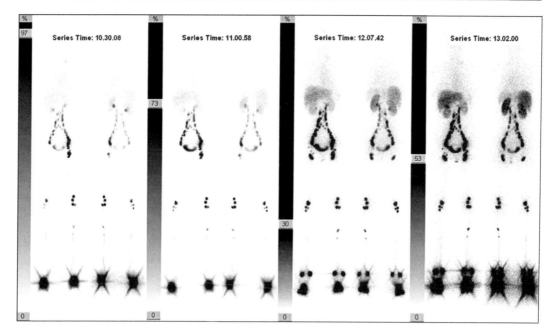

Fig. 28.7 Lymphangioscintigraphy with colloidal albumin: study of inferior limbs. Normal whole-body scan

causing functional damage that may exacerbate lymphedema), and, in extreme situations, may cause distant oily emboli, with the passage of the contrast medium into the blood stream. Taking into consideration these quite major problems, scintigraphy provides an alternative that is able to provide high-quality information and requires no special training. In addition, scintigraphy is not invasive, harmless to the lymphatic endothelium, devoid of collateral adverse effects (and therefore well tolerated by the patient), economic, repeatable, and especially reproducible (Fig. 28.7).

The investigation consists of administering a preparation of micelles of purified human albumin, with very low immunogenic power, in colloidal form, radiolabelled with an artificial radioisotope with a low energy and a reduced half-life, intradermally or subcutaneously. The substance has a very high biocompatibility and is filtered and degraded at the hepatic level and removed by urinary course in the hours immediately following administration. Furthermore, the very low dose of radioactivity makes its use absolutely safe, even for the study of congenital pathologies in infants [7, 8]. This test is

repeatable and can be prolonged for another 24 h, allowing lymphovenous shunt evaluation.

From a methodological point of view, various approaches have been proposed: most of them aim to evaluate the capacity of the lymphatic circulation to transport the radiolabelled substance (and then, indirectly, the lymph) in a centripetal sense and to verify transit times and the percent of substance "purified" from the injection point (a rather liberally concept of clearance), the maintenance of a "throbbing" flow inside the manifolds, the display, the number and percent quantification of lymph node capitation, and the passage in the main blood stream. There are several trends of thought about the "type" of circulation that can be analyzed: deep or superficial.

The investigation represents the necessary complement of an evaluation of "lymphedema without further exploration"; diagnosis is itself already within the reach of the clinical exam and of a careful anamnesis.

Independent of the type of evaluation, we have found that for the evaluation of malformative alterations, it is preferable to distinguish between the deep and the superficial circulation,

Fig. 28.8 Two cases of unexpected pathological lymphatics of the lower limbs. Both patients demonstrate dysplasia and hypertrophy of the superficial lymphatic system with noticeable dermal diffusion (*backflow*) and a normal appearance of the deep system. (**a**) The first patient shows also a star-shaped "lymphatic lake" on the anterior side of the right calf. (**b**) The second patient has a manifest failure of the deep circulation, compensated by the superficial one. A persistent faint drainage of the para-aortic lymphonodal chain coexists

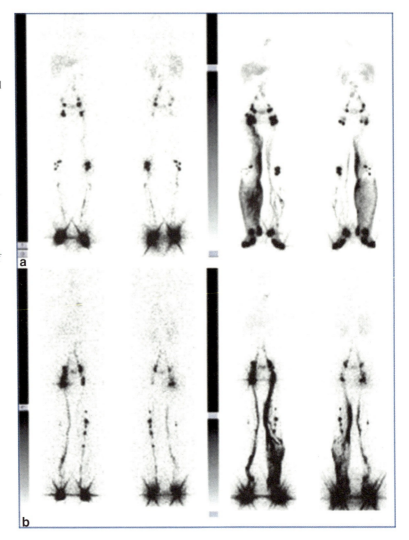

as frequently, alterations in the deep circulation are totally offset by a superficial circulation that functionally corrects an insufficience of primary or secondary nature.

In fact, only about 20 % of the lymphatic circulation starts in the muscle-fasciae compartment, in continuity with the deep lymph nodes. This explains why it difficult to see a normal alteration of the deep manifold, as it is masked or hidden by a superficially normal or differently pathological lymphoscintigraphic pattern (Fig. 28.8) [9].

This is even more true in the study of the complex alterations where subversion of the normal vascular anatomy frequently results in somatic alterations, such as corporeal segment gigantism, alterations in the number and morphology of skeleton segments, secondary cardiac and circulation alterations, or, on the contrary, hypotrophy and hypoplasia as a consequence of a growth defect (Fig. 28.9) [10].

Such alterations often involve the formation of anomalous ectasias of the lymphatic trunks and of preferential escape courses, the development of "lymphatic lakes" dependent on the presence of concomitant muscular alterations or on aberrant dysplastic venous masses, and, finally, shunting in the venous circulation [11]. Therefore, it is preferable to evaluate the draining capacity of deep manifolds using a single deep injection at

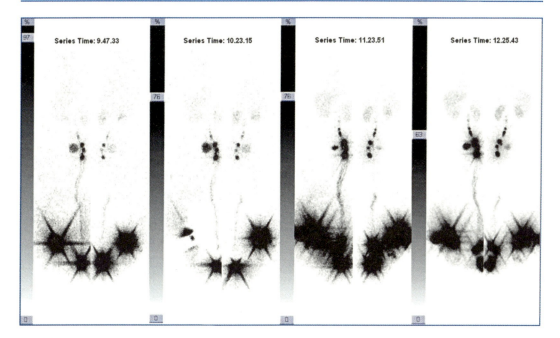

Fig. 28.9 In this patient, the same as in Fig. 28.2, a clear deficit of the lymphatic system of the right leg, both deep and superficial, is observed. On the left side, progression of the tracer is prevalently superficial but with an optimal compensation. No edema or swelling is visible. On the right side, there is no evidence of dermal backflow or venous commission: the examination excluded the presence of lymphovenous shunt and gave evidence of monolateral lymphatic agenesia

the level of the plantar arc (or palmar, in the case of a superior limb study), followed by an early scintigraphic scanning (within 10 min) to highlight the main deep lymphatic trunk and the deep lymph nodal stations. In normal situations, after a few minutes, the high capacity of extraction of the radioactive tracer from the injection point allows a clear visualization of the intermediate (popliteal, inguinal, iliac, para-aortical) lymph nodal stations.

In the case of a lack of conformity of the highlighted pattern with respect to the normal picture, multiple whole-body scans are recommended after centripetal stimulation, obtained by prolonged walking or with an isometric exercise (hand grip), which acts by "squeezing" the deep tissues. It is also possible in some cases to perform a manual draining massage of the area of interest.

With this methodology, it is possible to observe the behavior of a lymphatic flow altered by obstructive phenomena, by the presence of ectatic trunks, by the development of anomalous escape courses, by the presence of dermal diffusion ("backflow"), by crossover with retrograde tracer backflow (reflux), or by delayed tracer transport due to inversion of the flow direction.

After this first phase of study, a multiple subcutaneous injection between the fingers or toes is carried out, followed by an early scan followed by later ones, which are able to highlight with sufficient precision the superficial downflow course [11].

Also, in this case, it is the direct study of lymphoscintigraphic pattern that guides the clinician in deciding the timing of the subsequent observations. These can be prolonged until the following day if the presence of low-speed spare alterations is suspected (Fig. 28.10).

The final diagnostic option is the injection of radiotracer near cystic lesions that have been demonstrated with other methods in order to identify the tributary territories of the lesions themselves or, alternatively, the direct injection of radiocolloid inside the lesion itself, to identify any escape course (Fig. 28.11).

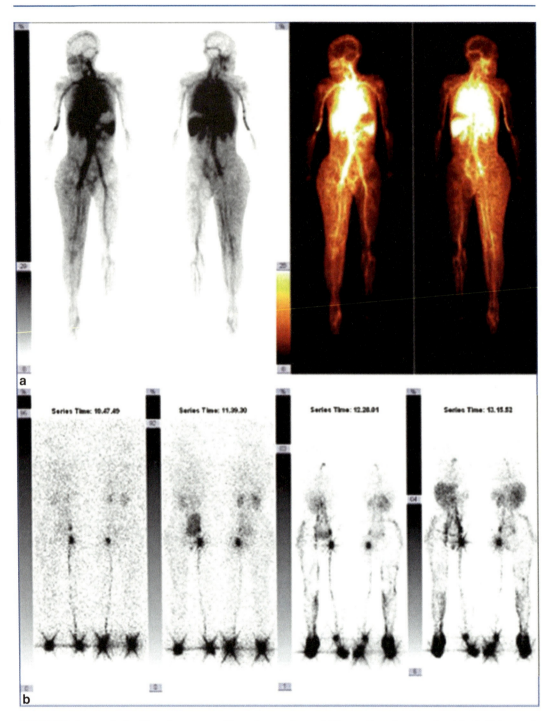

Fig. 28.10 A case of mixed lymphovenous malformation in a female patient. (**a**) The angioscintigraphy study demonstrates a volumetric asymmetry of the limbs, with an essentially preserved vascular tree and no evidence of AVM. Noticeable is the increased caliber of the iliac vessels. (**b**) In the lymphoscintigraphic study, lack of right main lymphatic manifolds, in particular the deep one, is observed. The centripetal progression of colloidal tracer is evident with slender superficial vessels, in part in marginal position. Notice the presence of dermal diffusion ("backflow") in the calf and gluteal region. On the left side too, the lymphatic flow is mainly superficial. This agrees with the RBC study

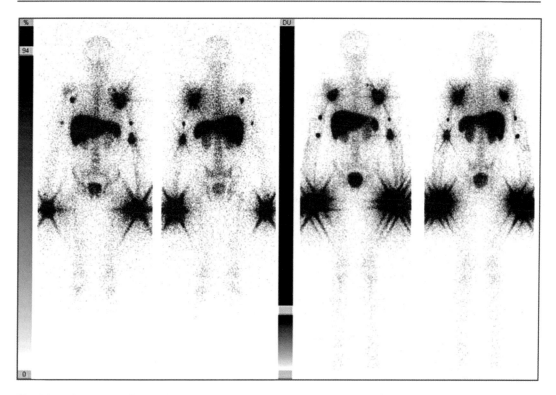

Fig. 28.11 Post-traumatic lymphovenous shunt of the right arm, persistent after repeated surgical treatments. Notice the quick, intense visualization of liver and reticuloendothelium of the bone marrow (not because of erroneous intravein injection!), patent proof of mixing. Consequent lymphatic theft and faint drainage into axillary nodes. The whole lymphatic circulation of both arms is normal

In our studies, we noticed several times the existence of an abnormal draining lymphatic, sited on the lateral edge of the limb. While in the first cases it was demonstrated in patients with a marginal vein, later also patients without venous anomalies had the same defect. We called this abnormal lymphatic "marginal lymphatic." In a case, we observed a tendency to lymphedema after surgery of marginal vein; performing lymphoscintigraphy, we noticed a marginal lymphatic occluded at the point where surgery was done. The suspicion was that an unsuspected marginal lymphatic was injured by surgery. In a lymphoscintigraphic study performed in 23 cases affected by truncular venous malformations, we found 14 (61 %) cases with a normal lymphatic system, 5 (22 %) cases with a marginal lymphatic, and 4 (17 %) cases with defects of the deep lymphatic system. None of the patients with abnormal deep lymphatics or marginal lymphatic has signs of lymphedema. The conclusion was that surgery of marginal vein should be preceded by lymphoscintigraphy to recognize marginal lymphatic (Fig. 28.12).

Recently, a new diagnostic technique to study lymphatic system has been proposed: dynamic magnetic resonance lymphangiography (MRL), based on interdigital injection of a paramagnetic contrast agent, like gadobenate dimeglumine, and MR imaging [12, 13]. That technique is today less performed, but some reports indicate that it seems to offer more precisely about data of structural and functional abnormalities of lymph vessels and nodes than lymphoscintigraphy [14].

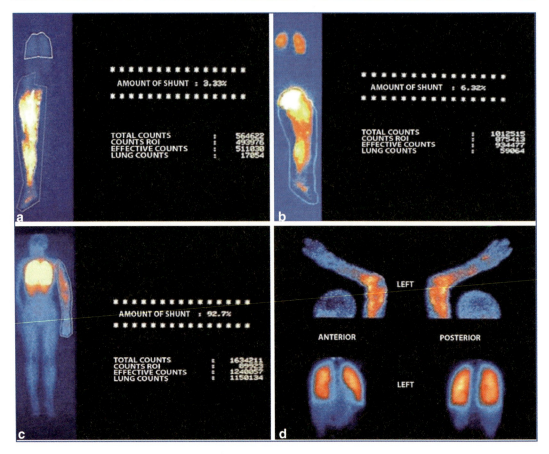

Fig. 28.12 Three cases of transarterial perfusion study ("microspheres test"). Clockwise from *top left*: a normal picture with shunted quote of <4 % (**a**); a slight positive picture, with shunted quote of ≅7 % (**b**); a frank positive picture with clear blood theft and shunted quote of 92 % (**c**); spot images of the last case with evident ischemia of the forearm and hand (**a**) (Figure 28.12a is reproduced from Dentici et al. [3])

Transarterial Lung Perfusion Scintigraphy (TLPS) (or "Microspheres" Study)

The study of AV shunts by nuclear medicine techniques has long been abandoned because other methods (duplex scan, angiography) are considered far more effective and precise [15–17]. However, in complex congenital vascular malformations (CVM), shunts may be multiple, differently located, and of the microshunt variety, detectable with difficulty. To recognize those fistulas, a time-consuming duplex scan examination or an invasive catheter angiography with multiple contrast injection is necessary. In this situation, a simple and effective nuclear medicine technique is able to give a quick response about existence or not of a shunt, and, if the response is negative, avoid an unnecessary angiography. The method is also capable of evaluating in semiquantitative terms both the functional impact of the fistula in the malformation system and the arterial and capillary outflow.

The method is based on the same principle used in pulmonary perfusional scintigraphy and consists of intra-arterial injection of microaggregations (more commonly called microspheres) of purified human albumin radiolabelled with 99 m technetium [15]. The examination is possible in the upper and lower limbs. The injection is made in the most easily accessible artery afferent to the malformative area to be examined (femoral artery for the lower limb, axillary, brachial, or, in some cases, the

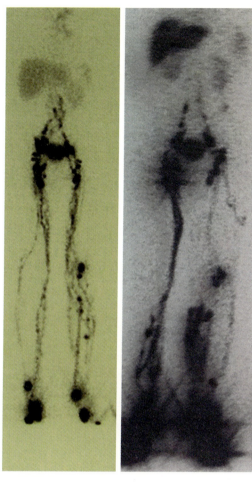

Fig. 28.13 Two cases demonstrating a marginal lymphatic (ML) vessel. In the *left picture*, a long ML is visible on the lateral edge of the right limb; in the *left picture*, in a complex lymphatic defect, an ML is visible on the lateral side of the left calf

the anomalous circuit: application of a simple mathematical formula indicates the shunted microspheres' quote at the pulmonary level. Moreover, a "morphologically" significant aspect also exists: with optimal arterial injection, whole-body spot scans, and high-speed tomographic acquisition, it is possible to notice the capillary flow distribution "visually," demonstrating poor or preferential perfusion areas.

The quantification of the shunt can be estimated as more precise as more tracer is injected near the shunt site; the faster the injection, the greater the bolus dispersion in the capillary circle and therefore the shunted quote will be more of an underestimate. Theoretically, an injection through a catheter placed on the afferent artery would give the most precise data, but in this way, the method becomes invasive, like angiography.

The three-dimensional rebuilding of the vascular district improves clinical and instrumental information about the physiopathological effect on the tissues by the "blood theft" due to the shunt.

TLPS is effective also as a control of treatment in terms of shunting volume reduction and also as a long-term follow-up of the spontaneous evolution of an AV malformation [21].

It should be considered that arterial puncture is normally not included in the technical skills of the nuclear physician and this may explain the tendency to ignore this procedure. Training by an angiography specialist or by a vascular surgeon is recommended.

ulnar artery if the superior limb is to be studied). The tracer, owing to the size of particles (<100 μm), is normally kept at the capillary circle of the limb (first filter); it is estimated that about one capillary in every 1,000 temporarily becomes embolized, a sufficient quantity to recognize and evaluate the blood flow. If fistulas exist, microspheres bypass the capillary circle of the limb (first filter), enter the venous circulation, and get trapped at pulmonary capillaries (second filter) (Fig. 28.13) [18–20].

To confirm or rule out the existence of a shunt, a comparative analysis of the perfusion curves is performed. It is also possible to quantify in percentage terms the amount of blood diverted by

References

1. Barton DJ, Miller JH, Allwright SJ, Sloan GM (1992) Distinguishing soft-tissue hemangiomas from vascular malformations using technetium-labeled red blood cell scintigraphy. Plast Reconstr Surg 89:46–52; discussion 53–55
2. Dubois J, Garel L, Grignon A et al (1998) Imaging of hemangiomas and vascular malformations in children. Acad Radiol 5:390–400
3. Dentici R, Mattassi R, Vaghi M (2002) La diagnostica per immagini in medicina nucleare. In: Mattassi R, Belov S, Loose DA, Vaghi M (eds) Malformazioni vascolari ed emangiomi. Testo-atlante di diagnostica e terapia. Springer, Milano, pp 32–39

4. Kim YH, Choi JY, Kim YW, Kim DI, Do YS, Choe YS, Lee KH, Kim BT (2014) Diagnosis and whole body screening using blood pool scintigraphy for evaluating congenital vascular malformations. Ann Vasc Surg 28:673–678

5. Yun WS, Kim YW, Lee KB, Kim DI, Park KB, Kim KH, Do YS, Lee BB (2009) Predictors of response to percutaneous ethanol sclerotherapy (PES) in patients with venous malformations: analysis of patient self-assessment and imaging. J Vasc Surg 50(3):581–589, 589

6. Witte CL, Witte MH (2000) An imaging evaluation of angiodysplasia syndromes. Lymphology 33:158–166

7. Dubois J, Garel L (1999) Imaging and therapeutic approach of hemangiomas and vascular malformation in the pediatric age group. Pediatr Radiol 29:879–893

8. Williams WH, Witte CL, Witte MH, McNeill GC (2000) Radionuclide lymphangioscintigraphy in the evaluation of peripheral lymphedema. Clin Nucl Med 25:451–464

9. Sloan GM, Bolton LL, Miller JH et al (1988) Radionuclide- labeled red blood cell imaging of vascular malformations in children. Ann Plast Surg 21:236–241

10. Lee BB, Mattassi R, Kim BT et al (2004) Contemporary diagnosis and management of venous and arteriovenous shunting malformation by whole body blood pool scintigraphy. Int Angiol 23:355–367

11. Solti F, Iskum M, Banos C, Salamon F (1985) Arteriovenous shunts in peripheral lymphedema: hemodynamic features and isotopic visualization. Lymphology 18:187–191

12. Liu N, Wang C, Sun M (2005) Noncontrast three-dimensional magnetic resonance imaging vs lymphoscintigraphy in the evaluation of lymph circulation disorders: a comparative study. J Vasc Surg 41:69–75

13. Liu NF, Lu Q, Jiang ZH, Wang CG, Zhou JG (2009) Anatomic and functional evaluation of the lymphatics and lymph nodes in diagnosis of lymphatic circulation disorders with contrast magnetic resonance lymphangiography. J Vasc Surg 49:980–987

14. Liu N, Wang C, Ding Y (1999) MRI features of lymphedema of the lower extremity: comparison with lymphangioscintigraphy. Zhonghua Zheng Xing Shao Shang Wai Ke Za Zhi 15:447–449

15. Inoue Y, Ohtake T, Wakita S et al (1997) Flow characteristics of soft-tissue vascular anomalies evaluated by direct puncture scintigraphy. Eur J Nucl Med 24: 505–510

16. Inoue Y, Wakita S, Yoshikawa K et al (1999) Evaluation of flow characteristics of soft-tissue vascular malformations using technetium-99m labelled red blood cells. Eur J Nucl Med 26:367–372

17. Ennis JT, Dowsett DJ (1983) Radionuclide angiography: intraarterial studies. In: Vascular radionuclide imaging: a clinical atlas. John Wiley, London, pp 122–123

18. Dentici R, Mattassi R, Vaghi M (2002) La diagnostica per immagini in medicina nucleare. In: Mattassi R, Belov S, Loose DA, Vaghi M (eds) Malformazioni vascolari ed emangiomi. Testo-atlante di diagnostica e terapia. Springer, Milano, pp 32–39

19. Solti F, Iskum M, Banos C, Salamon F (1986) Arteriovenous shunt-circulation in lymphoedematous limbs. Acta Chir Hung 27:223–231

20. Lee MJ, Dowsett DJ, Ennis JT (1990) Peripheral arteriovenous malformation: diagnosis and localization by intraarterial injection of technetium-99m-MAA. J Nucl Med 31:1557–1559

21. Lee BB, Mattassi R, Kim YW et al (2005) Advanced management of arteriovenous shunting malformation with transarterial lung perfusion scintigraphy for follow-up assessment. Int Angiol 24:173–184

Imaging of Vascular Malformations

29

Andrea Ianniello, Roberta Giacchero,
Massimo Vaghi, Alberto Cazzulani,
and Gianpaolo Carrafiello

Although almost 90 % of congenital vascular malformations (CVM) can be diagnosed based on the anamnesis and clinical history [1], imaging (conventional radiology [CR], ultrasound [US], magnetic resonance imaging [MRI], eventually computed tomography [CT], angiography, and venography) is not only an essential element for the ultimate diagnosis but it is also critical to assess the extent of the malformation and to plan the most appropriate treatment [1, 2]. Ultrasound diagnostic is discussed in Chap. 25 and CT and MRI in Chap. 26.

Conventional Radiology

Because of limited soft tissue contrast resolution, CR has little role for the evaluation and diagnosis of CVM; however, it plays an important role

A. Ianniello, MD (✉) • A. Cazzulani
Department of Radiology, "G. Salvini" Hospital,
Milan, Italy
e-mail: ianand@libero.it

R. Giacchero
Department of Pediatrics, San Paolo Hospital,
Milan, Italy

M. Vaghi
Department of Vascular Surgery, A.O.G. Salvini
Hospital, Garbagnate Milanese, Italy

G. Carrafiello
Department of Interventional Radiology, Macchi
Foundation Hospital, University of Insubria,
Varese, Italy

when there are clinical signs of involvement of the bones and joints. The radiographic examination is able to detect the presence of dystrophic calcification that can commonly occur in venous malformations (VM) and more rarely in lymphatic malformations (LM). Typical of the VM is the finding of phleboliths, caused by phenomena of thrombosis and calcification (Fig. 29.1a). If a CVM is sufficiently large, it can show a mass effect or distortion of adjacent bone [3]. Congenital vascular malformations close to the bone can cause hypoplasia, thinning of cortical bone, demineralization, and sometimes osteolysis (especially in high-flow vascular malformations) [3]. CVM may alter long bone growth originating a limb length difference; bone overgrowth is the best known mechanism, but also, hypotrophy is possible [4, 5]; a CR study in standing position of *both* involved limbs with comparative measures is useful to recognize and quantify the defect [6, 7].

A typical finding, present in the 70 % of cases of Klippel-Trénaunay syndrome, is mild limb length discrepancy due to increased longitudinal growth in the affected limb; this aspect can be easily assessed with long-standing radiograph (Fig. 29.1b) [3].

Other radiographic findings can be identified within VM-containing syndromes: plain film findings of Maffucci's syndrome include the sine qua non finding of multiple enchondroma phlebolith formation; because a high percentage of enchondromas can undergo malignant degeneration to

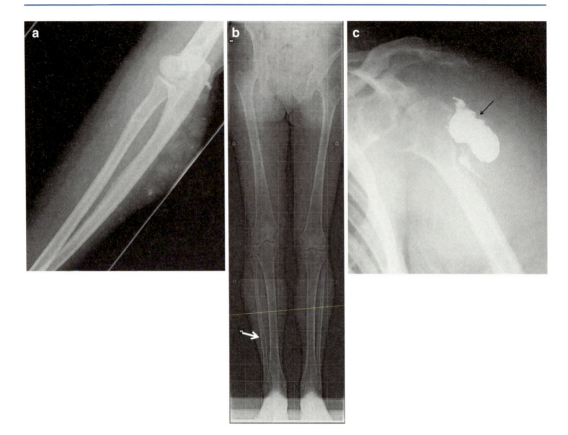

Fig. 29.1 (**a**) Plain film radiograph reveals multiple phleboliths identified within an extensive infiltrative VM of the forearm with thickening and mass effect on cutaneous and subcutaneous soft tissue. (**b**) Long-standing radiograph of Klippel-Trénaunay syndrome. 14-year-old girl with typical limb length discrepancy due to increased longitudinal growth in the affected right limb; the CVM also causes thinning of cortical bone at the distal third of peroneal diaphysis (*white arrow*). (**c**) Plain film radiograph of an AVM involving the left shoulder. Plain film radiograph shows the involvement of glenohumeral junction with osteolysis of inferior glenoid labrum and of the head of the humerus. Black arrow indicates radiopaque material (Onyx®) due to previous endovascular treatment

chondrosarcoma, clinical and radiographic vigilance is required. Gorham-Stout syndrome, or disappearing bone disease, is a rare skeletal disorder that is associated with diffuse VMs. The disease is characterized of progressive relentless osteolysis usually within the skull, shoulder, or pelvis that may be preceded by trauma. Intramedullary and subcortical lucent foci coalesce to diminish the diaphyses resulting in tapered ends of the long bone creating a cone-like or "sucked candy" appearance [3].

Vascular malformations may alter bone structure and bone growth. Arteriovenous malformations (AVM) may be sited inside the bones showing some typical images in plain film radiograph pictures of bone. The precise study of these defects, especially the areas of thinning of cortical or even the aspects of cortical "holes," is useful in order to detect specific bone point where direct puncture may be attempted if an intraosseous direct injection in the malformation (coils, glue, alcohol, etc.) is planned (Fig. 29.1c).

Venography

The phlebographic techniques (ascending or descending venography and direct percutaneous venography [DPV]) are by far less performed than in the past because other noninvasive methods like US, MR, and CT give excellent results [8]. However, in some specific conditions, when noninvasive tests failed to confirm the diagnosis, they may be effective to complete diagnosis or in the preoperative planning in low-flow CVM [9].

Ascending phlebography is mainly performed to study the deep venous system of the lower limbs: *anomalies of the deep venous system in fact occur in almost one half of congenital vascular malformations of venous predominance* [10]. *The correct diagnosis of these anomalies represented by avalvulia, aplasia, hypoplasia, phlebectasia, and venous aneurysms* (Fig. 29.2a–e) *is important to prevent serious therapeutic consequences* [10].

This apparently easy technique requires specific knowledge about CVM and skills to be really useful, as wrong results are common. Missing to visualize deep venous system which is hypoplastic (but not aplastic) in some segment is not uncommon because preferential outflow alternative ways may canalize contrast media to superficial vessels. Normal deep venous system may be failed to contrast because of abnormal large perforants to the superficial veins, like in cases of marginal vein (Fig. 29.2f).

Venipuncture is performed via the dorsal vein of the great toe using a size 22-gauge cannula; for venous cannulation, the patient then sits on the edge of the bed or chair with the legs dependent. Before cannulation, the feet are bathed in warm water for 5 min, allowing the veins to become dilated and more prominent. The warm water has the additional effect of softening the skin and may also provide a mild analgesic effect. The dorsal vein of the great toe has the advantage of being easily located, even in an edematous foot, by gently squeezing the dorsum of the toe with both thumbs; a more proximally and laterally located venous cannulation results in inadequate filling and opacification of the deep venous system with contrast more likely to pass into the dorsal venous arch, which then drains into the long and short saphenous veins.

To prevent superficial vein filling and to aid deep vein filling, two tourniquets are used: the first tourniquet is placed tightly above the ankle malleoli, whereas the second is placed 5–10 cm above the patella. Repeated injections and different projections may allow to get the best results. Ideally, the procedure should be carried out with the patient in the erect position to allow maximum mixing of contrast and blood, with subsequent filling of the deep venous system.

Descending phlebography is today rarely performed as duplex ultrasound is the gold standard exam to study venous reflux. However, in some specific cases of abnormal deep reflux, like persistence of sciatic vein, the technique may be useful. Descending phlebography requires venous catheterism *of the common femoral vein* on a tilting radiological table in order to perform the examination with the patient in partially standing position (at least 60° semi-upright position). Subsequent contrast injection, during a Valsalva maneuver, is observed fluoroscopically and recorded on plain radiography. Abnormal incompetence, extent, and level of contrast material reflux are evaluated in order to classify venous insufficiency (Fig. 29.2g).

The *DPV* involves the direct puncture with a fine needle (20–21 gauge) of the lesion and the subsequent injection of a contrast agent under fluoroscopic guidance. Three different phlebographic pattern [2] can be seen with opacification of the VM: the "cavity" pattern (Fig. 29.2h), the most common aspect in VM, is characterized by late venous drainage without evidence of abnormal vein, the "sponge" (Fig. 29.2i) appearance with small cavities until the "honeycomb" aspect with a late venous drainage, and the third pattern with rapid opacification of dysmorphic veins (Fig. 29.2j) [10]. After sclerotherapy, the best results are achieved in the VM that show "cavity"; the "sponge" VM, especially if intramuscular, is more difficult to treat.

Another classification [9] that correlates the pattern of phlebography (in particular assessing the morphology and venous drainage) with the results and the risk of complications after sclerotherapy has been proposed identifying four different patterns: type I (Fig. 29.2k) VM shows negligible venous drainage into normal venous circulation, type II (Fig. 29.2l) VM anatomy reveals normal venous outflow into general venous circulation, type III (Fig. 29.2m) anatomy demonstrates drainage from the VM by way of abnormally ectatic or dysplastic veins, and type IV (Fig. 29.2n) lesions are composed entirely of ectatic or dysplastic veins. The sclerotherapy treatment can be carried out, but with caution, in patients with VM of types III and IV, while it can run safely in patients with malformations of type I and type II (low-risk lesions).

Arteriography

Currently, there is no role for diagnostic angiography in the diagnosis or follow-up of low-flow vascular malformations [2, 3]. At angiographic study, both the VM and LM did not show any pathological importance in the majority of cases; sometimes only in the later stages after the injection of a contrast agent, it is possible to detect the presence of dilated dysmorphic veins [3].

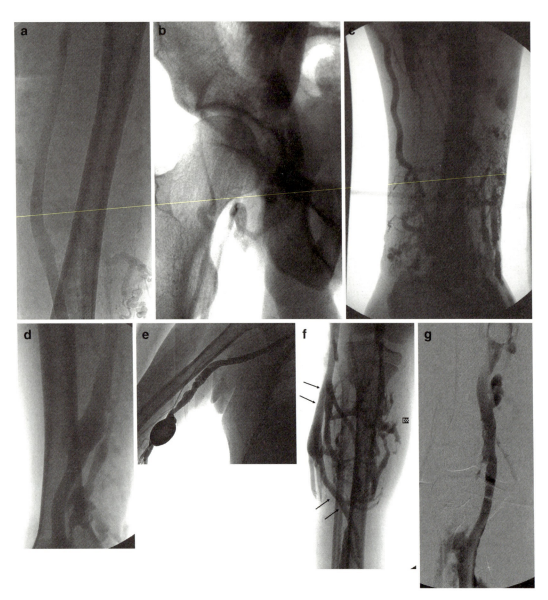

Fig. 29.2 (**a–f**) Ascending phlebography performed after cannulation of the dorsal vein of the great toe shows different type of deep venous system anomalies such as avalvulia (**a**), aplasia (**b**), hypoplasia (**c**), phlebectasia (**d**), and venous aneurysms (**e**); marginal vein (**f**: *arrows*), type II according to Weber classification. (**g**) Descending phlebography shows severe incompetence of venous system (Grade IV) with reflux into the calf veins. (**h–j**) Direct percutaneous venography: Dubois classification of phlebographic appearance of VMs: cavitary pattern illustration (**h**), spongy pattern (**i**) and dysmorphic illustration (**j**). (**k–n**): Puig classification of VMs based on venous drainage pattern. (**k**): Type I VM showing negligible venous drainage into normal venous circulation. (**l**) Type II VM anatomy revealing normal venous outflow into general venous circulation. (**m**) Type III anatomy demonstrates drainage from the VM by way of abnormally ectatic or dysplastic veins. (**n**) Type IV lesions are composed entirely of ectatic or dysplastic veins

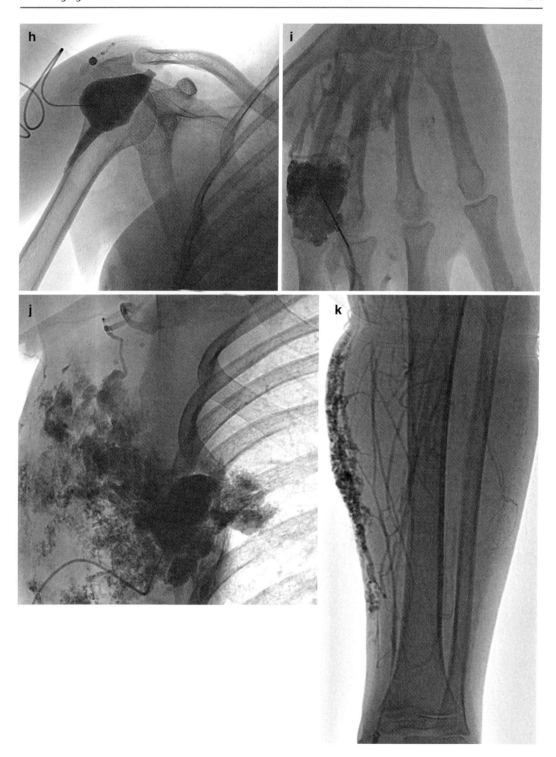

Fig. 29.2 (Continued)

Angiography is diagnostic, rather than essential, for treatment planning in high-flow AVM [3]. The pathognomonic findings of AVM at angiography are represented by enlarged afferent arteries with an early opacification (shunting) of the efferent veins, dilated. Selective injections and superselective are essential to assess the extent of the AVM and have the exact vascular map, with a

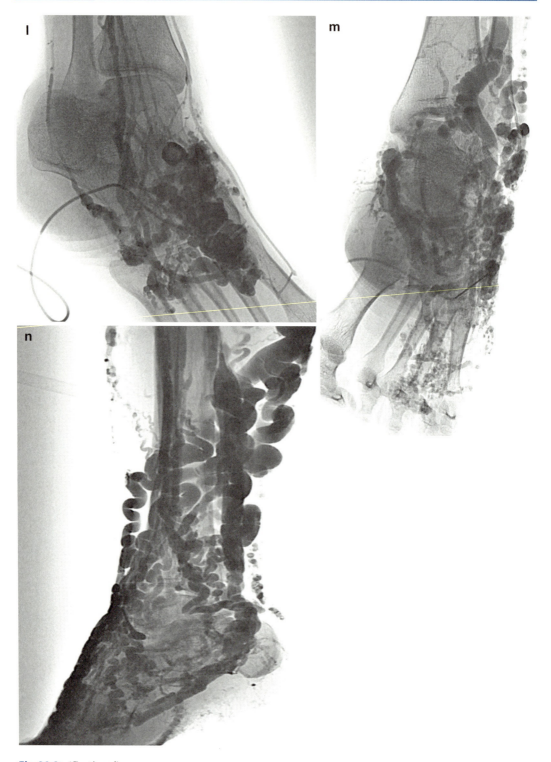

Fig. 29.2 (Continued)

focus on "feeding arteries" in order to properly plan the treatment [11]. Different classifications of AVM based on their arteriographic appearance have been proposed, resulting in the classification of Houdart and collaborators for the intracranial malformations and fistulae, the most simple and accurate [11]. This classification has distinguished the AVM into three different groups, based solely on the evaluation of the shunts, visible on arteriography, as a "nidus," which is the main target of the embolic treatment: the arteriovenous, arteriolovenous, and arteriolovenulous fistulae. This classification, which makes no reference to congenital or

acquired nature of the lesion, indicates the type of approach in the endovascular treatment according to the group they belong to. More recently, the classification of Houdart has been modified and adapted to the peripheral AVM of the body; in this new classification, other aspects were evaluated—such as the presence of subtle blush or streaks. Peripheral body AVM, depending on the appearance on angiography, was divided into 4 different types [12]: type I (arteriovenous fistulae; Fig. 29.3a), type II (arteriolovenous fistulae; Fig. 29.3b), and type III (arteriolovenulous fistulae; Fig. 29.3c–d). If the fistula that joined the

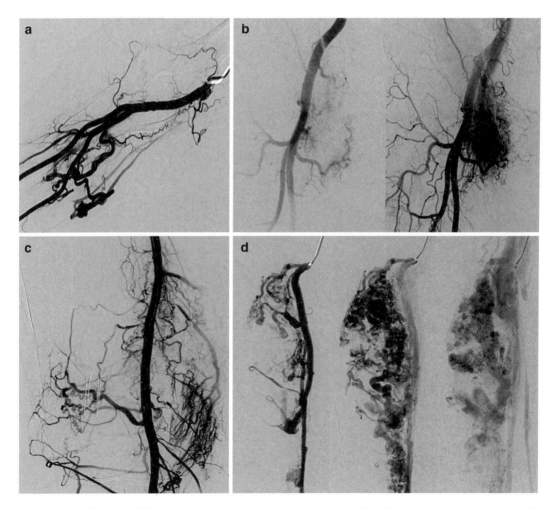

Fig. 29.3 (a–c) Types of AVMs based on nidus morphology. (a) Type I (arteriovenous fistulae). No more than three separate arteries shunt to the initial part of a single venous component. (b) (Arterial and venous phase) Type II (arteriolovenous fistulae). Multiple arterioles shunt to the initial part of a single venous component, in which the arterial components show a plexiform appearance on

angiography. (c) Type IIIa (arteriolovenulous fistulae with non-dilated fistula). Fine multiple shunts are present between arterioles and venules and appear as a blush or fine striation on angiography. (d) Type IIIb (arteriolovenulous fistulae with dilated fistula). Multiple shunts are present between arterioles and venules and appear as a complex vascular network on angiography

nidus is seen at angiography as a blush or as a thin streak, it is subcategorized as type IIIa (not dilated fistula), while if the fistula that joined the "nidus" appears as a dense vascular network, it is classified as IIIb (dilated fistula) [6, 12]. In this last classification, Cho and collaborators correlate approach and therapeutic outcome after ethanol embolization [11]. More details about classification of AVM are discussed in Chap. 32.

References

1. Hyodoh H, Hori M, Akiba H et al (2005) Peripheral vascular malformations: imaging, treatment approaches, and therapeutic issues. Radiographics 25(Suppl 1):S159–S171
2. Dubois J, Alison M (2010) Vascular anomalies: what a radiologist needs to know. Pediatr Radiol 40(6):895–905
3. Legiehn GM, Heran MK (2008) Venous malformations: classification, development, diagnosis, and interventional radiologic management. Radiol Clin North Am 46(3):545–597
4. Servelle M (1985) Klippel and Trenaunay syndrome. 768 operated cases. Ann Surg 201(3):365–376
5. Belov S (1990) Haemodynamic pathogenesis of vascular-bone syndromes in congenital vascular defects. Int Angiol 9(3):155–161
6. Mattassi R, Vaghi M (2007) Vascular bone syndrome – angio-osteodystrophy: current concepts. Phlebology 22(6):287–290
7. Lee BB, Bergan J, Gloviczki P, Laredo J, Loose DA, Mattassi R, Parsi K, Villavivencio JL, Zamboni P (2009) Diagnosis and treatment of venous malformations. Consensus document of the International Union of Phlebology. Int Angiol 28(6):434–451
8. Lee BB, Baumgartner I (2013) Contemporary diagnosis of venous malformations. J Vasc Diagn 1:25–34
9. Puig S, Aref H, Chigot V et al (2003) Classification of venous malformations in children and implications for sclerotherapy. Pediatr Radiol 33(2):99–103
10. Eifert S, Villavicencio JL, Kao TC et al (2000) Prevalence of deep venous anomalies in congenital vascular malformations of venous predominance. J Vasc Surg 31(3):462–467
11. Konez O, Hopkins KL, Burrows PE (2012) Pediatric techniques and vascular anomalies. In: Rubin GD, Rofosky NM (eds) CT and MR angiography. Lippincott, Philadelphia, pp 1118–1187
12. Cho SK, Do YS, Shin SW et al (2006) Arteriovenous malformations of the body and extremities: analysis of therapeutic outcomes and approaches according to a modified angiographic classification. J Endovasc Ther 13(4):527–538

Principles of Treatment

30

Raul Mattassi, Dirk A. Loose, and Massimo Vaghi

Introduction

The decision process about the best treatment in congenital vascular malformations (CVM) should consider several factors: symptoms, possible complications of treatment, hemodynamic correction expected, invasivity of the procedure and others (see Chap. 24 for more details about clinical conditions and treatment). In other words, a balance between risks and advantage of the treatment is mandatory, as in any therapy. However, that decision may be much more difficult in CVM, due to the great variability of the disease. Several techniques are available, and often, best result is obtained by a combination of those procedures and also by a correct timing.

Truncular vascular dysplasia of veins and arteries is mainly treated by conventional vascular techniques, like revascularization surgery or reflux control surgical techniques in venous truncular dysplasia. Specific reconstructive techniques are available for some cases of truncular lymphatic defects (see Chap. 51). In arteriovenous truncular fistulas, complex devascularization techniques or, sometimes, endovascular procedures can be used.

Extratruncular forms are much more frequent and variable and have a tendency to recur because they are composed by a remnant of embryonic cells. To prevent recurrence, the ideal treatment should be a radical surgical removal, rather than a simple occlusion, that close the lumen of the dysplastic vessels but let the abnormal cells in site. Limited forms can be treated by surgery or by occlusion. In extensive infiltrations of organs, surgical resection is performed according to general surgical techniques. Occlusion techniques, by catheter or percutaneous, are available as an alternative or a combination with surgery.

R. Mattassi (✉)
Center for Vascular Malformations "Stefan Belov",
Department of Vascular Surgery,
Clinical Institute Humanitas "Mater Domini",
Castellanza (Varese), Italy
e-mail: raulmattassi@gmail.com

D.A. Loose
Section Vascular Surgery and Angiology,
Facharztklinik Hamburg, Hamburg, Germany
e-mail: info@prof-loose.de

M. Vaghi
Department of Vascular Surgery, A.O.G. Salvini
Hospital, Garbagnate Milanese, Italy
e-mail: vaghim@yahoo.it

Truncular CVM

Treatment of truncular CVM should be addressed to the correction of the hemodynamic disorder. Treatment options are the following [1, 2]:

Revascularization techniques (repair of a vascular defect), mainly surgical, (bypass, vascular plastics) are indicated in cases of congenital aneurysma, hypoplasia, or aplasia of the arteries and veins. Endovascular techniques, like covered stent implantation or balloon techniques, are also useful in these instances.

R. Mattassi et al. (eds.), *Hemangiomas and Vascular Malformations: An Atlas of Diagnosis and Treatment*,
DOI 10.1007/978-88-470-5673-2_30, © Springer-Verlag Italia 2009, 2015

Devascularization techniques (removal of dysplastic vessels) can be based on surgery or on endovascular occlusion.

Extratruncular CVM

Extratruncular malformations are much more common and variable than truncular forms. Several treatment techniques are available: surgery, catheter embolization, percutaneous occlusion, and laser. These methods can be combined in order to improve results.

According to the site, extension, and infiltration of structures, the best approach for the single case is selected.

Limited forms can be treated by occlusion, percutaneous or by catheter, resected surgically or vaporized by laser application [3–5]. Decision between surgery and occlusion depends mainly on the site of the defect: by superficially, easy accessible locations, surgery can be more radical than occlusion as a complete removal of an embryonic remnant should probably guarantee more against recurrence. Laser treatment is best applied in superficial, limited forms.

Infiltrating forms can be treated by steps, sometimes best combining occlusion and surgery, like partial surgical resection and completion by occlusion or also by laser. The contrary is also possible: occlusion by embolization of an atriovenous malformation followed by surgical resection. Partial resection can be performed also by transfix suture of the mass without removal, if that would be too difficult. Some instruments are available for the surgeon for resections, like radiofrequency implemented clamps for resection+hemostasis and ultrasound aspirators to prepare vessels.

Occlusion of vessels can be done by injecting different substances in the vessels like glue, ethanol, particles, bleomycine, coils, and others. Selection of the best product to treat the single case is extremely important (see Chap. 32). Nonsurgical occlusion can be performed also by using intralesional laser or radiofrequency (see Chap. 35)

Crucial point in treatment selection is available in all procedures (surgery, embolization, percutaneous occlusion, and laser) in the group that intend to treat the patient. Moreover, a large panel of specialists should collaborate in order to be available in specific cases, especially if surgical knowledge and specific skills are required by a treatment of a CVM in a difficult location. Availability of all techniques and of specialists may be the difference between finding a solution or refusing the patient [6]. Another point which is of significant importance is the presence of a leader of the group which has the knowledge of all the procedures and techniques and may be decisive for the best procedure and for the selection of a specialist that should join the team of the treatment of a specific case.

In conclusion, approach to CVM is not a job for a one-tool man.

Support Therapy

Beside direct approach to the defect, support medical therapy to treat specific symptoms is often indicated.

Pain

Pain control is mandatory for a good life quality of patients. Many types of pain drugs are available. However, pain origin in the single case should be known in order to treat the case in the best manner.

In arteriovenous extratruncular malformations, pain is mainly due to compression of structures. Pain drugs are effective.

Pain is common in extratruncular venous malformations because of thrombosis inside the defect. Elevated D-dimer indicates an activation of the clotting system [7, 8]. In these cases, anticoagulant therapy will be more effective than simple painkiller drugs. However, if pain in these venous cases is due to phlebolythes, which are painful at compression, best treatment is surgical removal rather than heparin or painkiller drugs.

Pain in extratruncular lymphatic defects is generally due to inflammation and infection; antibiotic therapy is the best option.

Neuritic pain may be due to nerve compression or infiltration of the nerve by the malformation. In these cases, treatment of the defect itself may be more effective than simple pain drugs. In severe pain due to non-treatable venous malformations infiltrating nerves, spinal cord stimulation may be the only effective option to control pain.

Edema

Venous and lymphatic edema may reduce significantly by wearing elastic stockings. Patients with arteriovenous malformations and limb edema may also have advantage from elastic stockings. However, in case of painful phlebolythes or inflammation of extratruncular lymphatic malformation, compression may be not tolerated by the patient.

Phlebotonic drugs may be an effective adjunctive treatment in venous forms.

Lymph drainage is the key therapy for lymphedema (see Chap. 50).

References

1. Belov S (1994) Surgical treatment of congenital vascular defects. In: Chang JB (ed) Modern vascular surgery. Springer, New York/Berlin/Heidelberg, pp 383–397

2. Mattassi R, Loose DA, Vaghi M (2009) Principles of treatment of vascular malformations. In: Mattassi R, Loose DA, Vaghi M (eds) Hemangiomas and vascular malformations. Springer, Milan/New York, pp 145–151

3. Lee BB, Baumgartner I, Berlien HP, Bianchini G, Burrows P, Do YS, Ivancev K, Kool LS, Laredo J, Loose DA, Lopez-Gutierrez JC, Mattassi R, Parsi K, Rimon U, Rosenblatt M, Shortell C, Simkin R, Stillo F, Villavicencio L, Yakes W (2013) Consensus Document of the International Union of Angiology (IUA)-2013. Current concept on the management of arterio-venous management. Int Angiol 32(1):9–36

4. Lee BB, Baumgartner I, Berlien P, Bianchini G, Burrow P, Gloviczki P, Huang Y, Laredo J, Loose DA, Markovic J, Mattassi R, Parsi K, Rabe E, Rosenblatt M, Shortell C, Stillo F, Villavicencio L, Zamboni P (2014) Diagnosis and treatment of venous malformations Consensus document of the International Union of Phlebology (IUP) updated 2013. Int Angiol, PMID: 24566499 (Ahead of print)

5. Lee BB, Andrade M, Antignani PL, Boccardo F, Bunke M, Campisi C, Damstra R, Flour M, Forner-Cordero I, Gloviczky P, Laredo J, Partsch H, Piller N, Michelini S, Mortimer P, Rabe E, Rockson S, Scuderi A, Szolnocky G, Villavicencio JL (2013) Diagnosis and treatment of primary lymphedema. Consensus document of the international union of phlebology UIP. Int Angiol 32(6):541–574

6. Lee BB, Do YS, Yakes W, Kim DI, Mattassi R, Hyon WS (2004) Management of arteriovenous malformations: a multidisciplinary approach. J Vasc Surg 39(3):590–600

7. Dompmartin A, Acher A, Thibon P et al (2008) Association of localized intravascular coagulopathy with venous malformations. Arch Dermatol 144:873–877

8. Mazoyer E, Enjolras O, Bisdorff A et al (2008) Coagulation disorders in patients with venous malformation of limbs and trunk: a study in 118 patients. Arch Dermatol 144:861–867

Surgical Techniques in Vascular Malformations

31

Raul Mattassi, Dirk A. Loose, and Massimo Vaghi

Introduction

Surgery was the only available technique to treat congenital vascular malformations (CVM) for a long time. However, even after progress by technique and equipments in the last century, results of surgical approach were often disappointing. The well-known publication of Szylagyi in 1976, which reported about negative results in a group of arteriovenous malformations (AVM) treated surgically, discouraged many physicians to approach these diseases [1]. After introduction of catheter embolization several decades ago, main tendency was to send all patients to the interventional radiologist, without considering surgery.

However, more recent experiences have shown that surgery has still a significant role in the approach of CVM [2, 3]. In several cases, it is the main or even the only possible treatment. In other patients, surgery is required as an important step in a integrated, multidisciplinary treatment program, which is today considered as the correct approach to CVM [4, 5]. In a modern multidisciplinary CVM-oriented group, surgeons of different specialties are crucial components. As CVM are vascular diseases, vascular operations are common; a vascular surgeon experienced in the application of vascular techniques to CVM should exist in the group and could also have a leading role if he has a general overview of all treatment options and techniques.

Surgical Techniques

Stefan Belov proposed a classification of surgical techniques applicable in CVM [6, 7]. His schema is based on the type of correction of the hemodynamic defect, as follows:

1. *Devascularization techniques*: operations to remove an area of abnormal blood vessels. These are the most often performed procedures. Different technical skills can be applied:
   - "En bloc" resection by complete removal of the vascular area, separating dysplastic vessels from normal tissues. This technique is normally used in extratruncular forms and is especially effective in limited defects that do not infiltrate non-resectable structures. Complete removal of CVM is crucial, as these dysplastic vascular areas are the result of a remnant of embryonic cells that have

R. Mattassi (✉)
Center for Vascular Malformations "Stefan Belov",
Department of Vascular Surgery,
Clinical Institute Humanitas "Mater Domini",
Castellanza (Varese), Italy
e-mail: raulmattassi@gmail.com

D.A. Loose
Section Vascular Surgery and Angiology,
Facharztklinik Hamburg, Hamburg, Germany
e-mail: info@prof-loose.de

M. Vaghi
Department of Vascular Surgery, A.O.G. Salvini
Hospital, Garbagnate Milanese, Italy
e-mail: vaghim@yahoo.it

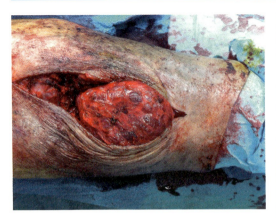

Fig. 31.1 Surgical removal of a venous limited malformation of the calf. Complete removal "en bloc" was possible because the mass was well delimited

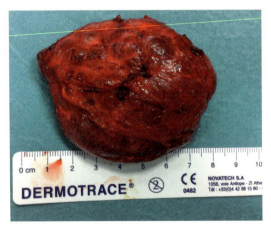

Fig. 31.2 Removed mass of Fig. 31.1

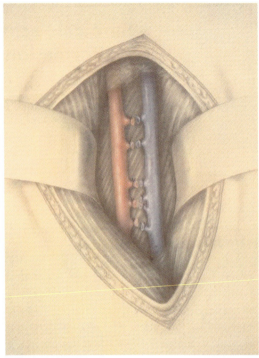

Fig. 31.3 Resection of direct A-V communications

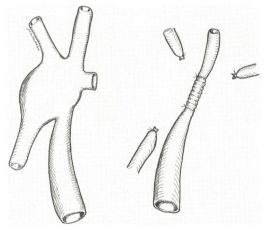

Fig. 31.4 Removal of a direct A-V fistula with prosthetic reconstruction of the artery and vein ligation

the tendency to recur if not completely removed [8] (Figs. 31.1 and 31.2).

- Resection of abnormal vessels which communicate a main artery with a main vein, eliminating an arteriovenous malformation (Figs. 31.3 and 31.4). This procedure is the ideal, curative operation of an A-V fistula [10]. However, it is rarely possible because much more common is the fistula were connections between artery and vein happen through a fistulous "nidus." In this case, the former procedure is required.

- Removal of abnormal vessels. This procedure is performed mainly to remove abnormal veins, like marginal vein, sciatic vein, or superficial, dilated dysplastic veins

(Fig. 31.5). Operation can be not always easy, as these vessels may be sometimes very fragile, with a high tendency to bleed, or have very large perforators in the limbs, which should be recognized before surgery and cautiously ligated to avoid bleeding. Very often in addition, small A-V fistulas are present which should be ligated.

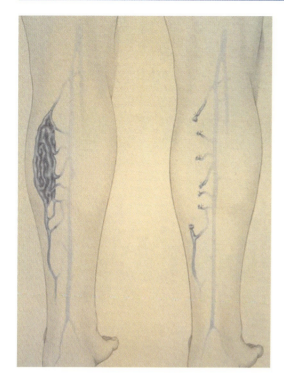

Fig. 31.5 Resection of superficial abnormal veins

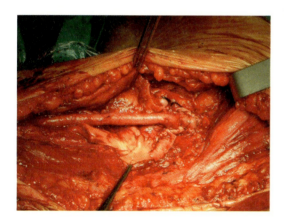

Fig. 31.6 Replacement of a congenital femoral artery aneurysm by a saphenous vein prosthesis

2. *Revascularization techniques*: operations to correct conditions of a reduced or altered blood flow due to the malformation. This group includes:
   - Resection of a stenosis or of an aneurysm and direct vascular surgical reconstruction of the vessel (Fig. 31.6).
   - Bypass techniques in case of aplasia or hypoplasia of main vessels.
   - Reconstructive plastic of venous aneurysms, like a tangential resection of the aneurysmatic vein with reconstruction to a normal diameter of the vessel [11].
   - Patch plastic in main arteries or in venous stenosis.
   - Prosthetic replacement of congenital aneurysms of arteries or veins. Prosthetic material selection is crucial, according to the case. Synthetic material, like Dacron or PTFE, is implantable in arteries of adults. In veins, the first option is authologous veins, like saphenous vein. In case of unavailability, other material for vein replacement can be biological grafts, like homograft (limited availability: only in vessel banks) or umbilical vein graft. A main problem could be an artery replacement by a graft in a child, like in the rare case of an aortic aneurysm.
   - Vein valves reconstruction in case of valve dysplasia or aplasia (for more details, see Chap. 48).

3. Hemodynamic techniques: operations to reduce the hemodynamic effect of a malformation in cases where radical surgery is impossible. These procedures are usually required in infiltrating extratruncular forms. Some technical skills are effective:
   - Tangential clamping of a part of the mass by a Satinsky clamp and suture of the basis below the clamped area, in order to exclude all clamped part of the mass, which is resected after the Blalock suture (Fig. 31.7). During the same operation, the procedure can be repeated in order to increase the quantity of excluded/removed malformed mass [12].
   - Transfix trespassing stitches through the dysplastic vascular area, occluding the abnormal vessels. By this method, a dangerous and difficult dissection is avoided. A Doppler intraoperative guidance is useful [13] (Fig. 31.8).
   - Skeletonization of artery in the area of A-V malformations [8, 12]. This technique means to resect all efferent vessels from the arteries sited in the area involved by the

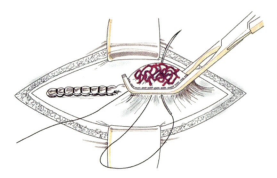

Fig. 31.7 Tangential clamping of a dysplastic area with a Satinsky clamp. Trespassing sutures are given on the basis of the clamped area to exclude a part of the malformation

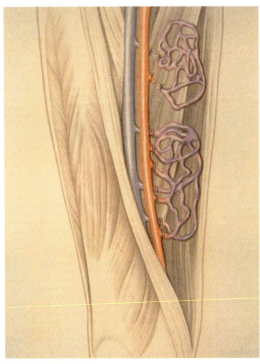

Fig. 31.9 Skeletonization of the main artery and vein in an area with extratruncular A-V malformations. Aim of the procedure is to occlude all feeding vessels to the malformed area. However, that technique exposes to early recurrence (see text)

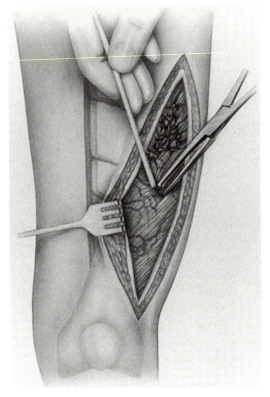

Fig. 31.8 Trespassing stitches through an area with A-V malformations (*upper part* of the picture). An intraoperative Doppler examination is useful to recognize site of the malformations and result of the technique

malformation in order to cut off the feeding vessels to the malformation (Fig. 31.9). However, as the "nidus" of the defect remains, recurrence is the rule. It is considered today an obsolete procedure. An

exception is the skeletonization of the marginal vein in case of multiple, small A-V fistulas entering the vein itself. This rare condition has been recommended in a persistence of the marginal vein by aplasia of the deep venous system. Removal of the fistulas by skeletonization of the vein means to reduce the hemodynamic overloading of the valveless, nonremovable (as the only outflow vessel in deep aplasia) vein [14] (Fig. 31.10)

• Ligation of one or more main feeding vessels of the A-V malformation. This procedure, unfortunately even today sometimes performed, has negative results because of immediate recurrence through collaterals and because the main accessible vessels for catheter embolization will no more be available. It is reported that sometimes, a ligated artery has been reconstructed in order to get catheter access to the A-V malformation.

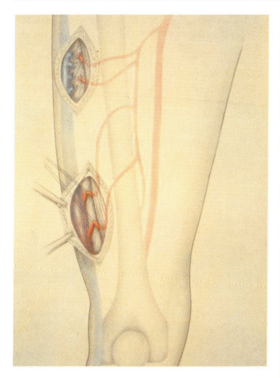

Fig. 31.10 Ligature of small afferent fistulas to a marginal vein

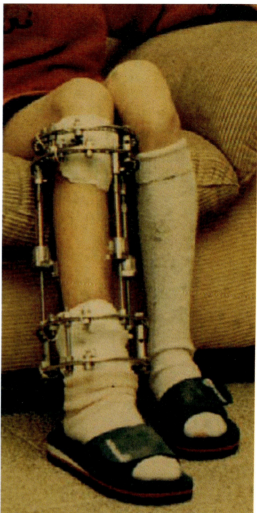

Fig. 31.11 Ilizarov technique for limb elongation

- Resection of superficial secondary dilated veins in an A-V malformation. As these veins are only some of the outflow ways of the malformation, it is often a useless procedure which only may result in a temporary cosmetic result. If the "nidus" of the AVM remains inside, no improvement could be expected by removal of superficial veins. An exception is the surgical resection of a dilated vein in an A-V malformation with several, small arteries entering directly the dilated vein. In this case, surgical resection is curative, as the fistulas are removed together with the vein. The recognition of this condition by a precise diagnosis is mandatory.

4. Other nonvascular operations: surgical nonvascular procedures to correct secondary effects of the CVM:
   - Orthopedic techniques to correct limb length discrepancy, like bone elongation techniques (Ilizarov technique) (Fig. 31.11) or bone growth blockage (epiphysiodesis)

   - Amputations. The real necessity of an amputation should be carefully evaluated by an expert multidisciplinary group, which is aware of the possibility of all techniques available to treat the disease. Unfortunately, amputations are sometimes performed without this prior evaluation, often because of nonavailability of the expertise group.

Conclusion

These surgical techniques should be considered as a part of the treatment options in CVM, as other procedures are available. However, each time a treatment for a simple or complex case of CVM is planned, they should be kept in mind, considering their possibility. An equilibrated evaluation, based on a knowledge of the possibilities of surgery as much as of embolization, laser, alcohol, and foam sclerotherapy, is the key of the best treatment plan for the patient. A decision based on the experience with a single technique with limited knowledge of the others may condition the selection of the best procedure.

References

1. Szylagyi DE, Smith RF, Elliott GP, Hageman JH (1976) Congenital arteriovenous anomalies of the limbs. Arch Surg 11:423–429
2. Belov S, Loose DA, Mattassi R, Spatenka J, Tasnadi G, Wang Z (1989) Therapeutical strategy, surgical tactics and operative techniques in congenital vascular defects (multicentre study). In: Strano A, Novo S (eds) Advances in vascular pathology, vol 2. Excerpta Medica, Amsterdam, pp 1355–1360
3. Loose DA (2000) Combined treatment of vascular malformations: indications, methods and techniques. In: Chang JB (ed) Textbook of angiology. Springer, Berlin/Heidelberg/NewYork, p 1278ff
4. Mattassi R (2009) Multidisciplinary treatment of vascular malformations. In: Mattassi R, Loose DA, Vaghi M (eds) Hemangiomas and vascular malformations. An atlas of diagnosis and treatment, 1st edn. Springer, Milan
5. Loose DA, Weber J (1992) Indications and tactics for a combined treatment of congenital vascular defects. In: Balas NP (ed) Progress in angiology 1991. Edizione Minerva Medica, Torino, pp 373–378
6. Belov S (1990) Surgical treatment of congenital vascular defects. Int Angiol 9(3):175–182
7. Belov S (2000) Vascular malformations and hemangiomas: surgical treatment. In: Chang JB (ed) Textbook of angiology. Springer, Berlin/Heidelberg/New York, pp 1284–1293
8. Malan E (1974) Vascular malformations (angiodysplasias). Carlo Erba Foundation, Milan
9. Belov S, Loose DA, Weber J (eds) (1989) Vascular malformations. Einhorn Presse Verlag, Reinbeck
10. Vollmar J (1967) Rekonstruktive Gefäßchirurgie. Thieme, Stuttgart
11. Loose DA (2005) Die chirurgische Therapie venöser Aneurysmata. Gefäßchirurgie 6:143–152
12. Belov S (1992) Operative-technical peculiarities in operations of congenital vascular defects. In: Balas P (ed) Progress in angiology. Minerva Med, Torino, pp 179–382
13. Loose DA, Funck I (1995) Angeborene Venenfehler – Diagnostische und therapeutische Möglichkeiten. Aktuelle Chir 30:329–340
14. Belov S (1972) Congenital angenesis of the deep veins of the lower extremity: surgical treatment. J Cardiovasc Surg 13:594–598

Interventional Treatment in AVM

32

Friedhelm Brassel, Dan Meila,
and Martin Schlunz-Hendann

Due to growing understanding of pathophysiological relationships and the continuing progress in the development of endovascular materials, the prevalence, significance, and need of interventional treatment in AVM have continued to increase. This chapter first presents the techniques and materials employed in interventions of AVM. Based on this description, the application of endovascular procedures for vessel occlusion is explained. In this context, particular attention is given to the treatment of peripheral AVM and those in the head and neck region.

Treatment Methods

Mastering different vessel occluding techniques is mandatory for the interventional treatment of AVM. In particular, we speak about endovascular

F. Brassel (✉) • M. Schlunz-Hendann
Department of Radiology and Neuroradiology,
Klinikum Duisburg GmbH, Duisburg, Germany
e-mail: friedhelm.brassel@sana.de;
martin.schlunz-hendann@sana.de

D. Meila
Department of Radiology and Neuroradiology,
Klinikum Duisburg GmbH, Duisburg, Germany

Institute for Diagnostic and Interventional
Neuroradiology, Medical School Hannover,
Hannover, Germany
e-mail: dmeila@yahoo.de

embolization procedures that can be performed with the use of different liquid embolic materials or mechanical embolic materials like coils. The treatment with liquid embolic agents requires maximum carefulness and should be performed only with the exact knowledge of the specific anatomy, angioarchitecture, and hemodynamics. Coiling is nowadays a well-established treatment method for intracranial aneurysms but has also a specific role in the treatment of AVM. Endovascular coiling on both the arterial and venous sides must be equally managed with the highest accurateness.

Approaches

Depending on the specific angioarchitecture (Fig. 32.1) and on the localization of the vascular lesion a sole transarterial or transvenous approach or the combination of both is required [1]. In most cases, the groin is punctured. Alternatively, a transbrachial approach can be performed when the passage through the femoral artery or vein is obstructed. Usually, a sheath available in different sizes according to the age of the patient and to the vessel and its size secures the vascular approach. Following, a guiding catheter is placed selectively as near as possible to the AVM for a better stability. The therapeutic catheter, that is, in most cases, a pushable or flow-guided microcatheter, is then forwarded coaxially through the lumen of the guiding catheter ideally intra-nidal. The correct position of the microcatheter tip is

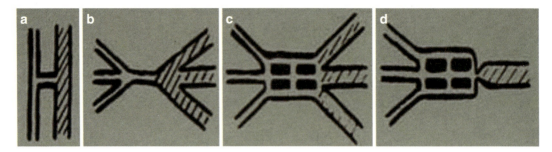

Fig. 32.1 Hemodynamic classification of AVM [2]. (**a** and **b**) Arteriovenous fistulas with one fistula between one (**a**) or multiple (**b**) artery/arteries and vein/veins. (**c**) Arteriovenous malformation (av angioma) with multiple communicating shunting vessels (nidus). (**d**) Vascular malformation (as in dural av fistula) with one or more feeding arteries and a collateral vascular network, shunting directly – fistulous type – into one draining vein

checked via the microcatheter by performing superselective angiography in series. A special difficulty turns out when dealing with AVM that do not (more) have feeding arteries that can be reached by the microcatheter. In those particular cases, being mostly diffuse and extensively plexiform and tiny AVM or micro-AVM, embolization can be performed only after a percutaneous direct puncture.

Material

Microcatheters and Microwires

Microcatheters used for the endovascular treatment of AVM are available between 1.2 and 3.0 F. Depending on the intended purpose, pushable or flow-guided microcatheters can be used. The placement of pushable microcatheters requires the use of coaxial microwires. On the other hand, flow-guided microcatheters are maneuvered passively with the use of the blood flow into the area of the AVM. The tip of the flow-guided microcatheter is floppy and, without restoring force, easily formable. Flow-guided microcatheters favor the strongest blood flow and hence can be used for atraumatic catheterization and superselective proximate embolization of the AVM nidus. Recently, new microcatheters are available that are optionally pushable and flow-guided.

Embolic Materials

Different embolic agents are used in the endovascular treatment of vascular malformations and highly vascularized tumors since the past decades [1]. Numerous methods have been developed in order to sclerotize AVM based on the endovascular injection of embolic and/or sclerosing substances. Basically, two different groups of embolic materials are employed. On the one hand, this includes so-called liquid embolic and sclerosing materials like acrylates, fibrin glues, Ethibloc®, ONYX®, strong alcohol, and Aethoxysklerol® (polydocanol). On the other hand, mechanical embolic materials can be used, for example, in the form of small particles such as polyvinyl alcohol and collagen fibers, metal spirals of platinum, tungsten or stainless steel, suture material pieces, and detachable balloons, all of which leading to a mechanical obliteration of the vessel associated with flow deceleration and subsequent thrombosis.

Liquid Embolic Materials

Acrylates like Histoacryl (n-BCA) and Glubran polymerize in contact with blood while Ethibloc®, a protein derived from maize and dissolved in alcohol, precipitates. Depending on the particular pathophysiology, Ethibloc® may be diluted with Lipiodol and, in particular, with Lipiodol plus additional alcohol [2]. Nowadays, the use of

Onyx® is widely accepted in neuroradiologic interventions, and it becomes more and more important for other interventions as well [3–5]. Onyx® is a liquid embolic material consisting of ethylene vinyl alcohol copolymer dissolved in various concentrations of dimethyl sulfoxide (DMSO) and suspended micronized tantalum powder to provide contrast for fluoroscopy. The use of ethanol in the treatment of AVM will be discussed in the following chapter by another author.

Coils

Pushable coils were used in the endovascular treatment of arterial bleeding in different vascular territories since the past decades. The disadvantage of the first generation of these coils was if once deployed, retrievement was no longer possible. The next generation of coils, the electrolytic detachable coils, has been invented and introduced in the endovascular treatment of intracranial aneurysms by Guglielmi and colleagues [6]. Nowadays, we have a vast range of coils that can also be detached mechanically. Apart from the originally bare coils, we can work with hydro coils, liquid coils, fibered coils, and different types of bioactive coils. Moreover, different sizes, shapes, and forms are available from very large coils over volume coils to very small and very soft coils.

Both liquid and mechanical embolic materials have their specific fields of application. Generally speaking, liquid embolic materials may permit a vascular area to be homogeneously filled. This means that a secondary reopening of the embolized area can hardly take place. Moreover, a vascular short circuit in an area previously embolized by means of a liquid embolizate can hardly reopen by a secondary dilatation of neighboring collateral vessels. This is the reason why liquid embolizates are excellently suited for the treatment of complex plexiform AVMs. Compared to the use of particulate embolizates, they offer the advantage that the recanalization risk and frequency is significantly reduced due to the fact that the AVM is filled more completely.

However, too fast injection of liquid embolic materials may result in retrograde embolization, in the worst case of normal vessels and may furthermore lead to a glued microcatheter tip in the vessel. This risk is more often seen when using acrylates. In contrast, a passage of the embolizate into the draining vein or veins without complete occlusion of the AVM nidus may compromise physiologic venous drainage with possible complications like venous congestion with the risk of venous infarcts and bleeding. Passage of embolic material to the heart or lungs is a major feared adverse effect when dealing with uncontrollable liquid materials. Very rare but disastrous complications have been reported leading to fatal cardiovascular collapse during ethanol therapy of a venous malformation [7].

Particles like PVA are nowadays used solely for the preoperative embolization of high-vascularized tumors in order to diminish the perioperative bleeding risk and to induce a tumor necrosis. Due to their composition and size, particles do not reach and bridge the fistulous connections with their inflow zone, nidus, and outflow zone. They can occlude arterial feeders at the inflow zone only. Thus, they are not eligible in the treatment of the AVM nidus.

Indication and Safety Aspects of Embolization Procedures

As the general basis of safety aspects in any embolization procedures, mastering functional vascular anatomy and choosing the proper materials is mandatory. Specific technical complications in the interventional treatment of AVM can occur nonetheless. This might be in particular vessel perforation, undesired embolization of normal vessels that do not feed the AVM, and passage of embolic materials away from the target, for example, into the lungs or heart or into the intracranial circulation when dealing with head and neck AVM. The latter is a very feared and serious complication that may lead to stroke or hemorrhagic infarction of the brain. Therefore, highest selectivity and accuracy is performed when treating any AVM. The external carotid artery territory is linked embryological to the intracranial arteries, and thus, knowledge of functional vascular anatomy and embryology is mandatory. When treating AVM in the face or neck area, the interventionalist must know all anastomoses and supply to the cranial nerves. Usually or most of the time, extracranial-intracranial anastomoses are not visualized on serial global angiographies, but nevertheless, they do always exist. They may open under following circumstances as Geibprasert and colleagues [8] summarized: (1) with increased intra-arterial pressure, for example, during superselective injections, (2) in the presence of high-flow shunts as a consequence of the "sump effect," or (3) as collateral routes when occlusions of the major intracranial arteries occur. These principles also apply to peripheral AVM in a similar fashion. Hence, superselective placement of the microcatheter as close as possible to the nidus or best intra-nidal, is one of the most important preventive measures to avoid embolic material passage into an undesired circulation. Another safety aspect is the continuous observation of the embolization procedure during fluoroscopy. It is important to visualize the antegrade flow of the embolic agent and to realize immediately when retrograde flow occurs.

Concerning the indication and need for treatment, meticulous consideration between risk of endovascular treatment and risk of natural history is mandatory. The therapeutic goal must always be defined by clinical symptoms and not just by angiographic pictures. The main goal is never just the occlusion of a vessel or the reduction of flow but rather the reduction of AVM-related risks and symptoms like bleeding, pain, and necrosis, for example, [9]. Therefore, the indication for treatment has always to be made interdisciplinary taking into account any therapeutic alternatives.

Endovascular Embolization

The interventional treatment in AVM uses different endovascular embolization techniques. The theoretical aim should be the closure of the nidus, ideally with both its in- and outflow zone, but without occluding vessels feeding normal tissue. However, in large peripheral AVM and multiple nidus, "complete cure" is rather the exception. The main therapeutic goal in the endovascular treatment of AVM is superselective microcatheter embolization using liquid embolic agents with different viscosities to achieve a casting of the whole nidus. Depending on the angioarchitecture, a sole transarterial or transvenous approach or the combination of both might be necessary. A combined transarterial and transvenous method using a so-called kissing microcatheter technique can be chosen in very special and difficult cases. This technique has been proven to show good results even in the treatment of pediatric vein of Galen malformation, being equally AVM [10]. We transferred this neuroradiologic technique to the treatment of AVM in other regions [9]. Krings et al. recently described the technique and term of partial "targeted" embolization, albeit in the treatment of brain AVM. They stated that, in acutely ruptured AVM where the source of bleeding can be identified, targeted embolization of this compartment may be able to secure the AVM prior to definitive treatment. In unruptured symptomatic AVM, targeted treatment may be employed if a defined pathomechanism can be identified that is related to the clinical symptoms and that can be cured with an acceptable risk via an endovascular approach depending on the individual AVM angioarchitecture and hemodynamics [11]. A sole transarterial approach can be successful only when reaching superselectively the vascular network (Fig. 32.2). It fails when the feeding arteries are not reachable by microcatheter. Embolization would lead in these non-exceptional cases to proximal occlusion of the feeding arteries, which is an undesired effect leading to angioneogenesis and revascularization of the AVM by new more tiny and more tortuous collateralizing vessels. In contrast,

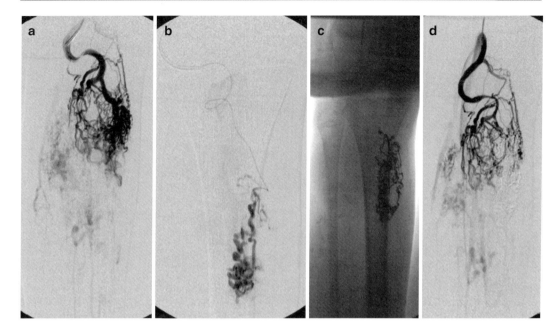

Fig. 32.2 Transarterial endovascular embolization of a congenital AVM of the left leg in a young man (frontal projection). (**a**) DSA pre-embolization. Selective injection of left popliteal artery showing the AVM. (**b**) DSA pre-embolization. Superselective microcatheterization of the AVM feeding artery. (**c**) Non-subtracted image post-embolization. Note the ONYX cast in the AVM nidus. (**d**) DSA post-embolization. Selective injection of the left popliteal artery showing a significant reduction of shunting AVM

when many or most of the arterial feeders reach one fistula point or few points where the venous drainage begins, a transvenous approach and retrograde embolization might be favored. In case of an AVM nidus with a single outflow vein, retrograde transvenous coil embolization of that vein directly at the nidus can induce complete retrograde thrombosis and occlusion of the nidus. Transvenous retrograde intranidal microcatheter embolization into the nidus allows a complete AVM nidus casting with liquid embolic material like Onyx® (Fig. 32.3).

Percutaneous Direct Puncture

The application of embolizing and sclerosing agents by percutaneous direct puncture is predominantly indicated for the treatment of low-flow vascular malformations like venous or lymphatic malformations. However, in difficult cases of tiny and plexiform AVM with very small and tortuous vessels, a superselective endovascular approach by microcatheter is not always feasible. When neither the transarterial nor the transvenous approach succeeds, one should think about percutaneous direct puncture with very small cannulas (Fig. 32.4). Before injecting liquid embolic agents, the correct position of the tip of the needle must be controlled by an angiographic run. It must be ensured that the tip of the needle is located within the nidus and not in the vein or in the adjacent tissue before deployment of the liquid embolic agent.

Results

Long-term results in large series are still lacking, and due to the rarity of the disease, there are no prospective clinical trials in literature. However, we believe that patient satisfaction and quality of

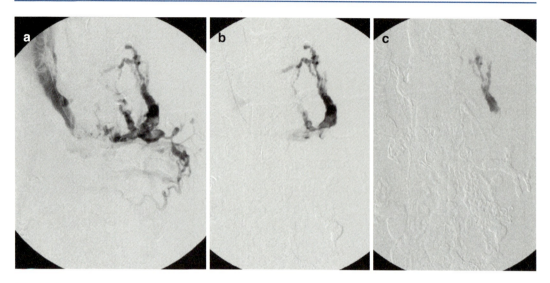

Fig. 32.3 Transvenous embolization of a congenital AVM in a young female (frontal projection). (**a**) DSA pre-embolization. Transvenous catheterization and injection of the deep femoral vein. (**b**) DSA pre-embolization. Superselective retrograde microcatheterization of an AVM draining vein. (**c**) DSA post-embolization. ONYX cast in the very beginning of the draining veins

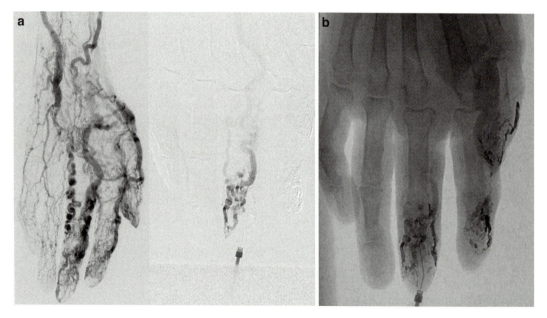

Fig. 32.4 Percutaneous direct puncture of a congenital AVM of the right hand of young female (frontal projection). (**a**) DSA pre-embolization. Serial angiographic run of the right forearm/hand showing a diffuse AVM involving mainly the first three digits. (**b**) DSA demonstrating the percutaneous direct puncture of the AVM nidus in the distal phalanx of digit III. (**c**) Non-subtracted image showing the direct puncture with the ONYX cast in the nidus of digit III. Note other ONYX casts in the previously treated first two digits

life are the most important outcome scores. We share with others the opinion that it should not be the first aim to occlude the vessels but rather to improve or at least stabilize patients' physical comfort [9, 12–14]. Reduce of pain and other AVM-related symptoms like functional impairment is the main goal in the treatment of AVM taking into consideration the less of possible treatment-related complications. Multiple treatment sessions are nearly always required, and a complete "cure" of this disease is only the exception.

References

1. Brassel F, Meila D, Papke K (2011) Vascular interventions in the head and neck region. Part 2: procedures for vessel occlusion. Radiologe 51(6):519–533
2. Brassel F (1997) Entwicklung und Erprobung eines Gefäßmodells zur Simulation einer Embolisation mit Ethibloc® bei spinaler duraler arteriovenöser Malformation. Bremen, Germany: H.M. Hauschild GmbH. ISBN: 3-931785-34-3
3. Numan F, Omeroglu A, Kara B, Cantaşdemir M, Adaletli I, Kantarci F (2004) Embolization of peripheral vascular malformations with ethylene vinyl alcohol copolymer (Onyx). J Vasc Interv Radiol 15(9):939–946
4. Thiex R, Wu I, Mulliken JB, Greene AK, Rahbar R, Orbach DB (2011) Safety and clinical efficacy of Onyx for embolization of extracranial head and neck vascular anomalies. AJNR Am J Neuroradiol 32(6):1082–1086
5. Wetter A, Schlunz-Hendann M, Meila D, Rohde D, Brassel F (2012) Endovascular treatment of a renal arteriovenous malformation with Onyx. Cardiovasc Intervent Radiol 35(1):211–214
6. Guglielmi G, Viñuela F, Sepetka I, Macellari V (1991) Electrothrombosis of saccular aneurysms via endovascular approach. Part 1: electrochemical basis, technique, and experimental results. J Neurosurg 75(1):1–7
7. Chapot R, Laurent A, Enjolras O, Payen D, Houdart E (2002) Fatal cardiovascular collapse during ethanol sclerotherapy of a venous malformation. Interv Neuroradiol 8(3):321–324
8. Geibprasert S, Pongpech S, Armstrong D, Krings T (2009) Dangerous extracranial-intracranial anastomoses and supply to the cranial nerves: vessels the neurointerventionalist needs to know. AJNR Am J Neuroradiol 30(8):1459–1468
9. Brassel F, Greling B, Schlunz-Hendann M, Schmitz T, Loose DA, Meila D. Endovascular treatment of congenital peripheral vascular malformations. Clinical and radiological long-term results (to be published)
10. Meila D, Hannak R, Feldkamp A, Schlunz-Hendann M, Mangold A, Jacobs C, Papke K, Brassel F (2012) Vein of Galen aneurysmal malformation: combined transvenous and transarterial method using a "kissing microcatheter technique". Neuroradiology 54(1):51–59
11. Krings T, Hans FJ, Geibprasert S, Terbrugge K (2010) Partial "targeted" embolisation of brain arteriovenous malformations. Eur Radiol 20(11):2723–2731
12. Bowman J, Johnson J, McKusick M, Gloviczki P, Driscoll D (2013) Outcomes of sclerotherapy and embolization for arteriovenous and venous malformations. Semin Vasc Surg 26(1):48–54
13. van der Linden E, Pattynama PM, Heeres BC, de Jong SC, Hop WC, Kroft LJ (2009) Long-term patient satisfaction after percutaneous treatment of peripheral vascular malformations. Radiology 251(3):926–932
14. Tan KT, Simons ME, Rajan DK, Terbrugge K (2004) Peripheral high-flow arteriovenous vascular malformations: a single-center experience. J Vasc Interv Radiol 15(10):1071–1080

Classification of Arteriovenous Malformation and Therapeutic Implication

33

Wayne F. Yakes and Alexis M. Yakes

Introduction

Vascular malformations constitute one of the most challenging entities in the history of medicine to diagnose and treat effectively by whatever endovascular or surgical approaches are employed. These congenital vascular lesions can involve any tissue in the body. The rarity of vascular malformations in the population compounds the problem of treating them. If a physician rarely encounters patients with vascular malformations, it is difficult to gain enough experience to optimally treat them and effectively eradicate them. High-flow arteriovenous malformations (AVMs) are extremely challenging to surgically extirpate or to endovascularly cure. The world's literature certainly verifies the extreme challenges in the diagnosis and treatment of AVMs. The purpose of this chapter is to advance a new AVM Classification System that has proven therapeutic implications to effectively treat complex AVMs in any anatomical area. By employing the Yakes AVM Classification System, a physician is now able to accurately classify AVMs and determine specific endovascular treatment strategies to consistently treat AVMs, and patients can enjoy the long-term excellent outcomes. Defining the angioarchitecture of the high-flow AVM determines accurately the endovascular management strategy to best permanently ablate the AVM requiring treatment. Further, employing this new Yakes AVM Classification will lower complication rates in treating these complex congenital vascular pathologies.

Overview

The Houdart Classification of Intracranial Arteriovenous Fistulae and Malformations of high-flow lesions and the Cho-Do Classification of AVMs of the peripheral arterial circulation are strikingly similar despite their anatomic locational differences (CNS vs. peripheral vasculatures) [1–3]. Both authors also suggest similar therapeutic approaches based on their arteriographic classification. Houdart et al. Classification states the following types of AVMs: Type A as multiple arterial connections flow into a large aneurysmal vein with single outflow drainage, Type B as multiple microfistulae into an aneurysmal vein with single outflow vein, and Type C as multiple shunts between many arterioles and venules connected to each other. The Cho-Do et al. Classification based on "nidus morphology" provides the following types: Type I being arteriovenous larger fistulae with no more than

W.F. Yakes, MD, FSIR, FCIRSE (✉) • A.M. Yakes, BA
Department of Neuroradiology and Radiology,
Vascular Malformation Center, 501 E. Hampden
Avenue, Suite 4600, Englewood,
Colorado 80113, USA
e-mail: wayne.yakesf@vascularmalformationcenter.com

R. Mattassi et al. (eds.), *Hemangiomas and Vascular Malformations: An Atlas of Diagnosis and Treatment*,   263
DOI 10.1007/978-88-470-5673-2_33, © Springer-Verlag Italia 2009, 2015

three separate arteries shunt to the initial single venous outflow component, Type II as "arteriovenous smaller fistulae with multiple arterioles shunt to the initial part of a plexiform appearance" into a single venous component, Type IIIa as "arteriovenous fistulae with non-dilated fistulae with multiple fine shunts are present between arterioles and venules," and Type IIIb being "arteriovenous fistulae with dilated fistulae with multiple shunts are present between arterioles and venules."

Houdart Type A is the same as the Cho-Do Type I; Houdart Type B is the same as the combination of the Cho-Do types IIIa and IIIb. Therapeutic implications are also similar as well. The Houdart Type A and Type B and Cho-Do Types I and II proffer retrograde approaches to occlude the vein aneurysm outflow as being a potential for curative treatment of these AVM types. I proposed and illustrated the retrograde vein occlusion techniques for high-flow malformations first published and three cases illustrated in my manuscript published in 1990 [4]. Later, Jackson et al. published the retrograde vein approach in 1996 [5]. The Do group in Seoul, Korea (also the publishers of the Cho-Do AVM Classification), published the retrograde vein approach in 2008 after collaboration with our group demonstrated its efficacy to them in patients at their Seoul, Korea, Samsung Medical Center [6].

The Yakes AVM Classification System has some similarities to both classification systems and some stark differences. The Yakes AVM Classification System consists of the following: Type I is characterized by a direct arteriovenous fistula, a direct artery to vein connection (e.g., typified by pulmonary AVF and renal AVF). This angioarchitecture type is not described in the Houdart or Cho-Do Classification Systems. Type II is an AVM characterized by usually multiple inflow arteries into a "nidus" pattern with direct artery-arteriolar to vein-venular structures that may, or may not, be aneurysmal. Type IIIa consists of multiple arteries-arterioles into an enlarged aneurysmal vein with an enlarged single outflow vein. Type IIIb consists of multiple arteries-arterioles into an enlarged aneurysmal vein with multiple dilated outflow veins. Type IV comprises microfistulous innu-

merable arteriolar structures to innumerable venular connections that diffusely infiltrate a tissue (typified by ear AVMs that infiltrate the entire cartilage of the pinna). What is different in this lesion is that there are admixed among the innumerable fistulae capillary beds within the affected tissue. If the affected tissue only had AVFs, the tissue could not survive as capillary beds are required for tissue viability. No other AVM angioarchitecture has this duality [7]. This angioarchitecture is not described in the world's literature.

Comparing Houdart's CNS Classification and the Cho-Do Peripheral Vascular Classification to the Yakes Classification has some parallels, as has been described, but has several distinct differences.

Houdart Type A and Cho-Do Type I are the same and compare to the Yakes Type IIIa. Houdart Type B and Cho-Do Type II are the same and again are placed in the Yakes Type IIIa. Whether the arteriovenous (Type A/Type I) or arteriolar-venular connections (Type B/Type II) are present is not important as the same arterial physiology is present that the "nidus" being present in the vein wall itself, regardless of the size of AVF on the vein wall, as they are both treated endovascularly in the same way. Therefore, the AVF size is irrelevant. Further, even when larger AVF are present, microfistulae are also present as well admixed with the larger connections. It never is purely one microsize only or one macrosize only.

The Houdart Type C is the same as bundling Cho-Do Types IIIa (arteriovenous) and IIIb (arteriolar venular). This is similar to the Yakes Type II. Both authors do not explain in their classifications the Yakes Type IV. The angioarchitecture of arteriovenous and arteriolar-venular innumerable fistulae, totally infiltrating a particular tissue, is another vascular phenomenon that is present that is not explained by the Houdart nor the Cho-Do Classifications. Being that arteriographically these innumerable microfistulae are proven to infiltrate a tissue, one has to also consider that despite the innumerable microfistulae, there is interspersed within these abnormal fistulae vascularity that is normal with capillary beds that is nutrient to the infiltrated tissue as well, or the tissue itself would be

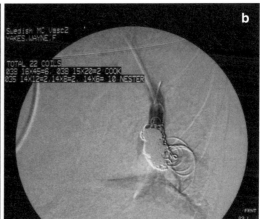

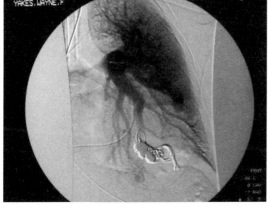

Fig. 33.1 Yakes Type I AVM (AVF) typified by a single inflow artery connected to a single outflow vein. (**a**) Ventilator Dependent 30 Year-Old Female with HHT and Massive Left Pulmonary AVM Causing O2 Sats of 35% on 100% Oxygen Through the Ventilator; Patient Sent By Air Ambulance Emergently For Treatment. Left Pulmonary Artery angiogram demonstrating a massive AVF shunt with single aneurysmal vein drainage. This single arterio- venous connection is Yakes Type I AVM (AVF). (**b**) Post- embolization selective Left Pulmonary Artery angiogram after placement of 22 fibered coils of .038 & .035 sizes in the AVF totally occluding the massive AVF. (**c**) Main Left Pulmonary Artery angiogram demonstrating closure of the massive AVF post-coil placement. Mechanical closure devices will permanently close and treat this Yakes Type I AVM (AVF)

devitalized and forced to necrose. Normal capil- laries must be present admixed with the innu- merable AVF in the infiltrated tissue, or it would not be viable and could not survive. Venous hypertension is usually the culprit in the injury that occurs in that infiltrated tissue, and this phe- nomenon as a vascular etiology for pathologic tissue changes was first elucidated by Jean Jacques Merland, M.D., and Marie Claire Riche, M.D [8]. Thus, the "normal" vascularity with capillary beds in the infiltrated tissue to allow it to exist is not discussed in the Houdart or in the Cho-Do Type Classifications or is the angioar- chitecture characteristics described.

The Yakes Type I Classification is a direct AV macro-connection that is characteristic of pulmonary AVF and renal AVF, but can also occur in other tissues. This direct AV connection is not described in the Houdart Classification or in the Shin-Do Classification. The Yakes Type I AV connection can also be present and inter- spersed in complex AVMs as well (Fig. 33.1).

The Yakes Type II Classification possesses an angioarchitecture synonymous with the classical "nidus" pattern commonly seen in AVMs with multiple inflow arteries of varying sizes coursing toward a "nidus" (a complex tangle of vascular structures without any intervening capillaries and exiting from this "nidus" into multiple veins from this "nidus"). The Houdart Type C and the Cho-Do Type IIIa/Type IIIb most resemble this angioarchitecture pattern. Thus, the Yakes Type II and Yakes Type IV further define the Houdart Type C and Cho-Do Type IIIa/IIIb patterns (Fig. 33.2), much more specifically.

As an aside, the term "nidus" is rampant in the medical literature (AVM nidus, nidus of infection, etc.). Unfortunately, the initial author was only partially familiar with the Latin language. "Nidus" means "nest" in Latin, and indeed it does. However, "nidus" with the ending "us" denotes male gender. In the Latin language, the true term meaning "nest" is, in fact, "nidum." The ending "um" denotes the neuter gender which a "nest" truly is. Thus, the original author accurately describing "nest-like" conglomeration of vascular structure was woefully inaccurate penning the words as "nidus" (masculine) instead

of the true word "nidum" (neuter). Being rife in the literature for decades, there is no possibility of any correction of this term.

In summary, Yakes Type I is the simplest macro direct AV connection. Yakes Type II is the common "nidum" (nest-like) AV connection. Yakes Type IIIa has multiple AV connections (arterial and arteriolar into an aneurysmal vein: "nidum" is in the vein wall) with single outflow vein physiology (Fig. 33.3). Yakes Type IIIb has multiple arterial inflow connections (arterial and arteriolar) into an aneurysmal vein ("nidum" is in the vein wall) with multiple outflow veins that is more difficult to treat by retrograde vein approaches (Fig. 33.4).

Yakes Type IV angioarchitecture has innumerable micro-AV connections (with lowered vascular resistance) infiltrating an entire tissue but with concurrent normal vascular structures possessing nutrient capillary beds (with normal

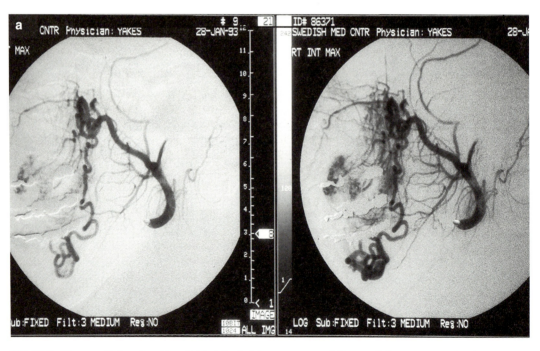

Fig. 33.2 24 year old female with painful right facial AVM also causing right facial swelling. (**a**) Example of Yakes Type II AVM with typical AVM "nidus". This type AVM can be treated by trans-arterial embolization (easiest approach usually), and direct puncture into the nidus (more difficult). Retrograde vein approaches are usually not successful. Lateral Right Internal Maxillary Artery arteriogram demonstrating arterial supply from a terminal Internal Maxillary artery branch arising from the Pterygo-Palatine fossa area. Note the typical AVM "nidus pattern"

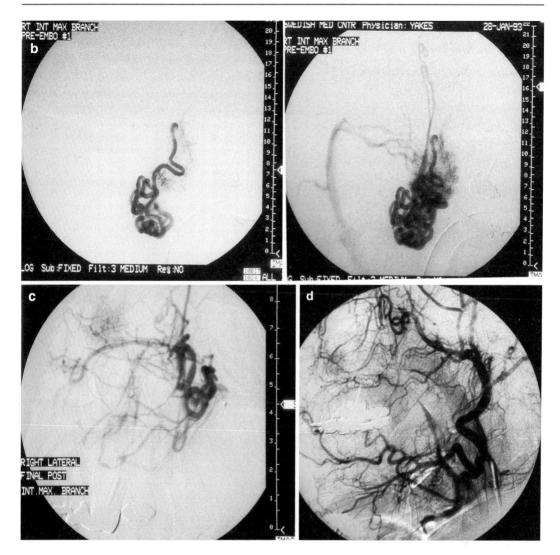

Fig. 33.2 (continued) (**b**) Lateral selective Right Internal Maxillary Artery branch arteriogram pre-embolization. A micro-catheter is required to obtain superselective arterial positioning for ethanol embolization of the AVM. This is required to ONLY embolize the AVM and spare all the normal tissues and capillary beds from ethanol arterial embolization. If not done this way, there will be total tissue devitalization and necrosis that will occur with inad-vertant embolization of ethanol of the normal tissues. (**c**) Lateral Right Internal Maxillary Artery arteriogram immediately post-embolization demonstrating total occlusion of the right face AVM with all normal branches remaining intact. (**d**) Lateral Right External Carotid Artery arteriogram at 2 year follow-up. No residual AVM is identified. Note that the normal arterial vascularity remains intact

vascular resistance) to supply and drain the tissue that is diffusely infiltrated to allow this tissue to survive and not be devitalized. The postcapillary veins compete with AVF outflow veins that are arterialized (hypertensive) (Fig. 33.5) and cause the resultant nonhealing pathology. This entity has not been described in the world's literature [9–22].

Therapeutic Implications of the Yakes Classification

Determining a classification system based on the AVM angioarchitecture is of little use without a practical application. For example, the Spetzler-Martin Brain AVM Classification is of importance to determine the surgical morbidity for treating brain AVMs [23]. The higher the Spetzler-Martin grade, the higher the morbidity. This allows the neurosurgeon to inform his/her patient accurately of the risks for treatment. The Schobinger AVM Classification for peripheral AVMs (non-neuro) is useful to quantify the degrees of symptomatology a patient possesses regardless of the AVM's angioarchitecture. The Yakes Classification is utilized to determine endovascular approaches and embolic agents that will be successful to ablate these peripheral AVMs.

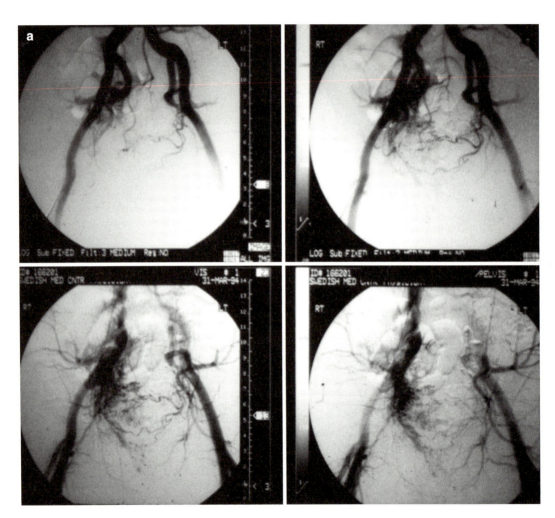

Fig. 33.3 Example of Yakes Type IIIa AVM angioarchitecture with multiple in-flow arteries/arterioles and single out-flow vein physiology. The vein wall is the "nidus" in this AVM type. Multiple Right Internal Iliac Artery branches supply this right pelvic AVM. (**a**) 32 year old male with right pelvic AVM with single outflow vein drainage towards Right Internal Ilaic Vein. Arterial supply is from multiple Right Internal Iliac Artery branches. Because of the diffuse innumerable small arteries supplying the AVM vein aneurysm wall, transarterial ethanol embolization is not possible. Normal structures could potentially be embolized and resultant nerve damage, pelvic organ damage, tissue necrosis, etc., could result

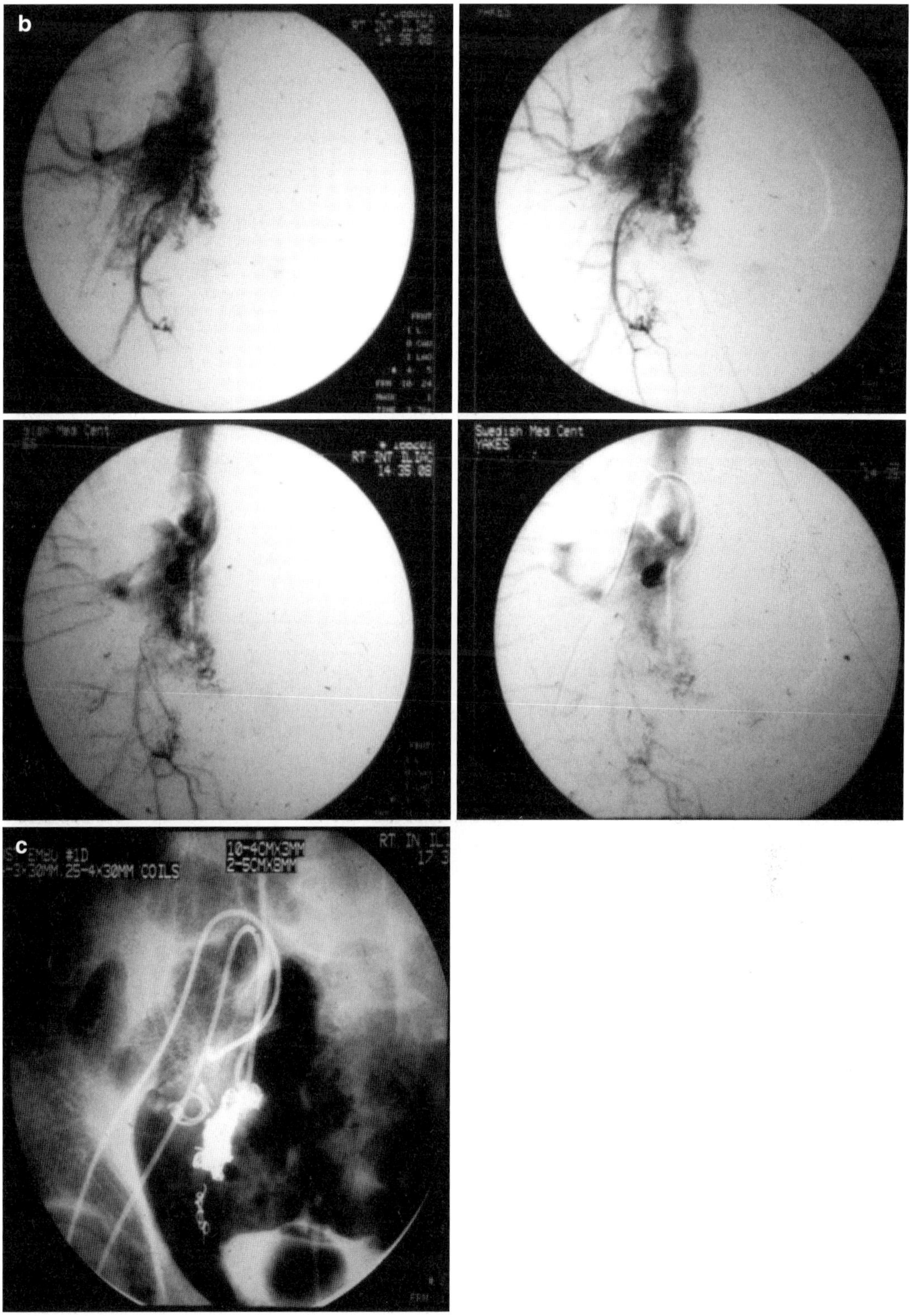

Fig. 33.3 (continued) (**b**) AP selective Right Internal Iliac Artery arteriogram demonstrating innumerable small arterial connections to the single out-flow aneurysmal vein. Superselective catheter positioning for transarterial embolization is not possible. A retrograde venous approach must be employed to treat this Yakes Type IIIa AVM. (**c**) AP pelvis spot film demonstrating arterial catheter in Right Internal Iliac artery, and the retrograde vein catheter placed centrally within the AVM vein aneurysm with the resultant deposition of multiple coils in the vein aneurysm to treat this Yakes Type IIIa AVM

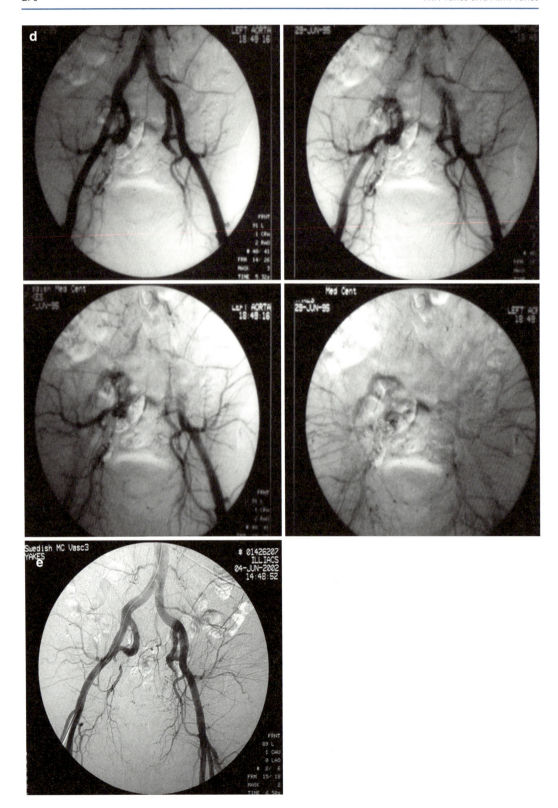

Fig. 33.3 (continued) (**d**) AP pelvis arteriogram immediately post-coil embolization demonstrating total occlusion of the right pelvic AVM. No residual arteriovenous shunting is present. All normal arteries remain intact post-coil emboliza-tion without complication. (**e**) AP pelvis follow-up arterio-gram 7 years post-retrograde vein coil embolization demonstrating long-term cure of the right pelvic AVM. Again, this technique is curative in Type IIIa and Type IIIb AVMs

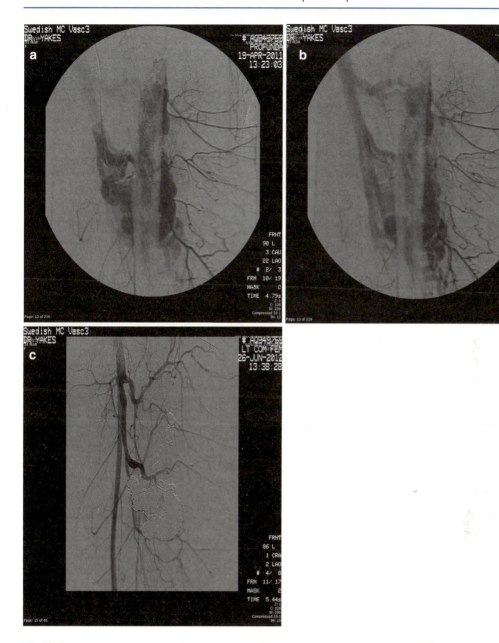

Fig. 33.4 Example of Yakes Type IIIb AVM typified by multiple inflow arteries/arterioles shunting into the aneurysmal vein with multiple out-flow veins. The "nidus" is the vein wall with the innumerable AV connections. (**a**) Left soft tissue and intraosseous left Femur AVM. Multiple arterial inflow branches from the Left Profunda Femoris Artery into the AVM. The arterial/arteriolar inflow has many parenchymal branches and also provides vascular supply to the AVM. (**b**) Venous phase of the Left Profunda Femoris arteriogram demonstrating the vein aneurysms and multiple out-flow vein physiol-ogy. To treat this Yakes Type IIIb AVM, multiple veins must be occluded to completely treat this AVM. Transarterial embolization is difficult to perform in that tissue necrosis could occur due to the many parenchymal arterial branches also arising from these multiple AVM feeding branches. (**c**) Left Common Femoral arteriogram at over one year follow-up demonstrating cure of the soft tissue and intraosseous AVM components. Note the multiple coil placements required to treat the multiple out-flow vein compartments that are present in Yakes IIIb AVMs

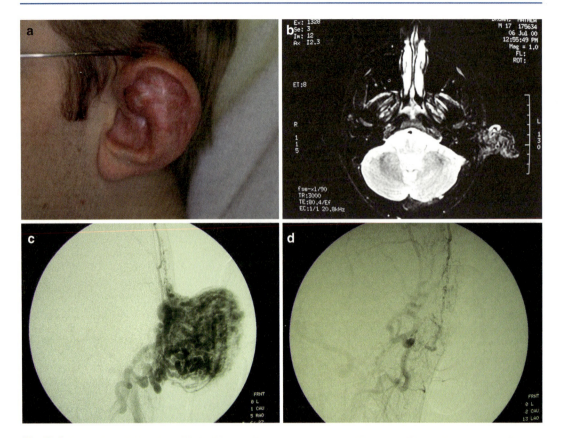

Fig. 33.5 Example of Yakes Type IV AVM typified by total infiltration of a tissue with innumerable micro-fistulas and innumerable outflow-veins. Capillaries are admixed with the innumerable fistulas throughout the tissue involved with this "infiltrative" form of AVM. (**a**) 19 year old male with progressively enlarging left ear over the last 5 years. Now has developed intermittent ulcerations, infections, and hemorrhages (Shobinger III stage). (**b**) T-2 weighted axial MR demonstrating an enlarged left ear with flow-voids totally infiltrating the entire ear and cartilages. The enlargement of the abnormal ear tissues is apparent. (**c**) AP External Carotid arteriogram demonstrating diffuse vascular infiltration of the left ear with innumerable micro-fistulae shunting into abnormal arterialized veins. The arteriogram mirrors the findings noted on the MR with ear enlargement and total micro-fistulous AVM infiltration and AV shunting evidenced by the MR flow-voids. (**d**) AP Left External Carotid arteriogram at 4 year follow-up demonstrating persistent cure of the left ear AVM. Note the normal vascularity that is now present and the total absence of any residual AV shunting post-endovascular ethanol sclerotherapy

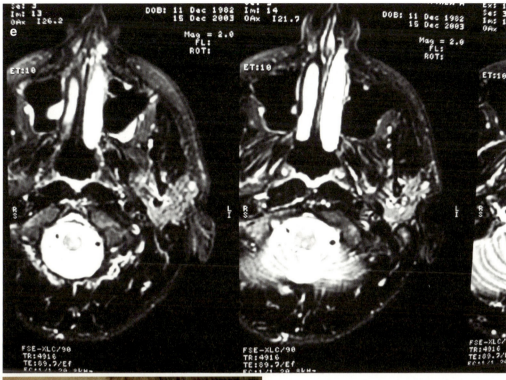

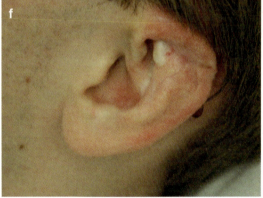

Fig. 33.5 (continued) (**e**) Axial MR T-2 weighted at 3 year follow-up demonstrating shrinkage of the left ear and normalization of the vascularity with total absence of the innumerable flow-voids previously present on the pre-treatment MR. (**f**) 4 year clinical follow-up of the left ear. A successful plastic surgery procedure was performed on the superior aspect of the left ear after the ear AVM was totally ablated and cured. The ear now has a more normal contour. Note the normalization of the skin color, no residual ruborous venous hypertensive skin changes are present

Embolic Agents Employed in the Yakes AVM Classification

Yakes Type I direct AV connections, as typically seen in pulmonary AVF and renal AVF, can be permanently ablated by occluding mechanical devices. Coils, Amplatzer plugs, occluders, detachable balloons, and the like are universally successful to cure Yakes Type I AVMs.

Yakes Type II AVMs with the "nidum" nest-like angioarchitecture can be permanently ablated with absolute ethanol from a superselective transcatheter/trans-microcatheter arterial approach. Also, a direct puncture into the artery(ies) supplying the

AVM immediately proximal to the AVM "nidum" and distal to any parenchymal arterial branches and then a superselective ethanol injection can be employed to circumvent catheterization obstacles when a transcatheter/trans-microcatheter positioning to achieve the same position to deliver ethanol into the "nidum" is not possible. These two transarterial approaches allow ethanol to sclerose and permanently ablate the "nidum." The "nidum" itself can be directly punctured, and ethanol (undiluted) can be injected to sclerose the "nidum" directly to effect cure in its multiple compartments as well.

Yakes Type IIIa AVMs (multiple inflow arteries into an aneurysmal vein with single enlarged vein outflow) and Yakes Type IIIb AVMs (multiple inflow arteries into an aneurysmal vein with multiple enlarged outflow veins) can be curatively treated by several endovascular approaches. The "nidum" in this type of angioarchitecture with an aneurysmal vein is in the vein wall itself. Superselective transarterial ethanol embolization distal to all parenchymal branches via transcatheter/trans-microcatheter and direct puncture endovascular approaches can be curative. An additional curative endovascular approach for Type IIIa AVMs is to coil embolize the aneurysmal vein itself with, or without, concurrent ethanol injection into the coils within the aneurysmal vein. This is also curative when the aneurysmal vein is totally and densely packed with coils. The aneurysmal vein can be endovascularly approached by direct 18 g needle puncture and by retrograde vein catheterization to achieve the same position within the aneurysmal vein to pack it with coils. The retrograde vein approach to curatively treat high-flow vascular lesions was first published and illustrated in 1990 by Yakes et al. The second article articulating the vein approach to AVM treatment was subsequently published in 1996 by Jackson et al. Cures were documented in these published patient series. Yakes et al. described cures of posttraumatic and congenital high-flow lesions, and Jackson et al. described cures of congenital AVMs by way of the retrograde vein approach in these publications [4, 5].

The Yakes Type IIIb AVMs (aneurysmal vein with enlarged multiple outflow veins) can be cured by transarterial transcatheter ethanol embolization and by direct puncture and retrograde vein coiling techniques. However, the aneurysmal vein portion and the immediate adjacent segments of each outflow vein must also be packed with coils completely to achieve cure. Yakes Type IIIb AVMs are more challenging to cure than the Yakes Type IIIa AVMs due to the more complex vein outflow morphology.

Yakes Type IV AVMs presented a unique challenge to determine curative endovascular treatment. AVMs, by definition, are direct AV connections without an intervening capillary bed (Yakes Types I–IV). Thus, superselective catheter and direct puncture needle positioning distal to *ALL* branches supplying parenchyma and immediately proximal to the AVM itself will obviate tissue necrosis being that the capillary beds are not embolized and only the abnormal AV connections are sclerosed. However, Yakes Type IV AVMs infiltrate an entire tissue, thus termed by the authors as an "infiltrative" form of AVM. Being that the "infiltrated" tissue (e.g., auricular AVMs) is viable proves that capillary beds are undoubtedly interspersed along with the innumerable microfistulae throughout the involved tissue as well. Injection of ethanol by transcatheter/trans-microcatheter and direct puncture approaches will sclerose the innumerable microfistulae, but also would flood the capillary beds with ethanol devitalizing that infiltrated tissue. Necrosis of that tissue would then ensue with occlusion of the capillary beds. Thus, Yakes Type IV AVMs were a conundrum to treat with endovascular approaches. Polymerizing agents would also occlude AVFs, but also capillary beds causing a massive necrosis.

Thinking through this conundrum, one could rightly conclude that the only option is total surgical resection of that entire tissue as the only treatment option. After further reflection, an endovascular option for curative treatment, not palliative treatment, was considered a possibility. Capillary beds have normal peripheral resistance which is a somewhat restrictive vascular flow pattern from artery to capillary to veins. AVMs/AVF has abnormally lowered peripheral vascular resistance with rapid stunting into arterialized veins. The arterialized AVM outflow veins are hypertensive. In AVMS, the normotensive post-capillary venules compete with the arterialized hypertensive post-AVF veins/venules for outflow of the blood. This then further restricts normal vein outflow, which in turn increases the systemic vascular resistance (SVR) of the normal arterioles immediately proximal to the capillary beds, further restricting arteriolar inflow to the capillary beds. The increased SVR into the capillaries coupled with abnormally low-resistance shunting into the admixed innumerable AVF allows preferential flow into the AVFs.

Mixing nonionic contrast with absolute ethanol changes the viscosity and specific gravity of ethanol in this mixture. Being "thickened" and diluted, this allows for preferential flow to the AVFs and further restricts flow into the capillaries. Despite being 50 % diluted with contrast, the ethanol can still effectively sclerose the innumerable microfistulae, due to the small luminal diameters. This combination of preferential flow into the innumerable AVFs, the increased SVR into the capillaries restricting flow, and the increased viscosity and changing the specific gravity of the contrast and ethanol 50 % mixture all work to spare the capillaries and sclerose the innumerable AVFs. Using pure ethanol would not have this capillary sparing effect, and the AVFs and capillaries would both be sclerosed and occluded. This does cure the AVFs, but devitalizes the tissue itself with occlusion of the capillaries. Use of various polymerizing embolic occlusive agents (NBCA, Onyx) would also cause the same devitalization of the tissues with occlusion of the capillaries. Particulate embolic agents (PVA, Contour Embolic, Embospheres, etc.) cannot permanently occlude the AVFs and will make the capillaries ischemic with the proximal occlusion in the inflow arterioles, but will not devitalize the tissues.

Summary

Yakes Type I: Can be permanently occluded, with mechanical devices such as coils, fibered coils, Amplatzer plugs, and other occluding devices.

Yakes Type II: Can be permanently occluded with undiluted absolute ethanol. At times slowing the arterial inflow in the "nidum" with occlusion balloons, tourniquets, and blood pressure cuffs does allow for less ethanol to be used to treat the AVM compartments. Direct puncture techniques into the inflow artery or AVM "nidum" allow ethanol to embolize the AVM as well.

Yakes Type IIIa: Can be permanently occluded with transarterial embolizations with ethanol of the "nidum" the same way as in the Yakes Type II AVM. They can also be permanently occluded by dense coil packing of the vein aneurysm with or without ethanol embolization. This can be accomplished via direct puncture of the vein aneurysm or by retrograde vein catheterization of the vein aneurysm.

Yakes Type IIIb: Can be permanently occluded via transarterial approach as in Yakes Type II AVMs. They can be permanently occluded by treating the vein aneurysm and the multiple aneurismal outflow veins by coil embolization.

Yakes Type IV: Can be permanently occluded via transarterial superselective 50 % mixture of nonionic contrast and ethanol that treats the micro-AVFs and spares the higher-resistance capillaries. Direct puncture with 23 gauge needles into the microfistulous AV connection itself (thus bypassing any capillaries) with pure undiluted ethanol injections is also curative.

References

1. Houdart E, Gobin YP, Casasco A, Aymard A, Herbreteau D, Merland JJ (1993) A proposed angiographic classification of intracranial arteriovenous fistulae and malformations. Neuroradiol ogy 35:381–385
2. Cho SK, Do YS, Shin SW, Kim DI, Kim YW, Park KB et al (2006) Arteriovenous malformations of the body and extremities: analysis of therapeutic outcomes and approaches according to a modified angiographic classification. J Endovasc Ther 13:527–538
3. Park KB, Do YS, Kim DI, Kim YK, Shin BS, Park HS et al (2012) Predictive factors for response of peripheral arteriovenous malformations to embolization therapy: analysis of clinical data and imaging findings. J Vasc Interv Radiol 23:1478–1486
4. Yakes WF, Luethke JM, Merland JJ, Rak KM, Slater DD, Hollis HW, Parker SH, Casasco A, Aymard

A, Hodes J, Hopper KD, Stavros AT, Carter TE (1990) Ethanol embolization of arteriovenous fistulas: a primary mode of therapy. J Vasc Interv Radiol 1:89–96

5. Jackson JE, Mansfield AO, Allison DJ (1996) Treatment of high-flow vascular malformations by venous embolization aided by flow occlusion techniques. Cardiovasc Intervent Radiol 19:323–328

6. Cho SK, Do YS, Kim DI, Kim YK, Shin SW, Park KB, Ko JS, Lee AR, Choo SW, Choo IW (2008) Peripheral arteriovenous malformations with a dominant outflow vein: results of ethanol embolization. Korean J Radiol 9:258–267

7. Yakes WF, Yakes AM (2014) Arteriovenous malformations. The Yakes classification and its therapeutic implications. Egyptian Journal of Vascular & Endovascular Surgery 10:19–23

8. Merland JJ, Riche MC, Chiras J (1980) Intraspinal extramedullary arteriovenous fistula draining into medullary veins. J Neuroradiol 7:271–320

9. Enjolras O, Wassef M, Chapot R (2007) Introduction ISSVA classification: color atlas of vascular tumors and vascular malformations, 1st edn. Cambridge University Press, New York, pp 1–12

10. Legiehu GM, Heran MKS (2006) Classification, diagnosis and interventional radiologic management of vascular malformations. Orthop Clin North Am 37:435–474

11. Puig S, Aref H, Chigot V, Bonin AB, Bruenelle F (2003) Classifications of venous malformations in children and implications for sclerotherapy. Pediatr Radiol 33(2):99–103

12. Lee BB, Laredo J, Lee TS, Huh S, Neville R (2007) Terminology and classification of congenital vascular malformations. Phlebology 22:249–252

13. Do YS, Yakes WF, Shin SW, Lee BB, Kim DI, Liu WC, Shin BS, Kim DK, Choo SW, Choo IW (2005) Ethanol embolization of arteriovenous malformations: interim results. Radiology 235:674–682

14. Yakes WFJ (2008) Endovascular management of high flow arteriovenous malformations. Chin J Stomatol 43:327–332

15. Yakes WF, Pevsner P, Reed M (1986) Serial embolizations of an extremity arteriovenous malformation with alcohol via direct percutaneous puncture. Am J Roentgenol 146:1038–1040

16. Vinson AM, Rohrer DB, Wilcox CW et al (1988) Absolute ethanol embolization for peripheral arteriovenous malformation: report of 2 cures. South Med J 81:1052–1055

17. Yakes WF, Haas DK, Parker SH, Gibson MD et al (1989) Symptomatic vascular malformations: ethanol and embolotherapy. Radiology 170:1059–1066

18. Yakes WF, Parker SH, Gibson MD et al (1989) Alcohol embolotherapy of vascular malformations. Semin Intervent Radiol 6:146–161

19. Mourao GS, Hodes JE, Gobin YP, Casasco A, Aymard A, Merland JJ (1991) Curative treatment of scalp arteriovenous fistulas by direct puncture and embolization with absolute alcohol. J Neurosurg 75:634–637

20. Vogelzang RL, Yakes WF (1997) Vascular malformations: effective treatment with absolute ethanol. In: Pearce WH, Yao JST (eds) Arterial surgery: management of challenging problems. Appleton and Lange Publishers, Norwalk, Connecticut, pp 553–560

21. Yakes WF, Rossi P, Odink H (1996) Arteriovenous malformation management: how I do it. Cardiovasc Intervent Radiol 19:65–71

22. Doppman JL, Pevsner P (1983) Embolization of arteriovenous malformations by direct percutaneous puncture. AJR Am J Roentgenol 140:773–778

23. Spetzler RF, Martin NA (1986) A proposed grading system for arteriovenous malformations. J Neurosurg 65:476–483

Sclerotherapy in Vascular Malformations with Polidocanol Foam

34

Juan Cabrera Garrido, Maria V. Rubia, and Dirk A. Loose

Introduction

Sclerotherapy is performed mainly in venous and lymphatic malformations using different substances. In arteriovenous (AV) forms, it is contraindicated because an erroneous intra-arterial injection may produce extensive necrosis. Classical sclerosis is mainly performed in venous dysplasias with polidocanol, sodium tetradecyl sulfate, and ethanol, among others, while in lymphatic malformations, OK-432 is preferred [1]. Sclerotherapy with our patented foam and original technique significantly improves the results of these lesions.

Indications

Currently, the greatest therapeutic challenges in congenital vascular malformations are posed by venous or low-flow vascular malformations and diffuse lymphatic vascular malformations of a large size or extent and those that show infiltration of mus-

J.C. Garrido
Surgical Unit, Vascular Clinic, Granada, Spain
e-mail: juan@drjuancabrera.com

M.V. Rubia
Unit of Phlebology and Intensive Care dr. JC Cabrera
Vascular Clinics, Barcelona, Spain
e-mail: mrubia@drjuancabrera.com

D.A. Loose (✉)
Section of Vascular Surgery and Angiology,
Facharztklinik Hamburg, Hamburg, Germany
e-mail: info@prof-loose.de

cle masses. Because of their invasion of proximal structures, venous malformations usually have a complex morphology and are often associated with anomalies of the deep venous system of the extremities, therefore limiting the possibilities of complete excision by surgery. For these lesions, sclerotherapy is the treatment of choice [2–6].

Vascular malformations associated with arteriovenous fistulae are contraindicated for liquid and foam sclerotherapy because an accidental intra-arterial injection can produce extensive necrosis. It must also be taken into account that head and neck veins lack valves and that those in the upper two-thirds of the facial region communicate directly with the cavernous sinus via the superior and inferior ophthalmic veins. Consequently, sclerotherapy has to be performed with caution at this level, insuring that the volume injected is equal to the volume of the malformation (Figs. 34.1 and 34.2).

Sclerosing Agents

The sclerosing agents used currently in the treatment in sclerotherapy include sodium morrhuate, sodium tetradecyl sulfate, polidocanol, ethanolamine oleate, ethanol, hypertonic saline, amidotrizoic acid, bleomycin, dextrose, tetracyclines, and OK-432. The selection of the specific agent depends upon the balance efficacy/side effects. In our opinion, the best is polidocanol as a specific kind of patented foam, approved in the USA as Varithena® [7–9].

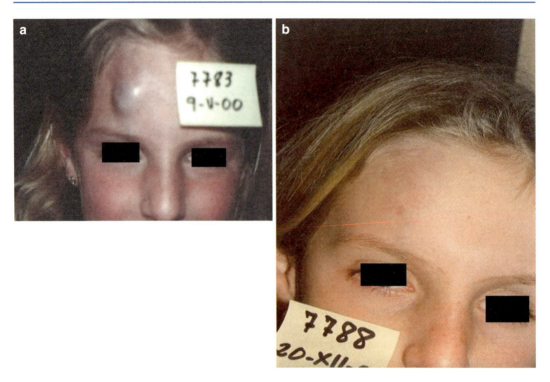

Fig. 34.1 Limited venous malformation of the right forehead. (**a**) Before and (**b**) 6 months after sclerotherapy with microfoam

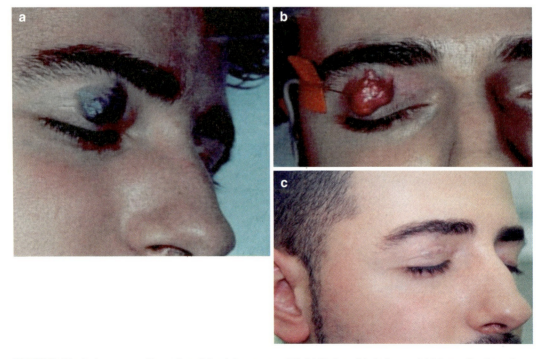

Fig. 34.2 Limited venous malformation of the right upper eyelid. (**a**) Before, (**b**) during, and (**c**) 3 months after sclerotherapy with microfoam

Sclerotherapy with ethanol, the most widely used agent in the treatment of these lesions, is highly aggressive and associated with major complications due to the lack of control over the injected liquid. In fact, adverse effects have been reported including necrosis of skin and mucosa, deep venous thrombosis in extremities, pulmonary embolism, sensory and motor neurologic lesions, superficial cellulitis, and cardiorespiratory collapse due to bronchial spasm [7]. Moreover, ethanol treatment is not readily repeatable, and this is essential for sclerotherapy, since partial recanalization after the intravascular thrombosis is frequent. Finally, sclerotherapy with ethanol is contraindicated in children and high-risk areas such as eyelids, mucosa, genital area, etc. [10].

Technique of Classic Sclerotherapy

The technique of sclerotherapy must ensure that a precise dose is administered and that the agent is homogeneously distributed on the entire endothelial perimeter of the treated venous segment [9]. It must also ensure that the intravascular concentration of the sclerosing agent is not reduced by dilution in the blood or that this dilution is minimal and always known. Finally, the sclerosant must remain in contact with the endothelium for the necessary time period. In short, the requirements for a successful sclerotherapy are the following:

Knowledge of the intravascular concentration of the sclerosant.
Homogeneous distribution within the vessel.
Control over the time of contact between agent and endothelia.
Sclerotherapy must be selective, i.e., limited to the targeted venous area.

These requirements are not met by conventional liquid sclerosants. By using these, beside their less safety, the correct dosage on the endothelia and therefore the sclerosing action are highly difficult to control. In addition, in vessels exceeding a certain volume or flow, the therapeutic effect is generally confined to a short segment.

Ethanol sclerotherapy, given its local and systemic secondary effects, is mostly indicated before surgery as a preoperative support to reduce the size of the lesion or as a postoperative complement [4, 8]. In contrast, conventional sclerotherapy of large malformations is ineffective because of the intrinsic limitations of the injected liquids including the following:

Dilution and progressive deactivation of the liquid in a large blood volume
Irregular distribution of the sclerosant on the endothelia of the treated area
Difficulties in manipulating and controlling the injected sclerosant
Imperceptibility of the liquid sclerosant in the vessel by duplex ultrasonography

The general complications of this technique vary according to the agent and the dose used. They include allergic reactions (especially with sodium tetradecyl sulfate), brain intoxication (especially with ethanol, which must never exceed a maximum volume of 1.2 ml/kg in patients of about 70 kg) [7], hemoglobinuria with possible renal damage, cutaneous necrosis by extravasations or reflux [11], and neurapraxia due to extravascular injection near a motor or sensory nerve.

Sclerotherapy with Microfoam

The introduction of sclerosants in the specific pharmaceutical form of microfoam has transformed the scenario depicted above. Microfoam physically displaces the blood contained in the vessels and minimizes dilution, allowing better knowledge of the intravenous concentration. Micronization of the injected sclerosant dramatically reduces the diameter of the bubbles and thus exponentially increases its surface area, enhancing its therapeutic action and allowing a major reduction in the total dose injected. Moreover, microfoam facilitates a more homogenous distribution of the sclerosant on the endothelial surface and prolongs sclerosant-endothelium contact time. The echogenicity of the microbubbles makes them indirectly visible and the easy manipulability of the injected microfoam allows it to be steered to areas distant from the injection site. In this way, microfoam allows the intravascular administration of a more precise dose of sclerosant [12–15].

Apart from its safety, a further benefit of the sclerosing microfoam is its manageability. The high internal cohesion of microfoam means that it can be aspirated and reinjected after its initial injection. The color of the aspirated microfoam, visible in the catheter, reveals the degree of dilution or intravascular occupation; it ranges from white, when the occupation is exclusive to pink or red, when there is moderate or major dilution, respectively. Furthermore, since microfoam can be steered within the vessels, the filling can be intensified or attenuated according to the sensitivity of the venous area under treatment.

Microfoam is made with 60 % O_2 and 40 % CO_2 which are physiological gases. A priori injection of a gas into the bloodstream raises alarm about the possibility of a gas embolism. However, CO_2 has been intravenously injected without adverse effects at doses of 50–100 cc as a contrast in radiological diagnosis since the 1950s.

Among the advantages of CO_2 are its fluidity, allowing the use of fine catheters; the absence of toxicity, even at high doses; and its low cost. Thus, on the one hand, the high solubility of the gases facilitates there metabolism in blood and pulmonary diffusibility, and on the other hand, the micronization increases exponentially the surface of the gas and facilitates its solubility in the corporal liquids. The sclerosant has a greater active surface area for making contact with the endothelium in comparison with the small surface area available to the liquid form. In this way, the dosage of sclerosants in microfoam is more precise and its action more predictable compared with the liquid form. The microfoam does not mix immediately with the blood but displaces it from within the vessel and fills its lumen, so that the sclerosant contacts the endothelia of the veins

homogeneously without dilution and at a known intravascular concentration. Because the vessel can be kept full of microfoam, the sclerosant-endothelium contact time can also be controlled at will [13, 14]. Finally, the blood solubility of the injected gases is very important, especially for patients with permeable oval foramen.

Technique of Treatment with Microfoam in Vascular Malformations

First of all, a precise and extensive anatomic and functional evaluation (MRI, CT angiography, and duplex ultrasound) must be performed to define the characteristics of a predominantly venous malformation or of a combined type. Thus, according to Puig et al. [16], the lesions can be divided into four groups:

Limited malformations without peripheral drainage
Malformations that drain into normal veins
Malformations that drain into dysplastic veins
Malformations that drain into ectatic veins

The technique consists in the injection under ultrasound guidance of the patented polidocanol foam [14]. At each session, 20–100 ml of microfoam is injected, at concentrations ranging between 0.25 and 3 %, in accordance with the location of the malformation and the hemodynamic characteristics of the area to be treated. Thus, infiltrating malformations (Figs. 34.3, 34.4, 34.5, 34.6, 34.7, and 34.8) require higher concentrations (2–3 %), whereas malformed lateral veins such as the marginal vein (Figs. 34.9 and 34.10) are treated with lower concentrations (around 1 %). The procedure is performed without anesthesia and the number of sessions is variable, ranging from a single one to several sessions depending on the size, complexity, and number of the anomalous veins. The interval between sessions is 2 weeks, spacing them to 4 weeks as the treatment advances. Clinical and radiological

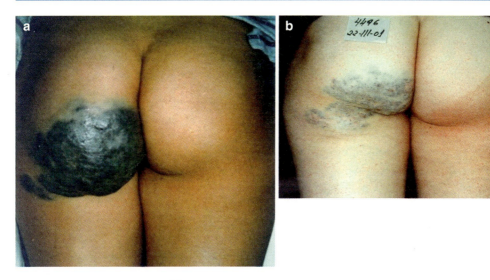

Fig. 34.3 Venous malformation of the left buttock, perineum, and genital region, extratruncular, infiltrating form. (**a**) Before and (**b**) 2 years after treatment with ten sessions of sclerotherapy with microfoam

improvement is usually possible in the great majority of patients (over 90 %).

The main adverse effects are skin pigmentations (which spontaneously disappear in nearly every case) and interdigital necrosis in one case. We have not observed deep venous thrombosis, pulmonary embolism, and neurologic lesions [17].

The benefits of polidocanol contrast with the aggressive effects of absolute alcohol and or sodium morrhuate on the malformation and on neighboring tissues. The injection of the latter agents is also very painful, requiring hospitalization, general anesthesia, and post-sclerosis analgesia [6, 7]. Furthermore, sodium morrhuate can produce allergic reactions. These two agents must therefore be administered with great caution.

The therapeutic efficacy of polidocanol microfoam depends on its mechanical action in displacing the blood within the vessel. If the blood flow is elevated, dilution of the injected microfoam can result in a reduction of foam's effect.

In routine practice, duplex ultrasonography often shows some areas in venous malformations with abnormal supplies of pulsatile blood delivered by small arteriovenous communications. Therefore, the existence of combined types of malformations (see Figs. 34.6, 34.7, 34.8, 34.10, and 34.11) is a reality (Table 34.1) or at least, the presence of high-flow areas in malformations that are considered low-flow. The presence of small arteriovenous fistulae reduces the efficacy of the treatment so that areas that initially thrombose after injection undergo early partial recanalization. Attempts can be made to counteract this considerable disadvantage by reducing the interval between sessions and using a higher concentration of sclerosant. For instance, hand malformations often show a radial artery of increased size and elevated blood flow connected to phlebectasias. In these cases, the high local flow reduces the response to the sclerosant injection and the technique must be adapted accordingly. For this purpose, we use duplex ultrasonography to identify the most hemodynamically active parts at the beginning of treatment, in order to compress the afferent arteries during the injection in close-up areas of the malformation. Once the lesion is compartmentalized and hemodynamically disconnected, it can be more easily closed up in its entirety by

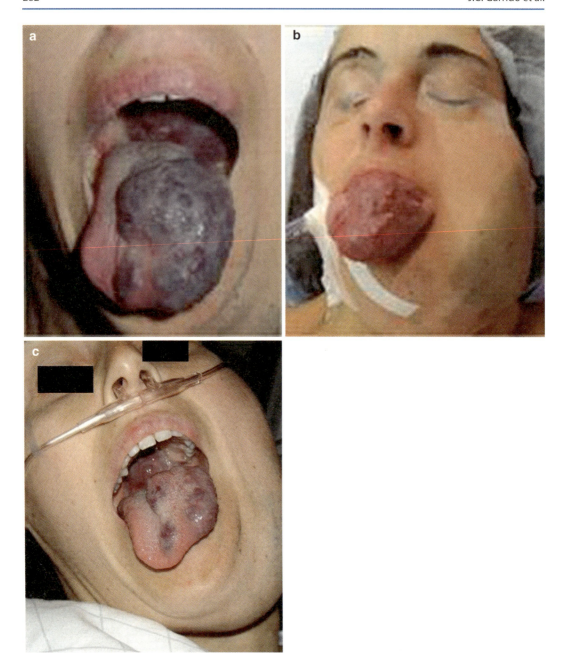

Fig. 34.4 (**a**) Tongue lesion before treatment. (**b**) Tongue lesion after two sessions of treatment with microfoam. (**c**) Tongue lesion and left half of the face, after four sessions of treatment

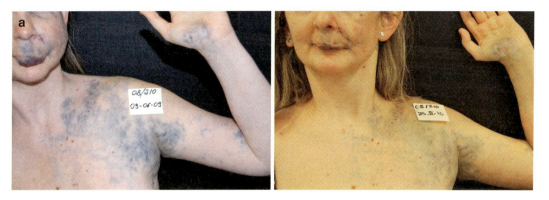

Fig. 34.5 Extensive venous malformation of the head, trunk, and upper left extremity. (**a**) Before and (**b**) 1 year after treatment with nine sessions

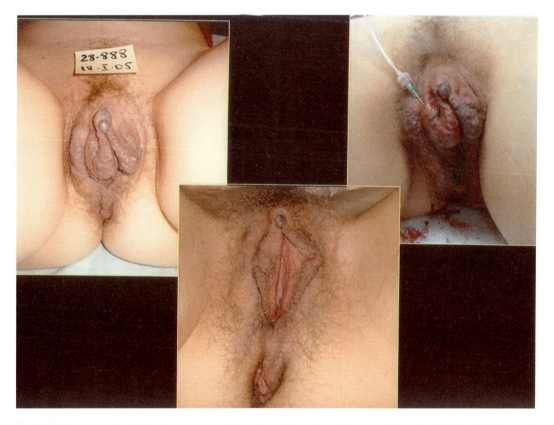

Fig. 34.6 Extratruncular infiltrating venous malformation of the vulva with recurrent thrombophlebitis. (**a**) Before and (**b**) after sclerotherapy with microfoam

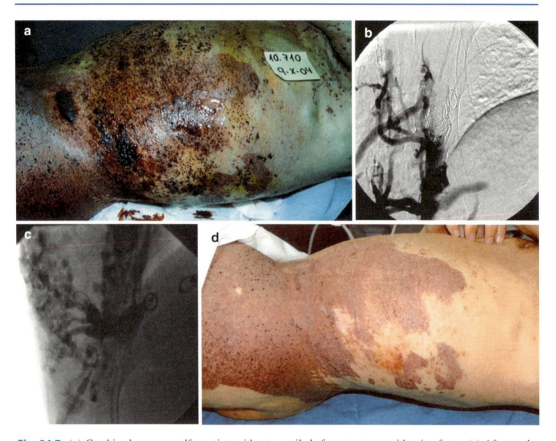

Fig. 34.7 (**a**) Combined venous malformation without AV shunt in the skin, extratruncular, with diffuse skin involvement. Important and recurrent hemorrhage in the wall of thorax and abdomen, leading to severe anemia and progressive general deterioration. (**b**) Endovascular occlusion of a large vein in the wall of the thorax with coils before treatment with microfoam. (**c**) After occlusion of the large veins, the vessels of the wall were treated with large volumes of microfoam over various sessions. (**d**) Good resolution at the skin level after the end of microfoam treatment

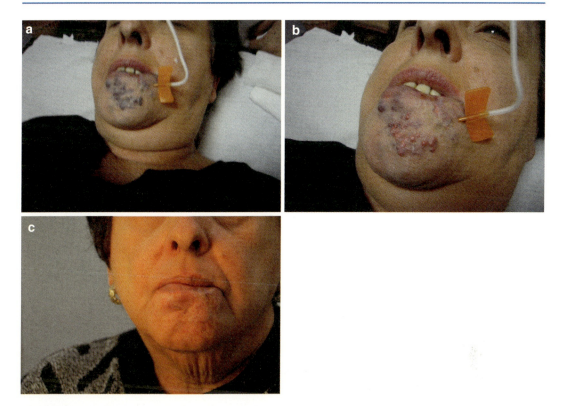

Fig. 34.8 (**a**) Venous malformation and scar in lip due to radiotherapy in childhood. (**b**) Broad spreading of the foam from just one point of injection. (**c**) After sclerotherapy, only the post-radiotherapy scar is visible.

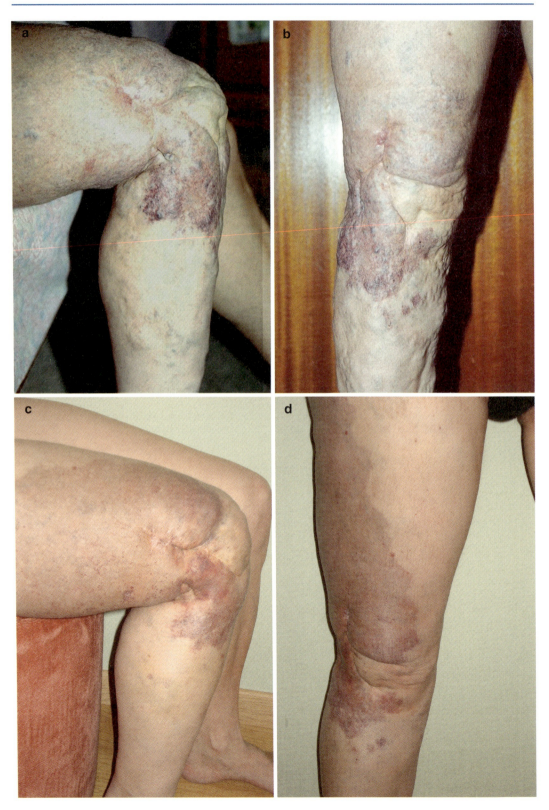

Fig. 34.9 *KTS* with linfovenous malformation. The patient suffered from weekly fever, which disappeared after sclerotherapy. Post treatment pictures show scars from previous failed surgery (**a**, **b**) before sclerotherapy (**c**, **d**) after sclerotherapyy

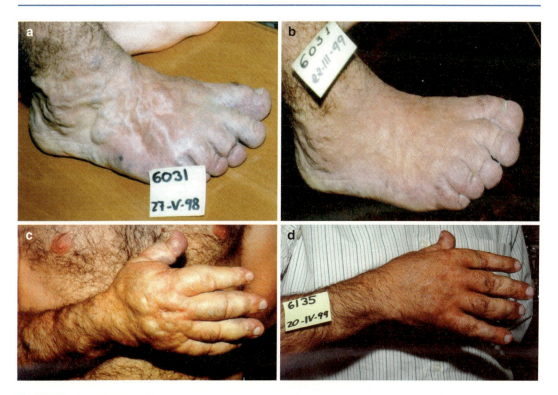

Fig. 34.10 Combined hemolymphatic malformation. The right foot (**a**) before treatment and (**b**) 10 months after sclerotherapy and the right hand (**c**) before treatment and (**d**) 9 months after sclerotherapy

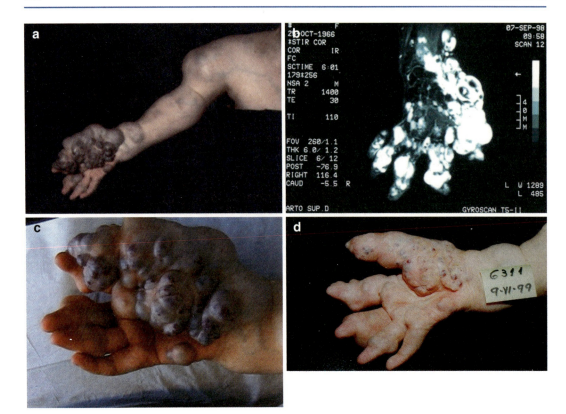

Fig. 34.11 Combined extratruncular hemolymphatic infiltrating malformation with extended involvement of chondrodystrophias and hemangiomatosis of the skin (Maffucci syndrome). (**a, b**) Before treatment, (**c**) MRI of the right hand with multiple venectasias, (**d**) 9 months after several sessions of treatment with sclerosant in microfoam form

Table 34.1 Classification of vascular malformations (Hamburg 1988)

Type of defect	Anatomical forms	
	Truncular	Extratruncular
Predominantly arterial	Aplasia or obstruction	Infiltrating
	Dilatation	Limited
Predominantly venous	Aplasia or obstruction	Infiltrating
	Dilatation	Limited
Predominantly lymphatic	Aplasia or obstruction	Infiltrating
	Dilatation	Limited
Predominantly AV shunting	Superficial AV fistulas	Infiltrating
	Deep AV fistulas	Limited
Combined defects	Arterial and venous (without AV shunt)	
	Hemolymphatic (with or without AV shunt)	Infiltrating hemolymphatic
		Limited hemolymphatic

Data from [1]

successive sessions. Nevertheless, the stability of the vascular occlusion achieved is more precarious than in predominantly venous malformations, and recanalization is frequent, so that a more rigorous follow-up is required.

The simplicity, reproducibility, low cost, safety, and strictly outpatient nature of microfoam sclerotherapy makes it the method of choice for the anatomical and functional elimination of a pathological venous area [17]. In low-flow malformations, sclerotherapy with microfoam is a therapeutic option that allows to moderate the progression of these lesions and to reduce their size. However, for large venous malformations, we can often only helplessly observe their natural evolution, unable to provide a definitive effective treatment.

Regarding the follow-up, it is evidently essential to differentiate between localized or limited (Figs. 34.1 and 34.2) and diffuse or infiltrating vascular malformations (Figs. 34.3, 34.4, and 34.5). The latter requires continuous and prolonged treatment, sometimes for years, at best controlling the lesion but never completely eradicating or curing it [10, 18].

References

1. Poldervaart MT, Breugem CC, Speleman L, Pasmans S (2009) Treatment of lymphatic malformations with OK-432 (Picibanil): review of the literature. J Craniofac Surg 20(4):1159–1162
2. Belov S, Loose DA, Weber J (1989) Vascular malformations. Periodica Angiologica, vol 16. Einhorn Presse Verlag, Reinbek, pp 25–27
3. Mulliken J, Young AE (1988) Vascular birthmarks: hemangiomas and malformations. WB Saunders, Philadelphia
4. Loose DA (2007) Modern tactics and techniques in the treatment of angiodysplasias of the foot. Chir del Piede 25:1–17
5. Lee BB, Mattassi R, Loose DA et al (2005) Consensus on controversial issues in contemporary diagnosis and management of congenital vascular malformation: Seoul communication. Int J Angiol 13:182–192
6. Loose DA (2007) Surgical management of venous malformations. Phlebology 22:276–282
7. Yakes WF, Luethke JM, Parker SH et al (1990) Ethanol embolization of vascular malformations. Radiographics 10:787–796
8. De Lorimier AA (1995) Sclerotherapy for venous malformations. J Pediatr Surg 30:188–194
9. Claesson G, Kuyelenstierna R (2002) OK-432 therapy for lymphatic malformation in 32 patients (28 children). Int J Pediatr Otorhinolaryngol 65:1–6
10. Villavicencio JL (2001) Primum non nocere: is it always true? The use of absolute ethanol in the management of congenital vascular malformations. J Vasc Surg 33:904–906
11. Belov S (1998) Late results in the treatment of vascular malformations. Int Angiol 7:136–143
12. Cabrera J, Cabrera J Jr, García-Olmedo MA (1997) Elargisement des limites de la sclerotherapie: Nouveaux produits sclerosants. Phlebologie 2: 181–188
13. Cabrera J, Cabrera J Jr, García-Olmedo MA (2000) Treatment of varicose long saphenous veins with sclerosant in microfoam form: long-term outcomes. Phlebology 15:19–23
14. Cabrera J, Cabrera J Jr (1997) BTG International Limited Assignee. Injectable microfoam containing a sclerosing agent. US patent 5676962
15. Bikerman JJ (1973) Foams. Springer, New York
16. Puig S, Casati B, Staudenherz A, Paya K (2005) Vascular low-flow malformations in children: current concepts for classification, diagnosis and therapy. Eur J Radiol 53(1):35–45
17. Cabrera J, Cabrera J Jr, García Olmedo MA, Redondo P (2003) Treatment of venous malformations with sclerosant in microfoam form. Arch Dermatol 139: 1409–141
18. Belov S (1990) Classification of congenital vascular defects. Int Angiol 9:141–146

Laser Treatment in Vascular Malformations

35

Hans-Peter Berlien

Introduction

Due to the potential for regression in congenital vascular tumors, the aim of laser therapy is only to induce this regression, while in vascular malformations the pathologic vessels must be destroyed. However, with exception of laser vaporization, all photobiological reactions have a delayed effect. On the other hand, the attitude is that a vascular malformation should be radically excised like a cancer with a high incidence of recurrence, and there is always the danger of massive bleeding and the need for extensive resection which may result in mutilation.

The wide variety of clinical presentations for these anomalies makes it difficult to outline specific management programs. It is important that the appropriate laser and application form be used. Therefore, treatment of these difficult vascular lesions must be carefully individualized. Whereas laser treatments in capillary malformations are the first choice therapy (Fig. 35.1 and Table 35.1), in arteriovenous (AV) malformations embolization is the first choice therapy. In venous and lymphatic malformations, laser therapy is a supplement to surgical excision and sclerotherapy.

H.-P. Berlien
Center for Laser Medicine, Elisabeth Hospital,
Berlin, Germany
e-mail: lasermed.elisabeth@pgdiakonie.de;
berlien@gmx.net

Capillary Malformations

Port-Wine Stains (PWS)

Capillary vascular malformations are the most frequent and the oldest indication for laser treatment in both children and adults [1].

With the introduction of the flash lamp-pumped pulsed dye laser (FLPDL), PWS can be treated in infancy and early childhood. The high pulse peak power of the pulsed dye laser disrupts the vessels. The energy fluency ranges from 4 to 10 J/cm^2 and is varied according to the age of the patient, the anatomic location, and the color of the lesion: 5.0–5.6 J/cm^2 in children less than 12 months of age, 5.6–6.4 J/cm^2 in children 12 months to 4 years of age, and approximately 7 J/cm^2 in children over 4 years of age. Energy is reduced over the eyelids and hands. If blanching or graying of the epidermis occurs during application, energy fluencies should be reduced in order to avoid blistering of the epidermis. Treatments start at the lowest energy density that shows an adequate primary reaction. The lighter the lesion, the higher the energy density for the age range. The darker the lesion, the lower the energy density. Immediately after treatment the area characteristically becomes blue gray and turns purpuric in a few hours with surrounding erythematous flare: this takes 7–14 days to resolve. Some edema, especially in the periorbital area, is possible. As the purpura disappears, the area

R. Mattassi et al. (eds.), *Hemangiomas and Vascular Malformations: An Atlas of Diagnosis and Treatment*,
DOI 10.1007/978-88-470-5673-2_35, © Springer-Verlag Italia 2009, 2015

291

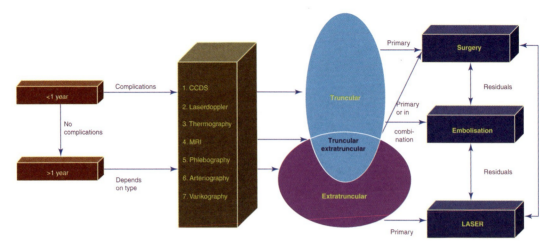

Fig. 35.1 Therapeutic algorithm of vascular malformations. Only the simple form of port-wine stain does not need any further diagnostics. In all other cases, the visible part of the vascular malformation may be the tip of the iceberg of underlying affections

Table 35.1 The choice of laser types depends on the depth, the thickness, and the kind of malformation

Superficial cutaneous	
Flat findings	Flash lamp-pumped dye laser
Telangiectatic findings	Argon laser, KTP
Tuberous findings	Pulsed Nd:YAG laser
Hyperkeratotic findings	CO_2 laser
Intra- and subcutaneous to a depth of 1–15 mm	
Impression technique with bare fiber	
Transcutaneous Nd:YAG laser with ice cube cooling	
Subcutaneous, voluminous up to a depth of 10 mm	
Nd:YAG laser interstitial or intraluminal	
Hollow organs, body cavities	
Nd:YAG laser endoscopic in air/water	

In general more superficial and smaller vessels are an indication for short pulse duration; the deeper and the larger the vessel size and volume, the longer the pulse duration up to CW exposure

KTP potassium-titanyl-phosphate

lightens progressively for up to 6 weeks. After treatment, the treated areas are covered with panthenol ointment. In case of blistering, parents are instructed to cleanse the area with polyvidone-iodine solution, even if a crust has formed. To avoid postoperative irritation of the treated areas, we instruct the parents to keep their children's fingernails short or that the children wear gloves to avoid trauma to the treated areas. Treatments are usually repeated at 6 week intervals until the desire degree of lightening is achieved.

Adult and teenage patients can often be treated without anesthesia, although this is dependent on the size and anatomic location of the lesion. General anesthesia is necessary for children with extensive lesions or in case of central facial PWS because of the need for eye protection (Fig. 35.2). A significant reduction of pain as well as skin protection during laser treatment can be achieved using a fluid cooling cuvette or cold air. Some authors use cryogen spray cooling. This can lead to patient discomfort, especially near the nose, eye, mouth, or ear.

The incidence of complete clearing is variable. PWS in dermatome V2 centrofacial regions involving the medial portion of the cheek, upper lip, and nose show less lightening than PWS in other locations. Furthermore, lesions on the hand and arm respond less well than lesions on the face, neck, and torso.

Patients younger than 4 years of age require fewer treatments [2]. Treatment of children at the earliest possible age may prevent considerable psychosocial impairment and result in a more complete response. Early treatment of these lesions is expected to prevent the progression of the vessels in the PWS to more ectatic structures that make the lesions dark purple, raised, and nodular in many adults. It is hoped

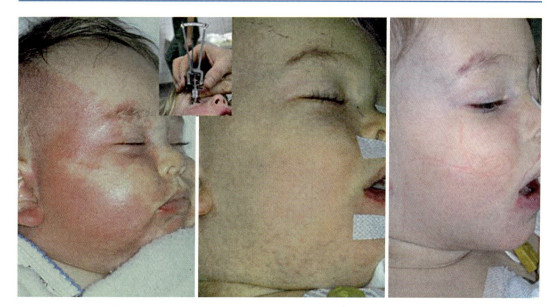

Fig. 35.2 Treatment of port-wine stains using the flash lamp-pumped pulsed dye laser. LPDL therapy of port-wine stain in early childhood. The earlier the therapy begins, the better the results. Due to intraoperative eye protection in facial lesions, general anesthesia is mandatory. In case of Sturge-Weber syndrome, anesthesia can be used for further clinical investigations such as ophthalmotonometry

that hypertrophy of affected areas, a common complication of extensive PWS, and permanent deformity associated with these lesions can be mitigated. The argon- or potassium-titanyl-phosphate (KTP) laser (power 2 W, pulse duration 0.1 s, interval 0.1 s, spot size 0.05–1 mm) is useful for telangiectatic PWS and dark purple and nodular PWS of adults, with a good response and a low risk of scarring.

Capillary-Lymphatic Malformation

Capillary-lymphatic malformations may be discriminated from the classical PWS by light staining and can be bluish red to black in color. Due to the lower erythrocyte concentration, the basic absorption for the FLPDL is reduced so the results of dye laser therapy are generally worse than for PWS. However, the ectatic venules in the epidermis are a good indication for the KTP, pulsed Nd:YAG, or chopped CW Nd:YAG with fluid cooling cuvette (Fig. 35.3). However, in these lesions the birthmark is only the tip of the iceberg. In nearly all cases, there is a mixed venous-lymphatic malformation in the underlying organs. Capillary-lymphatic malformations are observed either in association with Klippel-Trenaunay syndrome or alone. So the general anesthesia needed for the laser therapy in childhood may also be used for clinical examinations if necessary.

Hyperkeratotic Capillary Malformation

Angiokeratomas are usually known by their eponyms, matched with the predilection of the lesions: Mibelli for lesions on the hands or feet, Fordyce for lesions on the scrotum, and Fabry for lesions on the trunk or thighs. If only the lymphatic capillaries are affected, this is known as "lymphangioma circumscriptum" [3], but the subcutis may also be affected. Often these lesions bleed easily and weep, either spontaneously or following trauma. Another risk is the high rate of spontaneous erysipelas. The complications provide the indication for laser therapy. KTP laser is mostly not useful due to the high surface absorption. In punctual lesions a pulsed Nd:YAG laser coagulation is helpful, but the popcorn effect

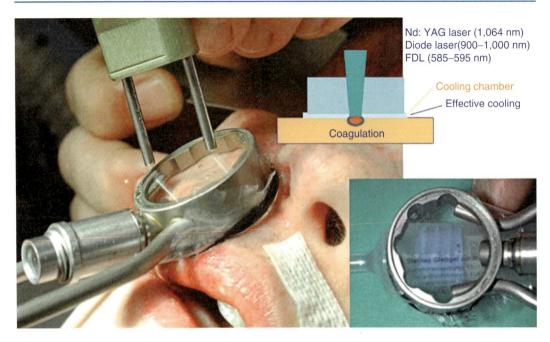

Nd: YAG laser (1,064 nm)
Diode laser(900–1,000 nm)
FDL (585–595 nm)

Cooling chamber
Effective cooling
Coagulation

Fig. 35.3 Cooling chamber. The flexible membrane on the patient side of the fluid cooling cuvette can follow all ana-tomical contours. This allows complete protection of the skin even in difficult regions

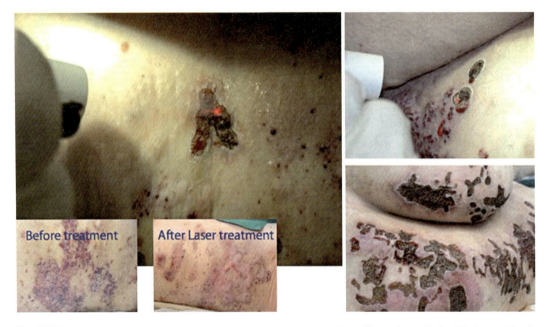

Before treatment   After Laser treatment

Fig. 35.4 CO_2-laser vaporization. In hyperkeratinization of mixed vascular malformation with the CO_2 laser, a blood-less ablation is possible. Due to depth of the disease, scar-free healing is not possible

due to high energy should be avoided because this can cause bleeding. In disseminated exces-sive bleeding areas, a homogeneous CW Nd:YAG laser coagulation through ultrasound jelly is necessary to avoid carbonization. However, this is followed by scarring. In more hyperkeratotic lesions CO_2-laser vaporization is possible, but even this results in scarring (Fig. 35.4).

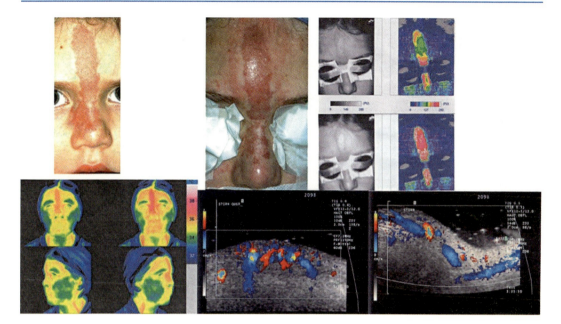

Fig. 35.5 Arteriovenous malformation. Centrofacial port-wine stains may be only an overlying symptom of a deep vascular malformation. As a screening method, thermography is an important investigation. The simple PWS show normotemperature, whereas a hyperthermia is a sign of an AV malformation. In this case no embolization was possible, so transcutaneous Nd:YAG laser therapy with ice cube cooling was started to occlude the microfistulas. The result is seen in the CCDS investigation with a decrease in perfusion

Port-Wine Stains with Associated Vascular Malformations (Neurocutaneous Syndromes or Phakomatoses)

Capillary or dermal vascular malformations are occasionally associated with deeper vascular anomalies. The key point is that these cutaneous signs permit early diagnosis, thus helping in further recognition of more complex syndromes. Sturge-Weber syndrome is the most well-known vascular malformation complex associated with port-wine staining. The same malformation affects the soft tissue of the face with the risk of subsequent hypertrophy. This can be detected early by color-coded duplex sonography (CCDS) and especially by thermography with hyperthermy. If this is shown despite the FLPDL therapy, the growing tissue will be treated in cases of dermal hypertrophy with a double pulsed Nd:YAG/pulsed dye laser or in cases of more subcutaneous or soft tissue hypertrophy with the transcutaneous ice cube-cooled Nd:YAG laser, as for infantile hemangioma but with a higher power of 60 W.

The large PWS of the extremities in Klippel-Trenaunay syndrome sometimes need the same combination of pulsed dye laser, transcutaneous ice cube-cooled Nd:YAG laser, or, in cases with hyperkeratinization, CO_2 laser. In Proteus syndrome with patchy PWS of the hands or feet, the effectiveness of pulsed dye laser therapy is limited, just as it is for other mixed capillary-lymphatic malformations. However, even here the treatment of ectatic vessels with pulsed Nd:YAG or KTP laser is possible.

In Wyburn-Mason syndrome/Bonnet-Dechaume-Blanc syndrome, the facial PWS may be the sign of unilateral arteriovenous malformation of the retina and the intracranial optic pathway (Fig. 35.5). This means that before FLPD laser starts, embolization of the feeding artery is helpful [4].

Nonfading Telangiectasias

Nonfading telangiectasias have been subcategorized under capillary malformations. These present in a spectrum, from the classical spider nevus to the

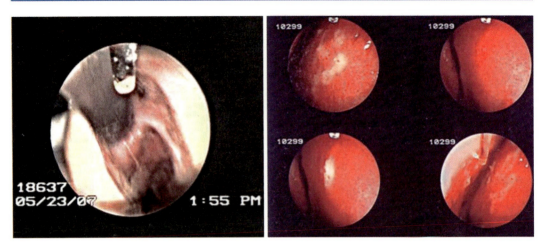

Fig. 35.6 Osler-Rendu-Weber (HHT). The glass spatula compression or rinsing of the blood is necessary during laser therapy of bleeding Osler spots to prevent vaporization and septum perforation. Nd:YAG laser, CW; upper septum

maculopapular punctate anomalies of Osler-Rendu-Weber syndrome to the characteristic reticulated marbling and cutaneous hypoplasia seen in cutis marmorata telangiectatica congenita (CMTC).

Cutis Marmorata Telangiectatica Congenita (Van Lohuizen Syndrome)

The characteristic lesion of CMTC has a distinctive deep purple color and is depressed in a serpiginous reticulated pattern. In some cases of CMTC-associated deep venous anomalies, ulceration of the reticulated purple areas and hypotrophy of the involved limb and subcutaneous tissue have been reported. The skin atrophy and deep vascular staining can persist into adulthood, along with diffuse ectasia of the veins in the involved extremities. If the steal effect of these pathological vessels causes skin atrophy, coagulation can enhance the microcirculation to avoid further trophic defects. Spider vascular lesions can be obliterated by KTP laser directed at the central artery under compression.

Osler-Rendu-Weber Syndrome (Hereditary Hemorrhagic Telangiectasia)

This disease is classified with the extratruncular capillary malformations and can appear as telangiectasias in the skin and AV malformations

widely distributed throughout the body with a predilection for the gums, lips, mucosa of the nose, face, and fingers [5].

The major complication is recurrent bleeding, especially of the nasopharyngeal cavity and the gastrointestinal tract with secondary iron deficiency. Besides this manifestation, the most important secondary involvement is the lung [6] and the liver with AV shunts. Cardiac failure, hepatic portosystemic encephalopathy, embolic abscesses, and a variety of neurologic symptoms are complications, resulting in the need for some of these patients to have organ transplantation.

For gastrointestinal bleeding spots, argon beamer electrofulguration is easier to handle endoscopically than side fire laser fiber. However, for all other manifestations, Nd:YAG laser therapy is the treatment of choice. For nasal or intraoral spots, including tongue mucous membranes, CW Nd:YAG laser with 600 μ bare fiber in near contact with 12–15 W at 300–400 ms in the repetition mode can be used. Higher power can induce vaporization with opening of the central shunt artery, and longer exposure times can cause a popcorn effect with massive bleeding. If acute bleeding has occurred, one has to remove the blood with continuous saline rinsing during lasering (Fig. 35.6). Here the power must increase to 20–25 W and CW mode. Another option is to compress the bleeding vessel with the Hopf/Jovanovic glass spatula during lasering. Here, even with 20–25 W, the exposure time has to be reduced to prevent carbonization under the glass

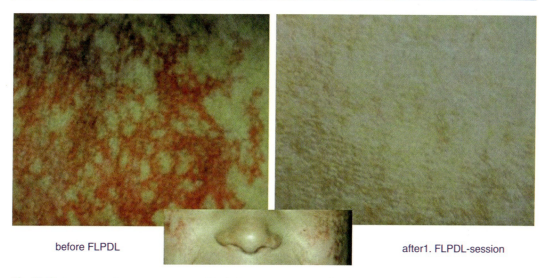

before FLPDL   after1. FLPDL-session

Fig. 35.7 Rothmund-Thomson syndrome. FLPD laser. One can immediately see the effect of pulsed dye laser on the halo-spaced clearance. A side effect can be long-term persistence of hyperpigmentation due to hemosiderin

spatula. For skin lesions including the face, finger, or subungual areas, pulsed Nd:YAG laser with intermittent ice cube cooling is the first choice. The parameters vary depending on the laser system, mainly between 50 and 100 J/cm². For micro AV shunts, CCDS-guided interstitial coagulation with 5 W and in CW mode is necessary. In larger AV shunts with life threatening bleeding on the face, additional arterial embolization is indicated.

Other Telangiectasias

Widespread telangiectasias as a component of other syndromes should also respond to pulsed dye laser treatment [7]. Patients with diffuse telangiectasias as a component of the Rothmund-Thomson syndrome or telangiectasia macularis eruptiva perstans demonstrate dramatic clearing following treatment with pulsed dye laser (Fig. 35.7). Other spider vascular lesions with a central artery show better results with pulsed Nd:YAG laser treatment.

Lymphatic Malformations

Pure lymphatic malformations are only found in the newborn period, but even here the majority of patients show additional venous malformations

as mixed malformations [8]. The older the patient, the more the venous part will be important for the complications, e.g., bleeding and overgrowth. The aim of early laser therapy is to reduce this secondary hypertrophy and above all manage these risks.

Truncular Lymphatic Malformation
Cystic Hygromas

The isolated single cystic lymphangioma of the neck is a truncular lymphatic malformation and as a rule is better to treat primarily by surgical excision because a previous interstitial Nd:YAG laser coagulation causes fibrosis which affects surgical preparation.

Extratruncular Lymphatic Malformation

If there is an early recurrence after surgery, the lesion was not an isolated truncular lymphatic malformation, but an extratruncular malformation. In extratruncular lymphatic malformations, the discrimination between micro- and macrocystic is not precise, but rather like a screenshot. By changing of resorption or production, the size of the cysts can change in short time periods. Furthermore, due to spontaneous rupture of the

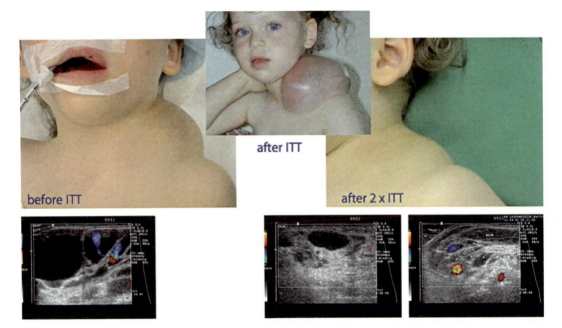

before ITT | after ITT | after 2 x ITT

Fig. 35.8 Interstitial Nd:YAG laser coagulation (ITT). The CCDS shows the intraseptal pathological veins which cause recurrent bleeding. During interstitial or intracystic Nd:YAG laser coagulation, one has to avoid direct puncture of these veins to reduce the risk of intraoperative bleeding

interseptal pathologic veins, massive bleeding can occur. Only a pure microcystic malformation, called solid lymphangioma, is its own entity and is indicated for surgical resection. In all other cases, depending on the actual local situation, different combinations of CW Nd:YAG laser techniques are used.

Intraluminal (Intracystic) Technique

Larger cysts are punctured under CCDS control to prevent a direct puncture of interseptal veins and to string several cysts. If the diameter is more than 2 cm, it is helpful to reduce the size by suction of the lymph fluid. In cases of previous hemorrhage, flushing with saline is necessary until the fluid is clear (Fig. 35.8). The kind of puncture cannula depends on the lesion. If possible, 16 or 18 G Teflon vein cannulas are preferred because this material has no heat conduction risk from the heated tip. In larger lymphangiomas or in anatomically difficult regions where the puncture directions must change, a steel cannula is easier to handle but carries the risk of skin burning.

As there is a lower basic absorption without erythrocytes, a power of approximately 10 W CW Nd:YAG laser is used [9]. The coagulation is stopped when an extensive color bruit is seen on the CCDS. Near the interseptal veins, the power must be reduced to prevent a vein perforation. If there is no risk of communication with vessels or body cavities, additional sclerotherapy can be helpful, e.g., with Picibanil [10]. The aim of laser coagulation in this combination is to destroy the lymph cyst's epithelium in order to enhance the effectiveness of the sclerotherapy. The puncture direction must never cross the nerve direction to avoid direct nerve palsy. However, due to postoperative swelling, an increasing hypesthesia or dysesthesia can occur within the next few days. This is transient and heals without any defects within a few weeks.

Microcystic (Solid) Lymphatic Malformation "ITT"

If a surgical resection due to the infiltrative growth or other risks is not possible, interstitial

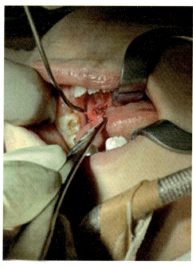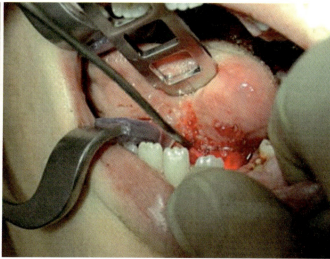

Fig. 35.9 Nd:YAG laser treatment with direct bare fiber or impression. In contrast to the case described in Fig. 35.10, with impression coagulation with a higher power of approximately 30 W and pulse of 0.5 s, contact vaporization of the small lymphatic cysts occurs. For larger cysts with risk of bleeding, a precoagulation with lower power and longer pulse duration is helpful

laser coagulation is possible. The biophysical basis is that the thin lymph cyst walls are transparent for the Nd:YAG laser near-infrared radiation. This means that not only the direct punctured cyst will be irradiated but also the surrounding areas. In contrast to the above or to the intraluminal techniques described later in venous malformations, here there exists a direct contact of the 600 μ bare fiber with the adjacent tissue. This means that power of more than 5–7 W leads to a carbonization at the fiber end which absorbs all laser energy. The effect is that vaporization occurs at the fiber, but no radiation can transmit to the tissue to perform large volume coagulation. Here additional sclerotherapy makes no sense and is dangerous.

Bare Fiber Contact Vaporization

What was described in the previous section as something to be avoided must immediately be induced in the treatment of mucous membrane hyperkeratotic cysts, such as intraoral or anogenital cysts, with a high power of 30 W and chopped mode carbonization of the fiber end to prevent uncontrolled deep coagulation and to perform bloodless vaporization.

Especially in the mouth, there are mixed venous-lymphatic vesicles which have a high risk of recurrent bleeding, superinfection, and fetor ex ore (Fig. 35.9). Postoperatively there is no specific treatment necessary, only continuous rinsing with fluid [11].

Endoscopic Coagulation

Palatinal, hypopharyngeal, and laryngeal and urethral, bladder, and intravaginal lymphatic cysts are coagulated with the noncontact method comparable to the methods described in the chapter on laser therapy of hemangiomas. In the oropharynx, direct coagulation in the near contact procedure is possible with 15–20 W and chopped mode. The more venous the parts with higher basic absorption, the greater the risk of the popcorn effect or direct vaporization. In a frog egg situation on the larynx, the Werner ice water technique gives a good overview of the malformation and prevents carbonization of the surface. The power has to be increased to 20–25 W, depending on the venous component.

In the bladder or in the genital tract, endoscopic coagulation is performed under continuous saline rinsing. Even here, the greater the venous component, the greater the risk of popcorn effect.

Often the lymphatic malformations are combined with a chylothorax and chylopericardium and a pleural adhesion and are called Gorham-Stout syndrome (or disappearing bone disease). Here an endoscopic CW Nd:YAG laser coagulation of the ectatic lymph vessels to reduce the chylous extravasation is possible.

Venous Malformations

Venous malformation of the head and neck region presents in a wide spectrum, from circumscribed venous anomalies in which the venous lacunae are connected to the venous circulation by capillaries to localized venous anomalies connected by veins to the venous circulation and diffuse venous ectasias. Furthermore, multiple venous lesions tend to coexist with venous ectasias and deep vein anomalies [12]. In principle the laser procedures are similar to the lymphatic treatments or the congenital vascular tumor protocols. However, in contrast to lymphatic malformations, here there is a high absorption of the Nd:YAG laser near-infrared radiation in the blood, so the parameters have to be adapted to this absorption.

Truncular Venous Malformation

Laser coagulation is, in contrast to sclerotherapy, a local and not a regional procedure. This is not good or bad: it is a fact. This means that no systemic or distant side effects can occur, but it also means that an effect can occur only where the laser hits the tissue. Furthermore, blood is a perfect absorber so the laser radiation does not hit the vessel wall, but cooks the blood. To prevent this effect, one has to remove all blood completely by rinsing the fiber. This explains why in simple varicose veins, which can be treated easily with foam or radiofrequency, intraluminal laser therapy is not used. So laser is an ideal tool for diseases that cannot be treated with easier techniques.

Large truncular venous malformations, such as enlarged persistent marginal veins, are a better indication for surgery or sclerotherapy. However, in a difficult anatomical situation such as after previous surgery or in incomplete marginal veins, an intraluminal procedure is indicated. Comparable to the macrocystic lymphatic malformation, under CCDS control the vessel is punctured, and a saline rinse is installed to clean up the fiber tip. With a maximum power of 10 W under CCDS, the coagulation is performed, while any direct contact of the fiber end with the vessel wall has to be avoided (Fig. 35.10) [13]. This would immediately cause a perforation with bleeding. Another option is the use of diffuse

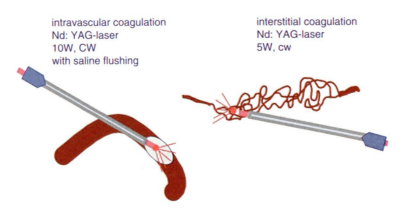

intravascular coagulation
Nd: YAG-laser
10W, CW
with saline flushing

interstitial coagulation
Nd: YAG-laser
5W, cw

Fig. 35.10 Interstitial coagulation. In principle the technique of intraluminal and interstitial Nd:YAG laser coagulation is the same, only the parameters have to be changed. In endovascular laser application, the blood has to be removed completely from the fiber end with rinsing, so the power has to be increased up to 10 W. In all other cases of interstitial laser application, the maximum power for coagulation is 5 W; otherwise, vaporization starts immediately

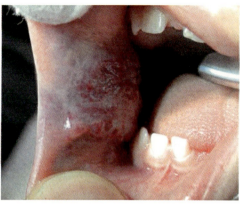
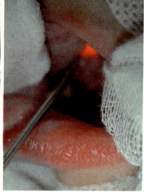
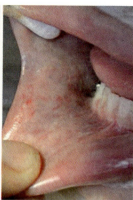

Fig. 35.11 In smaller lesions or in endangered regions, besides the ITT technique, the impression technique is another option for under surface coagulation. Only on the contact point of the bare fiber with the mucosa is there a fast healing coagulation point. The power is the same as in ITT; the coagulation volume underneath depends on the exposure time

irradiating interstitial applicators, which are used for the therapy of interstitial malignancies, such as liver tumors. The advantage is that vessel wall coagulation is more homogeneous; the disadvantage is that the puncture is larger and more difficult to handle. A string maneuver in kinked vessels is nearly impossible.

Extratruncular Venous Malformation

Similar to extratruncular lymphatic malformations, all tissues can be affected by extratruncular venous malformations, and so all the above-described laser techniques are in use. In the following paragraphs, only specific parameters that are different from the above will be described.

Soft Tissue Phlebectasias

Because the vessel wall as opposed to the blood is the target, if possible the ectatic vessel will not be punctured, but irradiated paravasally, as with perforator vein laser coagulation (Fig. 35.11). In cases where a paravasal application is not possible, but only an intraluminal application similar to the truncular procedure, the fiber tip has to be rinsed with saline solution to prevent carbonization followed by perforation. If there is no direct drainage over larger veins, an additional sclerotherapy can be performed. Postoperatively a compression bandage is obligatory for 24 h. Localized intravascular coagulopathy (LIC) is not a contraindication for this technique because a thrombus formation can be avoided with this procedure.

Cutaneous/Subcutaneous Malformation

The combination of cutaneous and subcutaneous malformation, also known as the blue rubber bleb nevus syndrome, can be treated like a congenital vascular tumor, with the transcutaneous ice cube-cooled Nd:YAG laser technique (Fig. 35.12). However, here a higher power of at least 50–60 W is needed because induction of regression and also direct coagulation is necessary. In cases of intracutaneous lesions, a scar formation in the affected region is not always avoidable.

Mucous Membrane Affection

The main localization for a mucous membrane affection is the oropharynx, followed by the vagina and the rectum. In case of hypopharyngeal or laryngeal lesions, the Werner procedure is obligatory in order to avoid any popcorn effect with massive bleeding (Fig. 35.13). In case of laryngeal localization, it is important to coagulate step-by-step over several sessions to lessen the risk of an airway obstruction necessitating a postoperative intubation. In tracheal lesions the procedure is similar to tracheal infantile hemangioma. Vaginal lesions are coagulated endoscopically under water; treatment depends on the extent of the lesion.

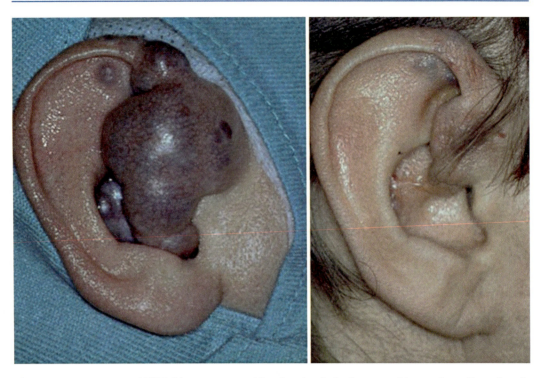

Fig. 35.12 Transcutaneous Nd:YAG laser treatment with ice cube cooling. Comparable to the technique in vascular tumors, the transcutaneous ice cube cooling Nd:YAG laser irradiation is even used in vascular malformations. In case of enlarged vessels, one must take before treatment after six treatments care to prevent a popcorn effect

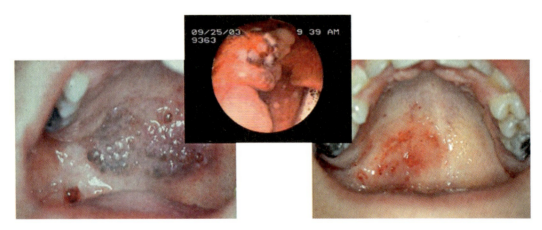

Fig. 35.13 Transmucosal Nd:YAG laser treatment under ice water protection. In mucous membrane lesions in the oropharynx, Nd:YAG laser irradiation through ice water can prevent vaporization with subsequent bleeding. These small coagulation points on the mucosa will heal without any scars

Glomuvenous Malformation ("Glomangioma")

Cases of large raised, soft, and compressible glomangiomas have been mistakenly diagnosed as blue rubber bleb nevus syndrome [14]. Glomangiomas are less likely to be painful than solitary glomus tumors. An effective therapy for multiple glomangiomas (glomangiomatosis) is treatment with Nd:YAG laser with continuous surface cooling. In solitary lesions the interstitial puncture technique is used as for microcystic lymphangiomas.

Arteriovenous Malformations

At present, the first choice therapy for the management of troublesome AV malformations is embolization, either alone or following laser therapy. The therapeutic principle in embolization is to deliver the embolic material into the center of the vascular anomaly (the nidus) in an attempt to block the smallest vessels first, from the inside out. For extensive lesions, interstitial Nd:YAG laser coagulation may help by obliterating all microfistulas in order to collapse the AV malformation permanently, or collateral vessels can develop very slowly.

Truncular Arteriovenous Fistula

In general the pure truncular AV malformation is successfully treated with embolization. However,

in some cases the peripheral smaller vessels remain and are an indication for laser therapy. Depending on the size and origin, the pulsed dye laser, the KTP laser, the pulsed Nd:YAG laser, or the CW Nd:YAG laser chopped with the fluid cooling chamber is used. For fistulas which are not treated by embolization, a paravasal or intraluminal Nd:YAG laser coagulation is performed (Fig. 35.14) [15]. The surrounding pathological vessels are treated in the same session with high-power transcutaneous ice cube-cooled Nd:YAG laser. Depending on the size of the lesion, multiple punctures with the afterloading technique and several sessions are necessary.

Combined Truncular/Extratruncular Arteriovenous Malformation

Besides the case of the capillary malformations described earlier, the most important malformation for laser therapy is the hamartous AV malformation (angioma racemosum). Even in AV fistulas, the first choice is embolization. However,

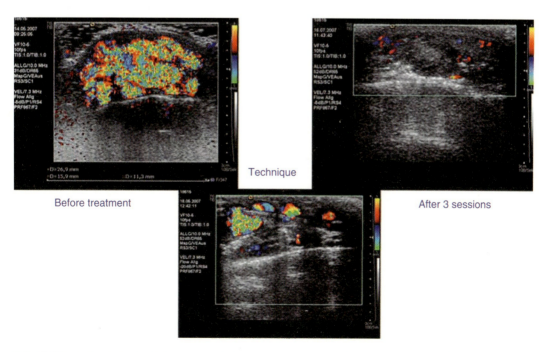

Before treatment   Technique   After 3 sessions

Fig. 35.14 Scalp-AV-fistula Nd:YAG-laser-ITT technique. Arteriovenous fistula on the scalp. Due to different feeding arteries, even from the ophthalmic artery, there was no possibility for previous embolization. After three sessions of paravasal interstitial coagulation of the nidus, the perfusion decreased

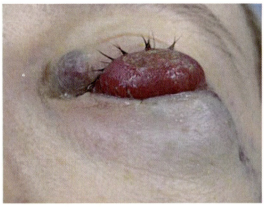
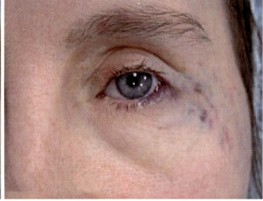

Before treatment   After 3 sessions

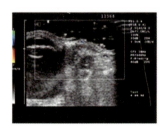

Technique

Fig. 35.15 Nd:YAG laser treatment transconjunctival. Mixed vascular malformation with secondary arterialization. Due to risk of uncontrolled emboli in the ophthalmic artery, the impression technique allows a precise application of laser energy to subcutaneous volumes. Even though no scattering can occur, near the eye, the bulb, and the cornea must be protected by a metal spatula

this is not always possible, and even after successful embolization in the periphery, small fistulas remain. Here an interstitial laser therapy or a transcutaneous ice cube-cooled Nd:YAG laser therapy is needed (Fig. 35.15). Mucous membrane bleeding is directly coagulated because here scar formation is not a concern.

References

1. Noe JM, Barsky SH, Geer DE, Rosen S (1980) Port wine stains and the response to argon laser therapy: successful treatment and the predictive role of color, age, and biopsy. Plast Reconstr Surg 65:130–136
2. Poetke M, Philipp C, Urban P, Berlien HP (2001) Interstitial laser treatment of venous malformations. Med Laser Appl 16:111–119
3. Whimster IW (1976) The pathology of lymphangioma circumscriptum. Br J Dermatol 94:473
4. Yakes WE (1989) Alcohol embolotherapy of vascular malformation. Semin Intervent Radiol 6:146–161
5. Menefee MG, Flessa HC, Glueck HI, Hogg S (1985) Hereditary hemorrhagic telangiectasia (Osler-Weber-Rendu disease): an electron microscopy study of the vascular lesions before and after therapy with hormones. Arch Otolaryngol 101:246–251
6. Wirbelauer J, Thomas W, Darge K, Singer D (2007) Zentrale Zyanose und Verdichtungen im Thoraxröntgenbild bei einem Säugling. Monatsschr Kinderheilkd 155:789–792
7. Bekov V, Bonsmann G, Kuhn A (2007) Kollagenosen. Monatsschr Kinderheilkd 156:122–133
8. Vogt R, Gillessen-Kaesbach G (2007) Das Noonan-Syndrom. Pädiatr Praxis 69:719–726
9. Poetke M, Bültmann O, Urban P, Berlien HP (1998) Vaskuläre Malformationen im Kindes- und Erwachsenenalter. Therapie mit dem Nd: YAG-Laser. Vasomed 10:338–347
10. Helmstaedter V, Quante G, Roth B et al (2007) Behandlung lymphatischer Malformationen mit Lysat attenuierter Streptokokken (Picibanil/OK-432). Monatsschr Kinderheilkd 155:1077–1082

11. Poetke M (2003) Laser treatment in haemangiomas and vascular malformations. In: Berlien H-P, Müller G (eds) Applied laser medicine. Springer, Berlin/New York
12. Sürücü O, Sure U, Stahl S et al (2007) Neue CCM1-Mutation bei einem 2-jährigen. Monatsschr Kinderheilkd 155:1161–1165
13. Urban P (2006) Vaskuläre Malformationen. In: Kubale R, Stiegler H (eds) Farbkodierte Duplexsonographie. Thieme, Stuttgart
14. Höger P (2005) Kinderdermatologie, Differenzialdiagnostik und Therapie bei Kindern und Jugendlichen. Schattauer, Stuttgart
15. Poetke M, Philipp C, Großewinkelmann A et al (2001) Die Behandlung von Naevi flammei bei Säuglingen und Kleinkindern mit dem blitzlampengepumpten Farbstofflaser. Monatsschr Kinderheilkd 32:405–415

Possibilities and Limits of Medical Treatment

36

Jennifer Fahrni and Iris Baumgartner

Medical management of vascular malformations is focused on prevention of symptoms and complications. There is currently no medical option to cure the vascular malformation in itself, unlike in vascular tumors. Progress, however, has been made in the use of drugs specifically targeting the vessels of the malformations themselves, such as antiangiogenic drugs. These are promising approaches, but not yet in widespread clinical use, and they are discussed at the end of this chapter.

Thrombosis and Bleeding

Slow-flow vascular malformations are associated with an increased risk for thrombosis as well as bleeding [1, 2]. The pathogenesis of coagulopathy in vascular malformations is still poorly understood. Thrombocytopenia which can be severe in vascular tumors (e.g., Kasabach-Merritt syndrome in giant hemangiomas) is usually mild, if present at all. However, in extensive venous malformations, ectatic vessels can lead to stasis with activation of the coagulation cascade as one component of the classic Virchow's triad. Additional factors might be abnormalities of the

endothelium within the malformed vessels resulting in a local disruption of the regulation of coagulation, and several studies have been able to demonstrate this localized intravascular coagulopathy (LIC) [3–6]. Laboratory assessments show low levels of fibrinogen and elevated D-dimers. Severity of LIC seems to be related to the extent of the malformation [5]. LIC rarely results in serious complications, but it can be aggravated by different stimuli such as surgery, endovascular therapy, or trauma, resulting in disseminated intravascular coagulopathy (DIC). It is especially important to bear this in mind in the perioperative management of patients with vascular malformations, and diligent prophylaxis with low molecular weight heparin (LMWH) is the recommended [7]. It seems reasonable to assume that large malformed draining veins, such as the marginal vein which is frequently ectatic and typically valveless, can be a source of pulmonary embolism [8, 9]. Elimination of such veins should be considered in patients who have suffered a pulmonary embolism. In general, any extensive venous malformation should be assumed to be a risk factor for venous thromboembolism, and prophylactic measures should be contemplated in any situation with increased risk.

Patients with venous malformations frequently suffer from painful episodes of local thrombosis within the malformed veins. These can often be successfully treated – minimizing intensity and duration of pain – with short courses of LMWH, similar to the treatment of superficial

J. Fahrni • I. Baumgartner (✉)
Department of Angiology,
Swiss Cardiovascular Center, Bern, Switzerland
e-mail: Jennifer.fahrni@insel.ch;
Iris.baumgartner@insel.ch

R. Mattassi et al. (eds.), *Hemangiomas and Vascular Malformations: An Atlas of Diagnosis and Treatment*,
DOI 10.1007/978-88-470-5673-2_36, © Springer-Verlag Italia 2009, 2015

vein thrombosis in patients without vascular malformations [3]. In patients who experience such episodes very frequently and in whom this treatment has proven beneficial, self-administration of LMWH at the onset of symptoms should be discussed. Continuous long-term heparinization can be considered in patients with severe and chronic pain that has responded to LMWH treatment. With the increasingly widespread use of novel oral anticoagulants, an alternative to treat superficial thrombosis might be emerging, although at this point there is very little experience in this setting, and the use of these agents is off-label.

Depending on the site of the malformation, recurrent bleeding can cause chronic anemia. It is often not possible to completely eliminate the lesion to prevent bleeding. Anemia in these patients should be treated the same as chronic anemia by other causes. This might require iron replacement therapy or even regular red blood cell transfusions. As vascular malformations can predispose patients to bleeding as well as thromboembolic events, a particularly challenging clinical problem can occur when there is recurrent bleeding and an indication for anticoagulation, and risk and benefits must be carefully weighed.

Infections

Malformations with a lymphatic component carry a risk of infection. These patients need to be aware of this risk and instructed on how to act appropriately to prevent infection, how to recognize early signs, and when to seek medical attention or, in select cases, initiate self-medication. Preventive measures include good skin care and treatment of possible sources of infection (e.g., athlete's foot in malformations of the lower extremities). When an infection occurs, prompt treatment with an appropriate antiinfective agent is important. Choice of the specific antibiotic does not differ from similar infections in patients without vascular malformations. If infections are recurring, patients should be given the option to initiate treatment themselves at the first sign of infection. In patients with frequent infections, a long-term antibiotic prophylaxis should be considered.

Medications to Avoid

In extratruncular malformations, oral contraceptives containing estrogen should be used with caution. They can stimulate proliferation of malformed vessels (in particular in arteriovenous malformation), similar to endovascular or surgical trauma, and precipitate worsening of symptoms. Additionally, especially in patients with extensive venous malformations, risk of thromboembolic disease is increased, and this risk could be substantially heightened by the addition of estrogen-containing drugs.

Nonmedical Conservative Treatment

For the large majority of patients with vascular malformation, the most important conservative treatment by far is compression therapy. Adequate compressive treatment can minimize symptoms and prevent complications and progression of the vascular malformation. The specifics of compression therapy do not differ from those for chronic venous insufficiency or lymphedema.

A considerable number of patients with vascular malformations report signs of anxiety, depression, and somatic or psychological distress if specifically prompted [10]. Treating physicians should be aware of the psychological impact that a vascular malformation can have and should offer appropriate support.

Future Developments

Thalidomide has been shown to reduce bleeding in patients with hereditary hemorrhagic telangiectasia, possibly by promoting vessel maturation [11]. Additionally, several reports about positive effects of thalidomide in gastrointestinal bleeding due to vascular malformations have been published [12–14]. The drug is also known to have an antiangiogenic effect by suppression of endothelial growth factor (EVGF) [15]. A combination of thalidomide and interferon-α has been used in extensive CVMs with acceptable results [16]. In another case, the use of a combination of thalidomide, interferon, and zoledronate has been described [17]. The most important adverse effect of thalidomide is peripheral neuropathy which occurs in about 20 % [18, 19]. In summary, the efficacy of this drug in CVM has yet to be demonstrated, and data exists mainly on the effect in gastrointestinal bleeding, but not in other VM, LM, or AVM.

Sildenafil selectively inhibits phosphodiesterase 5, decreasing the contractility of vascular smooth muscle and resulting in vasodilation [20]. The drug has been approved for the treatment of pulmonary hypertension in adults and is used off-label in children for the same pathology [21]. Some positive effect of this drug on complex lymphatic malformations has been reported [22–24]. This effect could be due to smooth muscle relaxation in lymphatic cysts which in turn might facilitate either relaxation of the cysts themselves or draining of the cysts. However, no randomized study exists to assess effectiveness of sildenafil in this setting.

Sirolimus (also known as rapamycin), a macrolide produced by *Streptomyces hygroscopicus* bacteria, was originally developed as an antifungal agent [25]. After exhibiting immunosuppressive and antiproliferative effects [26], it was then used to prevent kidney transplant rejection [27] and to improve results of coronary stenting by applying it in drug-eluting stents [28]. Additionally, sirolimus demonstrated an anticancer effect by inhibition of angiogenesis [29] and has been utilized with good results in tumors [30, 31]. Recent reports indicate a possible positive effect in the treatment of vascular malformations, mainly of the lymphatic variety [32, 33]. A phase II clinical trial on different types of vascular malformations – mainly lymphatic, but also venous and kaposiform hemangioendothelioma – was presented at the ISSVA (International Society for the Study of Vascular Anomalies) 20th International Workshop in Melbourne, Australia, in 2014. Eighty-two percent of malformations demonstrated a partial response, and 5 % were stable, while a progression was noted in 12 % [34]. Treatment with sirolimus had a positive effect in three cases of Gorham-Stout syndrome [35]. Blue rubber bleb nevus syndrome has been treated successfully in an 8-year-old patient with massive gastrointestinal bleeding. A treatment with low doses of sirolimus completely halted bleeding during the 20-month follow-up and reduced venous masses [36]. Toxicity leading to interstitial pneumonitis and decreased glucose tolerance has been reported in other settings, but so far has not arisen in any reported cases of use of sirolimus in vascular malformation.

Octreotide is a somatostatin analogue which has been used for the treatment of gastrointestinal bleeding due to CVM. The drug may have an antiangiogenic effect [37] in addition to gastrointestinal effects like reduction of gastrin and pepsin and decrease in duodenal and splanchnic blood flow [38, 39]. Some series demonstrate a reduction of necessary transfusions after octreotide therapy [40]. It can be considered as an adjunctive treatment for gastrointestinal bleeding due to CVM or as the sole treatment if other, more aggressive options are not possible. No data exists about the usefulness of octreotide on CVM outside the gastrointestinal tract.

Estrogen and *progesterone* have been widely investigated in the treatment of gastrointestinal bleeding caused by vascular malformations. This was based on the observation that epistaxis in HHT improved in pregnancy and worsened after menopause [41]. Case reports showed positive results [42, 43]. However, a randomized multicenter study failed to demonstrate an advantage over placebo [44].

In summary, there are very promising developments in medical treatment of CVM, but further investigations are necessary to assess the efficacy and safety of the different drugs in this specific setting.

References

1. Oduber CE, van Beers EJ, Bresser P, van der Horst CM, Meijers JC, Gerdes VE (2013) Venous thrombo-embolism and prothrombotic parameters in Klippel-Trenaunay syndrome. Neth J Med 71(5):246–252. Epub 2013/06/27
2. Barbara DW, Wilson JL (2011) Anesthesia for surgery related to Klippel–Trenaunay syndrome: a review of 136 anesthetics. Anesth Analg 113(1):98–102
3. Dompmartin A, Acher A, Thibon P, Tourbach S, Hermans C, Deneys V et al (2008) Association of localized intravascular coagulopathy with venous malformations. Arch Dermatol 144(7):873–877. Epub 2008/07/23
4. Dompmartin A, Ballieux F, Thibon P, Lequerrec A, Hermans C, Clapuyt P et al (2009) Elevated D-dimer level in the differential diagnosis of venous malforma-tions. Arch Dermatol 145(11):1239–1244. Epub 2009/11/18
5. Mazoyer E, Enjolras O, Bisdorff A, Perdu J, Wassef M, Drouet L (2008) Coagulation disorders in patients with venous malformation of the limbs and trunk: a case series of 118 patients. Arch Dermatol 144(7):861–867. Epub 2008/07/23
6. Mazoyer E, Enjolras O, Laurian C, Houdart E, Drouet L (2002) Coagulation abnormalities associ-ated with extensive venous malformations of the limbs: differentiation from Kasabach-Merritt syn-drome. Clin Lab Haematol 24(4):243–251. Epub 2002/08/16
7. Lee BB, Baumgartner I, Berlien P, Bianchini G, Burrows P, Gloviczki P, et al (2014) Diagnosis and treatment of venous malformations consensus docu-ment of the International Union of Phlebology (IUP): updated 2013. Int Angiol. Epub 26 Feb 2014
8. Mattassi R, Vaghi M (2007) Management of the mar-ginal vein: current issues. Phlebology 22(6):283–286
9. Kim YW, Lee BB, Cho JH, Do YS, Kim DI, Kim ES (2007) Haemodynamic and clinical assessment of lat-eral marginal vein excision in patients with a predom-inantly venous malformation of the lower extremity. Eur J Vasc Endovasc Surg 33(1):122–127
10. Fahrni JO, Cho E-YN, Engelberger RP, Baumgartner I, von Känel R (2014) Quality of life in patients with congenital vascular malformations. J Vasc Surg Venous Lymphat Disord 2(1):46–51
11. Lebrin F, Srun S, Raymond K, Martin S, van den Brink S, Freitas C et al (2010) Thalidomide stimulates vessel maturation and reduces epistaxis in individuals with hereditary hemorrhagic telangiectasia. Nat Med 16(4):420–428
12. Garrido A, Sayago M, Lopez J, Leon R, Bellido F, Marquez JL (2012) Thalidomide in refractory bleed-ing due to gastrointestinal angiodysplasias. Rev Esp Enferm Dig 104(2):69–71. Epub 2012/03/01
13. Tan HH, Ge ZZ, Chen HM, Gao YJ (2013) Successful treatment with thalidomide for a patient with recur-rent gastrointestinal bleeding due to angiodysplasia
diagnosed by capsule endoscopy. J Dig Dis 14(3):153–155. Epub 2012/11/09
14. Kamalaporn P, Saravanan R, Cirocco M, May G, Kortan P, Kandel G et al (2009) Thalidomide for the treatment of chronic gastrointestinal bleeding from angiodysplasias: a case series. Eur J Gastroenterol Hepatol 21(12):1347–1350. Epub 2009/09/05
15. Tan H, Chen H, Xu C, Ge Z, Gao Y, Fang J et al (2012) Role of vascular endothelial growth factor in angiodysplasia: an interventional study with thalido-mide. J Gastroenterol Hepatol 27(6):1094–1101. Epub 2011/11/22
16. Adam Z, Pour L, Krejci M, Pourova E, Synek O, Zahradova L et al (2010) [Successful treatment of angiomatosis with thalidomide and interferon alpha. A description of five cases and overview of treatment of angiomatosis and proliferating hemangiomas]. Vnitr Lek 56(8):810–823. Epub 2010/09/18. Uspesna lecba angiomatozy thalidomidem a interferonem alpha. Popis peti pripadu a prehled lecby angiomatozy a proliferujicich hemangiomu
17. Adam Z, Krikavova L, Krejci M, Mechl M, Pour L, Moulis M et al (2008) [Treatment of multiple angio-matosis involving the skeleton and the abdominal and thoracic cavities with interferon alpha, thalidomide and zoledronate]. Vnitr Lek 54(6):653–664. Epub 2008/08/05. Lecba mnohocetne angiomatozy postihu-jici skelet, brisni i hrudni dutinu interferonem alpha, thalidomidem a zoledronatem
18. Molloy FM, Floeter MK, Syed NA, Sandbrink F, Culcea E, Steinberg SM et al (2001) Thalidomide neuropathy in patients treated for metastatic prostate cancer. Muscle Nerve 24(8):1050–1057. Epub 2001/07/06
19. Ochonisky S, Verroust J, Bastuji-Garin S, Gherardi R, Revuz J (1994) Thalidomide neuropathy incidence and clinico-electrophysiologic findings in 42 patients. Arch Dermatol 130(1):66–69. Epub 1994/01/01
20. Lin CS, Lin G, Xin ZC, Lue TF (2006) Expression, distribution and regulation of phosphodiesterase 5. Curr Pharm Des 12(27):3439–3457. Epub 2006/10/05
21. Karatza AA, Bush A, Magee AG (2005) Safety and efficacy of Sildenafil therapy in children with pulmo-nary hypertension. Int J Cardiol 100(2):267–273. Epub 2005/04/13
22. Swetman GL, Berk DR, Vasanawala SS, Feinstein JA, Lane AT, Bruckner AL (2012) Sildenafil for severe lymphatic malformations. N Engl J Med 366(4):384–386. Epub 2012/01/27
23. Singh P, Mundy D (2013) Giant neonatal thoraco-abdominal lymphatic malformations treated with sildenafil: a case report and review of the literature. J Neonatal Perinatal Med 6(1):89–92. Epub 2013/11/20
24. Danial C, Tichy AL, Tariq U, Swetman GL, Khuu P, Leung TH et al (2014) An open-label study to evaluate sildenafil for the treatment of lymphatic malforma-tions. J Am Acad Dermatol 70(6):1050–1057
25. Vezina C, Kudelski A, Sehgal SN (1975) Rapamycin (AY-22,989), a new antifungal antibiotic. I. Taxonomy of the producing streptomycete and isolation of the

active principle. J Antibiot 28(10):721–726. Epub 1975/10/01

26. McAlister VC, Mahalati K, Peltekian KM, Fraser A, MacDonald AS (2002) A clinical pharmacokinetic study of tacrolimus and sirolimus combination immunosuppression comparing simultaneous to separated administration. Ther Drug Monit 24(3): 346–350. Epub 2002/05/22

27. Ponticelli C (2014) The pros and the cons of mTOR inhibitors in kidney transplantation. Expert Rev Clin Immunol 10(2):295–305. Epub 2014/01/01

28. Barbash IM, Minha S, Torguson R, Ben-Dor I, Badr S, Loh JP et al (2014) Long-term safety and efficacy of the everolimus-eluting stent compared to first-generation drug-eluting stents in contemporary clinical practice. J Invasive Cardiol 26(4):154–160. Epub 2014/04/11

29. Xue Q, Nagy JA, Manseau EJ, Phung TL, Dvorak HF, Benjamin LE (2009) Rapamycin inhibition of the Akt/mTOR pathway blocks select stages of VEGF-A164-driven angiogenesis, in part by blocking S6Kinase. Arterioscler Thromb Vasc Biol 29(8):1172–1178. Epub 2009/05/16

30. Rao RD, Buckner JC, Sarkaria JN (2004) Mammalian target of rapamycin (mTOR) inhibitors as anti-cancer agents. Curr Cancer Drug Targets 4(8):621–635. Epub 2004/12/08

31. Guba M, von Breitenbuch P, Steinbauer M, Koehl G, Flegel S, Hornung M et al (2002) Rapamycin inhibits primary and metastatic tumor growth by antiangiogenesis: involvement of vascular endothelial growth factor. Nat Med 8(2):128–135. Epub 2002/02/01

32. Hammill AM, Wentzel M, Gupta A, Nelson S, Lucky A, Elluru R et al (2011) Sirolimus for the treatment of complicated vascular anomalies in children. Pediatr Blood Cancer 57(6):1018–1024. Epub 2011/03/30

33. Reinglas J, Ramphal R, Bromwich M (2011) The successful management of diffuse lymphangiomatosis using sirolimus: a case report. Laryngoscope 121(9):1851–1854. Epub 2011/10/26

34. Adams D, Hammill A, Trenor C (2014) Phase II clinical trial of Sirolimus for the treatment of complicated vascular anomalies: initial results. In: Proceedings 20th international workshop on vascular anomalies, Melbourne, 1–4 Apr 2014, pp 20–21

35. Rossler JJ, Geiger J, Földi E (2014) Retrospective analysis of Sirolimus in the treatment of generalized lymphatic malformation and Gorham Stout disease. In: Proceedings 20th international workshop on vascular anomalies, Melbourne, 1–4 Apr 2014, pp 22–23

36. Yuksekkaya H, Ozbek O, Keser M, Toy H (2012) Blue rubber bleb nevus syndrome: successful treatment with sirolimus. Pediatrics 129(4):e1080–e1084. Epub 2012/03/07

37. Barrie R, Woltering EA, Hajarizadeh H, Mueller C, Ure T, Fletcher WS (1993) Inhibition of angiogenesis by somatostatin and somatostatin-like compounds is structurally dependent. J Surg Res 55(4):446–450. Epub 1993/10/01

38. Tulassay Z (1998) Somatostatin and the gastrointestinal tract. Scand J Gastroenterol Suppl 228:115–121. Epub 1998/12/29

39. Kubba AK, Dallal H, Haydon GH, Hayes PC, Palmer KR (1999) The effect of octreotide on gastroduodenal blood flow measured by laser Doppler flowmetry in rabbits and man. Am J Gastroenterol 94(4):1077–1082. Epub 1999/04/14

40. Nardone G, Rocco A, Balzano T, Budillon G (1999) The efficacy of octreotide therapy in chronic bleeding due to vascular abnormalities of the gastrointestinal tract. Aliment Pharmacol Ther 13(11):1429–1436. Epub 1999/11/26

41. Koch HJ Jr, Escher GC, Lewis JS (1952) Hormonal management of hereditary hemorrhagic telangiectasia. JAMA 149(15):1376–1380. Epub 1952/08/09

42. Moss SF, Ghosh P, Thomas DM, Jackson JE, Calam J (1992) Gastric antral vascular ectasia: maintenance treatment with oestrogen-progesterone. Gut 33(5): 715–717. Epub 1992/05/01

43. Granieri R, Mazzulla JP, Yarborough GW (1988) Estrogen-progesterone therapy for recurrent gastrointestinal bleeding secondary to gastrointestinal angiodysplasia. Am J Gastroenterol 83(5):556–558. Epub 1988/05/01

44. Junquera F, Feu F, Papo M, Videla S, Armengol JR, Bordas JM et al (2001) A multicenter, randomized, clinical trial of hormonal therapy in the prevention of rebleeding from gastrointestinal angiodysplasia. Gastroenterology 121(5):1073–1079. Epub 2001/10/26

Definition and Correlation of Syndromes Related to Congenital Vascular Malformations

Massimo Vaghi and Vittoria Baraldini

Introduction

The term "syndrome" (from the Greek "συνδρομή" meaning concurrence) is referred to a group of signs and symptoms that collectively indicates a specific disease. Often syndromes are named according to the physician that did the first description. Regarding vascular anomalies, syndromes often indicate not only blood vessel defects (venous, arteriovenous, and lymphatic) but also other related tissue anomalies, like the skin, bone, and others.

Syndromes represent in several cases the first description of vascular malformations and are derived from the age of the observational medicine when modern diagnostic instruments were not available. At these times, simple clinical description was possible without the possibility to get a precise data of the underlying vascular defect.

Today, with the modern equipments and molecular investigations, a diagnosis using a "syndrome" term, which is only a description of signs and symptoms, should be considered out of time, as precise recognition of the defects is possible.

However, the use of eponyms is widespread in the literature, and it has been adopted also for the database of rare diseases in Europe and across the world. Otherwise, it would be difficult to link the presence of a vascular defect with distant manifestations like in telangiectasia hemorrhagica hereditaria or the presence of malignant tumors like in PTEN anomalies or Maffucci syndrome without the summarizing effect of the use of eponyms.

In several cases, diagnoses by eponyms in vascular malformations (the most common is "Klippel-Trenaunay syndrome") are based only on a clinical examination without performing specific diagnostic tests. This incorrect behavior may avoid a true recognition of the disease and related treatment and create stress and anxiety in the patients and relatives.

Syndromes can be divided in two categories according to the hemodynamic characteristics of the involved vessels, high flow and low syndromes (Table 37.1) [1].

Table 37.1 Classification of the vascular syndromes according to the flow pattern characteristics of the involved vessels

Slow-flow malformations
Sturge-Weber, Klippel-Trenaunay, Proteus syndrome, cutis marmorata, Maffucci syndrome, Gorham-Stout, blue rubber bleb nevus syndrome, CLOVES (sometimes)
High flow
Bonnet-Dechaume-Blanc syndrome, Parkes Weber, Rendu-Osler, Cobb, Servelle-Martorell, CLOVES (sometimes)

M. Vaghi (✉)
Department of Vascular Surgery, A.O.G. Salvini Hospital, Garbagnate Milanese, Italy
e-mail: vaghim@yahoo.it

V. Baraldini
Hemangioma Malformations Centre – "V.Buzzi" Children's Hospital, Milan, Italy
e-mail: Vittoria.baraldini@tiscalinet.it

R. Mattassi et al. (eds.), *Hemangiomas and Vascular Malformations: An Atlas of Diagnosis and Treatment*, DOI 10.1007/978-88-470-5673-2_37, © Springer-Verlag Italia 2009, 2015

Sturge-Weber Syndrome (SWS)

SWS, called also "encephalotrigeminal angiomatosis," is a rare congenital disease characterized by port-wine stain of the face (in the forehead and upper eyelid, so-called VI area), glaucoma, mental retardation, and ipsilateral leptomeningeal vascular malformation.

The dermis of the V2 (maxillary) and V3 (mandibular) areas is made of cells from the mesencephalic neural crests, cells not forming leptomeninges: this is why SWS is not linked to a PWS occupying the V2 and V3 skin, without VI location [2] (Fig. 37.1).

The syndrome is likely caused by a somatic mutation in the anterior neural primordium [2]. A recent work identified a somatic activating mutation in GNAQ, a gene that encodes a mediator of the G-protein-coupled receptor cascade [3].

The same mutation was identified also in non-syndromic cases (Parkes Weber syndrome). This implies that the origin of PWS and SWS is related. PWS might represent a late development of the somatic mutation in endothelial cells, while the SWS can be the result of an early mutation in progenitor cells that are precursors to a larger variety of cell types and tissues [3].

Epilepsy is the most severe symptom and may be devastating; it usually starts very early in life, between birth and 1 year. About 10 % of infants with VI PWS actually have leptomeningeal vascular anomalies. Cognitive deficit and mental retardation, loss of developmental milestones, and motor deficit contralateral to the meningeal lesions follow the onset of epilepsy, with a correlation between prolonged seizure and further severe developmental, motor, and intellectual deficits [3].

Prevention of the first seizure by prophylactic antiepileptic treatment aims at avoiding these severe developmental deficits. The seizures decrease strongly after puberty [3]. Ocular follow-up is also mandatory because of the risk of choroidal vascular anomaly and of glaucoma. The PWS can be treated by pulsed dye laser after pharmacological control of epilepsy [4, 5].

Klippel-Trenaunay Syndrome (KTS) and Related Syndromes

KTS, described in 1900 by the French neurologist Maurice Klippel and Paul Trenaunay [6], is a complex vascular malformation sited in the limbs which has a classical triad of signs: nevus, limb overgrowth, and dilated, abnormal superficial veins. These are the characteristics of the syndrome:

1. Diffuse capillary malformation (CM) scattered over an extremity and adjacent trunk with apparently unsystematic spreading and nonassociated abnormality.
2. Hypertrophy of the same extremity, with proportionate overgrowth over the years (angio-osteo-hypertrophy).
3. A slow-flow combined and complex vascular malformation with venous (VM) and, very often, lymphatic malformations (LM), manifesting as either lymphedema or lymphatic vesicles (Fig. 37.2). KTS is associated with SWS in some patients [2].

Vascular anomalies in the pelvis and also in the gut can be sometimes combined with the limb anomalies (see Chap. 46).

Even if association of lymphatic defects is considered a part of the syndrome, there are no accordance if, in the absence of LM, the case should be included or not in KTS.

Moreover, it remains unclear at which degree of combination of the above signs a case should be defined KTS or not. Klippel and Trenaunay described "incomplete cases" with only two of the signs of the triad. The reality is that today, many cases of vascular malformations of the limbs (and also sited in other areas!) are defined KTS.

To increase confusion, several cases in the literature are presented as "Klippel-Trenaunay-Weber syndrome" which can be defined a nonsense. If the main differences between KTS and PWS should be the presence/absence of venous and AV malformations (VM and no AVM in KTS, no VM and AVM in PWS), there should be no reason for this further combination. However, slight AV communications exist also in VM and may vary in extension.

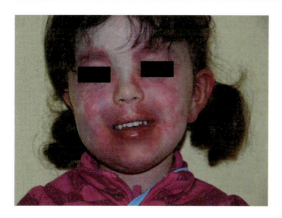

Fig. 37.1 Patient with Sturge-Weber syndrome and Port-wine stain involving the VI area. In this case the capillary malformation involves also the V2-V3 area and extends bilaterally

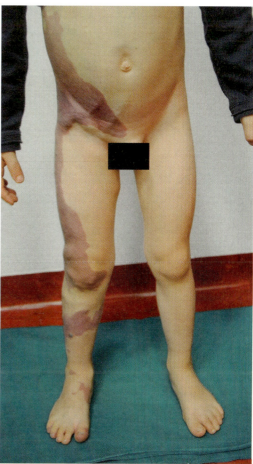

Fig. 37.3 Young patient affected by capillary malformation involving the lower limb and trunk associated to atresia of the ipsilateral common femoral vein. Compensatory dilated epigastric veins are visible on the lower part of the abdomen

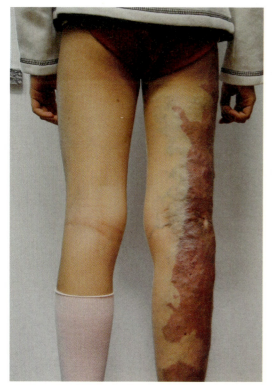

Fig. 37.2 Patient affected by Klippel-Trenaunay syndrome with Port-wine stain interesting the lateral aspect of the lower limb, associated superficial dysplastic varicose veins and mild hypertrophy of the involved limb

lymphoscintigraphy, and possible investigations for associated intestinal and urinary vascular anomalies [8, 9]. Anomalies of the deep veins of the limb (atresia, hypoplasia, or incompetence) can also be present and should be excluded (Fig. 37.3).

Patients with KTS and limb hypertrophy are not at higher risk of Wilms' tumor than the general population, as suspected before, and therefore, they do not need routine Wilms' tumor screening unless the patient has generalized hemihypertrophy [10].

Monitoring of limb length difference progression is mandatory in pediatric patients by ortho-

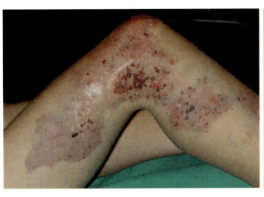
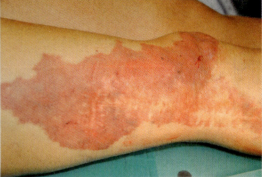

Fig. 37.4 Angiokeratoma Fig 37 B Result after laser treatment

pedic assessment once a year. Epiphysiodesis is considered at around 10–13 years of age, depending on the growth curve of the child, when leg discrepancy is more than 2–3 cm and is increasing. Elastic garments are useful on a lifelong basis if the defects are not treated.

Early surgical treatment of varicose veins and dilated marginal vein is advisable in order to prevent chronic progressive distal venous hypertension [11]. Laser photocoagulation (FPDL or Nd:YAG laser) is useful for treatment of bleeding angiokeratomas and PWS [11] (Fig. 37.4).

Parkes Weber Syndrome (PWS)

PWS includes the same clinical "triad" as KTS: nevus, dilated superficial veins, and limb overgrowth [12]. However, two main differences are typical of PWS: absence of venous anomalies and presence of AV shunts, often multiple small-caliber AV shunts.

Also this syndrome, as KTS, is unclear in the limits as several questions are open. The main one is if all or only some of the cases with AV malformations of the limb should be defined PWS or not.

The therapy is similar to that of KTS with the exception of intervention on the venous vessels. Embolization procedures are not always possible because of the small calibers of the affected vessels.

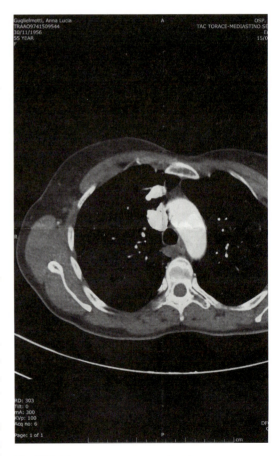

Fig. 37.5 Pulmonary av shunt in Rendu Osler syndrome

Servelle-Martorell Syndrome

This syndrome is characterized by diffuse venous malformations and inhibition of limb bone growth resulting in limb length difference (angio-osteo-hypotrophy) [13]. The venous malformations are often extratruncular and infiltrate the limb till bones with local compression and thinning of the bone itself. Often diffuse phlebolythes are visible on x-ray examination. Deep main veins may be normal.

Treatment is based by occlusion of the diffuse venous defects with foam sclerosis or alcohol. However, treatment can be very long as malformations are infiltrating and extended. Sometimes, some limited painful areas can be resected surgically.

This defect should not be confused with Klippel-Trenaunay syndrome in which there is a limb overgrowth instead of shortening.

Cutis Marmorata

This malformation is characterized by the presence of multiple dilated capillaries and veins in the reticular dermis. Atrophic cutaneous ulcerations may be present. Asymmetries of the limbs are described in some cases. The main clinical features of the syndrome are the presence of reticulated erythema without response to heat exposure. There is no treatment for cutis marmorata as it is a benign condition that improves with age. In 50 % of the patients, the erythema disappears in the first 2 years of age [14–16].

Blue Rubber Bleb Nevus Syndrome

Blue rubber bleb nevus syndrome is a venous malformation with mainly limited vascular lesions affecting the skin, the mucosae, and the bowel. Skin lesions may be dark blue keratotic spots, blebs of normal skin color, or large venous or lymphatic masses. Bleeding from intestinal lesions may lead to anemia.

Complications of the syndrome are intussusception, volvulus, and mesenteric venous ischemia. Diagnosis is possible by CT scan; however, the best way to demonstrate the presence of this disease in the bowel is capsule endoscopy.

Cutaneous malformations may be treated successfully by surgical ablation or sclerotherapy. In case of stable disease because of less gut bleeding, iron and vitamin supplementations are sufficient. In case of severe intestinal bleeding, octreotides, rapamycin, and thalidomide are effective. Single-lesion, surgical excision is curative. Otherwise, bleeding control may be obtained by sclerotherapy and/or laser treatment in localizations which are achievable by endoscopic approach [17–20]. Intestinal location is discussed in detail in Chap. 46.

Proteus Syndrome

Proteus syndrome is characterized by cutaneous nevi, venous malformations, and swelling of the soft tissue with asymmetric overgrowth of bones. The overgrowth becomes evident in adolescential time.

The malformation is caused by a genetic mosaic pattern (activating mutation in AKT1 kinase), but there is no genetic transmission [21]. In some patients, some evidence of a PTEN gene anomaly was found.

The differential diagnosis is to the Klippel-Trenaunay syndrome and the hemihyperplasia lipomatosis syndrome. The criteria for the diagnosis of Proteus syndrome are summarized in Table 37.2 [22–24].

Table 37.2 Criteria for the diagnosis of Proteus syndrome

Group A	Connective tissue nevus
Group B	Epidermal nevus
	Disproportionate area of overgrowth (one or more)
	Bilateral anexial cystadenomas or parotid adenoma
	Before the second decade of life
Group C	Lipomata or localized absence of fat
	Vascular malformations
	Lung cysts
	Facial malformations

A diagnosis of Proteus syndrome is made with the presence of one criterion of Group A, two criteria of group B, and three criteria of group C

Gorham-Stout Syndrome

This syndrome, also called "disappearing bone syndrome," was first described by Jackson in 1838 and successively published by Gorham and Stout in 1955 [25, 26]. It is typical of extreme osteolysis associated with lymphatic malformations. The cause of this disease is not known. Any bone may be involved, and in addition, pleural and abdominal effusions of the lymph and chyle are not uncommon. The pathological specimens of the involved bones show a hyperproliferation of lymphatic vessels which communicate with the blood vessels. The therapy is not well validated: some authors obtained good results using interferon and steroids, others injecting ethanol into the bone [27–29]. We had an excellent result with a Gorham-Stout case that has a large cyst on the distal femoral bone and extended smaller cysts along the whole bone. Repeated alcohol injections brought to a closure of the cyst and to a progressive strengthening of the whole bone which, at the beginning of treatment, was very easy to puncture.

Maffucci Syndrome

Maffucci syndrome is a rare, benign disease, which is characterized by the presence of multiple enchondromas (benign cartilage tumor, usually sited inside the bone) with involvement of short tubular bones, like in the hand, and firm blue nodules on the skin, which are venous malformations [30]. The syndrome becomes clinically evident between childhood and adolescence.

Often the disease causes no symptoms and does not require treatment. If however discomfort grows, surgical removal of the malformations may be necessary. Enchondromas may be treated by surgical removal and filling the bone with bone graft or other filling substances. There is a tendency to develop sarcomas, ovarian and pancreatic tumors, and also gliomas [31, 32].

Rendu-Osler Disease

HHT (hereditary hemorrhagic telangiectasia), also known as Rendu-Osler disease, is a genetic defect with abnormal blood vessel proliferation in the skin, mucosa, and sometimes in some organs, like the brain, lungs, and liver [33] (Fig. 37.5).

The disease is caused by derangements in the function of TGF beta, a protein that controls cell proliferation and differentiation.

According to the phenotypes, five types of HHT can be recognized, HHT1, HHT2, HHT3, and HHT4; the fifth type is juvenile polyposis associated with HHT.

HHT1 is caused by a mutation in the coding region of the ENG gene, which is the most common one and with the highest frequency of pulmonary AV malformations or AV fistulas [34, 35].

HHT is characterized by the presence of mucosal telangiectasia and AV shunts in the visceral organs. The most usual manifestations are epistaxis and bowel hemorrhages due to the rupture of superficial micro shunts. Complications are represented by the possible development of AV shunts in the lungs, in the liver, and in the brain.

Diagnostic criteria are summarized in Table 37.3.

The therapy is multimodal according to the complexity of the pathology. Iron and vitamin supplementation are requested. Topical therapy for the control of bleeding is indicated for the treatment of epistaxis and bleeding in the upper gastrointestinal system. Trans-arterial embolization is necessary in case of difficulty to control

Table 37.3 Diagnostic criteria for Rendu-Osler disease

Recurrent epistaxis
Multiple telangiectasias in the lips, oral cavity, fingers, or nose
Visceral lesions; cerebral, hepatic, and spinal AV shunt
A first-degree relative with HHT according to these criteria

The diagnosis of HHT is:
  Clear if three criteria are present
  Possible if two criteria are present
  Unlikely if only one is present

epistaxis. Radiological interventions are also indicated in pulmonary and cerebral AV shunts.

There are some reports of the possibility to use bevacizumab (Avastin) in the control of this pathology [36].

Cobb Syndrome

Cobb syndrome is a rare congenital disease sited in the trunk and characterized by association of metameric cutaneous (nevus but also angiokeratomas or lymphatic malformations), muscular, osseous, and medullary AV shunts or venous malformations [37]. The defects are usually sited on the same level of the affected skin. Progression of the disease may produce weakness, pain, and sensory or motor defects [38–40]. A complication is the so-called Foix-Alajouanine disease, which is an acute spinal defect syndrome due to a thrombosis of the sine malformation with subacute necrotic myelopathy [41]. Association with other malformation of the medulla is possible.

Bonnet-Dechaume-Blanc Syndrome

Also called Wyburn-Mason syndrome, Bonnet-Dechaume-Blanc syndrome is a metameric disease with unilateral arteriovenous malformations involving the face, the retina, and the intracranial vessels [42]. Symptoms are bleeding from the nose and mouth, unilateral blindness, and intracranial bleeding. Teeth extraction may provoke dangerous bleeding. Treatment is mainly catheter embolization. Retina bleeding may be treated sometimes by laser application [43].

Cloves Syndrome

CLOVES syndrome is a recently described rare disease. The term CLOVES stands for congenital, lipomatous, overgrowth, vascular malformations, epidermal nevi, and spinal/skeletal anomalies and/or scoliosis [44, 45].

Typically, fat overgrowth on the back or abdominal wall is visible with nevus on the skin. Vascular malformations, venous, lymphatic, or also arteriovenous, may be present in the involved area. Other features of the syndrome are representes, by hypertrophy of feet and hands, abnormalities in hip and knee joints and abscence of a kidney.

Till now, there are no genetic data about the origin of the disease.

Diagnosis is based on clinical and instrumental study of the involved area.

Treatment should be focused on the cause of the main discomfort.

References

1. Redondo R, Aguado L, Martinez-Cuesta A (2011) Diagnosis and management of extensive vascular malformations of the lower limb: part I – clinical diagnosis. J Am Acad Dermatol 65(5):891–906
2. Etchevers HC, Vincent C, Le Douarin NM, Couly GF (2001) The cephalic neural crest provides pericytes and smooth muscle cells to all blood vessels of the face and forebrain. Development 128:1059–1068
3. Shirley MD, Tang H, Gallione CJ, Baugher JD, Frelin LP, Cohen B, North PE, Marchuk DA, Comi AM, Pevsner J (2013) Sturge–Weber syndrome and port-wine stains caused by somatic mutation in GNAQ. N Engl J Med 21:1971–1979
4. Lo W, Marchuk DA, Ball KL, Juhàsz C, Jordan LC, Ewen JB, Comi A, Brain Vascular Malformation Consortium National Sturge-Weber Syndrome Workgroup (2012) Updates and future horizons on the understanding, diagnosis, and treatment of Sturge-Weber syndrome brain involvement. Dev Med Child Neurol 3:214–223
5. Hennedige AA, Quaba AA, Al-Nakib K (2008) Sturge-Weber syndrome and dermatomal facial port-wine stains: incidence, association with glaucoma, and pulsed tunable dye laser treatment effectiveness. Plast Reconstr Surg 4:1173–1180
6. Klippel M, Trenaunay I (1900) Du noevus variqueux et ostéohypertrophique. Arch Gen Med 3:641–672
7. Malan E (1974) Vascular Malformations (Angiodysplasias). Carlo Erba Foundation, Milan, p 17
8. Glovickky P, Driscoll DJ (2007) Klippel – Trenaunay syndrome: current management. Phlebology 22(6): 291–298
9. Cohen MM (2006) Vascular update: morphogenesis, tumors, malformations, and molecular dimensions. Am J Med Genet A 140(19):2013–2038

10. Greene AK, Kieran M, Burrows PE, Mulliken JB, Kasser J, Fishman SJ (2004) Wilms tumor screening is unnecessary in Klippel-Trenaunay syndrome. Pediatrics 113:e326–e329

11. Baraldini V, Coletti M, Cipolat L, Santuari D, Vercellio G (2002) Early surgical management of Klippel-Trenaunay syndrome in childhood can prevent long-term haemodynamic effects of distal venous hypertension. J Pediatr Surg 2:232–235

12. Weber FP (1908) Haemangiectati hypertrophies of the foot and lower extremity, congenital or acquired, vol 136. Med Press, London, p 261

13. Servelle M, Trinquecoste D (1948) Des angiomes veineux. Arch Mal Coeur 41:436

14. Devillers ACA, de Waard-van der Spek FB, Oranje AP (1999) Cutis marmorata telangiectatica congenita. Clinical features in 35 cases. Arch Dermatol 135:34–38

15. Kienast AK, Hoeger PH (2009) Cutis marmorata telangiectatica congenita: a prospective study of 27 cases and review of the literature with proposal of diagnostic criteria. Clin Exp Dermatol 34:319–323

16. Amitai DB, Fichman S, Merlob P, Morad Y, Lapidoth M, Metzker A (2000) Cutis marmorata telangiectatica congenita: clinical findings in 85 patients. Pediatr Dermatol 17:100–104

17. Femandes C, Silva A, Coelho A, Campos M, Pontes F (1999) Blue rubber bleb naevus: case report and literature review. Eur J Gastroenterol Hepatol 11(4):455–457

18. Nahm WK, Moise S, Eichenfield LF et al (2004) Venous malformations in blue rubber bleb nevus syndrome: variable onset of presentation. J Am Acad Dermatol 50(5 suppl):101–106

19. Wong CH, Chow WC, Tàn YM, Tàn PH, Wong WK (2003) Blue rubber bleb nevus syndrome: a clinical spectrum with correlation between cutaneous and gastrointestinal manifestations. J Gastroenterol Hepatol 18(8):1000–1002

20. Kassarjian A, Fishman SJ, Fox VL, Burrows PE (2003) Imaging characteristics of blue rubber bleb nevus syndrome. Am J Roentgenol 181(4):1041–1048

21. Lindhurst MJ, Sapp JC, Teer JK et al (2011) A mosaic activating mutation in AKT1 associated with the Proteus syndrome. N Engl J Med 7:611–619

22. Biesecker LG, Happle R, Mulliken JB et al (1999) Proteus syndrome: diagnostic criteria, differential diagnosis, and patient evaluation. Am J Med Genet 84(5):389–395

23. Cohen MM Jr, Hayden PW (1979) A newly recognized hamartomatous syndrome. Birth Defects Orig Artic Ser 15(5B):291–296

24. Wiedemann HR, Burgio GR, Aldenhoff P, Kunze J, Kaufmann HJ, Schirg E (1983) The proteus syndrome: partial gigantism of the hands and/or feet, nevi, hemihypertrophy, subcutaneous tumors, macrocephaly or other skull anomalies and possible accelerated growth and visceral affections. Eur J Pediatr 140(1):5–12

25. Gorham LW, Wright AW, Shultz HH, Maxon FC (1954) Disappearing bones: a rare form of massive osteolysis: report of two cases, one with autopsy findings. Am J Med 17:674–682

26. Gorham LW, Stout AP (1955) Massive osteolysis (acute spontaneous absorption of bone, phantom bone, disappearing bone): its relation to hemangiomatosis. J Bone Joint Surg 37-A:985–1004

27. Patel DV (2005) Gorham's disease or massive osteolysis. Clin Med Res 3(2):65–74

28. Kai B, Ryan A, Munk PI, Dunlop P (2006) Gorham disease of bone: three cases and review of radiological features. Clin Radiol 61(12):1058–1064

29. Ceroni D, De Coulon G, Regusci M, Kaelin A (2004) Gorham-Stout disease of costo-vertebral localization: radiographic, scintigraphic, computed tomography, and magnetic resonance imaging findings. Acta Radiol 45(4):464–468

30. Maffucci A (1881) Di un caso di encondroma ed angioma multiplo. Mov Med Chir Nap 3:399–412

31. Collins PS, Han W, Williams LR, Rich N, Lee JF, Villavicencio JL (1992) Maffucci's syndrome (hemangiomatosis osteolitica): a report of four cases. J Vasc Surg 16(3):364–371

32. Flemming DJ, Murphey MD (2000) Enchondroma and chondrosarcoma. Semin Musculoskelet Radiol 4(1):59–71

33. McDonald J, Baynak-Toydemir R, Fyeritz RE (2011) Hereditary hemorrhagic telangiectasia: an overview of diagnosis, management, and pathogenesis. Genet Med 13(7):607–616

34. Kl G, Blobe GC (2008) Role of transforming growth factor-beta superfamily signaling pathways in human disease. Biochim Biophys Acta 1782(4):197–228

35. Richards-Yutz J, Grant K, Chao EC, Walther SE, Ganguly A (2010) Update on molecular diagnosis of hereditary hemorrhagic telangiectasia. Hum Genet 128(1):61–77

36. Flieger D, Hainke S, Fischbach W (2006) Dramatic improvement in hereditary hemorrhagic telangiectasia after treatment with the vascular endothelial growth factor (VEGF) antagonist bevacizumab. Ann Hematol 85:631–632

37. Cobb S (1915) Haemangioma of the spinal cord associated with skin naevi of the same metamere. Ann Surg 62:641–649

38. Dilmé-Carreras E, Iglesias-Sancho M, Márquez-Balbás G, Sola-Ortigosa J, Umbert-Millet P (2010) Cobb syndrome: case report and review of the literature. Dermatology 221(2):110–112

39. Johnson WD, Petrie MM (2009) Variety of spinal vascular pathology seen in adult Cobb syndrome. J Neurosurg Spine 10(5):430–435

40. Krings T, Geibprasert S, Luo CB, Bhattacharya JJ, Alvarez H, Lasjaunias P (2007) Segmental neurovascular syndromes in children. Neuroimaging Clin N Am 17(2):245–258

41. Wirth FP, Post KD, Di Chiro G (1970) Foix-Alajouanine disease. Spontaneous thrombosis of a spinal cord arteriovenous malformation: a case report. Neurology 20:1114–1118

42. Bonnet P, Dechaume J, Blanc E (1938) L'aneurysme cirsoide de la retine, l'aneurysme racemeux, ses relations avec l'aneurisme cirsoide de la face et l'aneurysme cirsoid du cerveau. Bull Soc Ophtal Frac 51:521–524

43. Schmidt D, Pache M, Schumacher M (2008) The congenital unilateral retinocephalic vascular malformation syndrome (bonnet-dechaume-blanc syndrome or wyburn-mason syndrome): review of the literature. Surv Ophtalmol 53(3):227–249

44. Sapp JC, Turner JT, van de Ksamp JM, van Dijk FS, Lowry RB, Biesecker LG (2007) Newly delineated syndrome of congenital lipomatous overgrowth vascular malformations, and epidermal nevi (CLOVE syndrome) in seven patients. Am J Med Genet A 143A:2944–2958

45. Alomari A (2009) Characterization of a distinct syndrome that associate complex truncal overgrowth, vascular and acral anomalies: a descriptive study of 18 cases of CLOVES syndrome. Clin Dysmorphol 18:1–7

Part IV

Treatment of Problems According to Specific Localizations

Introduction

38

Raul Mattassi, Dirk A. Loose, and Massimo Vaghi

In part III of this atlas, a general approach to CVM has been extensively illustrated. However, every clinician who is involved in these pathologies continues to face cases that he never has seen before. Due to the well-known extreme variability, peculiar sites, variable extension, different morphology, and complex combinations, single case problems may require specific, adapted to the case, solutions. As general principles may sometimes be not sufficient to solve specific problems, the following chapters, dedicated to some difficult localization of CVM, will discuss the issues.

The head and neck are one of the most common location of CVM. Anatomical peculiarity and complex structures may create a difficult approach to CVM localizations. As functional but also esthetic problems should be solved, several specialists may be involved in the treatment of difficult cases: plastic surgeons, dermatologists, ophthalmologists, otorhinolaryngologists, maxillofacial surgeons, and radiologists. Surgeons must avoid visible scars and damage to branches of the facial nerves; ophthalmologists must avoid eye damage; and radiologists, the creation of ulcers and fistulas.

The thorax wall is an anatomical structure with a large surface covered by different layers of flat muscles, where surgery may be difficult, particularly in cases of infiltrating forms. Sclerosis and embolization may be good alternative therapies although not necessarily always possible.

The pelvis is also a particular anatomic area with a complex access containing many delicate structures that treatment of CVM should avoid to damage. A surgical approach is often difficult and dangerous. The buttocks are a muscular zone with some main nerves passing the area.

The limbs are cylindrical structures with bones, long muscles, nerves, and vessels in specific positions. Infiltrating malformations may involve one or more tissues contemporaneously, creating approach difficulties.

The hand is a very peculiar organ; fine and high functions are located in small spaces. Therapeutic approaches demand a high degree of skill and knowledge of anatomy and function.

The joints are structures with a specific anatomy and function. Involvement of joints by vascular malformations may create severe damage and demand treatment. Specific orthopedic techniques are used in this area.

Chapters 38–52 should provide some concepts of the specific techniques needed to approach these particular areas.

R. Mattassi (✉)
Center for Vascular Malformations "Stefan Belov",
Department of Vascular Surgery,
Clinical Institute Humanitas "Mater Domini",
Castellanza (Varese), Italy
e-mail: raulmattassi@gmail.com

D.A. Loose
Section Vascular Surgery and Angiology,
Facharztklinik Hamburg, Hamburg, Germany
e-mail: info@prof-loose.de

M. Vaghi
Department of Vascular Surgery, A.O.G. Salvini
Hospital, Garbagnate Milanese, Italy
e-mail: vaghim@yahoo.it

Surgical Management of Head and Neck Vascular Malformations

Graham M. Strub and Jonathan A. Perkins

Introduction

What Is a Vascular Malformation?

When examining a head and neck vascular lesion, it is helpful to remember that there are three types of vascular vessels in humans: arterial, venous, and lymphatic [1]. Each of these vessels transports a unique fluid, which is reflected in their structure. These factors affect the clinical appearance of a vascular lesion composed of one or more of these vessel types.

Arteries carry blood at high pressure and velocity but do not leak. As a result, vascular lesions composed predominantly of arteries are often pulsatile and warm, requiring diagnostic tests that detect rapid blood flow and rapid venous filling. Occasionally, increased blood flow through an arterial vascular lesion can cause high-output cardiac failure.

Veins carry blood passively at low velocity and are leaky. Venous malformations are

non-pulsatile, but they swell with increased blood volume or venous blockage. Diagnostic studies used for venous malformations detect slow blood flow and characteristics unique to abnormal veins (i.e., phleboliths). Venous malformations are frequently associated with pain thought to be secondary to lesion expansion.

Lymphatic vessels transport lymph passively at slow rates, enlarge with inflammation, and are very leaky. Purely lymphatic malformations transilluminate and swell with inflammation, but diagnostic studies show no fluid movement (Fig. 39.1). Determining the predominant vessel type in vascular lesions through imaging is important for accurate diagnosis, treatment planning, and prediction of treatment outcomes [2].

Vascular Malformation and Vascular Tumors

Vascular malformations have been separated from vascular tumors. Other vascular anomalies are seen in Table 39.1 [3]. Vascular tumors are lesions composed of vessels that demonstrate neoplastic growth. In the head and neck, this is most often a hemangioma of infancy [4]. While this discussion is limited to vascular malformations of the head and neck, many of the diagnostic and therapeutic dilemmas present in head and neck vascular tumors are also present in vascular malformations (Fig. 39.2). Vascular

G.M. Strub, MD, PhD
Otolaryngology/Head and Neck Surgery,
University of Washington, Seattle, WA, USA
e-mail: strub@uw.edu

J.A. Perkins, DO (✉)
Department of Otolaryngology/Head and Neck Surgery, University of Washington, Seattle, WA, USA

Children's Hospital and Regional
Medical Center, Seattle, WA, USA
e-mail: jonathan.perkins@seattlechildrens.org

R. Mattassi et al. (eds.), *Hemangiomas and Vascular Malformations: An Atlas of Diagnosis and Treatment*,
DOI 10.1007/978-88-470-5673-2_39, © Springer-Verlag Italia 2009, 2015

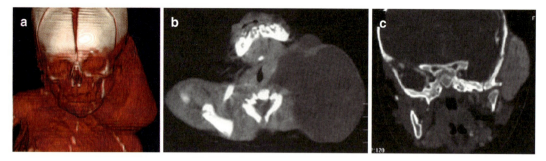

Fig. 39.1 Imaging characteristics of vascular anomalies. (**a**) Three-dimensional computerized tomography image of non-enhancing lymphatic malformation. (**b**) Axial section of same malformation. (**c**) Coronal section of pericranial hemangioma (*arrow*)

Table 39.1 Vascular anomaly classification

Vascular malformation	Vascular tumor
Single vessel type	*Hemangioma*
Capillary	Hemangioma of infancy
Venous	Congenital hemangioma
Lymphatic	Rapidly involuting congenital hemangioma (RICH)
Arteriovenous	Non-involuting congenital hemangioma (NICH)
Combined/complex malformations	*Vascular neoplasm*
Lymphaticovenous	Kaposiform hemangioendothelioma
Capillary-venous	Angiosarcoma
Capillary-lymphaticovenous	Hemangiopericytoma
Capillary-arteriovenous	Miscellaneous
	Tufted angioma
	Pyogenic granuloma

Binary classification system adopted by the International Society for the Study of Vascular Anomalies (ISSVA) in 1996

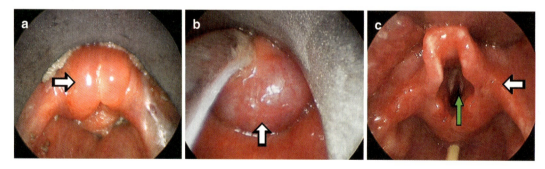

Fig. 39.2 Laryngeal involvement by vascular anomalies. (**a**) Epiglottis (*arrow*) swollen by lymphatic malformation in patient with bilateral upper neck lymphatic malformation. (**b**) Posterior laryngeal involvement by venous malformation (*arrow*). (**c**) Mucosal laryngeal involvement by hemangioma (white arrow), and subglottic narrowing by deep hemangioma (*green arrow*)

malformations are masses of abnormal vessels that can be present at birth or occur at any time during life. These abnormal vessels can have abnormal connections with other types of vessels, as seen in "arteriovenous" malformations (AVMs). In this situation, arteries are connected to veins prior to reaching capillaries. In lymphovenous malformations, there are abnormal connections between venous and lymphatic channels, thought to be a result of arrested separation of veins and lymph vessels. Venous and/or lymphatic malformations are often present at

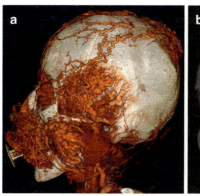
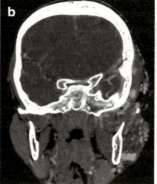
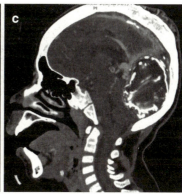

Fig. 39.3 Large low flow venous malformation involving the face and posterior cranial fossa. (**a**) Three-dimensional computerized tomography. (**b**) Coronal computerized tomography section demonstrating masticator muscle and skull base involvement. (**c**) Sagital computerized tomography section demonstrating large posterior cranial fossa venous malformation

birth and can be detected in utero. Following detection, these lesions enlarge with the patient throughout their life. AVMs are usually detected later in life and also slowly enlarge. Local trauma to the lesion or hormonal changes during puberty can be associated with rapid malformation growth. As in any region of the body, head and neck vascular malformations can be difficult to treat due to size and location.

Considerations in Head and Neck Vascular Malformation Treatment

During evaluation and treatment of head and neck vascular malformations (HNVM), the impact of the lesion on fundamental head and neck function must be considered. Of greatest importance is airway preservation [5]. Airway compromise from vascular lesions is most commonly seen in hemangiomas of infancy (Fig. 39.3). However, vascular malformations can distort or compress any aspect of the upper airway, inducing acute airway compromise or chronic sleep disturbed breathing. Evaluation of HNVM should always include a thorough assessment of the upper airway and trachea, as any malformation swelling can induce airway compromise. The management of upper airway involvement of HNVM will be discussed in detail in Chap. 40.

Intracranial vascular malformations are often associated with HNVM [6]. Occasionally, these

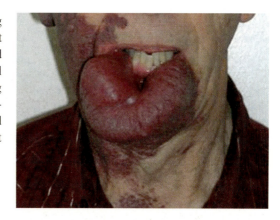

Fig. 39.4 Capillary malformation with progressive hypertrophy of soft tissue

lesions have direct intra-extracranial communication (Fig. 39.4). These communications can compromise cerebral function, and HNVM treatment can induce cerebral injury via these communications. This is especially apparent in orbital malformations, which can impair visual function, with and without treatment. Management of orbital HNVM will be discussed in detail in Chap. 41.

Skull base defects from the malformation or its treatment can cause leakage of cerebrospinal fluid, increasing the possibility of meningitis. The evaluation of HNVM with high-resolution imaging techniques can detect malformations that are high risk for neurologic compromise.

The pharynx and larynx provide us with swallowing and speech capabilities, which can be

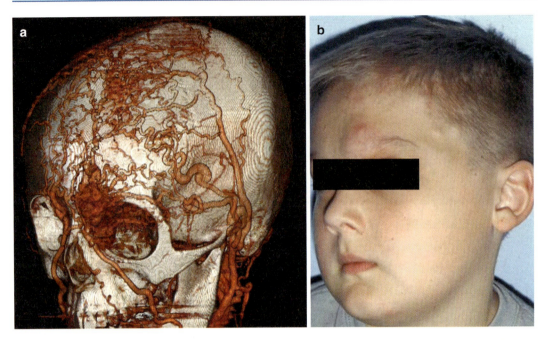

Fig. 39.5 High flow AVM of forehead, eyelid and orbit. (**a**) Three-dimensional computerized angiography of AVM (*arrow*). (**b**) Oblique clinical photo of affected patient

affected by HNVM. Again, this can be due to the HNVM itself or its treatment. Assessment of these functions is essential in the management of HNVM, as changes in lesion size can adversely affect swallowing and speech, necessitating treatment. One of the most problematic areas is the tongue, which can be affected by any malformation.

Our ability to interact with others in society is dependent on many factors; one of these is our physical appearance. In addition to causing functional changes, HNVM and their treatment often severely distort one's appearance (Fig. 39.5). This can have a major impact on an affected individual and their family. In evaluation and management of HNVM, it is essential to monitor and treat the psychological aspects of an individual's condition.

In addition to history and physical examination, HNVM need to be assessed with state-of-the-art imaging techniques, such as computerized angiography and/or magnetic resonance imaging with three-dimensional reformatting [7], to determine the full extent and physiology of the malformation (Fig. 39.6).

Specific HNVM

Lymphatic Malformations

The most common large HNVM are lymphatic [5]. These malformations are clinically apparent at birth approximately 70 % of the time and frequently occur in the posterior neck. The other 30 % occur at any time in life in association with infection or trauma. Lymphatic malformations are low-flow lesions usually not associated with any specific syndromes, with the rare exception of Gorham-Stout syndrome, where there is skull erosion which can lead to cerebrospinal fluid leak [8]. Depending on the lymphatic malformation location, they are variably associated with soft and bony tissue hypertrophy that can adversely impact breathing, swallowing, and speech (Fig. 39.7). While lymphatic malformations are frequently associated with bony abnormalities or other systemic disease, the molecular mechanisms linking these disorders are mostly unknown [9]. Oropharyngeal and/or laryngeal involvement of the malformation can cause airway narrowing

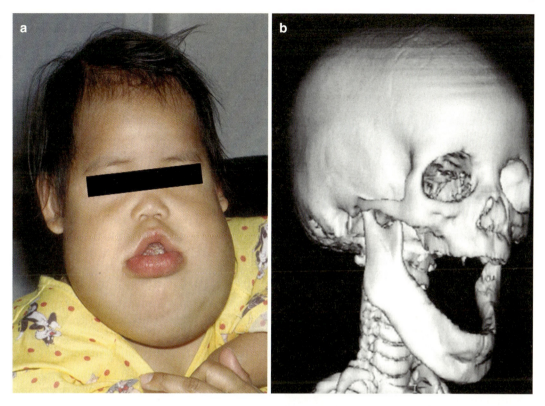

Fig. 39.6 Mandibular hyperplasia in setting of large bilateral upper neck lymphatic malformation. (**a**) Bilateral upper neck/ oral lymphatic malformation. (**b**) Three-dimensional CT of mandibular hyperplasia

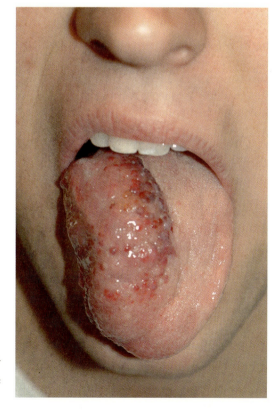

Fig. 39.7 Macroglossia from microcystic lymphatic malformation

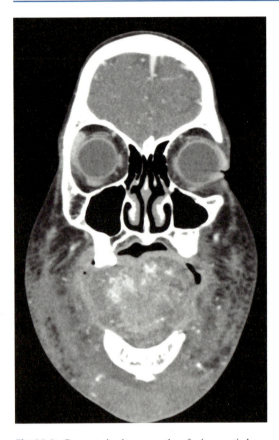

Fig. 39.8 Computerized tomography of microcystic lymphatic malformation

that is persistent or intermittent, as the malformation can swell intermittently with infection. When the malformation is in the orbit or near the skull base, any swelling can cause discomfort and potentially compromise function. Macroglossia is frequently associated with mandibular hypertrophy, both of which impair normal speech and swallowing function (Fig. 39.8).

In addition to clinical exam findings, lymphatic malformations are diagnosed with imaging studies that describe the extent and radiographic characteristics of the lesion. More extensive lesions involving the upper neck and oral cavity are more difficult to treat. Lesions can predominantly consist of large cystic spaces (i.e., macrocystic), small cysts (i.e., microcystic), or a mixture of both [10] (Figs. 39.1 and 39.9). Often, extensive lesions have a significant venous component. Determination of lesion extent and radiographic characteristics is essential in treatment planning and patient counseling.

Treatment of lymphatic malformations is guided by the presence of functional compromise and lesion extent and characteristic. When vision or breathing is affected by the malformation, orbital/ocular and/or oropharyngeal/laryngeal surgery may be necessary. For the common posterior neck lymphatic malformation, the major concerns are appearance and, occasionally, shoulder function. Malformations in this area can be cured with either sclerotherapy or surgery [11, 12]; a review of the efficacy of surgery vs. sclerotherapy did not show one modality as superior to the other [13]. However, if the malformation is in the oral cavity and upper neck, frequently treatment is partially effective, and lesion management, as opposed to cure, is necessary [14]. Upper aerodigestive lesions are particularly difficult to treat and cause significant functional compromise, with bilateral suprahyoid lesions requiring a staged approach [15]. Management consists of partial surgical resection, medical therapy (i.e., antibiotics, steroids) to treat intermittent malformation inflammation, good oral hygiene, and monitoring of immune function [16]. Excision of any lymphatic malformations in the vicinity of the facial nerve should be undertaken using preoperative facial nerve mapping combined with continuous intraoperative EMG and mapping to prevent damage to an aberrantly coursing facial nerve [17, 18].

Venous Malformations

Venous malformations are present in the head and neck at birth and involve any location in this region. Most commonly, they are in muscle tissue, where they temporarily enlarge and become painful with muscle use or trauma [19, 20]. These lesions consist of low-flow, blood-filled vessels. Just like lymphatic malformations, venous malformations can cause functional compromise based on their location. In the head and neck, venous malformations most commonly involve the mucosal surfaces, orbicularis oris, and muscles of mastication (Fig. 39.4); less frequently, they involve skin and neck. On occasion, they involve the facial bones and skull. Airway venous malformations may present with hemoptysis and/

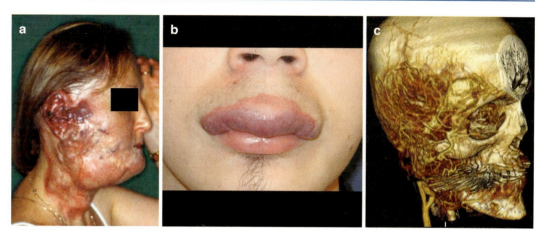

Fig. 39.9 Extensive AVMs. (**a**) AVM of ear and face. (**b**) AVM of upper lip and maxilla. (**c**) Computerized tomography angiography of AVM involving ear an d face

or dysphagia, differentiating them from the presentations of airway hemangiomas of infancy which typically present with stridor and cutaneous lesions [21]. Venous lesions next to skull bone can have direct communication with dural sinuses. When bone is involved, the venous malformation treatment can be complicated by bleeding. Tissue surrounding a venous malformation is frequently enlarged so that dental occlusion and facial symmetry are affected. In lesions that are incurable, long-term management must consider venous malformation persistence and the psychosocial aspects of this problem.

Treatment of venous malformations is done to alleviate functional compromise and improve appearance. Airway narrowing from a swollen venous malformation often requires staged procedures to avoid tracheotomy. Any mucosal surface in the upper aerodigestive tract can be involved, swell, and cause airway compromise. Most of these areas can be treated endoscopically through a combination of sclerotherapy, excision, and interstitial laser treatment. The use of preoperative glue embolization has also been demonstrated to be a safe and effective technique to minimize morbidity and facilitate surgical excision [22]. When the venous malformation is near the upper airway and a general anesthesia is required, careful induction of anesthesia and airway control are necessary, since the malformation will frequently swell with recumbency and the vasodilatory effect of some anesthetic agents.

This can be accomplished with awake and upright intubation. When there is pain associated with the venous malformation, treatment is necessary. Pain frequently occurs in adolescence when vessels within the malformation are occluded with thrombi. If this is a persistent problem, antiplatelet therapy or anticoagulation can be used for treatment. Surgical excision and chemical or laser sclerotherapy of the involved area can also be performed when the symptomatic area is well localized. When surgery is considered, preoperative occlusion of the malformation with glue is very helpful in reducing hemorrhage. Skin that is involved with venous malformations can be treated with excision and transcutaneous and interstitial laser therapy. Often, this does not completely solve the problem. In this situation, long-term management strategies must be employed.

Arteriovenous Malformations

AVMs can involve any region of the head and neck [23]. Most frequently, they involve the auricle (Fig. 39.10). These lesions are thought to arise from a nidus of blood vessels that have abnormal connections between arteries and veins. Due to excessive blood flow through these channels, surrounding blood vessels become dilated. Consequently, AVMs are pulsatile, may have a bruit, and slowly enlarge. During periods of

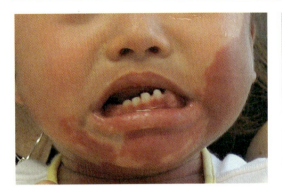

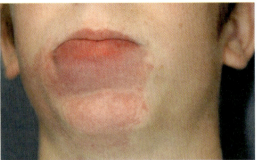

Fig. 39.10 Capillary Malformation with mandibular overgrowth

hormonal change (i.e., puberty, pregnancy) or trauma, these lesions can enlarge rapidly. Due to the expansion of AVMs, soft and bony tissue in the head and neck can become compromised. Intracranial AVMs can cause life-threatening bleeding. Most extracranial AVMs do not communicate with intracranial vasculature, but this is always possible. Large untreated AVMs can induce high-output cardiac failure due to increasing vascular area.

AVM treatment is determined by lesion extent, location, and functional compromise. Conceptually, treatment centers around complete excision of the lesion nidus. In reality, it is difficult to determine when the nidus has been completely removed, and as a consequence, surgical excision and reconstruction may be extensive. Small localized lesions can be treated with surgical excision alone. Larger AVMs are removed with a combination of preoperative embolization and surgery. Embolization is done to reduce intraoperative blood loss. Long-term follow-up is necessary to detect lesion recurrence. For large, unresectable lesions, periodic embolization may be necessary to control bleeding. Intraosseous AVMs can be controlled with endovascular placement of biologically tolerated glue.

Capillary Malformations

Capillary malformations, also known as port-wine stains, frequently involve the dermatomes of cranial nerve five [24]. When these lesions involve the V1 and V2, it is necessary to make sure the vascular malformation does not involve the meninges. When meningeal involvement is present with a capillary malformation, Sturge-Weber syndrome is diagnosed. Capillary malformations progressively thicken for unclear reasons [25] (Fig. 39.5). Soft and bony tissue around these malformations also hypertrophies (Fig. 39.11). It is thought that the skin nodules that develop in these lesions are neural hamartomas, reflecting a deficiency in neural control of capillary diameter. Occasionally, capillary malformations can be on the surface of AVMs, so careful assessment of all malformations is necessary (Fig. 39.12).

Treatment of capillary malformations is directed reduction of skin discoloration with serial pulsed dye laser treatments. For extensively thickened lesions and nodules, surgical excision can be performed.

Summary

HNVM arise from different types of vessels. All can adversely affect function, depending on their size and location. A primary concern is preserving or restoring normal function of breathing, vision, speech, and eating, if possible. After the HNVM impact on function has been determined, an accurate diagnosis of the lesion must be obtained with history, exam, and imaging studies; occasionally, a biopsy is necessary to solidify the diagnosis. Once the diagnosis is established, a variety of intradisciplinary treatment modalities are necessary for HNVM management, as

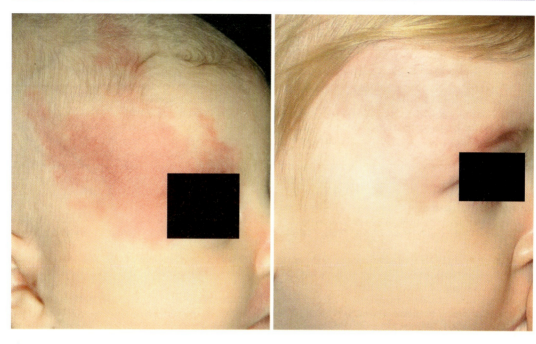

Fig. 39.12 Capillary malformation before and after four pulse dye laser treatment

often HNVM can be recalcitrant to cure. Paramount in any treatment is the need to preserve function and not induce further morbidity (i.e., motor nerve injury, scarring, stenosis, etc.). In general localized HNVM can be treated successfully, whereas more extensive lesions need long-term management.

Long-term management of HNVM needs to be focused on chronic problems that can be present in association with these lesions. These malformations can have intermittent swelling that is painful or induces functional compromise. Medical therapy directed at reduction of swelling and pain is essential. When functional compromise is present, therapeutic intervention may be required. Occasionally, these lesions become infected or reduce normal infection barriers predisposing patients to infection (i.e., meningitis from skull base erosion); judicious use of antibiotics is necessary in these circumstances. Chronic problems induced by HNVM morbidity and possibly by treatment complications can have significant adverse psychosocial impact on patients that must be addressed when caring for affected individuals.

References

1. North PE et al (2006) Vascular tumors of infancy and childhood: beyond capillary hemangioma. Cardiovasc Pathol 15(6):303–317
2. Konez O, Burrows PE (2004) An appropriate diagnostic workup for suspected vascular birthmarks. Cleve Clin J Med 71(6):505–510
3. Enjolras O (1999) Vascular tumors and vascular malformations: are we at the dawn of a better knowledge? Pediatr Dermatol 16(3):238–241
4. Frieden IJ et al (2005) Infantile hemangiomas: current knowledge, future directions. In: Proceedings of a research workshop on infantile hemangiomas, Bethesda, 7–9 April 2005. Pediatr Dermatol 2005; 22(5):383–406
5. Bloom DC, Perkins JA, Manning SC (2004) Management of lymphatic malformations. Curr Opin Otolaryngol Head Neck Surg 12(6):500–504
6. Burrows PE et al (1998) Cerebral vasculopathy and neurologic sequelae in infants with cervicofacial hemangioma: report of eight patients. Radiology 207(3): 601–607
7. Bittles MA et al (2005) Multidetector CT angiography of pediatric vascular malformations and hemangiomas: utility of 3-D reformatting in differential diagnosis. Pediatr Radiol 35(11):1100–1106
8. Cushing SL et al (2010) Gorham-stout syndrome of the petrous apex causing chronic cerebrospinal fluid leak. Otol Neurotol 31(5):789–792

9. Balakrishnan K, Majesky M, Perkins JA (2011) Head and neck lymphatic tumors and bony abnormalities: a clinical and molecular review. Lymphat Res Biol 9(4):205–212

10. Burrows PE, Mason KP (2004) Percutaneous treatment of low flow vascular malformations. J Vasc Interv Radiol 15(5):431–445

11. Claesson G, Kuylenstierna R (2002) OK-432 therapy for lymphatic malformation in 32 patients (28 children). Int J Pediatr Otorhinolaryngol 65(1):1–6

12. Riechelmann H et al (1999) Total, subtotal, and partial surgical removal of cervicofacial lymphangiomas. Arch Otolaryngol Head Neck Surg 125(6):643–648

13. Adams MT, Saltzman B, Perkins JA (2012) Head and neck lymphatic malformation treatment: a systematic review. Otolaryngol Head Neck Surg 147(4): 627–639

14. Raveh E et al (1997) Prognostic factors in the treatment of lymphatic malformations. Arch Otolaryngol Head Neck Surg 123(10):1061–1065

15. Perkins JA et al (2010) Lymphatic malformations: review of current treatment. Otolaryngol Head Neck Surg 142(6):795–803, 803 e1

16. Tempero RM et al (2006) Lymphocytopenia in children with lymphatic malformation. Arch Otolaryngol Head Neck Surg 132(1):93–97

17. Chiara J et al (2009) Facial nerve mapping and monitoring in lymphatic malformation surgery. Int J Pediatr Otorhinolaryngol 73(10):1348–1352

18. Lee GS et al (2008) Facial nerve anatomy, dissection and preservation in lymphatic malformation management. Int J Pediatr Otorhinolaryngol 72(6):759–766

19. Hein KD et al (2002) Venous malformations of skeletal muscle. Plast Reconstr Surg 110(7):1625–1635

20. Lee A et al (2005) Evaluation and management of pain in patients with Klippel-Trenaunay syndrome: a review. Pediatrics 115(3):744–749

21. Parhizkar N et al (2011) How airway venous malformations differ from airway infantile hemangiomas. Arch Otolaryngol Head Neck Surg 137(4):352–357

22. Tieu DD et al (2013) Single-stage excision of localized head and neck venous malformations using preoperative glue embolization. Otolaryngol Head Neck Surg 148(4):678–684

23. Kohout MP et al (1998) Arteriovenous malformations of the head and neck: natural history and management. Plast Reconstr Surg 102(3):643–654

24. Orten SS et al (1996) Port-wine stains. An assessment of 5 years of treatment. Arch Otolaryngol Head Neck Surg 122(11):1174–1179

25. Sanchez-Carpintero I et al (2004) Epithelial and mesenchymal hamartomatous changes in a mature port-wine stain: morphologic evidence for a multiple germ layer field defect. J Am Acad Dermatol 50(4): 608–612

Head and Neck Congenital Vascular Malformations: Sclerosis Treatment

40

Francesco Stillo and Giuseppe Bianchini

Indications

Percutaneous sclerotherapy of head and neck congenital vascular malformations (CVMs) was developed as a minimally invasive treatment and has become a widely accepted technique, alone or in combination with surgery, for all the types of vascular malformations, either low flow (VMs and LMs) or high flow (AVMs) [1].

The sclerosing treatment is preferable to surgery in many cases of infiltrating extratruncular CVMs of the head and neck: when the excision may result in severe tissue defects, leading to cosmetic and functional complications; when the lesions are poorly demarcated; when the walls of dysplastic vessels are thin and friable; and when there is a diffuse involvement of important anatomic structures making the surgical approach extremely difficult or dangerous.

Furthermore, sclerotherapy of cervical and craniofacial CVMs has proved helpful as a preoperative adjunctive treatment, leading to easy resection and increasing the success of surgery. In fact the scleroembolization causes swelling and hardening of the lesions, so delineating the surgical extent of resection and reducing the blood loss.

The indication to perform sclerosis in head and neck CVMs often depends on the presence of cosmetically severe deformity that cannot be camouflaged by clothing and significantly compromise the patient's social life. It is advisable to treat by scleroembolization the CVMs located at trauma-prone region of the face, such as the nose, chin, or cheekbones. Furthermore, the sclerosing treatment is recommendable when cranial CVMs induce severe symptoms and signs: pain, discomfort, heavy sensation, and swelling. Sclerotherapy is also indicated when the CVMs produce a breakdown of skin or mucosa with resultant hemorrhage, skin ulceration, and possible infection of surrounding tissues. Finally, sclerotherapy is mandatory in CVMs located in proximity to vital or sensorial organs, potentially life-threatening or compromising vital functions: breathing, seeing, eating, or hearing [2].

Methods

Sclerotherapy of cervical and facial CVMs is usually performed under general anesthesia, especially when ethanol is used as the sclerosing agent because of the pain it causes during injection.

The more common approach adopted is the percutaneous or peroral direct puncture of the

F. Stillo
Department of Surgery, Casa di Cura Guarnieri,
Center of Vascular Anomalies, Rome, Italy
e-mail: f.stillo47@gmail.it

G. Bianchini (✉)
Division of Vascular Surgery,
Istituto Dermopatico dell'Immacolata,
Center of Vascular Anomalies, Rome, Italy
e-mail: giuseppe_bianchini@yahoo.it

R. Mattassi et al. (eds.), *Hemangiomas and Vascular Malformations: An Atlas of Diagnosis and Treatment*,
DOI 10.1007/978-88-470-5673-2_40, © Springer-Verlag Italia 2009, 2015

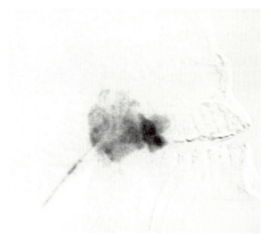

Fig. 40.1 Percutaneous sclerotherapy in a facial congenital vascular malformation

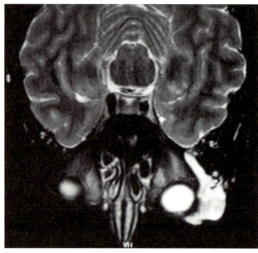

Fig. 40.2 Juxta-ocular venous malformation

lesion [3, 4]. According to this technique, a small-bore needle is inserted percutaneously into the lesion (Fig. 40.1), and its position is confirmed with aspiration of blood in VMs and AVMs or lymph in LMs. In most CVMs of the head and neck, the needle can be placed easily into a vascular channel just by palpation of the lesion. Preoperative magnetic resonance imaging is helpful in planning the best approach to puncture the lesion. Sometimes, when the CVM is too small and deep, it may be technically difficult to reach the nidus of the lesion. In these cases ultrasound guidance can be used to achieve needle placement.

It is very useful to perform a preoperative angiography before injecting the sclerosing agent. Contrast material is injected and imaging performed to confirm that the needle is within the lesion, to well evaluate the size of the malformation and to ensure that there is no extravasation into normal tissues. The contrast material in the abnormal vascular pool is then aspirated through the needle, to limit the dilution of the sclerosant. The volume of contrast material required to fill the space is then used to estimate the quantity of sclerosant needed.

Scleroembolization is preferably assisted by fluoroscopic guidance, injecting the sclerosing agent mixed with a contrast medium to control its spread within the vessels. Furthermore, it is advisable to perform the puncture of the lesion from multiple accesses and inject small doses of sclerosing agent at each point, in order to reduce the risk of local complications. The sclerosing agent should be slowly injected until the abnormal vascular structure is filled.

Simultaneous external compression, manual or mechanic, may also be required to occlude outflow vessels. Compression is recommendable especially in juxta-ocular lesions (Fig. 40.2), to avoid the risk of propagation of the sclerosant in the retinal vessels.

In the CVMs located in close proximity of the upper airway, it is highly recommended to perform a preoperative tracheostomy, to prevent the risk of asphyxiation from edema post-sclerosis and airway occlusion (Fig. 40.3).

Various sclerosing agents have been used in the treatment of CVMs of the neck and face, including sodium tetradecyl sulfate, polidocanol, morrhuate sodium, ethanolamine oleate, and ethibloc.

The foam of sodium tetradecyl sulfate or polidocanol has been proposed for VMs extended through or very close to the skin or mucous membranes, in order to reduce the risk of necrosis and ulceration.

In the LMs of the head and neck, both in microcystic and macrocystic forms, OK-432, bleomycin, doxycycline, and pingyangmycin are the more widely used sclerosants.

In craniofacial AVMs N-butyl-cyanoacrylate and ethylene-vinyl-alcohol copolymer have been

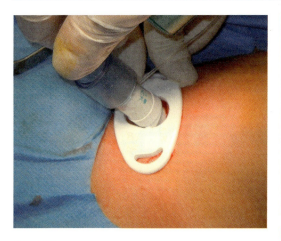

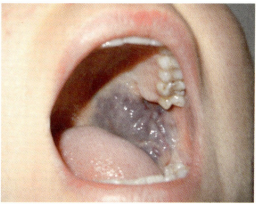

Fig. 40.4 Venous malformation of the oral mucosa

Fig. 40.3 Preoperative tracheostomy in a congenital vascular malformation involving the upper airways

proposed for preoperative scleroembolization, to achieve a more easily surgical excision.

Absolute ethanol is certainly the most effective and the most commonly used sclero-agent for all the types of cervicofacial CVMs, both low flow and high flow [5, 6]. In fact ethanol is the only sclerosant which is able to induce denaturation of tissue protein and to avoid regeneration of endothelial cells with subsequent permanent obliteration of the vessel lumen. The worst aspect of ethanol is its extremely dangerous toxicity, which induces a significant morbidity rate that is particularly high in CVMs located in the facial region. In most situations ethanol is injected in its dehydrated form (>98 % pure). The total amount used depends on the location and extent of the CVM lesion. Anyway it must not exceed the maximum allowable amount (1 mL/kg of body weight), to minimize its toxicity.

A multistaged treatment strategy is mandatory to obtain the best results minimizing the risks: it is possible to repeat the sclerosant treatment to the recurrent and incompletely controlled lesion as necessary.

Complications

Many adverse events are described after sclerotherapy of head and neck CVMs [7].

Usual collateral effects are pain, swelling, and hyperemia at the injection sites. These signs and

symptoms are very discomforting and troublesome in the area of the face, resulting in significant cosmetic disorders. Anyway they are transient, usually peaking at 48–72 h, and well controlled with oral steroids and nonnarcotic analgesics administered for a few days.

The skin or mucosal damage is a frequent adverse event of the sclerosing treatment of the head and neck CVMs. The lesions located in close proximity to the facial skin or oral mucosa (Fig. 40.4) carry a significant risk of ulceration. The risk of necrosis is particularly high for the lesions of the tongue, lip, and gum. Most of the acute lesions are simple erythema or vesicles confined to the skin or mucosa. Sometimes there is an involvement of the subcutaneous tissue with development of necrosis and ulcers. Most of these lesions heal spontaneously with or without minimal wound disposition or debridement.

Another adverse event is the thrombosis of the cervical deep veins such as internal jugular or brachiocephalic vein, sometimes complicated with acute pulmonary embolism. The risk of thromboembolic events is higher in CVMs with large outflow vessels directly connected with an internal jugular or brachiocephalic vein (Fig. 40.5). Furthermore arrhythmias, pulmonary hypertension and cardiovascular collapse are more frequently observed in these cases. For these reasons it is recommendable to perform in all patients a complete coagulation profile before treatment. Thromboembolic events require a treatment with low-molecular-weight heparin, subsequently replaced with warfarin

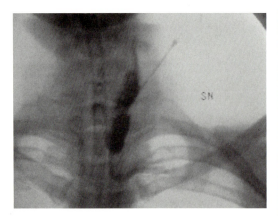

Fig. 40.5 Cervical venous malformation draining into the internal jugular vein

sodium, maintained for an average period of 6 months.

Peripheral nerve damage, either transient or permanent, is also described in cervical and cranial CVMs. The most frequent injuries involve the facial nerve, producing a paralysis of the mimic muscles of the face [8]. The risk is higher when the malformation is located in the parotid or masseter region, especially if it diffusely infiltrates the soft tissues and extends into the deep layers. In many patients it is observed a suffering of trigeminal nerve branches with hypoanesthesia of more or less extensive areas of the face. Rarely there may be a damage of the oculomotor, trochlear, or abducens nerves, which induces disorders of eye movements. There are some reports of recurrent laryngeal nerve injury with paralysis of the vocal cords. It has been also described the optic nerve damage with visual acuity deficits of varying severity, up to complete blindness. This risk is higher in CVMs located to eyelid, frontal, temporal, and nasal region, especially when there is an intraorbital outflow.

Finally, it is necessary to warn about the risk of airway occlusion in the cervical or maxillofacial CVMs located in close proximity to the soft palate, pharynx, and larynx (Fig. 40.6), caused by the compressive effects of edema post-sclerosis.

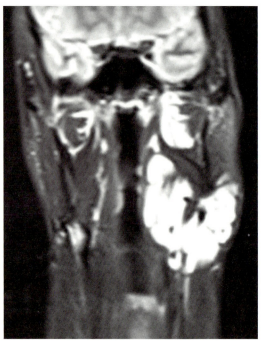

Fig. 40.6 Congenital vascular malformation located in close proximity to the pharynx and larynx

For all these reasons it is essential to perform an adequate preoperative assessment of the entire extent, the anatomical relationships, and the venous drainage of the malformation. A full investigation of all these aspects can be obtained by carrying out duplex scan, contrast-enhanced magnetic resonance, and direct-puncture venography. Scleroembolization must be used with great caution in head and neck CVMs when the preoperative investigations show conditions producing high risk of complications.

Results

The multistaged sclerotherapy of head and neck CVMs allows to obtain good outcomes in the most of cases, especially when ethanol is used as sclerosant. Shrinkage of CVMs of the cervicofacial region (Fig. 40.7) usually begins 1–2 weeks after the procedure. After 1 month, if the desired

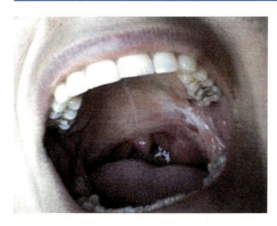

Fig. 40.7 Shrinkage post-sclerotherapy of oral venous malformation

degree of involution has not occurred, the procedure can be repeated.

Craniofacial CVMs are subject to a constant risk of recurrence because they are more often extratruncular forms with a high potential evolutionary power. Late recurrence is possible by two different ways: new expansion of the treated lesions or expansion of previously existing untreated lesions. Absolute ethanol has been accepted as the sclero-agent with the lower risk of recurrence.

The postoperative follow-up is based on the assessment of clinical findings, especially considering the quality of life. It is necessary to observe the subjective improvement of symptoms (pain, discomfort) and simultaneously the objective evidence of improved clinical signs (reduction of the size of lesion). A duplex scan assessment is recommendable in the immediate postoperative phase and subsequently after 1 week and 1 month. The long-term follow-up requires duplex sonography alternating every 6 months with magnetic resonance [9].

The postoperative evaluations should be made by a multidisciplinary clinic team, to confirm or modify the initial treatment strategy until the planned therapy is completed.

References

1. Buckmiller LM, Richter GT, Suen JY (2010) Diagnosis and management of hemangiomas and vascular malformations of the head and neck. Oral Dis 16:405–418
2. Zheng JW, Mai HM, Zhang L, Wang YA, Fan XD, Su LX, Qin ZP, Yang YW, Jiang YH, Zhao YF, Suen JY (2013) Guidelines for the treatment of head and neck venous malformations. Int J Clin Exp Med 6(5):377–389
3. Eivazi B, Werner JA (2013) Management of vascular malformations and hemangiomas of the head and neck: an update. Curr Opin Otolaryngol Head Neck Surg 21(2):157–163
4. Leung M, Leung L, Fung D, Poon WL, Liu C, Chung K, Tang P, Tse S, Fan TW, Chao N, Liu K (2014) Management of the low-flow head and neck vascular malformations in children: the Sclerotherapy Protocol. Eur J Pediatr Surg 24(1):97–101
5. Pekkola J, Lappalainen K, Vuola P, Klockars T, Salminen P, Pitkäranta A (2013) Head and neck arteriovenous malformations: results of ethanol sclerotherapy. AJNR Am J Neuroradiol 34(1):198–204
6. Su L, Fan X, Zheng L, Zheng J (2010) Absolute ethanol sclerotherapy for venous malformations in the face and neck. J Oral Maxillofac Surg 68(7):1622–1627
7. Odeyinde SO, Kangesu L, Badran M (2013) Sclerotherapy for vascular malformations: complications and a review of techniques to avoid them. J Plast Reconstr Aesthet Surg 66(2):215–223
8. Hu X, Chen D, Jiang C, Jin Y, Chen H, Ma G, Lin X (2011) Retrospective analysis of facial paralysis caused by ethanol sclerotherapy for facial venous malformation. Head Neck 33(11):1616–1621
9. Spence J, Krings T, terBrugge KG, da Costa LB, Agid R (2010) Percutaneous sclerotherapy for facial venous malformations: subjective clinical and objective MR imaging follow-up results. AJNR Am J Neuroradiol 31(5):955–960

Upper Airway Congenital Vascular Lesions

41

Teresa O and Milton Waner

Scope

The anatomical boundary of the upper airway extends superiorly from the oral cavity (lips) to the trachea (carina). However, we will confine our discussion from the oropharynx to the upper trachea. Vascular lesions in this area may cause dysphagia and, more concerning, upper airway obstruction.

The upper airway may be affected by:

Vascular tumors:

Infantile hemangioma (IH)

Vascular malformations:

Lymphatic malformation (LM)

Venous malformation (VM)

Capillary malformation (CM, port-wine stain)

In general, due to the risk of airway obstruction, regardless of the type of vascular anomaly, a staged approach is followed.

Airway Infantile Hemangioma (IH)

In the past, airway hemangiomas were referred to as "subglottic hemangiomas." This was inappropriate since not all hemangiomas were subglottic. Instead, the term "airway hemangioma" should be used to describe these lesions since they may occur anywhere in the upper airway [1].

The airway may be affected by focal or segmental hemangiomas. Focal lesions are almost always found in the subglottis, whereas segmental hemangiomas occur at all levels of the upper airway in a geographic or confluent pattern. This distinction is important since it will affect the treatment offered (Figs. 41.1 and 41.2).

Presentation

The clinical presentation is determined by the type of lesion. Focal lesions are solitary and not usually associated with cutaneous hemangiomas. Patients may present with stridor in the first 3 months of life, and diagnosis is made during laryngoscopy.

Segmental airway lesions will always have a cutaneous manifestation; depending on the study, 29–63 % of mandibular/beard or V3 segmental hemangiomas have laryngeal involvement [1, 2], while all patients with airway staining will have cutaneous involvement. Thus, it is essential that these patients be evaluated by an otorhinolaryngologist when the diagnosis of facial segmental IH is made.

Teresa O, MD, M. Arch (✉)
M. Waner, MB, BCh (Wits), FCS (SA), MD
Department of Otolaryngology, Center for Vascular Birthmarks, Vascular Birthmark Institute,
New York Head and Neck Institute,
Lenox Hill Hospital and Manhattan Eye, Ear, and Throat Hospital, New York, NY, USA
e-mail: to@vbiny.org; Mwmd01@gmail.com

R. Mattassi et al. (eds.), *Hemangiomas and Vascular Malformations: An Atlas of Diagnosis and Treatment,*
DOI 10.1007/978-88-470-5673-2_41, © Springer-Verlag Italia 2009, 2015

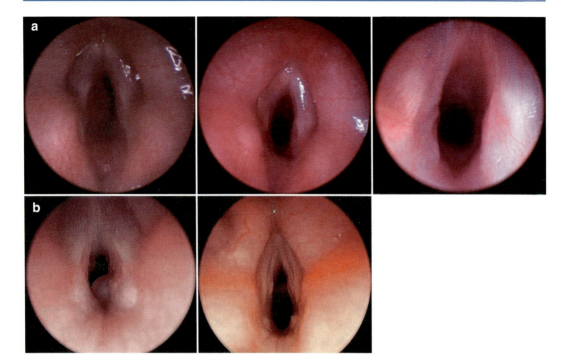

Fig. 41.1 (**a**) Focal airway infantile hemangioma of the left subglottis. (i) Initial presentation (ii) and (iii) after two CO_2 laser procedures. (**b**) Focal airway infantile hemangioma of right subglottis. (i) Initial presentation. (ii) After 6 months of oral propranolol therapy (Photos courtesy of Nancy Bauman, MD, Children's National Medical Center)

Management

The first-line treatment of airway infantile hemangioma is medical. Oral propranolol is used for both focal and segmental lesions and can often prevent tracheotomy [3–6].

Corticosteroids may be used as adjuvant therapy in cases of added airway edema, especially during surgical procedures.

Concerning focal lesions, intralesional corticosteroid injection (triamcinolone 40 mg/mL (latent effect) and betamethasone 6 mg/mL (fast acting), 1:1) is still popular among some otolaryngologists and may be performed at the time of laryngoscopy [7].

CO_2 laser may also be used to ablate and debulk IH. Complications such as subglottic stenosis from overaggressive laser treatment have been reported. As always, judicious use of the laser is still very helpful. Although the pulsed dye laser has a large role in the treatment of cutaneous IH, it does not have a role in the treatment of mucosal IH.

Surgical excision is possible for focal subglottic lesions. A direct translaryngeal approach was popular prior to the current propranolol era [3, 8, 9]. This method is still used by some and has its benefits as well as associated morbidity. In rare cases, tracheotomy is used as a temporary measure to bypass any subglottic obstruction.

Segmental IH are usually treated with propranolol. Because of the longer proliferative phase in segmental disease (2–3 years versus 1 year), longer treatment should be anticipated. In cases of poor response and significant obstruction, CO_2 laser ablation may be useful. In general, these lesions are followed with serial laryngoscopy. The staining may involve all levels of the endolarynx: supraglottis, glottis, and subglottis.

Airway Lymphatic Malformations

A large percentage (up to 73 %) of patients with head and neck LMs will have upper airway involvement. Areas most commonly

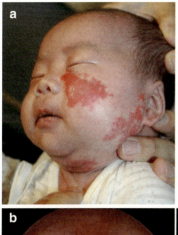

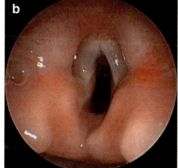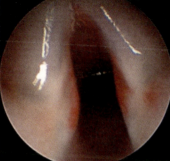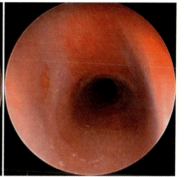

Fig. 41.2 (**a**) Child with a unilateral maxillary (V2) and mandibular (V3) segmental infantile hemangioma. (**b**) Direct laryngoscopy/bronchoscopy of the same child from Fig. 41.2a. (i) Note supraglottic staining of midline and right false vocal fold. (ii) Medial edges of bilateral true vocal folds are involved. (iii) Anterior tracheal wall staining toward carina

involved are the oral cavity (tongue), oropharynx (base of tongue), and supraglottis. Notably, the disease may extend to the supraglottis and not involve structures inferiorly such as the glottis, subglottis, and trachea [10]. Approximately, 30 % of patients will require tracheotomy for massive cervicofacial disease with associated airway involvement. Airway disease is often microcystic (less than 1–2 cm in diameter).

Presentation

The most common clinical presentation shows lymphatic malformation vesicles on the tongue surface which may be mucosal colored or hemorrhagic (Fig. 41.3). There is often accompanied swelling, pain, and malodor. The base of the tongue is often enlarged, and the epiglottis is omega shaped with or without LM involvement.

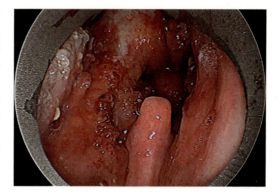

Fig. 41.3 Lymphatic malformation, mucosal and hemorrhagic vesicles involving bilateral tonsils, soft palate, and tongue

Glossoptosis may be caused by either macroglossia or floor of the mouth disease.

Severe cervicofacial LMs may be diagnosed in utero during routine prenatal screening. In cases of predictable airway obstruction, an EXIT

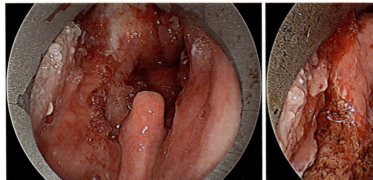
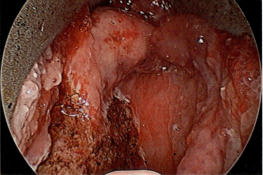

Fig. 41.4 Pre- and intraoperative CO_2 laser ablation of LM vesicles on mucosal surface or oropharynx

(ex utero intrapartum tracheotomy) procedure may be planned [11–14].

Management

Patients who present with extensive facial LM or with oral cavity LM should undergo an airway survey. MR imaging will delineate the extent of disease. Bilateral disease increases the risk of airway obstruction.

The treatment of LM as with all vascular anomalies is multidisciplinary.

Medical treatment is not curative and is used to control symptoms during acute exacerbations and remissions of lymphangitic episodes. High-dose corticosteroids and antibiotics are used with good effect.

Surgical intervention is staged and may incorporate various modalities of treatment.

CO_2 laser ablation is used to treat superficial mucosal disease (Figs. 41.4 and 41.5) [15, 16]. One must be cognizant of the risk of stenosis. Generally, one side at a time is treated.

Macroglossia is treated with surgical debulking of the tongue. A midline wedge excision decreases the width (Fig. 41.6). This may be followed by a second stage to address the vertical height of the tongue. Floor of the mouth disease may be treated with excision, with or without sclerotherapy.

Patients may require tracheotomy for impending obstruction or as a temporary measure during sclerotherapy of the airway.

Sclerotherapy is used to treat micro- or macrocystic LM. Traditionally, microcystic disease is not as responsive as macrocystic disease to sclerotherapy. However, recent advances in sclerosants (bleomycin) and techniques with a combined direct laryngoscopy with transmucosal bleomycin injection have offered excellent results and at times obviated the need for tracheotomy (Figs. 41.7 and 41.8).

Oral corticosteroids are given after all procedures or interventions. Surgical excisions are followed 4 weeks later with a local intralesional corticosteroid injection to address an inevitable and exuberant fibrotic reaction.

Airway Venous Malformations (VMs)

Presentation

Clinically, upper aerodigestive tract VMs present as a bluish, soft, and compressible mass in the lip, oral mucosa, tongue, palate, pharynx, and/or larynx. Patients often present later in life with dysphagia or dysphonia. Lesions expand in the dependent position and may reveal a history of obstructive sleep apnea.

Airway VMs may be either focal (isolated lip or tongue) or multifocal (Fig. 41.9). Laryngeal disease is usually part of a multifocal presentation and may affect all levels of the endolarynx (supraglottis, glottis, and subglottis). Up to 70 % of patients with facial cutaneous VM will also

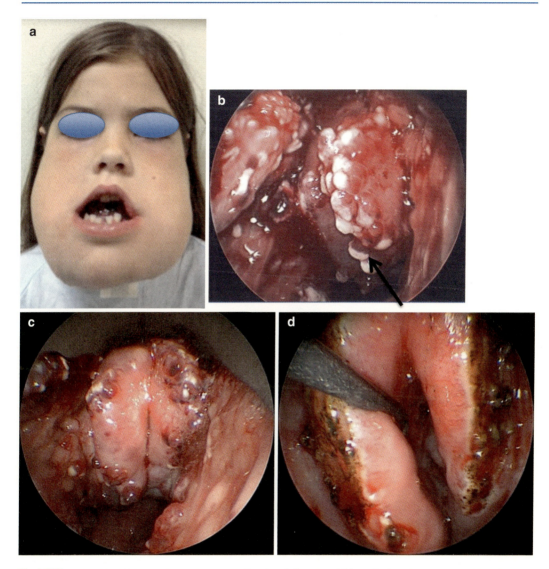

Fig. 41.5 (**a**) Child with bilateral massive cervicofacial LM. Note tracheotomy and anterior open mouth deformity. Patient is unable to vocalize. (**b**) Laryngoscopy at presentation. Epiglottis is omega shaped and collapsed with LM hemorrhagic vesicles and edema. *Black arrow* delineates midline of epiglottic opening. (**c**) 6 weeks after 1st laser treatment. Profile of epiglottis more defined. (**d**) Intraoperative view after CO_2 laser ablation of bilateral lingual surface of epiglottis. Midline is not treated

have airway involvement (poster presentation, ISSVA 2012).

MRI is the most informative imaging technique for documenting the nature and extent of VMs. Lesions are hyperintense on T2-weighted images, and the presence of phleboliths is diagnostic. Doppler ultrasonography also aids in diagnosis of a soft tissue VM. These lesions appear as hypoechoic, heterogeneous, and compressible masses with monophasic low velocity flow. Conventional angiography is usually reserved for pretherapeutic (sclerotherapy) evaluation.

Management

Due to the high incidence (70 %) of associated upper airway involvement with cutaneous facial

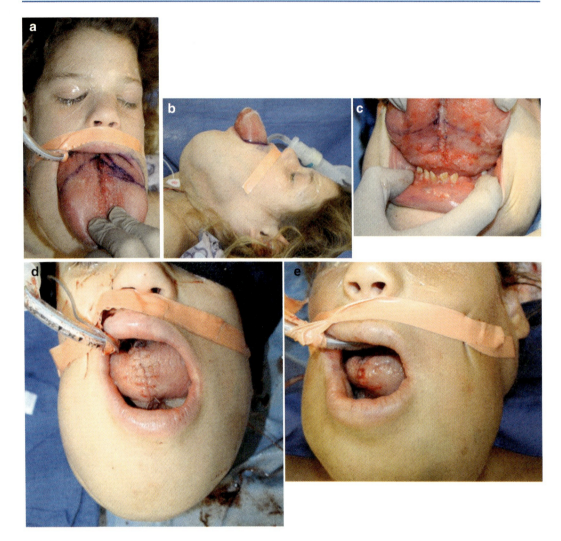

Fig. 41.6 (**a**) Child with macroglossia and glossoptosis secondary to tongue LM. Intraoperative wedge excision is marked. (**b**) Lateral view, note significant glossoptosis. (**c**) Ventral surface marking-distance allows for tongue protrusion. (**d**) Postoperatively, tongue is now inside the mouth. (**e**) Intraoperative second stage excision in horizontal vector addresses vertical dimension

disease, all patients should undergo an airway survey with flexible fiber-optic laryngoscopy in the office setting.

Treatment modalities will depend on several factors: whether the lesion is focal or confluent, the depth of the lesion (superficial, deep, or compound), and degree of impending or actual airway obstruction.

Superficial mucosal disease responds well to laser treatment. The neodymium:yttrium alumi-

num garnet (Nd:YAG) laser is a mainstay in the treatment of mucosal VM. The laser is used in a "snowstorm pattern" to prevent necrosis since the depth of penetration is approximately 1 cm [15].

Small focal lesions may be treated with laser, sclerotherapy, or surgical excision.

Large compound lesions may initially be treated with laser to create an intentional submucosal fibrotic plane to prepare the skin for subsequent surgical excision. Surgery or sclerotherapy

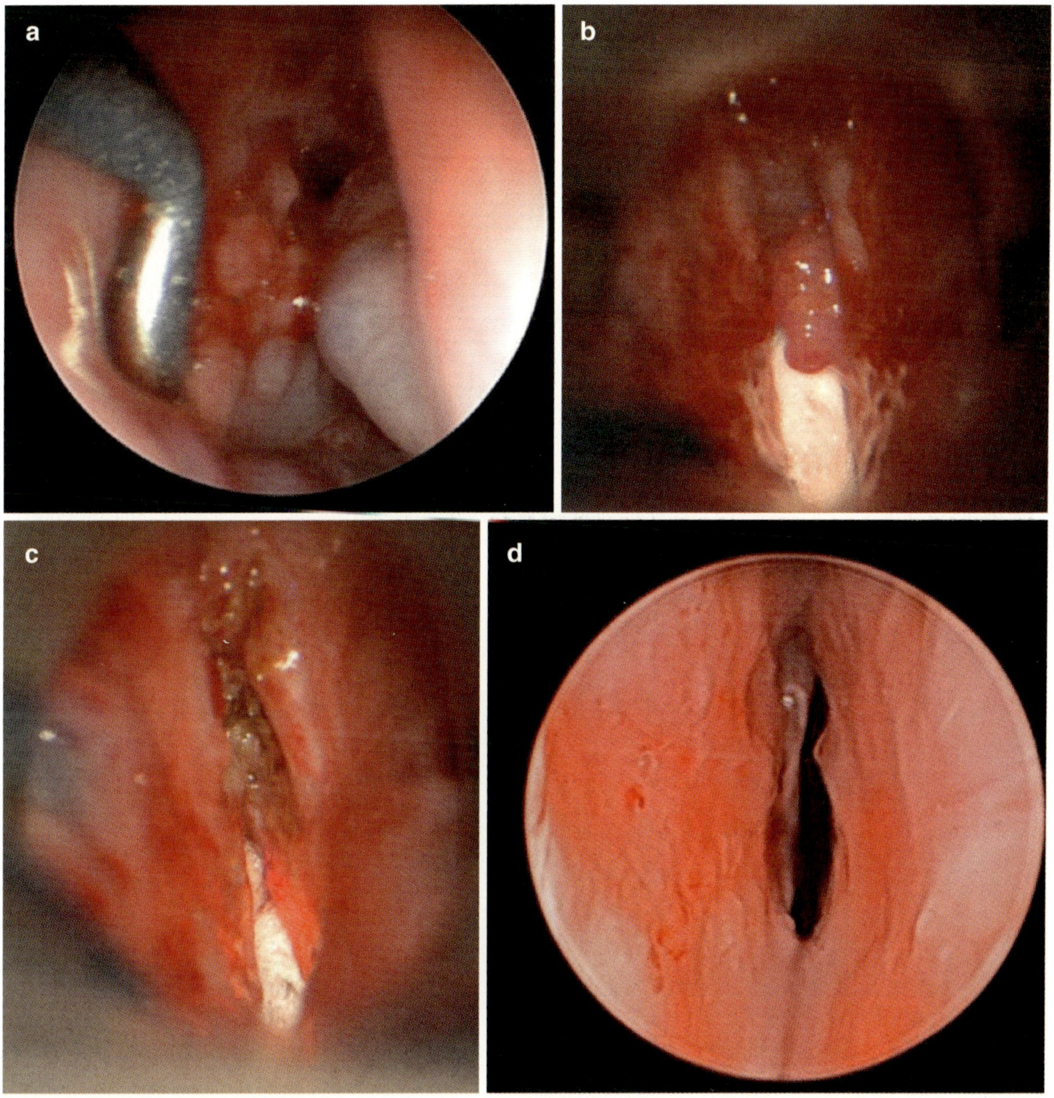

Fig. 41.7 Endolarynx of same patient as Fig. 41.5. (**a**) Left and right false vocal fold disease. (**b**) Patient with decreased bulk after one bleomycin injection to bilateral false vocal folds. (**c**) Intraoperative view after CO_2 laser ablation of left false vocal fold disease. (**d**) 6 weeks postop. Note resolution of supraglottic disease and opening of airway aperture

in a field of extensive mucosal VM will increase the risk of necrosis and poor flap healing. The surgical excision occurs approximately 4 weeks later.

Laryngeal disease is directly accessed via direct rigid laryngoscopy and microscopy. Laser (Nd:YAG laser with a fiber) (Fig. 41.10) or direct puncture transmucosal sclerotherapy may be used (Fig. 41.11). The choice of sclerosant will depend on whether the airway is secured. If the patient does not have a tracheotomy, bleomycin may be optimal since it induces minimal swelling. Another strategy of airway preservation is to only treat one side during each session.

If the disease is extensive and there is an anticipated risk of airway obstruction, a temporary tracheotomy may be placed during the treatment period.

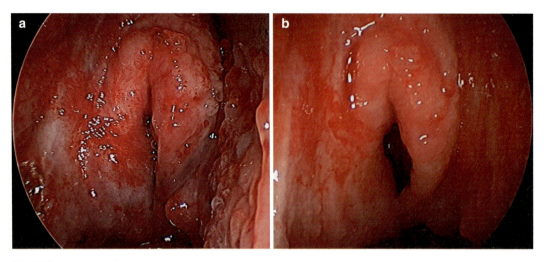

Fig. 41.8 (**a**) Epiglottis after one CO_2 laser treatment. (**b**) Epiglottis after one transmucosal direct puncture sclerotherapy with bleomycin. Patient's voice has now improved, and she is breathing with the tracheotomy capped

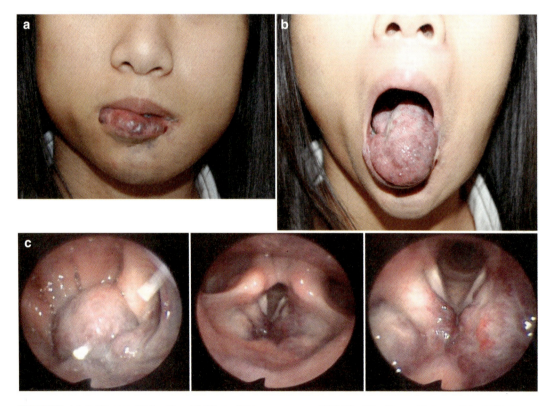

Fig. 41.9 (**a**) A 17-year-old female with bilateral lower lip and chin VM. (**b**) Tongue (L > R) and buccal mucosal involvement. (**c**) Same patient with multifocal airway VM. Patient presented with complaint of lower lip and tongue VM. Flexible fiber-optic nasopharyngolaryngoscopy revealed nasopharyngeal (i), oral cavity, and bilateral false vocal fold (ii, iii) VM as well

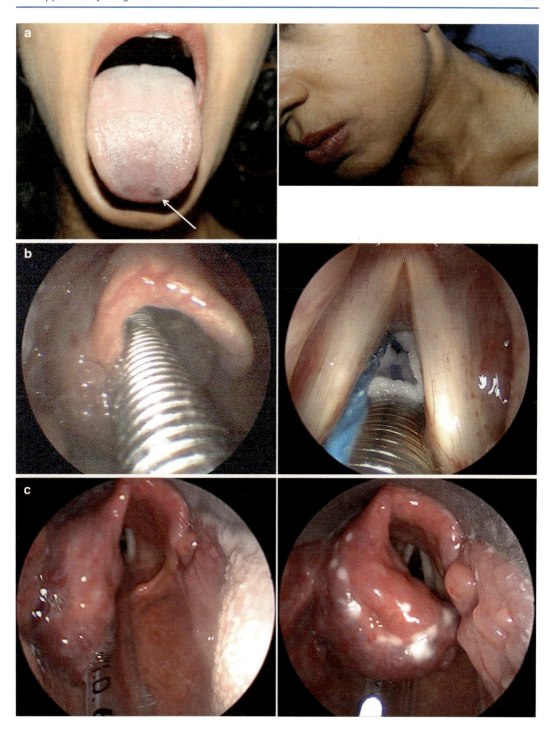

Fig. 41.10 (**a**) Adult female who presented with focal tongue VM (*arrow* points to lesion). Physical exam revealed left neck disease as well as left parotid disease. Flexible laryngoscopy showed further upper airway involvement. (**b**) Laryngoscopy images from same patient. (i) Left vallecula and lingual surface of epiglottis venous malformation. (ii) Right false vocal fold disease. (**c**) (i) 1 month postoperative after one Nd:YAG laser treatment. (ii) Note the tip of Nd:YAG laser fiber at the end of 0° telescope and resultant "snowstorm pattern" to VM

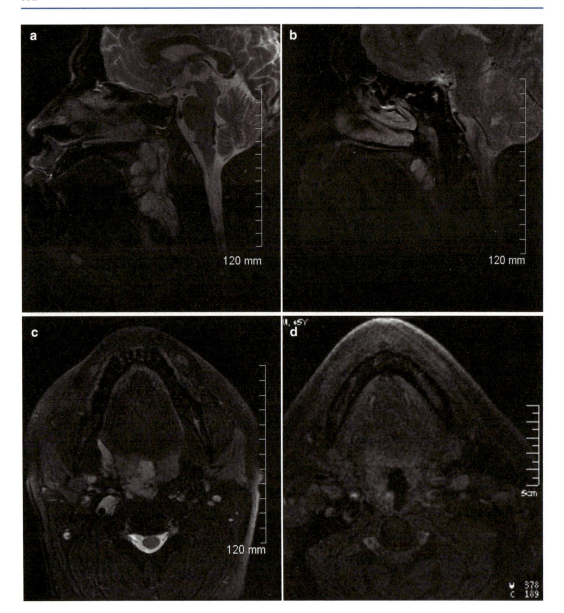

Fig. 41.11 A 35-year-old male with multifocal VM. Airway involvement includes nasopharyngeal, oral cavity, and oropharyngeal VM. (**a**) At initial presentation. Patient required urgent awake tracheotomy and Nd:YAG laser. (**b**) After combined direct laryngoscopy with direct puncture transmucosal sclerotherapy treatments. (**c, d**) Axial MRI images pre- and post-Nd:YAG laser and sclerotherapy treatments

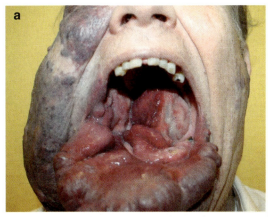
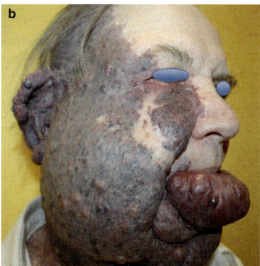

Fig. 41.12 Adult male with extensive capillary malformation/port-wine stain and obstructive sleep symptoms. (**a**) Intraoral view with right hemitongue, floor of the mouth, soft palate, and buccal mucosa soft tissue hypertrophy with overlying erythematous staining. (**b**) Lateral view showing cutaneous disease: right hemiface with massive ear, face, and lower lip hypertrophy

Airway Capillary Malformations/Port-Wine Stains

Presentation

Capillary malformation may involve the oral cavity and oropharynx. Typically, there is buccal mucosa, tongue, floor of the mouth, and palate staining. In long-standing cases, one can see soft tissue hypertrophy in the same distribution. It is not uncommon to have obstructive sleep apnea (Fig. 41.12).

Management

The only treatment for soft tissue hypertrophy is surgical excision—tongue, floor of the mouth, or uvula. Patients should be scoped in the office in the supine position. A Muller maneuver will help to assess pharyngeal collapse. Care must be taken during intubation since patients may obstruct secondary to redundant pharyngeal tissues. Traditional surgical methods for OSA may be employed: tonsillectomy or uvulopalatopharyngoplasty.

Airway Arteriovenous Malformations

No laryngeal arteriovenous malformations per se have been described. This may be explained by the absence of choke zones in the larynx [17, 18]. However, large AVMs adjacent to the airway (tongue, parapharyngeal space) may lead to obstructive symptoms and/or hemorrhage into the airway. Embolization with or without surgery is the preferred method of treatment (Fig. 41.13).

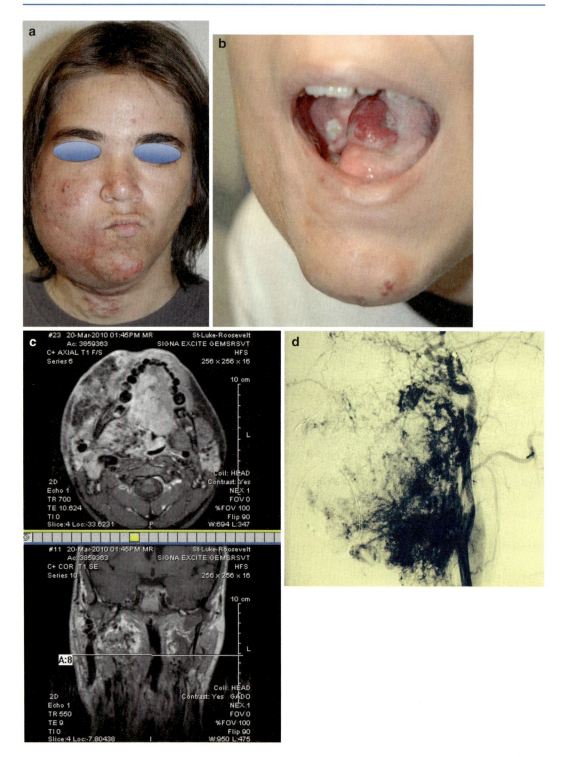

Fig. 41.13 (**a**) A 21-year-old male with history of right facial high-flow arteriovenous malformation. (**b**) Oral cavity/right tongue disease. (**c**) Axial and coronal T1-weighted MRI shows high-flow arteriovenous malformation involving the right face, oral cavity (tongue), and parapharyngeal space. (**d**) Lateral angiogram image shows large area of nidus/blush in tongue and parapharyngeal space. Patient has no obstructive symptoms; however, he has had a history of oral cavity hemorrhage treated with embolization

References

1. O TM, Alexander RE, Lando T et al (2009) Segmental hemangiomas of the upper airway. Laryngoscope 119:2242–2247
2. Orlow SJ, Isakoff MS, Blei F (1997) Increased risk of symptomatic hemangiomas of the airway in association with cutaneous hemangiomas in a "beard" distribution. J Pediatr 131:643–646
3. Van Den Abbeele T, Triglia JM, Lescanne E et al (1999) Surgical removal of subglottic hemangiomas in children. Laryngoscope 109:1281–1286
4. Denoyelle F, Garabedian EN (2010) Propranolol may become first-line treatment in obstructive subglottic infantile hemangiomas. Otolaryngol Head Neck Surg 142:463–464
5. Leaute-Labreze C, Dumas de la Roque E, Hubiche T, Boralevi F, Thambo JB, Taieb A (2008) Propranolol for severe hemangiomas of infancy. N Engl J Med 358:2649–2651
6. Buckmiller L, Dyamenahalli U, Richter GT (2009) Propranolol for airway hemangiomas: case report of novel treatment. Laryngoscope 119:2051–2054
7. Waner M, Suen J (1999) Treatment for the management of hemangiomas. In: Hemangiomas and vascular malformations of the head and neck. Wiley-Liss, New York, pp 234–239
8. Cotton RT, Evans JN (1981) Laryngotracheal reconstruction in children. Five-year follow-up. Ann Otol Rhinol Laryngol 90:516–520
9. Sharp HS (1949) Hemangioma of the trachea in an infant, successful removal. J Laryngol Otol 63:413
10. O TM, Rickert SM, Diallo AM et al (2013) Lymphatic malformations of the airway. Otolaryngol Head Neck Surg 149:156–160
11. Mychaliska GB, Bealer JF, Graf JL, Rosen MA, Adzick NS, Harrison MR (1997) Operating on placental support: the ex utero intrapartum treatment procedure. J Pediatr Surg 32:227–230; discussion 230–221
12. Stefini S, Bazzana T, Smussi C et al (2012) EXIT (Ex utero Intrapartum Treatment) in lymphatic malformations of the head and neck: discussion of three cases and proposal of an EXIT-TTP (Team Time Procedure) list. Int J Pediatr Otorhinolaryngol 76:20–27
13. Otteson TD, Hackam DJ, Mandell DL (2006) The Ex Utero Intrapartum Treatment (EXIT) procedure: new challenges. Arch Otolaryngol Head Neck Surg 132:686–689
14. Schwartz MZ, Silver H, Schulman S (1993) Maintenance of the placental circulation to evaluate and treat an infant with massive head and neck hemangioma. J Pediatr Surg 28:520–522
15. Waner M, Suen J (1999) The treatment of vascular malformations. In: Hemangiomas and vascular malformations of the head and neck. Wiley-Liss, New York
16. Glade RS, Buckmiller LM (2009) CO2 laser resurfacing of intraoral lymphatic malformations: a 10-year experience. Int J Pediatr Otorhinolaryngol 73:1358–1361
17. Houseman ND, Taylor GI, Pan WR (2000) The angiosomes of the head and neck: anatomic study and clinical applications. Plast Reconstr Surg 105:2287–2313
18. Mitchell EL, Taylor GI, Houseman ND, Mitchell PJ, Breidahl A, Ribuffo D (2001) The angiosome concept applied to arteriovenous malformations of the head and neck. Plast Reconstr Surg 107:633–646

Vascular Malformations of the Orbit

42

Aaron Fay, Vicky Massoud, and Milton Waner

Introduction

Orbital vascular malformations, like vascular malformations elsewhere in the body, can be categorized by vessel and flow type: arteriovenous malformation, venous malformation, and lymphatic malformation. Together they comprise approximately 15 % of all orbital lesions [1]. The appearance and behavior differ among these categories, from bright red to deep blue, from well-demarcated to infiltrative into orbital and periorbital tissues. Each has different clinical presentation, imaging characteristics, natural history, genetic etiology, and management strategies [2]. Clinical impact can vary greatly even within a single histologic category, and diagnosis is not always straightforward. Therefore, thorough clinical evaluation and specific ancillary testing are essential in making the diagnosis and eventually guiding the therapeutic alternatives. Current approaches range from serial observation to radical resection with many intermediate alternatives.

Clinical Evaluation

Patients with orbital vascular malformations come to clinical attention for a variety of reasons. Among these, exophthalmos, pain, and diplopia are most common. Patients presenting with these symptoms must undergo a thorough orbital and ophthalmic history and examination. Every patient should have a complete eye exam in order to document the type of the tumor and determine its clinical impact.

Careful history taking is one of the most important tools available to the ophthalmic clinician. Chief complaint typically includes periocular pain or retro-orbital headache, consistent or intermittent visual loss, double vision, or disfigurement. The duration, timing, and character of the complaint should be determined: Is the pain mild or severe? Is it intermittent or does it occur continuously? Is it exacerbated by supine or inverted positioning, physical activity, or extraocular motility? If proptosis exists, is it sudden onset or slowly progressive? Is it associated with pain? Is the proptosis exacerbated by Valsalva, sneezing or cough, physical activity, or inversion? Does the lesion change with ambient temperature or menstruation? On presentation is redness of the eye present? Does the patient hear a bruit or internal pulsations? All these questions

A. Fay (✉)
Department of Ophthalmology,
Harvard Medical School, Boston, MA, USA
e-mail: aaronfay@gmail.com

V. Massoud
Department of Otolaryngology, Massachusetts Eye and Ear Infirmary, Boston, MA, USA

M. Waner, MB, BCh (Wits), FCS (SA), MD
Department of Otolaryngology, Center for Vascular Birthmarks, Vascular Birthmark Institute, New York Head and Neck Institute, Lenox Hill Hospital and Manhattan Eye, Ear, and Throat Hospital,
New York, NY, USA
e-mail: Mwmd01@gmail.com

R. Mattassi et al. (eds.), *Hemangiomas and Vascular Malformations: An Atlas of Diagnosis and Treatment*,   357
DOI 10.1007/978-88-470-5673-2_42, © Springer-Verlag Italia 2009, 2015

aid the clinician in determining the type of lesion and indications for intervention.

Comprehensive orbital evaluation begins with visual acuity, but there are four critical parameters of optic nerve health that should always be measured whenever an orbital process is suspected: visual acuity, pupil function, color vision, and visual field. Pupils are inspected with the swinging flashlight for a relative afferent pupillary defect. Color vision is tested using standardized color plates, and visual field is inspected for scotomas using automated (static) or manual (dynamic) testing devices. Color vision is felt to be the most sensitive indicator of optic nerve compromise, while visual field assessment has greater capacity to indicate the nature of the optic nerve insult. In the absence of formal visual field testing, confrontational visual fields can help detect an optic neuropathy caused by orbital tumor. Pupillary function is an easy test to perform that provides general insight into optic nerve conditions. Other important parameters in cases of suspected orbital disease include extraocular motility, exophthalmometry, diplopia mapping, and intraocular pressure (a proxy measurement of orbital pressure). Clinical photos are strongly recommended to document appearance at presentation and for future comparison.

The eye examination should consist of the best corrected visual acuity and intraocular pressure detected by applanation tonometry (normal pressure raging between 9 and 21 mmHg). Slit lamp examination is used to inspect the conjunctiva for any dilated blood vessels, tortuosity, and chemosis (conjunctival swelling). "Corkscrew" vessels are indicative of carotid-cavernous fistula.

Inspection of the eyelids includes measuring the height of the palpebral fissure (distance between the upper and lower lids), the margin to corneal light reflex distance, and binocular comparison for asymmetry; orbital tumors can produce either eyelid ptosis or eyelid retraction. Exophthalmometry quantifies protrusion of the eyeball. Measurement above 21 mm or more than 2 mm difference between the eyes is considered abnormal. Ocular motility should be evaluated in all gazes: up, down, right, and left. One common scale is the 5-point scale with 4 indicating full motility in that direction and 0 indicating no movement at all. Extraocular motility will be affected depending on the specific location of the lesion within the orbit. Ocular motility disturbance can produce diplopia in various gazes or in primary position (looking straight ahead). Dilated fundus exam is another important component of the examination, allowing direct inspection of the retina and optic nerve. Pupils can be dilated safely using phenylephrine 2.5 % or tropicamide 1 %. The optic nerve head should be examined to evaluate its margins. Hazy borders, swelling, or hyperemia indicate acute or subacute processes; optic nerve pallor or atrophy indicates chronic disease. Choroidal folds or retinal striae indicate the presence of a space-occupying lesion in the orbit or posterior compression of the eyeball.

When a vascular lesion is suspected within the orbit, it is essential to inspect for pulsatile proptosis or the presence of a thrill. This can be done by simple auscultation. Examining the patient in sitting position and then asking her/him to cough or bend can help to highlight venous lesions that are sensitive to changes in venous pressure.

Important ancillary tests include ultrasonography, computed tomography (CT), magnetic resonance imaging (MRI), CT angiogram, MR angiogram, and dynamic CT. Each of the three major orbital vascular malformations has its own clinical characteristics, imaging modalities, and pathognomonic findings.

Arteriovenous Malformation (AVM)

Blood flows directly from the arterial circulation into the venous one without passing through intervening capillaries. Intraorbital AVMs are congenital anomalies with slow growth patterns [3]. They are supplied by branches of both the external and internal carotid artery. AVMs of the orbit can result from trauma or can appear spontaneously.

Diagnosis

Patients with orbital AVMs typically present with pulsatile proptosis. When the lesion is anterior in the orbit, a blue pulsating subcutaneous mass can be seen on physical exam (Fig. 42.1a, b). Other signs include epibulbar congestion and audible bruit.

Nonenhanced CT is helpful in visualizing the small foci of calcification often associated with arteriovenous malformations and foci of hemorrhage if any exist. Contrast-enhanced CT reveals enhancement of the vascular channels, whereas MRI demonstrates these lesions as vascular channels that appear as flow voids (Fig. 42.1c, d). More adequate evaluation is usually obtained by a magnetic resonance angiography or CT angiography, but the gold standard remains traditional angiography [4] (Fig. 42.1e).

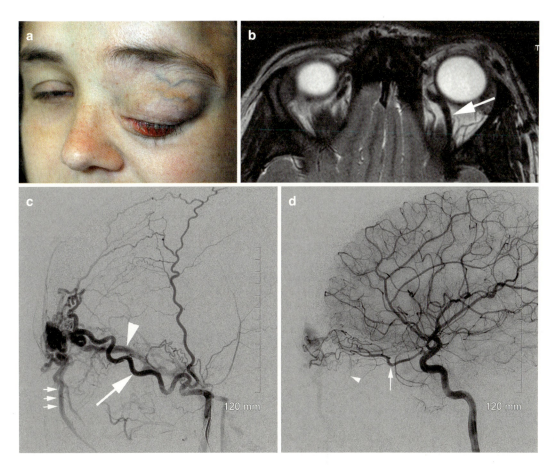

Fig. 42.1 Arteriovenous malformation of the orbit and eyelids. (**a**) Clinical photo demonstrates anterior displacement of the eyeball (proptosis), with upper eyelid ptosis and conjunctival swelling (chemosis). Arterialized veins can be seen in the eyelid. (**b**) Axial views of this T2-weighted MRI in a different patient with orbital AVM demonstrates multiple serpiginous flow voids in the preseptal soft tissues of the left orbit with a dilated left superior ophthalmic vein (*arrow*). (**c**) Left distal EXTERNAL carotid artery angiogram shows two branches of the superficial temporal artery, one of which is supplying blood to the AVM (*arrow*). Venous drainage can be seen posteriorly along the superior ophthalmic vein (*arrow head*) and inferiorly along the facial vein (*small arrows*). (**d**) Left INTERNAL carotid artery angiogram shows AVM with blood supply from supraorbital and ethmoidal branches of the ophthalmic artery (*arrow*). Choroidal blush can be seen identifying the outline of the retina (*arrow head*). (**e**) Left EXTERNAL carotid artery angiogram post-embolization shows complete elimination of the malformation with preservation of all the normal arteries including the maxillary branch (*arrow*) of the external carotid and two major branches of the superficial temporal artery (*arrow heads*). (**f**) Left INTERNAL carotid artery angiogram post-embolization. The supply to the AVM from the ophthalmic artery (*arrow*) has been completely eliminated. Choroidal blush remains (*arrow head*), indicating retained blood supply to the retina

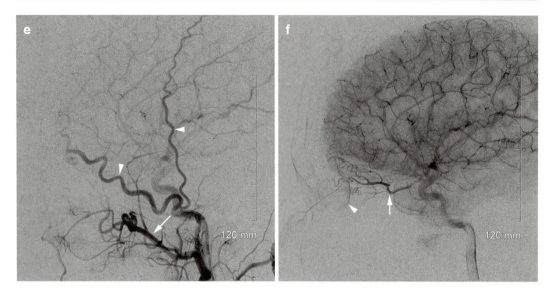

Fig. 42.1 (continued)

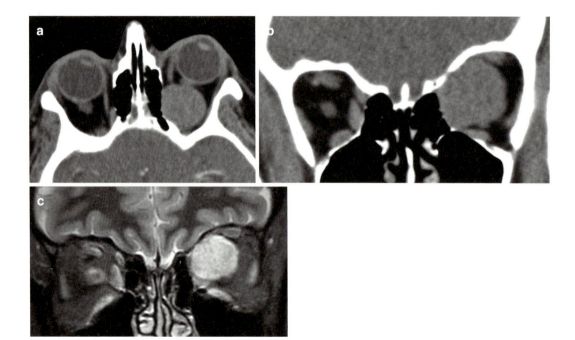

Fig. 42.2 Encapsulated venous malformation of the orbit. (**a**) Axial view of computed tomograph (CT) of the orbit without contrast demonstrates an ovoid, clearly delimited lesion of approximately 2 cm in the intraconal space. (**b**) Coronal view of the same CT shows the lesion abutting the medial wall and roof of the orbit in the super-omedial quadrant of the orbit. (**c**) This coronal view of this T1-weighted, gadolinium-enhanced, fat-suppressed MRI demonstrates numerous septations within the lesion but fails to highlight the relationship of the lesion to the thin bones of the orbit. Additional findings include displacement of the extraocular muscles and optic nerve sheath complex. (**d**) Histopathologic section of the lesion above demonstrates the general architecture of the lesion with numerous thick fibrous septa (hematoxylin and eosin, 20×). (**e**) Higher magnification view demonstrates large vascular spaces filled with erythrocytes, with flattened endothelial cells (hematoxylin and eosin 100×). D2–40 stain for lymphatic endothelial cells was negative (not shown)

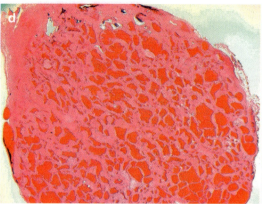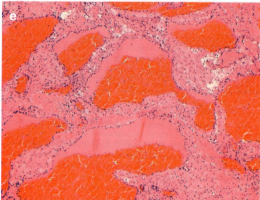

Fig. 42.2 (continued)

Treatment

Angiographic embolization can occlude the nidus and major bleeding vessels in an orbital AVM [4, 5] (Fig. 42.1f). The most serious risk of this treatment is ophthalmic artery or central retinal artery occlusion and is stratified according to specific location of the AVM. The effect of embolization is often temporary, however. Surgical resection, in contrast, can be definitive. Without embolization, surgical resection is possible but difficult due to the risk of massive bleeding. A combination of embolization and surgical excision offers better control and ultimately an optimal outcome. Gamma knife radiotherapy, according to Liscak et al., resulted in obliteration of AVMs in 74 % of cases after the first cycle and 69 % after the second [6].

Carotid-Cavernous Fistula

A carotid-cavernous fistula is an abnormal shunt between the carotid artery and cavernous sinus, or a directly related ophthalmic vein. These fistulae are sometimes categorized as arteriovenous malformations in the ophthalmic literature.

Direct carotid-cavernous sinus fistulae can be caused by trauma or spontaneous rupture of an aneurysm of the intracavernous carotid or an atherosclerotic artery [7]. Indirect carotid-cavernous sinus fistulae are characterized by arterial blood that flows through the meningeal branches of the internal or the external carotid arteries indirectly into the cavernous sinus [7].

Diagnosis

Carotid-cavernous sinus fistulae usually present with epibulbar injection, pulsatile proptosis, and a bruit or thrill. Blepharoptosis and hemorrhagic chemosis can also be seen. The patient can experience limitations of extraocular movements and complain of decrease in vision, headache, and eyelid swelling. The presence of increased intraocular pressure is typically caused by elevation in episcleral venous pressure, limiting outflow of aqueous humor. Anterior segment ischemia, characterized by corneal edema, iris atrophy, and rubeosis iridis, can be seen. Retinal hemorrhages are possible.

CT and MRI can detect a prominence of the superior ophthalmic vein. An arterial angiography helps in making the definitive diagnosis.

Treatment

In most cases, observation allows spontaneous resolution of the fistula. Selective embolization to occlude the fistula is usually done if visual impairment becomes progressive or in case of severe proptosis or if the patient is complaining of intolerable headache or bruit [8].

Venous Malformations

Venous malformations (VM) can be encapsulated or distensible. The former have been incorrectly called "cavernous hemangiomas," while the latter are sometimes referred to as "varices."

Encapsulated venous malformations are the most common orbital lesions found in adults. They are benign, slow-growing vascular lesions of the orbit [9].

Diagnosis

Patients with encapsulated venous malformations typically present with axial proptosis described as painless, slowly progressive protrusion of the eye associated with mild eyelid swelling. Axial proptosis (direct forward displacement of the eyeball) is produced most commonly, as these lesions tend to be found in the intraconal space defined by the four rectus muscles. Less commonly, the encapsulated venous malformation is seen extraconally, in which case the eyeball may be displaced vertically or horizontally. With direct observation alone, this can be difficult to distinguish from strabismus, a condition in which the eye is *rotated* vertically or horizontally. Alternate cover testing reveals the difference; in the strabismic condition, the uncovered eye rapidly rotates back into primary fixation, whereas the eye does not move back from horizontal or vertical translation. When located close to the orbital apex, encapsulated venous malformations can cause compressive optic neuropathy and decreased visual acuity. Diplopia, when present, is explained by distortion or distension of the extraocular muscles rather than by direct intramuscular involvement [1, 10]. Differential diagnosis usually includes schwannoma because of the similarity in size, shape, and location [11].

As with all orbital conditions, imaging studies are critically important. First, an orbital ultrasound, with the advantage of being a noninvasive technique, can detect a uniformly high-echogenic lesion with well-defined borders. A color Doppler US helps in detecting the blood flow and mapping the vasculature. Computed tomography should be performed with contrast. It shows an oval- or round-shaped, sharply demarcated homogenous lesion with slow contrast enhancement. On MRI, the lesion is seen isointense on T1 and hyperintense on T2; few internal septa can be seen, with a progressive accumulation of the contrast on late-phase images [12] (Fig. 42.2a).

Treatment

The treatment of orbital venous malformations is mostly conservative, but an intervention is needed in case of high orbital pressure or unbearable pain, deep orbital hemorrhage causing drop in vision, and cosmetic deformity [13].

In the cases in which surgical excision is indicated, the approach is dictated by the location of the lesion within the orbit. Most cavernous hemangiomas are found within the intraconal space between the extraocular muscles and the optic nerve. When the lesion is located lateral to the optic nerve, a lateral approach is used, either with or without temporary removal of the orbital rim. Inferior or inferomedial lesions can be removed endoscopically [14]. The medial intraconal space can also be accessed transconjunctivally, sometimes requiring temporary disinsertion of the medical rectus; occasionally the lateral orbital rim is removed to allow retraction of the eyeball during medial tumor removal. Inferiorly located lesions can be approached with a subciliary incision or transconjunctivally, while superiorly located lesions can be removed via an eyelid incision. Superior-posterior lesions may require cranio-orbitotomy for complete removal (Fig. 42.2b).

Distensible Venous Malformations

In contrast to encapsulated venous malformations, distensible venous malformations are meandering and poorly demarcated. They are more likely located outside the muscle cone and also tend to involve the eyelids. These lesions are not encapsulated and do not respect anatomic boundaries. Whereas the encapsulated lesions are almost always seen in isolation, the distensible lesions are more commonly associated with venous malformations of the hemiface including scalp, airway, buccal space, and masseter. These lesions have been described as a "bag of grapes" [1]. The most striking feature of distensible venous malformations, a feature starkly contrasted in encapsulated venous malformations, is a dramatic volumetric response to changes in venous pressure.

Diagnosis

Patients with distensible venous malformations of the orbit tend to complain of intermittent orbital pain, intermittent exophthalmos, or enophthalmos (sunken eye). The clinical scenario is dictated by the degree to which native orbital fat has been replaced by the malformation. When present, the pain is associated with physical activity and concomitant with exophthalmic episodes. One imagines that the pain results from rapid physical distortion of orbital soft tissues and venous congestion that raises the pressure in the orbit. Alternatively, direct neural tension or compression may be the painful stimulus. Importantly, when present, the exophthalmos is non-pulsatile and not associated with bruit. It is easily demonstrated with inversion, Valsalva maneuver, or other methods of raising venous pressure (Fig. 42.2a,b).

The patient experiences this change during athletic or vocational activities that may bring the lesion to medical attention. In cases with eyelid involvement, coughing or other raised venous pressure produces unsightly, externally visible irregularities of the lid structure and veins. The conjunctiva may house significant extensions of the primary lesion or may occur in complete isolation from an orbital venous malformation. Alternatively, conjunctival vessels may be secondarily enlarged and tortuous.

While most cases can be diagnosed clinically, imaging studies are important in order to define which anatomical structures are directly or indirectly involved, the specific anatomic location of the lesion, and to determine treatment alternatives planning. Orbital ultrasound can be extremely useful in detecting and measuring orbital masses. In the case of vascular lesions, ultrasound and color Doppler imaging can detect not only location of the lesion but also blood flow. In venous malformations, reversal of flow can be seen during Valsalva maneuver. (No such flow can be identified in cases of encapsulated venous malformations.) On computed tomography, distensible venous malformations may be entirely invisible, especially when the scan is performed in the usual supine position. In many cases an indistinct, small lesion may be visible with contrast-enhanced imaging. If the scan is performed in the prone position, or if the venous pressure is artificially raised during scanning, the lesion typically becomes obvious and potentially enormous within and around the orbit. Phleboliths within the lesion are pathognomonic. Any imaging of the orbit (computed tomography or nuclear magnetic resonance) must provide thin, 1–3 mm slices, with direct views in the axial and coronal planes. Sagittal views can also be helpful in some cases. While computed tomography is unsurpassed for anatomic location and, therefore, surgical planning, magnetic resonance imaging is preferred to identify tissue types and lesion characteristics. Magnetic resonance imaging, however, reveals the bony orbit only as unimaged space, and phleboliths can appear as flow voids. Magnetic resonance images should be ordered with gadolinium enhancement, and as in computed tomography, the venous pressure must be raised. The venous malformation appears with intermediate signal intensity on T1 and high signal intensity on T2, and it enhances strongly after the administration of a contrast material (Fig. 42.2c,d). This lesion, which intermingles with orbital fat, can be seen more easily with T1 fat suppression.

Treatment

Treatment of orbital venous malformations ranges from observation to complete surgical extirpation. Superficial lesions that involve primarily the eyelid can be treated with YAG laser, sclerotherapy, or surgical excision. Surgery is made easier if the lesion is pretreated with endovascular embolism. Laser treatment of the conjunctival component must be undertaken with extreme caution; the epibulbar conjunctiva should not be treated with laser. In many cases, surgical removal is more straightforward, safer, and definitive. Indeed, small conjunctival lesions can be cauterized using bipolar electrocautery.

More significant, space-occupying orbital lesions require greater treatment planning. In cases where exophthalmos is the chief complaint, a two-stage approach is needed. Endovascular sclerotherapy has become an excellent first-stage treatment to eliminate the mass of the malformation. Bleomycin is a safe and effective agent. Critical to successful treatment is containment of the sclerosant away from the cavernous sinus, where most of these lesions drain. Successful first-stage treatment is likely to produce enophthalmos, which requires surgical augmentation with soft tissue or alloplastic implants.

Surgical excision of orbital venous malformation alleviates any risk related to sclerosing agents but often still requires a two-stage approach. Excision of untreated lesions risks truly significant orbital hemorrhage that is difficult to control without risking injury to the optic nerve or other neural structures transiting the orbital apex. Therefore, preoperative endovascular embolization is preferred. These lesions can be embolized percutaneously or directly with surgical exposure of the lesion. Thrombin-gelatin slurries have been effective agents. The lesion is effectively thrombosed, making surgical removal technically simpler and safer. Bipolar electrocautery is indispensible during these orbital surgeries.

Lymphatic Malformations

Until recently, lymphatic malformations have been called "lymphangiomas" in the ophthalmic literature. These lesions represent between 1 and 8 % of all orbital lesions [15]. Periocular lymphatic malformations can involve the orbit, eyelids, and conjunctiva. They can be seen in isolation or associated with hemifacial lymphatic malformations. Another typical distribution involves the anterolateral scalp down to the superior orbit and eyelid. Within the orbit, these lesions do not respect tissue planes and tend to involve both intraconal and extraconal spaces [16, 17]. Rapidly expanding cystic segments due to hemorrhage have been called "chocolate cysts" and produce acute-onset exophthalmos, pain, and optic neuropathy.

Diagnosis

Lymphatic malformations of the orbit most commonly present in children ages birth to puberty. They may include visible components in the eyelid or conjunctiva. Diagnosis in these cases may be straightforward. Conjunctival involvement, however, can mimic the "salmon patch" typical of conjunctival lymphoma. Confusion can usually be resolved, however, by patient age; lymphoma is very rare in children, and new onset lymphatic malformation is exceedingly rare in adults. Anterior lesions appear as several soft bluish masses in the upper nasal quadrant associated with a cystic conjunctival element. Eyelid involvement can mimic venous malformation especially when the blue hue arises from intracystic hemorrhage. Deeper lesions, without a superficial manifestation, may be obvious at birth or may remain quiescent for years then suddenly become symptomatic, particularly at the onset of puberty [15]. Posterior orbital lesions usually induce slowly progressive proptosis of the eye, but sudden painful proptosis can be caused by spontaneous hemorrhage (Fig. 42.3a,b). Subacute presentation is seen in cases of upper respiratory infection or other immunologic stimuli. Rhabdomyosarcoma must be excluded with any rapidly evolving orbital lesion in the pediatric age group [18].

Ultrasound evaluation of orbital lymphatic malformations demonstrates large cystic areas in macrocystic areas and irregular lesions in microcystic regions. Flow is absent in these lesions, making color Doppler less useful. Computed tomography is the favored imaging technique in most orbital pathology, as it demonstrates the relationship of the lesion to the surrounding bony orbit and specific anatomic location of the lesion that is critical in surgical planning. Magnetic

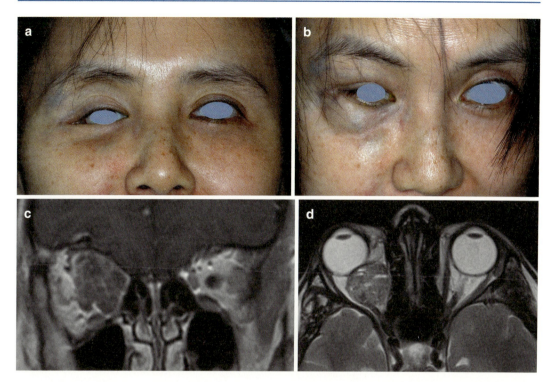

Fig. 42.3 Distensible venous malformation. (**a**) With the patient in the upright position, the right eyeball appears sunken (enophthalmos), and *blue discoloration* can be seen in the upper lateral eyelid. The lower lid shows incipient entropion that often accompanies severe enophthalmos. (**b**) With the patient in the inverted position, the lower eyelid component of the lesion is appreciated, the eyeball has moved forward, and the position of the lower eyelid has stabilized against the eyeball. The venous nature of the lesion can be appreciated in the increase blue discoloration of the upper eyelid. (**c**) This T1-weighted MRI in the coronal plain demonstrates the irregular nature of the lesion, with irregular septa and cystic spaces extending from the intraconal to the extraconal space. (**d**) The T2-weighted axial view demonstrates more discrete boarders with irregular internal cavities in the medial, retrobulbar orbit

resonance, however, is the gold standard for imaging orbital lymphatic malformations, as the tissue type, fluid type (e.g., lymph, new blood, old blood), and nature of the cysts are most exquisitely demonstrated with this technology. Hemorrhagic cysts appear hyperintense on T1-weighted images (Fig. 42.3c).

Treatment

Surgical excision of extensive orbital lymphatic malformations has been fraught with difficulty; the lesions tend to hemorrhage due to delicate vessels in the cyst walls, and complete extirpation is frequently impossible because of the meandering and stealthy projections of lesion well beyond the visible borders. "Recurrence" is better described as "continued proliferation" and may be anticipated in cases of incomplete resection [19] (Fig. 42.3d). One area in which surgical resection continues to be the optimal treatment is the conjunctival component. Quadrantic resection allows adequate healing and may involve amniotic reconstruction of the ocular surface [20].

More recently, endovascular sclerotherapy has become the treatment of choice for extensive or surgically inaccessible orbital lymphatic malformations. These lesions are extremely sensitive to bleomycin treatment. OK-432 is strongly discouraged due to uncontrolled inflammation and swelling that can produce an orbital compartment syndrome [21]. In this case, massive pressure develops from inflammatory swelling, with subsequent compression or stretching of the optic nerve. In the emergent situation, lateral canthotomy

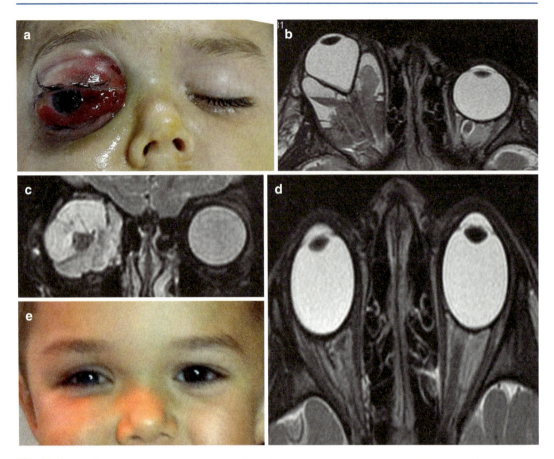

Fig. 42.4 Lymphatic malformation of the eyelids and orbit. (**a**) Severe anterior displacement of the eyeball (proptosis) of the right eye with exposed, hemorrhagic conjunctiva. (**b**) Axial views of this gadolinium-enhanced, T2-weighted MRI with fat suppression demonstrate massive proptosis of the eyeball with dramatic deformity of the globe and stretching of the optic nerve. The intra- and extraconal spaces are occupied with a multicystic lesion demonstrating characteristic fluid levels. (**c**) Coronal view of the same MRI demonstrates the lesion completely filling the orbit. (**d**) Axial view of this posttreatment, T2-weighted MRI demonstrates nearly complete resolution of the lesion. (**e**) One year after initial treatment, the eyeball has returned to normal position

and cantholysis can be vision-saving maneuvers. Alcohol sclerosants have reportedly been used effectively, but these agents are neurotoxic and also produce inflammation that is difficult to control [16] (Fig. 42.4).

by the specific ancillary tests, optimal management can be achieved.

Conclusion

Orbital vascular malformations including arteriovenous malformation, venous malformation, and lymphatic malformation demonstrate a wide spectrum of clinical presentation. The most urgent concern is protection of the optic nerve and visual acuity, followed by preservation of periocular functions such as eyeball and eyelid movements. Depending on the type and location of the lesion, and guided

References

1. Rodgers R, Grove SA (2000) Vascular lesions of the orbit. In: Albert D, Jakobiec F, Azar D et al (eds) Principles and practice of ophthalmology, vol 4, 2nd edn. WB Saunders Company, Philadelphia, pp 3144–3154
2. Yadav P, De Castro DK, Waner M, Meyer L, Fay A (2013) Vascular anomalies of the head and neck: a review of genetics. Semin Ophthalmol 28(5–6):257–266
3. Kaufman Y, Cole P, Dauser R et al (2007) Intraorbital arteriovenous malformation: issues in surgical management. J Craniofac Surg 18:1091–1093

4. Hayes BH, Shore JW, Westfall CT et al (1995) Management of orbital and periorbital arteriovenous malformations. Ophthalmic Surg 26(2):145–152

5. Dmytriw AA, Ter Brugge KG, Krings T et al (2014) Endovascular treatment of head and neck arteriovenous malformations. Neuroradiology 56(3):227–236

6. Liscak R, Vladyka V, Simonova G et al (2007) Arteriovenous malformations after Leskell gamma knife radiosurgery: rate of obliteration and complications. Neurosurgery 60:1005–1014

7. Kanski J (2007) Orbit. In: Kanski J (ed) Clinical ophthalmology: a systemic approach, 6th edn. Butterworth-Heinemann/Elsevier, Edinburgh;/New York, pp 180–185

8. Williamson R, Ducruet A, Crowley W et al (2012) Transvenous coil embolization of an intraorbital arteriovenous fistula: case report and review of the literature. Neurosurgery 72:130–134

9. Osaki TH, Jakobiec FA, Mendoza PR, Lee Y, Fay AM (2013) Immunohistochemical investigations of orbital infantile hemangiomas and adult encapsulated cavernous venous lesions (malformation versus hemangioma). Ophthal Plast Reconstr Surg 29(3):183–195

10. Jakobiec FA, Zakka FR, Papakostas TD, Fay A (2012) Angiomyofibroma of the orbit: a hybrid of vascular leiomyoma and cavernous hemangioma. Ophthal Plast Reconstr Surg 28(6):438–445

11. Andreoli CM, Hatton M, Semple JP, Soukiasian SH, Fay AM (2004) Perilimbal conjunctival schwannoma. Arch Ophthalmol 122(3):388–389

12. Lewin JS (2004) Low-flow vascular malformations of the orbit: a new approach to a therapeutic dilemma. AJNR Am J Neuroradiol 25(10):1633–1634

13. Rootman J (1988) Diseases of the orbit: a multidisciplinary approach. JB Lippincott, Philadelphia, pp 553–557

14. Chhabra N, Wu AW, Fay A, Metson R (2014) Endoscopic resection of orbital hemangiomas. Int Forum Allergy Rhinol 4(3):251–5

15. Wiegand S, Eivazi B, Bloch L et al (2013) Lymphatic malformations of the orbit. Clin Experim Otorhinolaryngol 6:30–35

16. Illif WJ, Green WR (1979) Orbital lymphangiomas. Ophthalmology 86(5):914–929

17. Vavvas D, Fay A, Watkins L (2004) Two cases of orbital lymphangioma associated with vascular abnormalities of the retina and iris. Ophthalmology 111(1):189–192

18. Fay A, Fynn-Thompson N, Ebb D (2003) Klippel-Trénaunay syndrome and rhabdomyosarcoma in a 3-year-old. Arch Ophthalmol 121(5):727–729

19. Eivazi B, Ardelean M, Baumier W et al (2009) Update on hemangiomas and vascular malformations of the head and neck. Eur Arch Otorhinolaryngol 266(2):187–197

20. Mehta M, Waner M, Fay A (2009) Amniotic membrane grafting in the management of conjunctival vascular malformations. Ophthal Plast Reconstr Surg 25(5):371–375

21. Suzuki Y, Obana A, Gohto Y et al (2000) Management of orbital lymphangioma using intralesional injection of OK-432. Br J Ophthalmol 84(6):614–617

Orthopedic Problems

43

Jürgen Hauert and Dirk A. Loose

Vascular malformations have an incidence rate of approximately 1.2 % [19]. These diseases manifest themselves mostly in childhood, with vascular malformation syndromes displaying a link to orthopedic diseases and diagnoses of, e.g., osteolysis, benign tumors and differing leg length [3, 15, 22, 29]. There is extensive literature on causal links, as well as the different phenotypes of these conditions [1, 2, 11, 23–28].

The vascular-bone syndrome with long-bone growth discrepancy, especially of the lower extremity, has been known to be an enigma among congenital vascular malformations, and it is interpreted by the intra-/extraosseous congenital vascular malformations as a secondary phenomenon (Tables 43.1 and 43.2) that results in abnormal intraosseous circulation (Fig. 43.1) [36].

The management of the length discrepancy requires an early removal of the hemodynamic and metabolic causes for the bone pathology because the likelihood of correction by this vascular operation to the primary lesion is much higher when done during infancy (Table 43.3) [12, 34, 35]. When, however, the long-bone length discrepancy is more than 4–5 cm, the combined approach of an orthopedic procedure and vascular surgery has been generally accepted as the primary strategy. When presented with severe length discrepancy, noninvasive and/or invasive diagnosis procedures should be started even before the age of 3 in order to perform the necessary vascular procedure to correct the pathologic hemodynamics first before it is too late [17]. However, if the vascular cause of the length discrepancy can be contained until the age of 7, orthopedic surgery may then be performed (Table 43.4). The policy of first performing vascular surgery to arrest further abnormal long-bone growth and then subsequent additional orthopedic correction is the treatment of choice. An early aggressive approach is mandatory [9, 30–32].

In the long run, length discrepancy may not represent the underlying problem in these patients. That is why a critical indication should be considered.

Children and young people with a congenital vascular malformation sometimes also suffer mono- or oligoarthralgia of the large joints, mainly of the lower limbs (Table 43.5) (Hauert Disease) [33].

What we notice here is that this includes cases in which destruction of the affected joints occurs early on in childhood, sometimes even before the age of 5, the considerable extent of which stands in extraordinary contrast to the usual complaint of moderate or slight pain. What is also striking is that this joint condition is accompanied only by very marginal inflammatory malformations and

J. Hauert
Department of Orthopedics and Emergency Surgery, Hospital "Dr.Guth" and Facharztklinik Hamburg, Hamburg, Germany,
e-mail: Dr.hauert@t-online.de

D.A. Loose (✉)
Section Vascular Surgery and Angiology, Facharztklinik Hamburg, Hamburg, Germany
e-mail: info@prof-loose.de

R. Mattassi et al. (eds.), *Hemangiomas and Vascular Malformations: An Atlas of Diagnosis and Treatment*,
DOI 10.1007/978-88-470-5673-2_43, © Springer-Verlag Italia 2009, 2015

Table 43.1 Pathogenesis of congenital circulatory-hypoxic hyperostosis

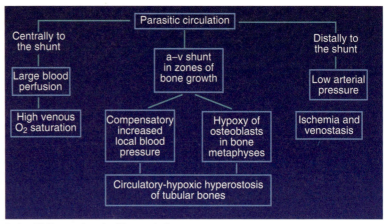

Belov [34] reproduced with permission

Table 43.2 Pathogenesis of congenital angio-osteohypotrophy

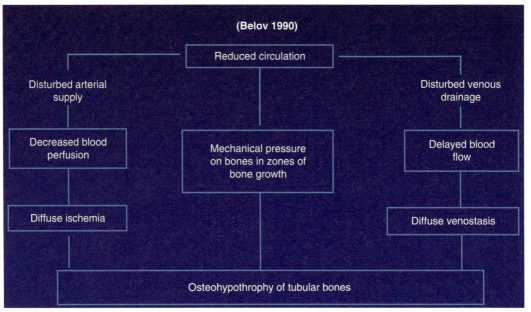

Belov [34] reproduced with permission

that, entirely unlike in primary degenerative joint changes, this type of destruction appears not to show any significant tendency of progression after longitudinal growth is complete. There are no signs of systemic inflammation; rheumatoid factors are consistently negative [5–8]. The vertebra joints appear to be recessed. Based on our experience and knowledge of international literature, this very unusual clinical phenotype is as yet undocumented, so we have provisionally opted for the descriptive term of angiodysplasia

arthropathy, or "Hauert disease," for this set of conditions, with the aim of having it acknowledged as a stand-alone entity.

Vascular malformation on the affected limb makes most patients seriously ill in any case, a major symptom being chronic bouts of phlebitis causing pain and restriction of movement. The clinically visible signs of vascular malformation explain why it is only in later examinations that joint disease is considered as a cause of the symptoms. The vascular malformation alone is

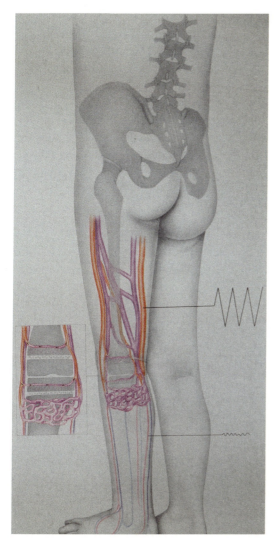

Fig. 43.1 Drawing explaining pathogenesis of congenital circulatory-hypoxic hyperostosis at the zones of bone growth in the region of the distal thigh and the proximal shank: large blood perfusion in the arteries of the thigh and hypotonia in the arteries of the shank. AV fistulas in the proximal shank lead to hypoxia of osteoblasts in bone metaphyses which signifies a stimulation to their activity resulting in hyperostosis of the tubular bone [35, 36]

Table 43.3 Therapeutic strategies in congenital vascular defects

To start in early childhood (at the age of 3–7)
To influence the pathophysiologic process and to abolish the hemodynamic dysfunction
To perform a harmonized individual treatment
To perform surgery radically without loss of function
To perform a stepwise surgical treatment
To practice a multidisciplinary therapy

Table 43.4 Indications for an additional orthopedic treatment to correct a length discrepancy of the legs in angiodysplasias

If in a distinct length discrepancy (even after vascular surgery) the correction is not satisfying.
After the end of growth (temporary epiphysiodesis being excluded).
If there is no indication for vascular surgery to correct the length discrepancy.

Table 43.5 Distribution patterns of angiodysplasia arthropathy

$N=53$	♂	♀
Knee	10	26
Hips	–	4
Ankle joint	1	2

capable of compromising joint function so much so that its typical symptoms such as limping, contractures, and painful movement can obscure an arthropathy, which shares the same symptoms. The most striking symptom in patients is a loss of function of the joint, a limp, and possibly a periarticular swelling. Effusion in the knee joint or hemarthrosis is key exceptions. There are generally no lab-based inflammation parameters.

A restriction in movement of the ankle and foot joints can already be detected in newborns. Clinical examination using duplex ultrasound (color-coded ultrasound of the vessels) can quickly diagnose vessel failure (vascular malformation).

We have divided the disease into three degrees of severity depending on the extent of the tissue malformations (Table 43.6).

Diagnostics

A plain radiological image in the early stages I and II shows almost no malformation. The earliest signs are irregularities in the subchondral plate (in a test comparison). A demineralization of the joint-adjacent bone may be detected – only rarely do we find signs similar to actual arthritic signs [2]. This recessed reaction in the bone may have contributed to the failure to diagnose during phlebographic examinations [20]. Subchondral sclerosis can occur from level II upwards which at level III leads to unmistakable malformations in the bones of the joint. Actual arthritic malformations with osteophytes etcetera are rare.

At the hip joint, the damage is localized mostly at the head with an extensive recess of the acetabular partner. We have never seen this develop into an ankylosis; the clinically detected movement restrictions were ligamentous and algogenic in nature. Phleboliths (calcifications in the malformed blood vessels) are a strong indicator of "Hauert disease" (HD).

MRT

MRT imaging presents the damage to the capsule, cartilage, and bone. At the same time, you can see the existing pathological vessels in the surrounding tissue (resolution up to 1 mm). Predominantly long, slow-flow vascular proliferations point to suspected vascular malformation. The sequences best suited to this are proton heavy with spectral fat saturation or, if not available, then turbo inversion recovery sequences. The proliferating giant-cell synovioma can be easily defined by proving blood degradation products such as hemosiderin of the venous malformations. The appearance of narrow-diameter venous malformations, partial thrombosis, or thromboses as well as by inflammatory changes in the walls requires the intravenous administration of contrast agents.

Arthroscopic Diagnosis

With level I malformations (Fig. 43.2), arthroscopy (Fig. 43.3) shows a highly irritated mucosa, part of which are the menisci. Vascular malformations can show through the synovial

Table 43.6 Diagnostic and therapeutic algorithm

$N=53$	Severity level I	Severity level II	Severity level III
Quantity	11	24	18
Substrate	Synovial fluid	Synovial fluid, cartilage	Synovial fluid, cartilage, bone
Plain X-ray	Unobtrusive, phlebolith	Irregularity of the subchondral plate, demineralization (in a comparison test)	Subchondral sclerosis, mutilations
MRT	Thickening of the synovial fluid + vascular malformation	Cartilage reduction, vascular malformation	Destroyed bone, vascular malformation
Symptoms	Limping, soft tissue inflammation (pain)	Reduced function, pain	Severe pain, contractures
Treatment	Conventional, diagnostic arthroscopy, partial synovial fluid resection	Debridement	Debridement, Quengel orthoses, joint replacement

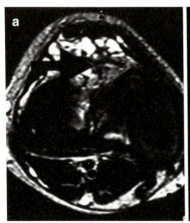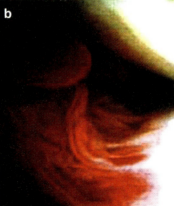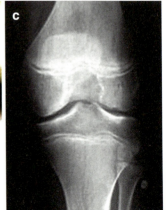

Fig. 43.2 Angiodysplasia arthropathy grade 1. (**a**) Subpatellar vascular malformation to be documented by MRI (*arrow*). (**b**) Transarthroscopic view of an intra-articular vascular malformation. (**c**) X-ray of the knee joint of the same patient 11 years after treatment without complaints and recurrences

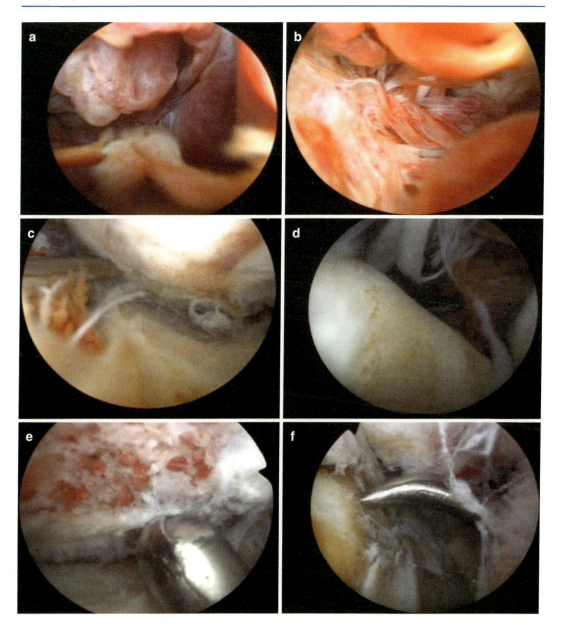

Fig. 43.3 Transarthroscopic aspect: (**a**) and (**b**) Intra-articular vascular malformation partially free floating. (**c**) and (**d**) Hemosiderin precipitation in the cartilage or in the bone. (**e**) Visible free bone under rudimentary arranged cartilage or (**f**) desquamated cartilage

fluid membrane. Rarely do you also find individual malformations as soft, vascularized tumors in the joint. Yellow/brown plaque points to hemosiderin deposits which must then be distinguished from a giant-cell tumor of the tendon sheath. The examination is often complicated by pronounced forming of adhesion. With level II malformations (Fig. 43.4), you can recognize the random cartilage destruction and the oversized menisci. With level III malformations, the exposed bone is seen with red spots. You can see the white of the bone showing through where it is almost entirely stripped. These malformations are independent of the stress zones. Overall, the experienced arthroscopist will conclude an "unseen image."

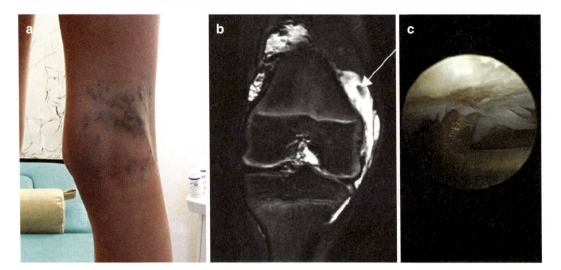

Fig. 43.4 Angiodysplasia arthropathy grade 2. (**a**) Clinical aspect of the vascular malformation in the right popliteal region. (**b**) MRI demonstrating a vascular malformation at the onset insertion of the lateral collateral ligament (*white arrow*). (**c**) Transarthroscopic view of free bone surface of the trochlea as well as underdeveloped cartilage in the peripheral part

Treatment

The treatment relies on interdisciplinary cooperation [9–11, 13, 14, 30]. Therapeutically we use the soft approach [16, 21]. Under the notion that there is little chance of regeneration of the diseased tissue, until now we have preferred the use of just transarthroscopic debridement to create optimal morphological conditions. As there is no medial hip joint capsule with angiodysplasia arthropathy, even after resecting, the remaining capsule fails to form neo-capsules (see Fig. 43.5).

With level III malformations – bone destruction and pronounced pain as well as lack of function (movement contracture) – the only route in most cases is endoprosthetic replacement. Here, the hemostasis is often extremely precarious, so we have to resort to unusual measures such as muscleplasty, leaving the tibial posterior in knee implantations, or retro-resection of the calcar femoris. The osseous integration of endoprosthetics is incredibly robust and enables true remodeling. Unfortunately we have not yet seen a safe indication for cartilage/bone grafts [18].

Naturally, we would recommend resectioning in the case of complaints about vascular malformation in the joint itself.

Progress

Progress has been followed up clinically and, in a few cases, also with the use of the abovementioned diagnostic procedures (MR, arthroscopy). We have not seen a rapid progression in malformation, as shown above. Checkup examinations should be performed at reasonable regular intervals for both the endoprosthesis and vascular/joint patients.

Complications

We have not experienced any real complications. It can be extremely difficult to provide endoprosthesis for malformations in the area itself. For example, we have left a posterior bony edge at the tibial plateau during a knee implant before, so as not to affect the area of malformation. Hip implants where the medial capsule has given

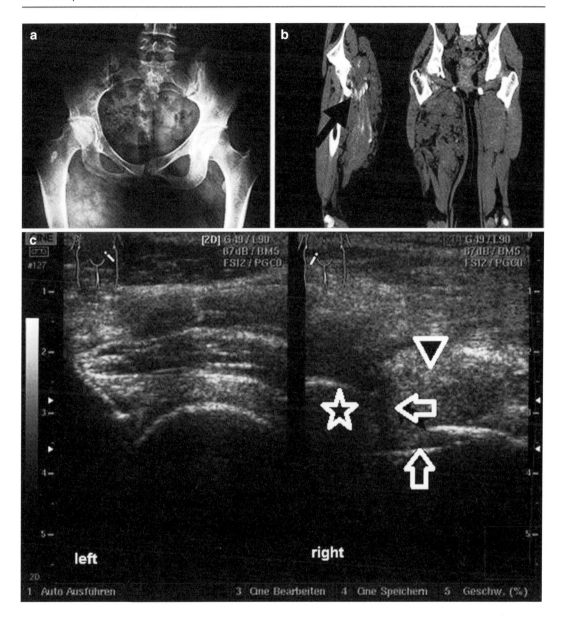

Fig. 43.5 Angiodysplasia arthropathy grade 3 (**a, b**) findings before surgery. (**a**) Plane X-ray of pelvis: narrowing of the intra-articular space without sclerosis of the joint partner. (**b**) MRI demonstrates vascular malformation of the dorsal part of the capsula of the hip joint (*arrow*). (**c**) Ultrasound of the hip joints comparing the left side to the right side: artificial socket (***); artificial prosthesis, *top* (*arrow*); muscle plastic (*triangle*), because of missing dorsal part of the capsula of the joint (*arrow*)

way to a malformation proliferation had to be followed up with a complex hemostasis with muscleplasty. With mobilization surgery, you have to consider the risk of overstretching the nerves.

Our Preliminary Results

Subjectively, all patients treated were happy with the treatment and results. Considering the disastrous defects, the results of the transarthroscopic,

Table 43.7 Differential diagnoses

Diagnosis	Treatment
Juvenile idiopathic oligoarthritis	MTX, anti-infl. therapy, Resochin
Seroneg. rheuma	MTX
Giant-cell tumor of the tendon sheath	60Gy
Intraosseous hemangioma	Cancellous bone filling
M. Ahlback	
M. Schlatter	
Osteoidosteom	
Osteochondrosis dissecans	
Atraumatic hemarthrosis	
Hemophilia	
Thrombophilia	
M. Perthes	
Coxitis fugax	
M. Reiter*	Anti-inflammation treatment
Sarcoidosis	
Borreliosis	Long-term antibiotics
Lyme arthritis*	
Reactive arthritis (with viral infection)	
Joint emphasis	
Brodie abscess	
M. Blouth	
Malformation pain	
Arthrosis	Realignment osteotomy
Valgus gonarthrosis	

Table of misdiagnoses of Hauert Disease in our cases (*externally treated) with the conducted non-indexed approaches

so far only resecting, treatments are better than expected [28]. The results of the endoprostheses (N=9) are good so far. We have not observed any complications. All nine implants are stable. The range of motion and pain-free capabilities are in the normal range.

We also saw patients provided externally with spongiosaplasty, radical synovectomies, realignment osteotomies, and one-off mobilizations with external fixation in the case of contractures. We were not convinced of the long-term results (Table 43.7).

Orthopedic Therapeutic Aspects of Vascular Malformation

The healing of bone fractures can be complicated, but our impression in providing endoprosthesis is that remodeling is so far advanced that the prosthesis is accepted without compromise. Endoprosthetics should avoid the use of cement, so as not to impede the osseous integration. Contractures can result from joint infection as well as independently. With muscle-infiltrating malformations, the affected muscle loses its elasticity and leads to a contracture of the affected joint (hamstring/calf muscles). The pain-inducing malformation should be treated surgically [4, 12, 20]. In the area of the Achilles tendon, the patient will also need considerable Z-plasty, beyond the plantigrade, as there is a risk of recurrence. Healing is usually straightforward, but there is a risk related to recurrence. The severing of tendons around the ischiocrural muscles (hamstrings) has been reported only in severe cases. Generally, the patient will improve with a Quengel orthosis. We can assume a high rate of "Hauert disease" in the area of the knee joint and treat it simultaneously along with the vascular malformation.

Defining angiodysplasia arthropathy will help to avoid errors in diagnosis and treatments and can contribute to the further development of meaningful therapy. Safe diagnosis protects sick children from additional stress and anxieties. Future systematic examinations of the resected tissue to find the characteristics of malformation in the nonvascular tissue and genetic studies of the affected part of the body, as well as the genetic makeup, could help to better understand these new symptoms with the ultimate aim of its inclusion in the Hamburg classification of vascular malformations.

References

1. Broillard P, Vikkula M (2007) Genetic causes of vascular malformations. Hum Mol Genet 16(Review issue 2):R140–R149

2. Diehlmann W (1987) Gelenke – Verbindungen: klinische Radiologie einschl. Computertomographie – Diagnose, Differentialdiagnose. Thieme, New York

3. Enjolras O, Ciabrini D, Mazoyer E, Laurian C, Herbreteau D (1997) Extensive pure venous malformations in the upper or lower limb: a review of 27 cases. Am Acad Dermatol 36:219–225

4. Gloviczki P, Hollier LH, Telander RL, Kaufmann B, Bianco AJ, Stickler GB (1982) Surgical implications of Klippel-Trenaunay syndrome – page 353. J.B. Lippincott Company, New York

5. Helmchen U, Loose DA, Weber J (1997) Zur Histopathologie congenitaler Angiodysplasien unter besonderer Berücksichtigung der Angiogenese, Angeborene Gefäßmissbildungen. Nordlanddruck GmbH, Lüneburg

6. Hochheim B, Sonntag M (1984) Tierexperimentelle Untersuchung zur Erzeugung einer Osteoarthrose durch venöse Stase – Vorläufige Mitteilung. Beitr Orthop Und Tramatol 31(H 4):S.177–S.185, Medizinische Akademie Erfurt

7. Yercan HS, Okcu G, Erkan S (2007) Synovial hemangiohamartomas of the knee joint. Arch Arthop Trauma Surg 127:281–285, Published online 12. April 2006, Springer Verlag 2006

8. Yoon KH, Bae DK, Kim HS, Song SJ (2005) Arthroscopic synovectomy in haemophilic arthropathy of the knee. Int Orthop 29:296–300

9. Lee BB, Mattassi R, Loose DA, Yakes W, Tasnadi G, Kin HH (2005) Consensus on controversial issues in contemporary diagnosis and management of congenital vascular malformation: Seoul communication. Int J Angiol 13:182–192

10. Lee BB, Laredo J, Lee TS, Huh S, Neville R (2007) Terminology and classification of congenital vascular malformations. Phlebology 22:249–252

11. Lee BB, Gloviczki P, Laredo J, Loose DA, Mattassi R, Parsi K, Villavicencio JL, Zamboni P (2009) Diagnosis and treatment of venous malformations – Consensus Document of the International Union of Phlebology (IUP)-2009. Int Angiol 28(6):434–451

12. Loose DA, Weber J (1987) Angeborene Gefäßmissbildungen – Interdisziplinäre Diagnostik und Therapie (Angiodysplasien) Periodica Angiologica Band 21. Verlag Nordlanddruck GmbH, Lüneburg. ISBN 3-922639-03-8

13. Mallick A, Weber AC (2007) An experience of arthroplasty in Klippel-Trenaunay-Syndrome. Ezr J Orthop Surg Traumatol 17:97–99, March 2006, Springer Verlag 2007

14. Mattassi R, Loose DA, Vaghi M (2009) Hemangiomas and vascular malformations. Springer, New York. ISBN 978-88-470-0569-3

15. Mulliken JB, Young AE (1988) Vascular birthmarks: hemangiomas and malformations. Saunders, Philadelphia

16. Obermayer B, Westphal F, Loose DA, Hauert J (2011) Hauert disease: Gelenkdestruktion bei angeborener Gefäßmalformation im Kindes- und Jugendalter. Indikation für Gelenkersatz – 60. Jahrestagung 2011 der Norddeutschen Orthopäden- und Unfallchirurgenvereinigung e.V./Juli 2011 CCH (Seite 97, 72 Kinder-Hüfte und Varia)

17. Peixinho M, Arakaki T, Toledo CS (1982) Correction of leg inequality in the Klippel-Trenaunay-Weber-syndrome. Int Orthop 6:45–47, Springer Verlag

18. Price NJ, Cundy PJ (1997) Synovial hemangioma of the knee. Lippincott-Raven Publishers, New York. ISSN: 0271–6798

19. Tasnádi G (2009) Epidemiology of vascular malformations. In: Mattassi R, Loose DA, Vaghi M (eds) Hemangiomas and vascular malformations. An atlas of diagnosis and treatment. Springer, Milan, Italy

20. Weber J (2010) Phlebographie, Bein-, Becken- und Abdominalvenen in Anatomie und Funktion, .4–7, 668 ff. Angeborene Gefäßfehler: Kongenitale vaskuläre Malformationen (CVM). Rabe Verlag, Bonn, ISBN: 978-3-940654-15-1

21. Westphal FM, Obermayer B, Loose DA, Hauert J (2009) Hauert disease: destruktive, angiodysplastische arthritis. Hamb Arztebl 05:12–16

22. Belov S (1989) Classification, terminology and nosology of congenital vascular defects. In: Belov S, Loose DA, Weber J (eds) Vascular malformations. Einhorn-Presse Verlag, Reinbek, pp 25–30

23. Hauert J, Betthäuser A, Loose DA (2000) Vascular malformation arthritis – transarthroscopic treatment – communication at the 13th Workshop of the International Society for the Study of Vascular Anomalies 10–13 May, Montreal, Canada

24. Laurian C (2002) Malformazioni venose intraarticolari del ginocchio. In: Mattassi R, Belov S, Loose DA (eds) Malformationi vascolari ed emangiomi. Testo atlante di diagnostica e terapia, 2003; Springer, Milan, Italy, pp 179–179

25. Breugem CC, Maas M, Breugem SJ et al (2003) Vascular malformations of the lower limb with osseous involvement. J Bone Joint Surg Br 85:399–405

26. Bonaga S, Bardi C, Gigante C, Turra S (2003) Synovial involvement in hemangiomatosis. Arch Orthop Trauma Surg 123:102–106

27. Breugem CC, Maas M, Reekers JA, van der Horst CM (2001) Use of magnetic resonance imaging for the evaluation of vascular malformations of the lower extremity. Plast Reconstr Surg 108:870–877

28. Moseley JB, O'Malley K, Petersen NJ et al (2002) A controlled trial of arthroscopic surgery for osteoarthritis of the knee. J Fam ract 51:813

29. Yakes WF (2009) Diagnosis in management of vascular malformations of bone. In: Mattassi R, Loose DA, Vaghi M (eds) Hemangiomas and vascular malformations. An atlas of diagnosis and treatment. Springer, Italia, pp 319–324

30. Loose, DA, Mattassi R, Vaghi M (2012) Gefäßmalformationen. In: Debus ES, Gross-Fengels W (Hrsg.) Operative und inverventionelle Gefäßmedizin. Springer, Berlin-Heidelberg, pp 769–791

31. Loose, DA, Belov S, Mattassi R, Vaghi M, Tasnadi G, Rehder A. Long follow-up results in active causal

treatment of vascular malformations. A review of 1378 cases (Multicenter Study). Proceedings of the 14th Congress of the European Chapter of the International Union of Angiology, Cologne (Germany) May 23–26, 2001, Monduzzi Editore International Proceedings Division (2001), pp 431–450

32. Loose DA (2007) Surgical management of venous malformations. Phlebology 22(6):276–282

33. Hauert J, Loose DA, Dreyer T, Obermayer B, Deibele A (2012) Angiodysplastische arthropathie ("Hauert disease"). Orthopäde 41:493–504

34. Belov S (1990) Hemodynamic pathogenesis of vascular bone syndromes in congenital vascular defects. Int Angiol 9:155–162

35. Belov S (1993) Correction of lower limbs length discrepancy in congenital vascular-bone diseases by vascular surgery performed during childhood. Semin Vasc Surg 6:245–251

36. Hauss WH (1973) Transport und Stoffwechsel in Bindegewebe. In: N. Klueken (ed) Aktuelle Angiologie, Folia Angiologica supp Vol II. Verlag Haupt & Koska AG, Berlin Wien, pp 174–191

Treatment of Vascular Malformations in the Hand

44

Piero Di Giuseppe

Introduction

The hand has a very complex function strictly related to its complex anatomy. It is of great interest to remember that sensorial and motor functions are interdependent [1].

CVMs in the hand may involve any structure and are atypically distributed [2, 3]. As many different tissues of high functional value are located in a small space, clinical pictures can be extended and complex and can involve the skin, bones, nerves, muscles, and tendons, posing special therapeutic problems. To surgically treat CVMs in the hand, the fourth Belov principle should be followed: a *functional radical operation* should be performed, meaning as radical as possible to avoid recurrences and as sparing as feasible in order to preserve or restore hand function [3, 4].

Surgical strategies can consist of single or multiple stage surgery, alone or associated with other procedures such as sclerotherapy, embolization, or laser treatment [5–7].

Surgical techniques should respect the general principles of hand surgery, including skin incisions and undermining, and the selection criteria of structures to be resected according

P. Di Giuseppe
Unit of Plastic and Hand Surgery,
Hospital of Magenta, A.O. Ospedale Civile di
Legnano, Magenta (MI), Italy
e-mail: chirurgiadellamano@fastwebnet.it;
piero.digiuseppe@ao-legnano.it;
http://www.chirurgiadellamano.it

to their function. Techniques and timing of hemostasis and postoperative bandage should also be performed correctly.

General Principles of CVM Surgery in the Hand

Considering that tissue involvement by different kinds of malformations is the most challenging problem in hand CVM surgery, and that combined CVMs are also possible, the Hamburg classification is currently used to elaborate our therapeutic program. Clinical examination does not always allow a complete diagnosis, so imaging and Doppler are essential as previously illustrated in this book. In the hand, plain x-rays are very useful.

Skin Incisions

The skin in the hand works like a distinct organ with its own passive motor function. The dorsal skin of the hand is more elastic, while the palmar skin is more adherent and sensitive. The elasticity of the skin allows movements; the web spaces allow independent movements of the fingers; scar contracture precludes mobility even if all other structures are normal.

When skin incisions are planned, scar lines should be broken mainly at the level of skin creases to avoid scar contracture.

R. Mattassi et al. (eds.), *Hemangiomas and Vascular Malformations: An Atlas of Diagnosis and Treatment*,
DOI 10.1007/978-88-470-5673-2_44, © Springer-Verlag Italia 2009, 2015

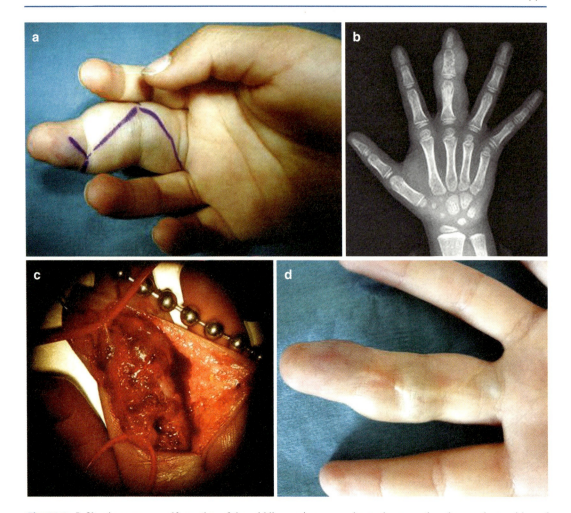

Fig. 44.1 Infiltrating venous malformation of the middle finger in a girl. (**a**) Drawing of incisions in the palmar aspect of the middle finger. (**b**) Bone infiltration evident in plain radiograms, (**c**) subdermal undermining under the microscope shows the avascular plane and exposition of the involved tissue (skin-sparing technique) and the nerve identified and isolated before tissue excision. (**d**) Late result showing scars without contracture

There are some typical incisions in hand surgery. Each of these incisions can be adopted alone or combined with others. CVMs may be sometimes difficult to approach through conventional incisions; atypical incisions may sometimes be necessary.

Incisions for hand surgery should respect some basic principles:

1. Limited undermining and preparing of flaps that offer a large exposure of the deep structures should be planned.
2. Web spaces and joint creases should be respected by broken incisions to avoid scar contracture (Figs. 44.1a and 44.7a).
3. Scars of previous surgery influence the choice of new incisions. A flap should not be performed with a previous scar at its base. In extended CVM, incisions should be planned in order to permit extensions, when necessary. Drawing the contour of the CVM mass on the skin before marking the incision lines is helpful in order to better approach the malformation.

Skin-Sparing Technique

Skin sparing is possible by subdermal undermining, which should be carefully done with a scalpel to preserve the subdermal vascular network. This allows minimal blood loss and saves skin flaps for coverage (Figs. 44.1c and 44.7b–c). It is best performed under a microscope or with loupe magnification.

Use of Tourniquet

A tourniquet reduces bleeding and is useful for microsurgical techniques, especially in venous malformations. In arteriovenous (AV) malformations, a tourniquet is best applied at the beginning to expose the tissue and removed to permit Doppler examination after preparation of the fistulous area, as fistulae may be difficult to recognize during ischemia [8].

Microscope

CVMs often enclose nerves and a direct approach may be difficult and risky. In these cases microsurgical techniques permit neurovascular pedicles to be isolated with extreme precision, following their course inside the vascular lesion. The resulting dissection is then much more precise and not only permits the integrity of the nerves to be respected but also can be used as a guide during the dissection of CVM (Figs. 44.1c and 44.6b).

This technique lengthens surgery time but allows a precise dissection which is essential in difficult cases [8].

Tissue Involvement: Clinical Pictures and Surgical Treatment

One of the main challenges in this surgery is the involvement of the surrounding structures, such as the bones, nerves, muscles, tendons, ligaments, and skin. CVM inside tissues may cause infiltration or compression [9, 10].

Skin Involvement

In venous CVM, the skin is thinned by compression. A subdermal dissection is possible, preserving skin flaps and reducing bleeding ("skin-sparing technique") (Figs. 44.1, 44.2, 44.3, 44.4, 44.5, 44.6, and 44.7) [10, 11].

In AV CVM, the subcutaneous tissue is involved, and the skin is damaged by ischemia or direct infiltration.

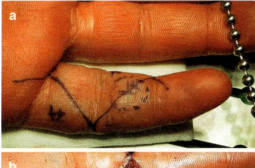
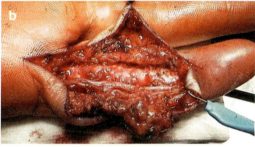

Fig. 44.2 Arteriovenous malformation in the volar aspect of the little finger. (**a**) Two fistulous areas detected guided by the choice of a Brunner incision. (**b**) The neurovascular bundles used as a guide for the dissection of the malformed tissue. Tourniquet and microscope control reduced bleeding and resulted in a safe radical excision

In lymphatic CVM, the subcutaneous tissue is firmly infiltrated, and the fatty tissue is hypertrophic.

The best procedure is an en bloc resection of the CVM after a precise skin drawing of the involved areas with a correct orientation of the final scars, which is the main procedure (Fig. 44.4).

However, the involvement of other tissues is the main challenge in the surgical treatment of CVM of the hand: the most difficult to treat are the bones and nerves. Tendons are seldom affected, while the synovia and muscles are commonly involved.

Bone Involvement

The bones can be affected in venous, AV, and also lymphatic CVM.

Standard radiograms are the best diagnostic methods and should be always performed before surgery of CVMs (Figs. 44.1b and 44.5a).

Percutaneous direct bone puncture and intraosseous pathological vessel occlusion by ethanol or

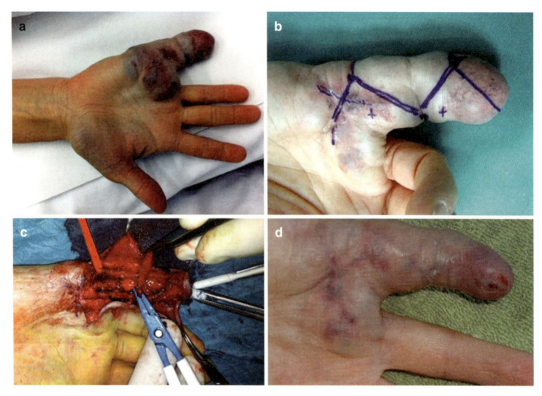

Fig. 44.3 Venous malformation in the palm and little finger. (**a**) Deformity of the involved area with the skin apparently damaged. (**b**) Skin incision of the second operation (the first was performed in the palm). Note the aspect of the skin after tourniquet inflation. (**c**) Excision of malformed tissue after isolation of neurovascular bundles. (**d**) Early result shows good wound healing

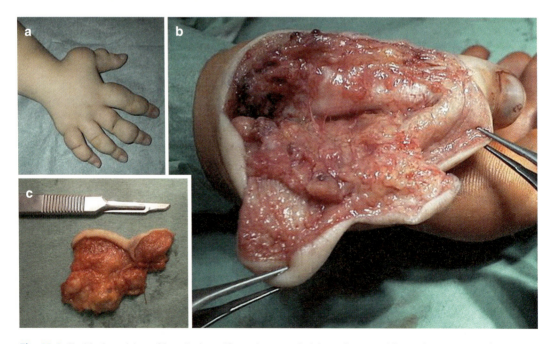

Fig. 44.4 En block excision of lymphatic malformation in the thumb of a young girl. (**a**) Clinical picture. (**b**) Radical resection of a planned segment of the skin and underlying hypertrophic subcutaneous tissue. (**c**) Specimen of the removed tissue

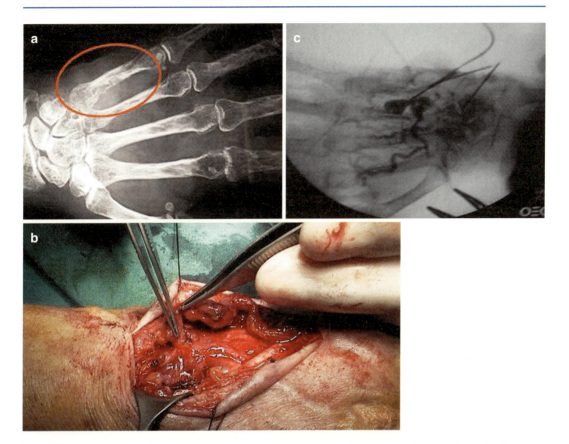

Fig. 44.5 Arteriovenous malformation with intraosseous fistulae. (**a**) Radiogram shows the extent and site of bone involvement. (**b**) Subcutaneous AV fistulae have been removed and communicating vessels to the bone are clearly seen. (**c**) Direct alcoholization of bone fistulae reduced the malformed tissue in a few minutes

glue injection seem to be the best treatment. In many cases, these procedures should be performed before surgery (Fig. 44.5) [10].

Nerves

Nerves may be surrounded or infiltrated by CVM. The main dilemma is to choose between resection of the surrounding malformed vessels only and to extend surgery inside the nerve. In our experience external decompression should be the first procedure used to reduce symptoms (Figs. 44.1c, 44.2b, and 44.6).

Internal, interfascicular neurolysis is a risky procedure and may lead to irreversible nerve damage, immediately or later as a result of scarring. Selective resection and nerve grafting should be the final option, performed only in case of severe pain and after failure of external resection of CVMs.

In case of nerve damage during surgery, immediate repair by suture or graft should be performed. To prevent damage, the best procedure is to follow the nerves as a guide through the malformation starting from a noninvolved area (Figs. 44.1c and 44.2). Direct approach can be risky [10].

Muscles

Total resection of expendable muscles is a common procedure, especially when they are extensively infiltrated. Partial resection of an important muscle or a group of muscles is also possible according to the severity of infiltration and the possibility of maintaining or restoring function. Non-resectable infiltrated muscles can be treated by foam sclerotherapy, direct alcohol injection, or echo-guided laser therapy [10, 11].

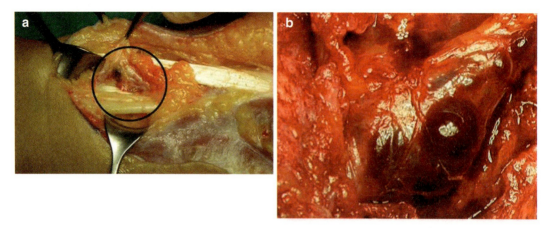

Fig. 44.6 Arteriovenous malformation involving nerves in the forearm. (**a**) External compression of the median nerve in the proximal forearm. (**b**) AV fistulae infiltrating the epineurium of the median nerve near the wrist

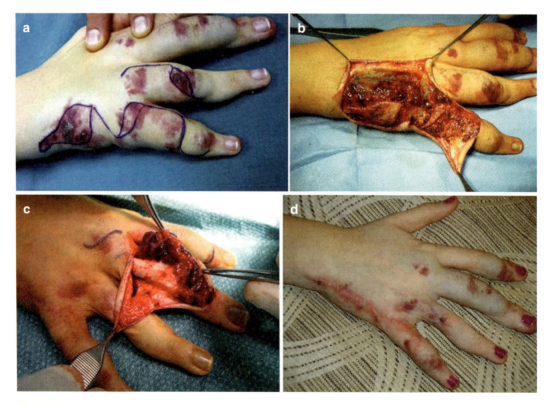

Fig. 44.7 Multistage excision of venous malformation. (**a**) Drawing of incisions includes excision of infiltrated areas. (**b**) First operation on the little finger and hand. (**c**) Second operation in the fourth finger. (**d**) Result at 1 year after last operation

Tendons

Tendons are generally not involved directly by CVMs. However tendon sheets are frequently invaded; synovectomy is a safe and effective operation (Fig. 44.8). Attention must be paid to important structures like pulleys of flexor tendons and complex extensor digital system [10].

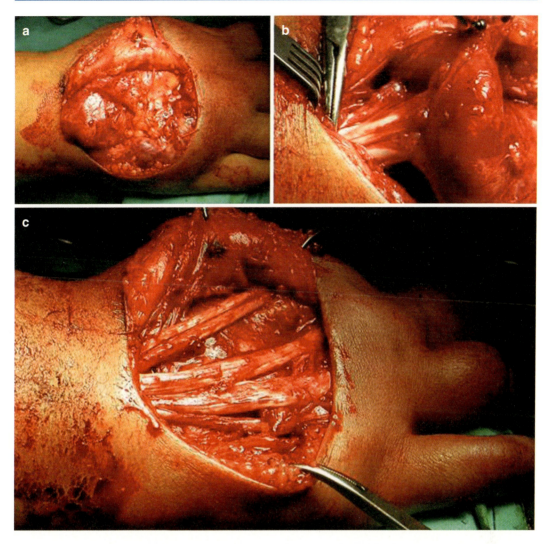

Fig. 44.8 Lympho-venous malformation in the dorsal aspect of the hand. (**a**) Malformed tissue well delimited within the tendon sheet permits an easy skin undermining. (**b-c**) Limited invasion of the tendons allows to perform a synovectomy with minimal bleeding

Results of Surgery

The extreme variability of vascular anomalies does not allow establishing comparable evaluation parameters. It is a difficult surgery and requires experience and multidisciplinary collaboration. The need for multiple operations is common. Recurrences are frequent in infiltrating venous and lymphatic CVMs, while in AVM they can appear suddenly as a consequence of opening of silent fistulae; the rate is different between the limited and infiltrating ones.

Results of treatment are considered good if there is a clinical and functional improvement, pain is reduced or absent, and major complications are avoided.

In our experience on 90 patients operated in the last 26 years, corresponding to 262 surgical procedures (Table 44.1), after long and sometimes difficult hemostasis, in no case did we observed postoperative bleeding or hematomas. In no case were plastic reconstructive procedures, flaps, or grafts necessary. Amputation of a finger was unavoidable in four cases of necrosis in AVM patients.

Table 44.1 Casuistic

Type of VM	
Venous	41
Arteriovenous	36
Lymphatic	13
Sex	
Male	46 %
Female	54 %
Age	
Median age	29.9
Age range	7–61
Site	
Fingers	65 %
Hand	28 %
Wrist	13 %

Our results confirm that, in the hand, surgery is more safe than sclerotherapy or embolization [12].

Conclusion

Surgical treatment of CVM of the hand is feasible. If properly planned, it can be effective and safe. A multistage and multidisciplinary approach is recommended. Some technical devices like the microscope and tourniquet can be used. Both devices allow a bloodless and accurate dissection of malformed tissues to be performed, particularly in the treatment of venous anomalies, which are the most common CVMs. The nerves can be used as a guide for dissection of CVMs, and the skin can be saved by a careful subdermal undermining.

Tissue involvement of VM is a major problem in the hand. The more difficult challenge is the infiltration of the nerves and bones. For the nerves, external neurolysis is our first choice; for the bones, direct sclerotherapy is useful. Muscles are frequently involved and can be totally resected if judged expendably. The tendons are seldom affected, but the synovial sheet is quite often involved and can easily be removed.

References

1. Levame J-H, Durafourg MP (1987) Reeducation des traumatises de la main. Maloine, Paris
2. Belov S (1989) Classification, terminology and nosology of congenital vascular defects. In: Belov S, Loose DA, Weber J (eds) Vascular malformations. Einhorn-Presse Verlag, Reinbeck, pp 25–30
3. Belov S, Loose DA (1990) Surgical treatment of congenital vascular defects. Int Angiol 9:175–182
4. Mattassi R (1993) Differential diagnosis in congenital vascular-bone syndromes. Semi Vasc Surg 6(4):233
5. Mattassi R (1993) Diagnosis and treatment of venous malformations of the lower limbs. In: Mattassi R (ed) Proceedings of the international conference on vascular surgery. Beijing, China, 21–24 October, 1993. International Academic Publishers, p 397
6. Lee BB, Do YS, Yakes W, Kim DI, Mattassi R, Hyon WS (2004) Management of arteriovenous malformations: a multidisciplinary approach. J Vasc Surg 39(3):590–600
7. Lee BB (2002) Advanced management of congenital vascular malformations (CVM). Int Angiolog 21(3):209–213
8. Upton J, Coombs CJ, Mulliken JB, Burrows PE, Pap S (1999) Vascular malformations of the upper limb: a review of 270 patients. J Hand Surg 24A(5):1019–1035
9. Breugem CC, Maas M, Breugem SJM, Shaap GR, van der Horst CMAM (2003) Vascular malformations of the lower limb with osseous involvement. J Bone Loint Surg 85(3):399–405
10. Di Giuseppe P (2006) Le angiodisplasie venose della mano ed il coinvolgimento dei tessuti. Riv Chir Mano 43(2):102–105
11. Hein KD, Mulliken JB, Kozakewich HPW, Upton J, Burrows PE (2002) Venous malformations of skeletal muscle. Plast Reconstr Surg 110(7):1625–1635
12. Park UJ, Do YS, Park KB, Kim YW, Lee BB, Kim DI (2012) Treatment of arteriovenous malformations involving the hand. Ann Vasc Surg 26(5):643–648

Thorax Wall

45

Francesco Stillo and Giuseppe Bianchini

Introduction

Congenital vascular malformations (CVMs) of the thorax wall are relatively rare but highly disabling as they cause severe functional and aesthetic disorders [1].

In most cases, these malformations are extratruncular type and infiltrate the soft tissues of the chest wall. Truncular forms are more rarely observed, which induce significant hemodynamic alterations because they have a direct drainage into the central vessels.

The treatment of thoracic CVMs is extremely difficult and dangerous because these malformations are often very extensive and have sometimes close relationships with vital organs.

The aims of the treatment are the partial or complete regression of the malformation, the reduction or disappearance of clinical symptoms, and the functional rehabilitation.

The therapeutic strategy must be planned for each patient on the basis of the clinical and instrumental findings, with particular reference to the site, the morphology, the extent, and the

F. Stillo
Casa di Cura Guarnieri,
Center of Vascular Anomalies, Rome, Italy
e-mail: f.stillo47@gmail.it

G. Bianchini (✉)
Division of Vascular Surgery,
Istituto Dermopatico dell'Immacolata,
Center of Vascular Anomalies, Rome, Italy
e-mail: giuseppe_bianchini@yahoo.it

hemodynamics of the malformation. A complete diagnostic picture can be obtained by carrying out a duplex scan, an MRI, and a transcatheter or direct puncture angiography.

The treatment options are different in the various types of thorax vascular malformations: venous malformations (VMs), lymphatic malformations (LMs), and arteriovenous malformations (AVMs) [2].

Venous Malformations

Thoracic venous malformations (VMs) are located on the anterior, lateral, or posterior thorax wall. These malformations are congenital but may show a progressive volume increasing in children and young patients. VMs are usually very large and deep with diffuse involvement of the thoracic wall muscles such as intercostals, latissimus dorsi, and trapezium. Sometimes it is possible to observe a costal bone or pleuric involvement [3] (Fig. 45.1).

Surgery is the elective choice in small and superficial VMs, located on skin and subcutaneous tissue [4]. The excision should be done by microinvasive techniques, using if possible a spiral purse-string suture. When the malformation is very large, a double-stage approach is preferable, performing the implant of a skin expander in the first step and the removal of the malformation followed by plastic reconstruction in the second step. The best positioning of skin expanders

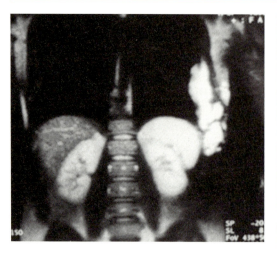

Fig. 45.1 Venous malformation of the thorax wall involving the pleura

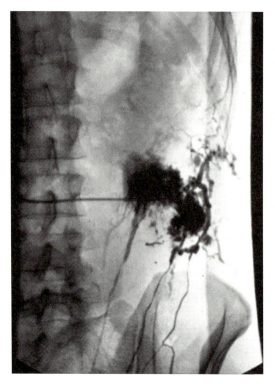

Fig. 45.2 Percutaneous sclerotherapy of a thoracic venous malformation

depends on the malformation site. In many cases, it is useful to implant the skin expander on the anterior abdominal or lumbar area, to perform a rotational flap after the exeresis of the thorax wall malformation.

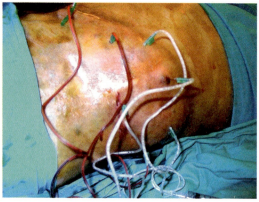

Fig. 45.3 Sclerotherapy of a chest wall venous malformation by multiple direct punctures

Sclerotherapy is useful in very extensive VMs with muscle or bone involvement, when a total surgical removal is impossible or dangerous [5]. It is recommendable to perform sclerotherapy under radioscopic guidance because these malformations often show a direct drainage in the azygos, hemiazygos, brachiocephalic, or superior cava veins. A preoperative direct puncture phlebography allows to confirm the needle position within the lesion and to evaluate the outflow veins. At this time, the scleroembolization is carried out injecting the sclerosing agent mixed with a contrast medium to control its spread within the vessels (Fig. 45.2).

Various sclerosing agents are commonly used. The choice will depend on the morphologic patterns, anatomical site, and extent of the malformation. For small-caliber VMs, it is possible to use 2–3 % polydocanol or 0.2–3 % sodium-tetradecyl-sulfate solution. For large-caliber VMs, it is preferable to use 95 % ethanol because a more powerful sclerosant is necessary. The dosage of the sclerosing agent will be established in proportion to the size of the malformation. The volume of contrast material required to fill the space is then used to estimate the quantity of sclerosant needed. Anyway, ethanol injected must not exceed a maximum dose of 2 ml/kg body weight. It is preferable to inject the sclerosant dose by multiple direct punctures of the malformation in different sites on the chest wall (Fig. 45.3). A low molecular weight heparin and steroid treatment is recommendable after sclerotherapy of thorax VMs in order to prevent thrombophlebitis, skin necrosis, or nerve damage.

A combined treatment is the preferred option in the majority of cases. The combination of percutaneous and surgical treatment offers the best clinical, morphological, and functional results. In cases of extensive thorax VMs, it is necessary to perform multiple sequential surgical or endovascular procedures to obtain a complete regression.

Lymphatic Malformations

Lymphatic malformations (LMs) of the chest wall are usually macrocystic extratruncular forms (cystic hygromas) arising from the subclavian or axillary regions. These malformations induce severe clinical symptoms because they are often very large and tend to gradually grow over the years, especially in concomitance with hormonal, traumatic, or infective events. Early treatment is recommendable to avoid the risk of a pleuric or mediastinal involvement with compression of vital structures such as trachea or central veins.

Surgical removal is considered the best cure for thorax LMs [6]. When the cystic sac is very large and deep with infiltration of muscle and peripheral nerves, it is very difficult to achieve a complete surgical excision. In these cases, it is possible to perform a multistaged surgical removal, so reducing the risk of hemorrhage or nerve injury.

Percutaneous sclerotherapy is accepted as safe and satisfactory treatment for LMs of the thorax wall, particularly in pediatric patients [7]. Intralesional injection of sclerosants is a low-invasive procedure which gives good clinical results with marked or complete shrinkage of the cystic mass and minimum recurrence (Fig. 45.4).

The size of the malformation dictates the choice of the sclerosing agent. Sodium-tetradecyl-sulfate solution is preferred for circumscribed forms. Ethanol is more effective in larger LMs of the thorax but induces a considerable risk of pleuric reactions or brachial plexus injuries. OK-432, bleomycin, doxycycline, and pingyangmycin are good alternative scleroagents

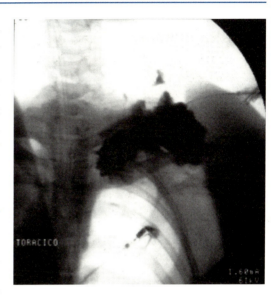

Fig. 45.4 Sclerotherapy of a macrocystic lymphatic malformation of the subclavian region

in these malformations, because they allow to achieve the mass shrinkage with a moderate inflammatory reaction.

Anyway, several sessions of sclerotherapy are required to obtain a complete reduction of the mass and to reduce complications or recurrence. In very large and deep lesions, it is useful to perform a percutaneous ultrasound-guided sclerotherapy. If possible, the sclerosing injection should be followed by a selective locoregional compression.

A combined treatment is very useful also in chest wall LMs. Intralesional sclerotherapy may be a preliminary treatment before performing the surgical excision of the lymphatic mass.

Arteriovenous Malformations

Arteriovenous malformations (AVMs) of the thorax wall take origin from the intercostal arteries or from the subclavian artery branches. The involvement of the thoracic wall muscles such as pectorals, intercostals, serratus, and latissimus dorsi is very frequent. In many cases, a costal bone infiltration is observed. These malformations are extremely dangerous because their natural history shows a fast growth and a high incidence of cardiac failure [8].

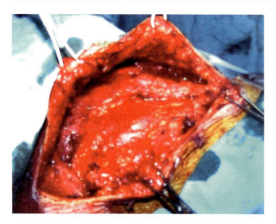

Fig. 45.5 Surgical excision of the nidus in a truncular arteriovenous malformation of the thorax wall

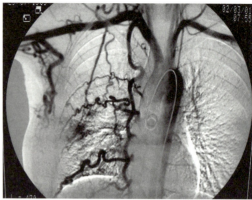

Fig. 45.6 Transcatheter embolization in an extratruncular arteriovenous malformation of the chest wall

For these reasons, the treatment of thorax AVMs is extremely difficult and controversial. Current international literature does not provide available scientific evidences in this field. Furthermore, an inappropriate therapy can be responsible for rapid growth of the malformation. The therapeutic strategy should be a multidisciplinary decision considering the type, extent, and localization of the malformation.

Surgery is indicated in truncular AVMs of the thoracic wall, especially in superficial and localized forms. Extensive ligation of all fistulas in the chest wall and skeletonization of the feeding arteries may obtain good early results but induce a high risk of late recurrence. Total excision of the nidus with surrounding soft tissues is recommendable when it is technically feasible (Fig. 45.5). A double-stage approach is also useful in these malformations, performing for the first time the implant of a skin expander to allow a more easy reconstruction in the second step. Surgery of thoracic AVMs leads to a very high risk of hemorrhage, because it is not possible to carry out an adequate intraoperative compression. For this reason, it is recommendable to perform a preliminary tissue infiltration by saline solutions and to achieve the control of bleeding by the use of autotransfusion system.

Endovascular treatments are preferred in extratruncular AVMs, particularly in deep, extensive, and infiltrating forms, using transcatheter or direct puncture techniques. The choice of different procedures or embolic materials depends on the anatomic configuration and hemodynamic patterns of the thorax AVMs [9].

Embolization of the afferent arteries by highly selective catheterization is a good choice in the AVMs showing a small number of large-caliber feeding arteries (Fig. 45.6). It is mandatory to release the sclerosing material directly into the nidus in order to prevent the recurrence of arteriovenous fistulas and to avoid the obliteration of normal vessels. The embolization of chest wall AVMs presents special problems related to inadvertent occlusion of important branches of the thoracic aorta, such as the spinal arteries with risk of paraplegia. In some cases, when the superselective catheterism is difficult or dangerous, it may be useful to perform a surgical access to the afferent arteries on the thoracic wall.

Retrograde venous sclerotherapy is an alternative way to treat the AVMs arising from multiple low-caliber feeding arteries, which are very frequent in the thorax wall and make the anterograde approach not feasible. The obliteration of dominant outflow veins is successfully obtained by direct puncture or transcatheter injection of the sclerosing agent. The vein occlusion using a balloon catheter may be helpful during the procedure.

Finally, when the malformation is superficial or easily accessible, it may be useful to perform the sclerosing treatment by direct puncture of the nidus.

Ethanol is certainly the most powerful and effective sclerosing agent. In fact, only ethanol is able to induce a permanent damage of the endothelium, which prevents the proliferation and recurrence especially in extratruncular forms. Polyvinyl alcohol and acrylic microspheres are solid agents useful to induce obliteration of the feeding arteries as pretreatment to surgery. N-butyl-2-cyanoacrylate glue and ethylene-vinyl-alcohol copolymer (Onyx) are fluid polymerizing materials which have been proposed in the last years for sclerosing treatment of chest wall AVMs. However, if on the one hand these agents give the advantage of a lower morbidity, on the other hand, they produce a higher rate of relapse in comparison to ethanol.

Endovascular treatments provide satisfactory early results with significant regression of the malformation and improvement of clinical features. However, the long-term follow-up shows a high recurrence rate. Furthermore, skin ulcerations and nerve injuries are relatively frequent complications in the scleroembolization of thorax wall AVMs.

A combined treatment is recommendable to improve the clinical outcome and to reduce morbidity and recurrence rate. In many cases, the scleroembolization should be a preliminary procedure to reduce the blood flow before subsequent surgical removal. Anyway, the most appropriate therapeutic strategy should be always based on clinical and instrumental picture of each individual case.

References

1. Maldonado JA, Henry T, Gutiérrez FR (2010) Congenital thoracic vascular anomalies. Radiol Clin North Am 48(1):85–115
2. Arneja JS, Gosain AK (2006) An approach to the management of common vascular malformations of the trunk. J Craniofac Surg 17(4):761–766
3. Demos TC, Posniak HV, Pierce KL, Olson MC, Muscato M (2004) Venous anomalies of the thorax. AJR Am J Roentgenol 182(5):1139–1150
4. Bianchini G, Nicodemi EM, Stillo F (2003) Thoraco-abdominal venous malformations: diagnostic and therapeutic strategies. Int Angiol 22(2 Suppl 1):69
5. Agus GB, Allegra C, Antignani PL, Arpaia G, Bianchini G, Bonadeo P, Botta G, Castaldi A, Gasbarro V, Genovese G, Georgiev M, Mancini S, Stillo F (2005) Guidelines for the diagnosis and therapy of the vein and lymphatic disorders. Int Angiol 24(2):107–168
6. Daya SK, Gowda RM, Gowda MR, Khan IA (2004) Thoracic cystic lymphangioma (cystic hygroma): a chest pain syndrome. Angiology 55(5):561–564
7. Kadota Y, Utsumi T, Kawamura T, Inoue M, Sawabata N, Minami M, Okumura M (2011) Lymphatic and venous malformation or "lymphangiohemangioma" of the anterior mediastinum: case report and literature review. Gen Thorac Cardiovasc Surg 59(8):575–578
8. Itano H, Lee S, Kulick DM, Iannettoni MD, Williams DM, Orringer MB (2005) Nontraumatic chest wall systemic-to-pulmonary artery fistula. Ann Thorac Surg 79(5):e29–e31
9. Uchida Y, Kawano H, Koide Y, Toda G, Yano K (2003) Arteriovenous fistula of internal thoracic vessels. Intern Med 42(10):987–990

Vascular Malformations in the Viscera

46

Nader Ghaffarpour

Introduction

Vascular malformations in connection with the digestive system may be diagnosed at any age. They may present with bleeding, anemia, protein deficiency, or if they form a mass lesion, with intussusceptions or mass effect on surrounding organs and functions. Many lesions remain asymptomatic. In a minority of patients, there are well-defined genetic conditions present, such as hereditary hemorrhagic telangiectasia (Mb Rendu-Osler). Vascular malformations may affect any section of the gastrointestinal tract, and occasionally there are vascular anomalies elsewhere, particularly in the skin.

Clinical Aspects

The patients with vascular malformation in the viscera are a heterogeneous group. They represent everything from the prenatally diagnosed infant with hydrops of the fetus to the elderly patient with an occult bleeding.

When confronted with a patient with vascular malformation in the viscera, some questions rises and must be addressed:

N. Ghaffarpour, MD
Department of Pediatric Surgery Q3:03,
Astrid Lindgren Children's Hospital,
Karolinska University Hospital,
Stockholm, Sweden
e-mail: nader.ghaffarpour@karolinska.se

1. What structures do the anomaly consist of?
   (a) The malformation may consist of venous, lymphatic, and arterial structures or a combination of all.
2. Is the malformation a high-flow or low-flow lesion?
   (a) High-flow malformation has AV shunts; the low-flow malformations are either venous or lymphatic.
3. What anatomical structures/ organs are involved?
   (a) The expansion of the malformation may compromise vital adjacent anatomical structures.
4. Is there evidence of impaired vital functions due to the malformation?
   (a) Obstruction of renal outlet, compression to central circulation, or in the infant it may impair the pulmonary function due to high abdominal pressure.
5. Do the clinical presentation require tissue sampling or biochemistry to make the accurate diagnosis?
   (a) If on imaging, there are solid tissue components the clinician must consider tissue sampling in order to rule out malignancies.
   (b) In large intra-abdominal cysts surrounding the viscera particularly in neonates, it may require biochemistry from cyst contents to rule out pseudo cysts from visceral organs, i.e., urinoma, ruptured choledochal cysts or pancreatic pseudo cysts.

6. Do the malformation bleed or is it loosing proteins?

  (a) Bleeding is a common sign of venous malformation, and protein deficiency may be associated with visceral lymphatic malformation.

Investigation Modalities

MRI

MRI is more sensitive than CT in detecting both venous and lymphatic malformations and their imaging manifestations such as bowel wall thickening, fat infiltration, dilated veins and associated soft-tissue masses, size of cysts in lymphatic malformations, and the expansion in to surrounding tissues.

Nuclear Scintigraphy

Nuclear scintigraphy can be useful to detect a venous or arterial malformation or to demonstrate a bleeding site. However, it cannot differentiate the various types of vascular anomalies nor differentiate to other bleeding causes such as bleeding from Meckel's diverticulum. It may be useful to confirm abnormal dilated lymphatic channels in the abdomen. The overall use of nuclear scintigraphy is limited in the investigation on visceral vascular malformations.

Angiography

Angiography is an invasive diagnostic modality that provides a treatment option by superselective microcoil embolization for the treatment of GI hemorrhage. The treatment by embolization is useful in AV shunts to the GI tract. Post embolization necrosis of the intestines is a risk and often this intervention is done as a presurgical procedure. Selective angiography is the most useful examination to establish the nature and extension of GI vascular anomalies.

Endoscopy: Esophagogastroduodenoscopy and Colonoscopy

Endoscopy: Esophagogastroduodenoscopy and colonoscopy are used for diagnosing vascular anomalies in the upper GI and lower GI tracts. In the upper and lower GI tract, these modalities provide both diagnostic and therapeutic solutions. The therapeutic solutions consist of local treatment with laser, heat coagulation or sclerotherapy. However, its role is limited in small-bowel venous malformation.

To be able to visualize the small intestine, intraoperative push-enteroscopy and balloon enteroscopy are the modalities if samples are required or if endoscopic intervention is aimed.

Wireless Capsule Endoscopy

Wireless capsule endoscopy is a noninvasive diagnostic technique with no radiation that involves the ingestion of a small video camera by the patient. Its advantage is the ability to detect mucosal involvement in small-bowel abnormalities. This technique is useful for obscure GI bleeding and in protein loosing enteropathy.

Diagnostic Laparoscopy

Diagnostic laparoscopy is a minimal invasive procedure that provides excellent access for differential diagnostics such as bleeding from Meckel's diverticulum and also provides the option of definitive surgical treatment.

Venous Malformations of the Viscera

Venous malformations are more common in the viscera than vascular tumors, i.e., hemangiomas. In the literature and in clinical practice, venous malformations in the GI tract are incorrectly often described as cavernous hemangiomas, angiodysplasias, or polyps. Patients with GI venous malformation often present with recurrent GI bleeding. Often the symptoms are rather iron-deficiency anemia than large GI bleeding. Intussusceptions and GI tract obstruction are much less common presentations although it may occur. Venous malformations can involve any portion of the GI tract. Careful clinical examination is necessary to uncover associated cutaneous or morphological anomalies such as in blue rubber bleb nevus syndrome (BRBNS) and Klippel-Trénaunay syndrome (KTS).

Venous malformations are vascular malformations of slow-flow; thus, it is associated with intralesional clotting and the formation of thrombophlebitis.

In more extensive venous malformations, the ongoing clotting within the malformation leads to consumption coagulopathy with a consumption of fibrinogen, platelets, and trombocytes ((LIC) Localized intravascular coagulopathy). This will add to the risk of bleedings from the intestinal lesions.

Blue Rubber Bleb Nevus Syndrome

Blue rubber bleb nevus syndrome (BRBNS) is a rare vascular anomaly syndrome consisting of multifocal venous malformations. The malformations are most prominent in the skin, soft tissues, and gastrointestinal tract but may occur in any tissue. The cutaneous lesions of BRBNS are generally small, measuring less than 1–2 cm, and blue to purple in color. At palpation, they have rubbery sensation. A common site is the sole of the feet (Fig. 46.1). A patient may have from several to hundreds of cutaneous and GI lesions [3].

Clinical Presentation

Patients usually exhibit GI bleeding at an early age that continues throughout their life. Massive sudden hemorrhage rarely occurs. Patients typically present with iron-deficiency anemia with the presence of blood in stool. They require lifelong iron replacement and repeated blood transfusions [3].

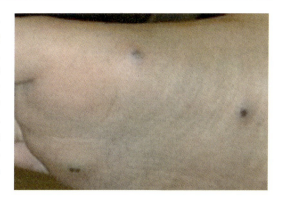

Fig. 46.1 Characteristic venous malformations on the sole of the foot of a blue rubber bleb nevus syndrome (BRBNS) patient. This skin manifestation on the sole of the foot is pathognomonic for BRBNS

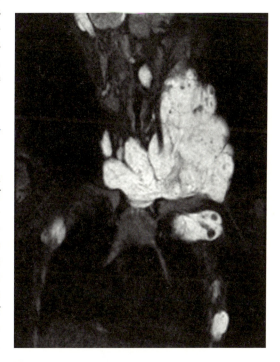

Fig. 46.2 BRBNS patient with a large venous malformation in the neck as the primary lesion. On MRI the muscle infiltrative VM is evident with multiple intralesional thrombophlebitis

Occasionally patients also present with a large primary lesion. The primary lesion consists of a large venous malformation (Fig. 46.2).

Patients with massive presence of VM at any location are associated with the risk of Localized intravascular coagulopathy (LIC). These patients are at risk of local pain due to thrombosis in the venous malformations and the formation of phlebolithes.

LIC leads to a consumption coagulopathy with consumption of fibrinogen, platelets, and thrombocytes due to ongoing clotting within the malformations.

Patients with elevated D-dimer levels associated with low fibrinogen levels (severe LIC) have a high risk of hemorrhage, and if GI lesions are present, bleedings from them increase [4].

Investigation

Patients with BRBNS do not differ from other patients presenting with iron-deficiency anemia with the presence of blood in the stool.

The investigation starts with an esophagogastroduodenoscopy and coloscopy.

If the clinical picture is mild, a wireless capsule endoscopy can be performed in order to investigate the small intestines.

Clinical presentation with typical skin lesions for BRBNS (Fig. 46.1) and iron-deficiency anemia with the presence of blood in stool require an investigation with diagnostic laparoscopy. The diagnostic laparoscopy will confirm the presence of venous lesions prior to converting to open surgery and also will rule out other more common bleeding sources in this age group such as Meckel's diverticulum.

The investigation of the small intestines is carried out with a push-enteroscopy where small incisions are made in the intestines and a sterile laparoscopic camera or a flexible gastro scope is inserted in the bowel and pushed through.

All patients are analyzed for coagulopathy. When there is evidence of LIC or severe LIC it is likely to be correlated with high presence of VM in the GI tract and often also a large primary lesion.

Treatment

The management of patients with BRBNS is built on several factors. Pharmacological treatment and aggressive surgical removals of lesions in the GI tract with multiple local resections will keep the patient free from bleeding. The management consists of extensive intestinal surgery with local excisions up to several hundred in one patient [3]. However the management also requires surgery or intervention to reduce the primary lesion.

If the lesions are within the reach of endoscopes, the treatment can be performed with endoscopic argon diathermia [11] (Fig. 46.3b, c).

Patients with high D-dimers as a sign of severe LIC and a presence of a large primary venous malformation must be treated with the aim to lower the overall presence of venous malformation. In these cases, the surgery and/or intervention is not limited to the GI tract but also to the primary venous malformation, in order to have less intralesional coagulation that causes LIC.

However BRBNS patients with severe LIC and ongoing bleedings that cannot be managed surgically or interventional are candidates for anticoagulation with low molecular heparin [4].

In addition to surgical and interventional treatment in severe cases of BRBNS with bleeding, there are some resent reports of the use of the immunosuppressant drug sirolimus also known as rapamycin that may be useful [2].

Klippel-Trénaunay Syndrome, GI Tract Aspects

Klippel-Trénaunay syndrome is a triad that consists of the following: (a) cutaneous port-wine capillary malformation, (b) mixed venous and lymphatic anomalies, and (c) hypertrophy of a limb.

The lower limbs are more commonly affected often with pelvic extension. This syndrome is present at birth, but progression of venous anomalies and limb hypertrophy is observed during growth. GI involvement in Klippel-Trénaunay syndrome due to the pelvic extension of both venous and lymphatic malformation usually takes place in the colorectal area. The lymphatic extension may expand in the pelvis and press on anatomical structures such as the bladder and the rectum. Treatments of these lesions are planned according to the symptoms that they cause. The venous malformation in the GI tract is often

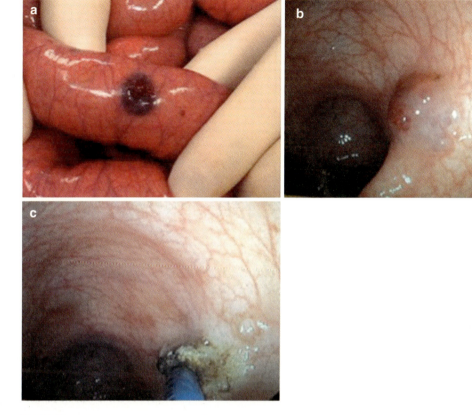

Fig. 46.3 (**a**) Intestines with venous malformation associated with BRBNS. (**b**) Endoscopic view of venous malformation associated with BRBNS. (**c**) Endoscopic APC (Argon Plasma Coagulation) of venous malformation associated with BRBNS

present as dilated submucosal veins and occasionally causes GI bleedings (Figs. 46.4, 46.5, and 46.6).

Patients with KTS in accordance to other patients with massive presence of VM such as patients with BRBNS also often have high D-dimers associated with low fibrinogen as an evidence of LIC.

High venous congestion in the affected limb and high D-dimers as an evidence of severe LIC is correlated to high risk of bleeding from the vascular lesions including the VMs present in the GI tract.

Treatment Aspects

KTS patients with venous malformations involving the GI tract can be treated locally with endoscopic sclerotherapy to the dilated submucosal veins. This will stop ongoing bleedings (Fig. 46.6). Resection of rectum is rarely indicated; thus, if there is severe bleeding with no possibility of medical treatment or surgical stepwise intervention, resection may be mandated [5].

The presence of large ecstatic veins surrounding the rectum that are in connection with the inferior mesenteric vein is a significant risk factor of pulmonary embolism (PE). In such case, interventional coiling or surgery is mandated to prevent PE.

The main treatment strategy however in the management of KTS patients with GI tract involvement is to lower the tissue congestion in the patients affected limb in order to lower the risk of consumption coagulopathy and thus to lower the venous pressure. Both these

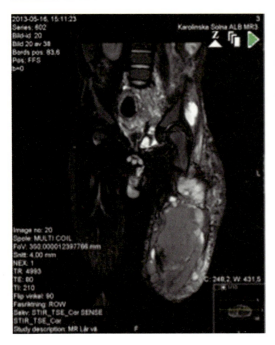

Fig. 46.4 MRI shows pelvic expansion of lymphatic and venous malformation in a patient with KTS

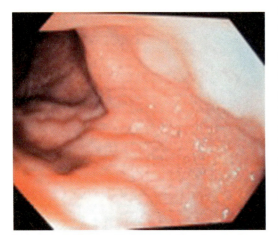

Fig. 46.5 Endoscopic view, dilated submucosal veins in patient with KTS

aspects will lower the risk of bleedings and thromboembolism.

In KTS patients with high risk of PE and evidence of consumption coagulopathy with severe LIC should be considered antithrombotic therapy with low molecular heparin [4].

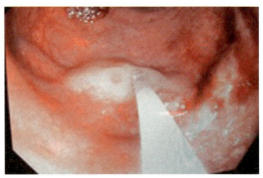

Fig. 46.6 Endoscopic sclerotherapy with microfoam in the rectum on a KTS patient with bleeding from dilated hypertensive veins

Lymphatic Malformations in the Viscera

Lymphatic malformations (LM) are defined as structural defects that occur because of defective lymphangiogenesis [6]. They may expand in the tissue with large cystic components (macrocystic LM) or infiltrative with small cysts (microcystic LM).

Histologically, LMs are benign lesions, but because of their localization and their size they can cause serious complications, i.e., compromise to vital anatomical structures. The incidence of abdominal lymphatic malformations is unknown; however, 75 % of all LMs occur in the head and neck region and the visceral LMs account for from 3 to 9 % of all pediatric LMs. LM recurrently get infected or inflamed causing peritonitis, pain, and septicemia. A sudden swelling within the malformation may also cause compromise to adjacent vital anatomical structures and functions [12].

Clinical Presentation

The majority of patients with LM in the viscera present in childhood. Abdominal cystic LM arise from the mesentery (59–68 %) (Fig. 46.7), omentum (20–27 %) (Fig. 46.8), and retroperitoneum (12–14 %) (Fig. 46.9) [13, 14].

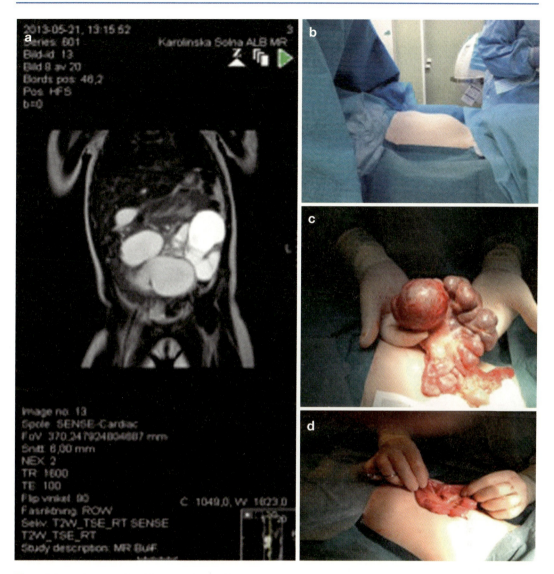

Fig. 46.7 A six-year-old girl, 1 week vomiting, and abdominal distension. Last days increasing abdominal pain and fever. (**a**) MRI showing mainly large cysts intra abdominally. (**b**) Preoperative view showing abdominal distention. (**c**) Operative view showing visceral LM involving the mesentery of a limited part of the small intestine. (**d**) End-to-end anastomoses after resection of 25 cm affected bowel with lymphatic malformation in the mesentery

Most cases of visceral LM are asymptomatic. However, patients may occasionally present with acute abdomen because of an intestinal obstruction or peritonitis caused by infected cysts, hemorrhaging, and/ or torsion or sudden distention of the abdomen with signs of compromise in adjacent organ functions.

The clinical presentation may also be more diffuse such as hypoproteinemia and failure to thrive due to chylus and protein-losing enteropathy such as in microcystic LM involving the mesentery or the mucosa of the bowel as in primary intestinal lymphectasia (PIL or mb Waldmann) [1] (Fig. 46.10).

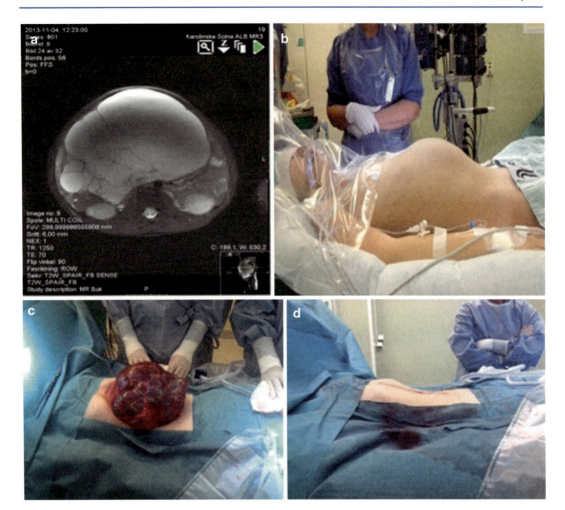

Fig. 46.8 An eleven-year-old girl previously healthy. One month history of gradually increasing abdominal circumference. Last 3 days dramatic distention of the abdomen and pain. Inflammatory signs elevated in serum. (**a**) Shows MRI findings with huge cystic expansion in the abdomen compromising the abdominal cavity. (**b**) Preoperative distention of the abdomen. (**c**) Huge cystic LM involving the lesser omentum (**d**) Postoperative view after resection

Lymphatic leakage into the intestinal lumen results in the hypoalbuminemia and lymphopenia, and the edema is a consequence of the hypoproteinemia, decreasing intravascular oncotic pressures.

A diagnostic challenge is to differentiate visceral macrocystic LMs from other asymptomatic abdominal cystic masses such as cystic teratomas (Fig. 46.11), mucinous cystadenomas (intestinal duplications), bronchogenic cysts, ovarian cysts, and pseudocysts, i.e., ruptured choledochal cyst (Fig. 46.12), ruptured pancreatic cysts, and urinoma (Fig. 46.13).

Investigation and Treatment

Ultrasound is a good screening modality, but in order to plan for treatment, a CT or MRI is required to investigate the extension of the malformation and the relationship to adjacent organs.

Prior to surgery or intervention, it is important to rule out differential diagnoses that may mimic the findings in imaging.

Laboratory work-up includes: Complete blood count, electrolytes, liver function tests, total Serum protein, Serum albumin and Serum triglycerids. AFP, hCG, CEA and CA-125 are the

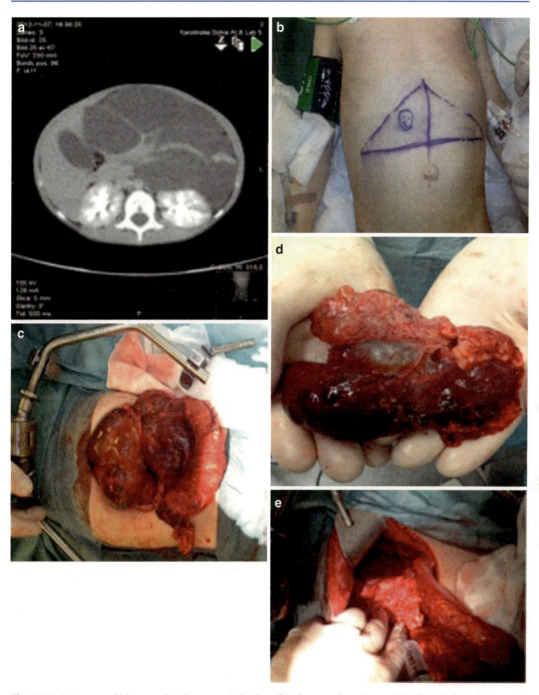

Fig. 46.9 A ten-year-old boy smaller than expected, −2 SD. Last month gradually distention of the abdomen. Last week aggravating symptoms with abdominal pain, peritonitis, fever, and respiratory distress. (**a**) MRI showing large retroperitoneal cystic LM surrounding the pancreas. (**b**) Preoperative view with distended abdomen. (**c**) Operative view with cystic LM expanding in the omental bursa. (**d**) Operative resection. (**e**) Intraoperative OK-432 sclerotherapy in the margins of the resection

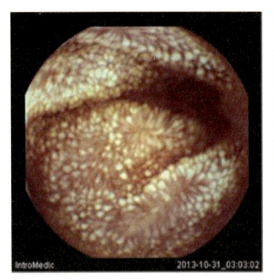

Fig. 46.10 Image from a wireless endoscope showing villi with characteristic lymphectasias associated with PIL (With permission from dr Charlotte Höög, Gastroenterologist Karolinska University Hospital)

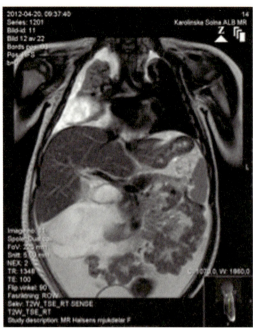

Fig. 46.12 Case of an infant with sudden abdominal distension and acute peritonitis. Initially suspected visceral LM. Evidence of bilirubin in the ascites liquid led to the accurate diagnose of ruptured choledochal cyst

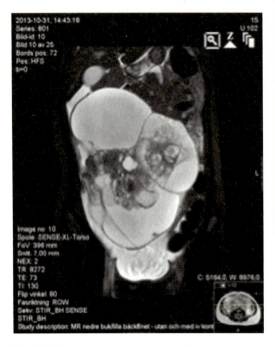

Fig. 46.11 Cystic teratoma (germ cell cancer) mimics visceral cystic LM

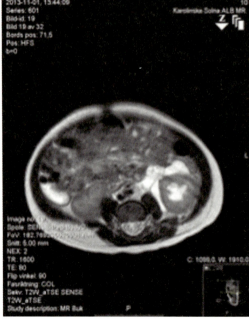

Fig. 46.13 Antenatal recognized hydronephrosis and suspected urinoma. Postnatal showed to be a retroperitoneal LM with compromise of the urethro-pelvic junction

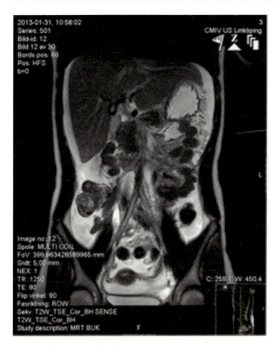

Fig. 46.14 An eighteen-year-old girl with recurrent abdominal swelling and pain on MRI with chylus ascites and microcystic LM in the mesentery

tumor markers which must be investigated for differential diagnoses.

FNAC from the cysts is used for cytology and chemical analysis to rule out pseudocysts such as urinoma (creatinine in cyst), ruptured choledocus cyst (bilirubin in cyst), and ruptured pancreatic cyst (amylase in cyst)

In cases of chylus ascites (evidence of chylomicrons in ascites) and MRI findings suggesting microcystic visceral LM, it may be mandated to further investigation with laparoscopy or open examination of the mesentery in order to visualize a lymphatic leak in to the abdominal cavity and thus evaluate the possibility to surgically close the lymphatic fistula or resect the affected mesentery (Fig. 46.14).

Children with failure to thrive or patients with protein-losing enteropathies may suffer from primary intestinal lymphectasia (PIL), a rare cause of protein-losing enteropathy, first described by Waldmann et al. [1]. PIL is according to LM classification a microcystic LM affecting the mucosa of the intestines.

PIL is investigated with endoscopies including wireless capsule endoscopy. If evidence of

limited intestinal involvement is made with signs of mucosal lymphatic leaks, a resection of affected bowel may be curable. However, the mainstay of treatment is a lifelong low-fat, high-protein diet supplemented with medium-chain triglycerides that, upon absorption, bypass the lymphatic system and directly enter the portal system, preventing engorgement of the lymphatic vessels of the intestines [1].

Cystic visceral LM may be treated with sclerotherapy. Several authors show evidence that OK-432 sclerotherapy is a safe and effective method and is suggested to be the first-line treatment for LMs. [9, 10]. However in the visceral LMs, OK-432 may be at some points hazardous to use due to additional swelling that the treatment causes. Other sclerosants such as doxycycline has been used in abdominal and retroperitoneal LMs [7]. Doxycycline gives less swelling; it is safe and may have a sclerosing effect [7].

Treatment Aspects for Cystic LM in the Viscera

Sclerotherapy:
> *OK-432*: if tolerated, gives additional swelling and may be hazardous
> *Doxycycline*: gives less swelling but also less chance of success

Surgery:
> *Elective surgery*:
>> Peritonitis caused by infection
>> Intracystic hemorrhage
>> Accelerated enlargement of cysts
> *Emergency surgery*:
>> Intestinal obstruction or volvulus
>> Torsion of cysts
>> Compromise of urinary tract or other vital functions

Watchful waiting:
> Visceral LM found as a secondary finding

In conclusion, it is necessary to deal with abdominal LMs on the basis of their symptoms. Emergency surgery should be considered for such pathological conditions as intestinal obstruction, volvulus, torsion of the cysts, rupture of the infected cyst, or obstruction of the urinary tract. In contrast, elective surgery may be acceptable after

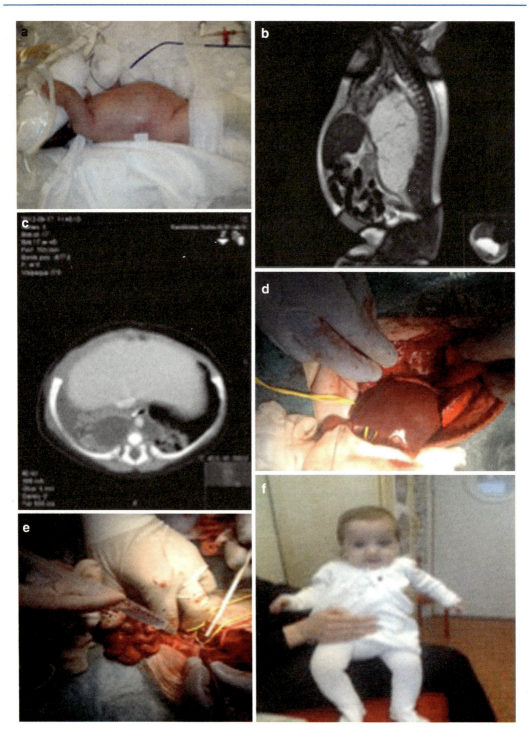

Fig. 46.15 Neonatal girl with respiratory distress, no possibility to wean of mechanical ventilation, high-pressure ventilation in spite of tube drainage of the malformation. (**a**) Preoperative view showing abdominal distention due to the retroperitoneal LM. (**b**) MRI showing huge prevertebral retroperitoneal LM. The malformation compressing the lung and preventing proper lung expansion, shifting the inferior vena cava anteriorly and compromising preload circulation. (**c**) CT follow-up after 9 sessions of doxycycline sclerotherapy. Due to risk of additional swelling, OK-432 sclerotherapy was not used preoperatively. (**d**) Retropleural and retroperitoneal debulking of the LM. (**e**) Intraoperative sclerotherapy with OK-432 after debulking surgery. (**f**) 3 weeks postoperatively, the baby was off mechanical ventilation; here on follow up in outpatient clinic 6 months postoperatively

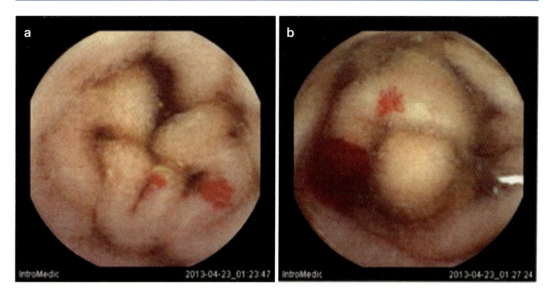

Fig. 46.16 Image from a wireless endoscope (**a**) showing HHT lesions in the bowel (**b**) showing ongoing bleeding from HHT lesions (With permission from dr Charlotte Höög, Gastroenterologist Karolinska university Hospital)

subsidence of symptoms by conservative therapy in cases of peritonitis caused by infection, intracystic hemorrhage, and an accelerated enlargement of the cysts, unless an intolerable condition occurs.

Since LMs are benign tumors, under these selective conditions a function-preserving operation is thus preferable to avoid any subsequent complications. After debulking surgery, intraoperative sclerotherapy is a safe option when radical resection is not possible.

It is important not to overlook the possible lethal complications such as intestinal and/or urological obstruction, aggressive peritonitis, and torsion of the cyst, which require emergency surgery. In neonates, increased abdominal pressure and the cystic expansion of the LM affect adjacent organ functions; thus emergency surgical debulking may be mandated (Fig. 46.15) [8].

Arteriovenous Malformations, GI Aspects

Arteriovenous malformations (AVMs) are abnormal communications between arteries and veins, bypassing the normal capillary bed. AVMs in the GI tract can be isolated as a result of an infection, trauma, and idiopathic or as a result of arterial surgery in the abdomen or retroperitoneum [15]. However, arterio-

venous shunts may also be associated with hereditary hemorrhagic telangiectasia (HHT).

HHT known as well as Rendu-Osler syndrome (mb Osler) is autosomal dominant inheritance disease with the worldwide prevalence of 1 case per 5,000–10,000 population and defines as follows: (a) diffuse malformation of the capillary system; (b) mucosal telangiectasia involving the nasopharynx, the GI tract, and sometimes the urinary and genital mucosa; (c) arteriovenous fistulas and arterial aneurysms involving the pulmonary, hepatic, and digestive arteries; and (d) high-flow intestinal arteriovenous fistula that can lead to portal hypertension and cirrhosis [16].

Clinical Aspects

Symptoms may start with clinical signs such as epistaxis and iron-deficiency anemia or massive GI bleeding.

Patients with arterio-enteric fistulas with massive GI bleeding often require emergency surgery in addition to intensive care of vital functions. In hospitals with a radio-interventional unit, the first line of treatment is arteriography with the possibility of superselective microcoil embolization (Fig. 46.16). Central embolization is usually not recommended in small-bowel and colonic lesions because of the risk of necrosis. Embolic therapy is sometimes considered preoperatively to lower the risk of operative bleeding.

In cases with intermittent epistaxis and iron-deficiency anemia, the management is esophago-gastroduodenoscopy, colonoscopy, and a wireless capsule endoscopy. If a limited segment of the bowel is confirmed with mucosal engagement, elective resection may be considered.

References

1. Waldmann TA, Steinfeld JL, Dutcher TF et al (1961) The role of the gastrointestinal system in "idiopathic hypoproteinemia." Gastroenterology 41: 197–207
2. Yuksekkava H et al (2012) Blue rubber bleb nevus syndrome: successful treatment with sirolimus. Pediatrics 129(4):1080–1084
3. Fishman SJ, Smithers CJ, Folkman J et al (2005) Blue rubber bleb nevus syndrome: surgical eradication of gastrointestinal bleeding. Ann Surg 241(3):523–528
4. Dompmartin A et al (2008) Association of localized intravascular coagulopathy with venous malformations. Arch Dermatol 144(7):873–877
5. Wilson CL et al (2001) Bleeding from cavernous angiomatosis of the rectum in Klippel-Trenaunay syndrome: report of three cases and literature review. Am J Gastroenterol 96(9):2783–2788
6. Zadvinskis DP, Benson MT, Kerr HH et al (1992) Congenital malformations of the cervico-thoracic lymphatic system: embryology and pathogenesis. Radiographics 12:175–1189
7. Chaudry G (2011) Burrows PE et al Sclerotherapy of abdominal lymphatic malformations with doxycycline. J Vasc Interv Radiol 22(10):1431–1435
8. Oliveira C, Sacher P et al (2010) Management of prenatally diagnosed abdominal lymphatic malformations. Eur J Pediatr Surg 20:302–306
9. Ogita S, Tsuto T, Nakamura K et al (1994) OK-432 therapy in 64 patients with lymphangioma. J Pediatr Surg 29:784–785
10. Claesson G, Kuylenstierna R (2002) OK-432 therapy for lymphatic malformation in 32 patients (28 children). Int J Pediatr Otorhinolaryngol 65:1–6
11. Ng WT et al (2003) Argon plasma coagulation for blue rubber bleb nevus syndrome in a female infant. Eur J Pediatr Surg 13(2):137–139
12. Wilson SR, Bohrer S, Losada R et al (2006) Retroperitoneal lymphangioma: an unusual location an presentation. J Pediatr Surg 41:603–605
13. Hebra A, Brown MF, MiGeehin KM et al (1993) Mesenteric, omental and retroperitoneal cysts in children a clinical study of 22 cases. South Med J 2:173–176
14. Muramori K, Zaizen Y et al (2009) Abdominal lymphangioma in children: report of three cases. Surg Today 39(5):414–417
15. Bergqvist D, Björck M (2009) Secondary arterioenteric fistulation – a systematic literature analysis. Eur J Vasc Endovasc Surg 37(1):31–42
16. Sharma VK, Howden CW (1998) Gastrointestinal and hepatic manifestations of hereditary hemorrhagic telangiectasia. Dig Dis 16:169–174

Pelvic Vascular Malformations

47

Raul Mattassi and Massimo Vaghi

Introduction

For practical purposes, the pelvic area can be divided into the pelvic cavity, including the pelvic floor and perineum, and the gluteal area.

Pelvic Cavity Vascular Malformations

Due to the anatomic peculiarity and the organs included, with differences in males and females, vascular malformations in the pelvic cavity may be the cause of severe disturbances, according to the extension and structures involved by the defect. Moreover, as the cavity is not easy to explore, diagnostic procedures and treatment techniques may be difficult and may require specific skills.

In the literature, several papers have described these malformations as related to malformations

R. Mattassi (✉)
Center for Vascular Malformations "Stefan Belov",
Department of Vascular Surgery,
Clinical Institute Humanitas "Mater Domini",
Castellanza (Varese), Italy
e-mail: raulmattassi@gmail.com

M. Vaghi
Deparment of Vascular Surgery,
A.O.G. Salvini Hospital,
Garbagnate Milanese, Italy
e-mail: vaghim@yahoo.it

of the lower limbs in the Klippel–Trenaunay syndrome [1–3]. However, pelvic vascular malformations may also exist as an autonomous entity, without any vascular defect of the lower limbs.

Truncular Anomalies

Arterial anomalies of the pelvic main vessels are rare. Congenital anomaly of the external iliac artery has been reported several times and has been classified in three types: (a) anomaly of course, (b) hypoplasia or atresia compensated by the persistent sciatic artery, and (c) isolated hypoplasia or atresia [4]. Group 1 is an asymptomatic curiosity; group 2 may develop acute symptoms because of the high incidence of atherosclerosis and aneurysm of the sciatic artery with thrombosis or embolization, while in group 3 symptoms of intermittent claudication may be manifested since childhood. Group 2 complications (aneurysm rupture, embolization, ischemia) require an endovascular repair by embolization, implant of a covered stent, or a ligation of aneurysm and bypass procedure [5, 6]. Iliac aneurysms have been reported in the Ehler–Danlos type IV defect. Rupture incidence is high and endovascular treatment by stent deployment is indicated [7] (Fig. 47.1).

Venous truncular defects are more common. Aplasia of the inferior vena cava is reported in 0.1–1 % of the general population and in up to

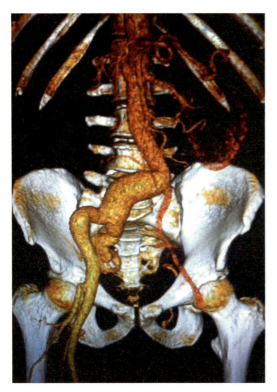

Fig. 47.1 3D CT demonstrating a congenital fusiform Congenital fusiform right iliac aneurysm, involving common and hypogastric artery. Asymptomatic patient

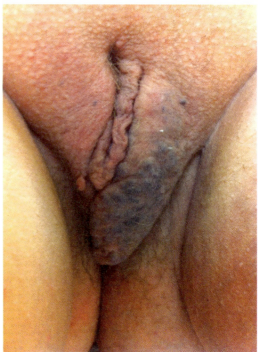

Fig 47.2 Venous malformation of labia majora

5 % in patients under 30 years [8]. Spontaneous DVT is not uncommon [9, 10]. A clinical picture of superficial abdominal dilated veins, as collateral cava–cava circulation, and duplex ultrasound investigation can suggest the diagnosis [11] which is confirmed by angio-CT or angio-MRI [12]. Aplasia of the common and/or external iliac vein is known [13]. Usually collateral circulation through suprapubic veins develops; in case of common iliac vein aplasia also, hypogastric vein-based collaterals compensate the defect which is mainly well tolerated. Aplasia of both external iliac veins is extremely rare [14].

Invasive treatment of inferior vena cava aplasia is not indicated, as collateral circulation often allows an almost symptom-free life. Some patients may develop thrombosis of collaterals, due to thrombophilia, and worsening of symptoms. DVT should be treated by anticoagulation; some authors suggest to precede anticoagulation by fibrinolysis [15]; we observed a case with DVT of collaterals in cava aplasia in which fibrinolysis was very painful for the patient without clinical advantages. In conditions that increase the risk of DVT, like trauma, pregnancy, or surgery, heparin-based prophylaxis is recommended. In deteriorating symptoms due to repeated DVT, ante- and retrograde thrombectomy of the iliac veins and IVC replacement by a ring-supported PTFE graft and temporary mono- or bilateral arteriovenous fistula in the femoral region were performed with 83 % long-term patency [16]. Iliac vein aplasia is also well compensated and does not require treatment.

Venous Extratruncular Malformations

The common site of venous malformations in the pelvis is the perineum, especially the labia majora in females [17, 18] (Fig. 47.2). Involvement of the vagina and also the cervix is possible [19]. Penis VM, sited mainly on the gland, is less common [20, 21].

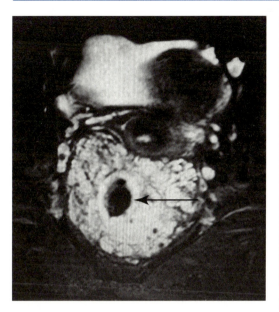

Fig. 47.3 Pelvic MR demonstrating a diffuse venous malformation (*bright irregular*) surrounding the rectum (*arrow*). Vagina and bladder are visible above

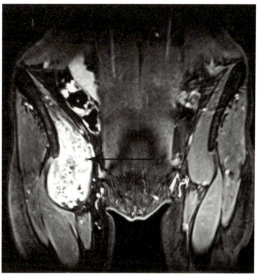

Fig. 47.4 Venous malformation infiltrating right iliopsoas muscle (*bright immage, arrow*)

Inside the pelvis, VM may develop venous masses involving the organs, like the rectum, bladder, uterus, prostate, and seminal vesicles (Fig. 47.3). Involvement of the hemorrhoidal veins may cause thrombosis and liver embolization [22]. A rare site of venous malformation is the iliopsoas muscle (Fig. 47.4).

Pure venous malformations of the uterus are rare [22]. A blue rubber-bleb nevus form in the uterus has been described [23]. Sometimes, VM may involve extensively the colon with single or diffuse mucosal VM that may cause repeated bleeding. Intestinal malformations limited to the gut wall are described in Chap. 43.

Ovarian or testicular venous malformations may be related to an insufficiency of nutcracker syndrome.

Female labia majora VM manifests with swelling and pain. Pelvic venous malformation may manifest with pain, due to episodic thrombosis inside the malformation or by rectal or ureteral bleeding.

Female genital VM is easily recognizable by a swelling, generally monolateral, which is compressible and fills out slowly. Duplex scan demonstrates a low-flow malformation. Pelvic VM is best diagnosed by MRI: typically VM are hyperintense in T2-weighted images and contain phleboliths [24]. The nutcracker syndrome is diagnosed by angio-CT or angio-MRI. Hemodynamic evaluation is done by Doppler ultrasound or by direct venous pressure measurement through a catheter introduced from the femoral vein. The higher the grade of the stenosis, the slower the blood flow velocity. In each case direct cannulation of the vein is mandatory in order to define the hemodynamic burden of the stenosis measuring the transvenous pressure gap. The pressure difference between the inferior cava and renal vein is in the range between 0 and 1 mmHg. Values between 1 and 3 mmHg indicate the presence of a compensated or chronic venous hypertension which may exist secondary to the development of collateral vessels. Values above 3 mmHg are typical of the presence of a high-grade stenosis [25].

The treatment of genital VM is mainly based on alcohol or foam sclerosis [22]. The alcohol sclerotherapy is preferred by us in labia majora malformation for the excellent result obtained, while foam sclerosis has a higher incidence of

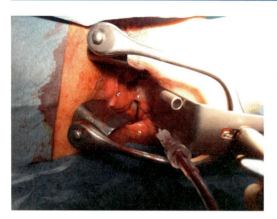

Fig. 47.5 Transrectal alcohol treatment of pelvic-infiltrating venous malformation in the case of Fig. 47.3. Patient was free of symptoms (pain and bleeding) after three sessions

recurrence. In rare cases with less response to alcohol, surgical resection is required. In penis malformations, foam sclerosis is preferred [26].

Symptomatic VM of the pelvis sited around the rectum and extended deeply can be treated by transrectal puncture and alcohol injection after a transrectal echographic study [27] (Fig. 47.5). However, as the complete occlusion of the dysplastic vessels is not possible, symptom recurrence may happen; new treatment should be planned.

In severe bleedings from the rectum nonresponding to sclerosis, surgical procedures are necessary which are difficult and with a high blood loss [28, 29].

VM localized in the site of the iliopsoas muscle can be treated by percutaneous alcohol injections with an inguinal, echo-guided approach. The treatment should be performed in several steps avoiding excessive ethanol injection in a single session because of the posttreatment edema of the muscle that may create painful irritation of the femoral nerve.

Arteriovenous Malformations

Arteriovenous malformations (AVM) are mainly located in a position between the bladder and

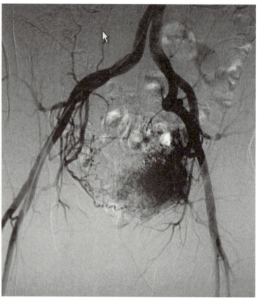

Fig. 47.6 Left-sided pelvic AVM in a male

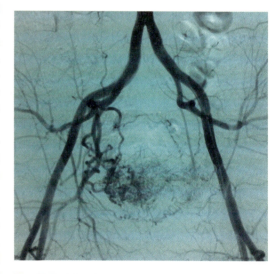

Fig. 47.7 After glue embolization of the AVM through the left feeding vessels, collateral feeders from right appeared

rectum with a tendency of a lateral prevalence that means a prevailing extension to one side. The feeding arteries are principally the branches of the hypogastric arteries with a prevalence of the vessels sited on the prevailing location. Other feeding vessels, which are commonly associated with the hypogastric branches, are

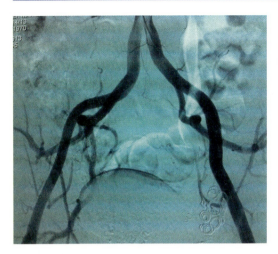

Fig. 47.8 After embolization of right feeders of AVM, the patient is free of fistulas

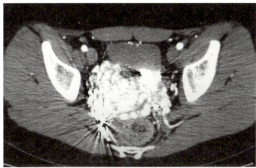

Fig. 47.9 Uterus AVM (*bright area*). Rectum is visible below and bladder above

collaterals of the contralateral hypogastric arteries and collaterals of the abdominal aorta, medial sacral artery, and superior rectal artery (Figs. 47.6, 47.7, and 47.8).

In males, the malformation may involve the posterior bladder wall, prostate, and seminal vesicles. Sometimes, the malformation may compress the ureters with hydronephrosis. Rarely, AVM may involve the rectal area [30]. In female, several papers refer to AVM located in the uterus [31] (Fig. 47.9). It has been reported that retained products of conception may simulate an endometrial AVM which regresses spontaneously after abortion completion [32].

The diagnosis of pelvic cavity AVM is not easy because of the deep location. Rectal exploration may reveal a pulsation in some areas near the rectum. By careful auscultation a slight vascular souffle may be recognized. Transrectal ultrasonography may show multiple anechoic areas with high flow. In females, high-flow areas in the myometrium may reveal the malformation. Angio-CT with 3D images may demonstrate clearly the malformation; angio-MRI is also effective for diagnosis.

Surgery was the only treatment available in the past. However, due to the peculiar anatomy of the area, surgical access revealed difficult and radical removal of the fistulous area and may be complex due to some important structures that may be involved, like the ureter, bladder, seminal vesicles, prostate, and nerves. A team approach together with a urologist is recommended. Careful interruption of the afferent vessels and radical removal of the dysplastic mass was reported in a case [33] and was successful also in one case in our experience.

Catheter embolization is mainly the best approach to pelvic AVM. As this area is fed by several vessels with high possibility of collateral circulation, it is crucial to avoid the occlusion of main branches by spirals or other materials but to focus on nidus closure with glue or alcohol. Treatment may require several steps, as after one apparently successful embolizing session, collaterals often develop (see Figs. 47.6, 47.7, and 47.8) [34].

Uterine AVM can be also treated successfully by the same technique. Fertility may not be compromised; 11 cases of pregnancy after successful embolization of uterine AVM have been reported [35].

A combination of catheter embolization and contemporary occlusion of the draining vein has been reported with excellent results: 83.3 % healed and 16.7 % on partial remission [36, 37].

The combination of embolization and surgery has also been performed, but today it is less frequently done [38].

A complex problem may represent patients who have been treated before by surgical or endovascular occlusion of the hypogastric artery, as the main arterial approach to the nidus is no longer available. Careful angiographic study of collaterals (contralateral hypogastric artery, medial sacral artery, hemorrhoidal arteries, and even deep femoral artery should be explored) often demonstrates other available feeding vessels to the fistula. Retrograde venous access is also an alternative approach to nidus embolization [33].

In the rare case of missing endovascular approach and severe symptoms, surgical treatment is the only possibility. Suture by trespassing stitches into the fistulous area with the aid of an intraoperative Doppler to localize fistulas and immediate control of the effect of the procedure may be the best solution. The collaboration with a urologist is mandatory to avoid damage to the ureters, seminal vesicles, bladder, and nerves. The placement of a catheter in the ureters before operation is recommended. Uterus AVM, if not treatable by embolization, which is rare, can be resolved by hysterectomy.

Lymphatic Malformations

Lymphatic malformations of the vulva are the most common lymphatic dysplasias of this area [39, 40]. Lymphatic cysts of the scrotum are by far rarer [41]. Lymphatic cysts inside the pelvis may be sited in different locations, as the bladder [42]. Macrocystic or microcystic varieties or a combination of both is possible.

MRI exam demonstrates shape, extension, and variety, microcystic or macrocystic.

Macrocystic LM can be treated by direct puncture, aspiration of fluid, and injection of sclerosant substance, like alcohol, OK-432, polidocanol foam, or others [43]. In our experience, we prefer ethanol as it reveals very effective, cheap, and with rare secondary effects because of the lack of outflow vessels in lymphatic cysts, unless venous or AV malformations. Surgical resection has also been performed with good results.

Microcystic LM can be treated by laser with good results.

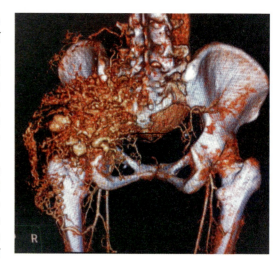

Fig. 47.10 3D CT (*posterior view*) demonstrating an extended AVM sited in the *left* gluteal area (*arrow*)

Gluteal Vascular Malformations

The gluteal area is a prevalent muscular district that contains vessels and nerves. VM in this area may be located intramuscularly or subcutaneously and symptoms depend from the effect of the abnormal vascular mass. Endovascular and percutaneous access are not difficult.

Venous Malformations

VM localized in the buttocks are always of the extratruncular type and may be limited to the subcutaneous level or may infiltrate gluteal muscles; extended forms may involve both areas. Usually only one side is involved: bilateral gluteal venous malformations are extremely rare. Clinically, a nevus and/or multiple bluish small masses may be visible with variable enlargement of the involved buttock (Fig. 47.10).

The patient may complain of swelling and sense of heaviness. Sudden pain may be due to local thrombosis into the malformed vessels. Hemorrhage is rare.

Diagnosis is based first on clinical data: skin aspect and a depressible, slow-filling area, mainly corresponding to the skin signs, may be the first data indicating a VM. Duplex scan may show low-flow areas. MRI (much better than CT) will confirm the diagnosis.

Treatment of gluteal VM is mainly based on percutaneous alcohol sclerosis [44, 45]. In deep forms, duplex mapping is useful to reach the dysplastic area by a long needle; echo-guided procedure is also possible. Several sessions may be required in diffuse forms. In case of cutaneous involvement of the defect, appearance of ulcers due to necrosis of a thin skin after treatment may be possible. Healing of ulcers by medication is always the end result but in extended necrosis may require a long time. In our early experience we got some large, slow-healing ulcers after alcohol treatment, but by reducing the quantity of injected alcohol in the superficial layers of the lesion and immediate removal of ethanol by aspiration after injection, the incidence and extension of skin necrosis reduced dramatically and is no more a problem now.

Foam sclerosis revealed by far less effective in our experience and with a high incidence of recurrence, especially in extended forms. Surgical removal of the dysplasia should be considered only as a second option in case of failure of the alcohol treatment: operation may be difficult, often incomplete, and with poor aesthetical results.

Arteriovenous Malformations

Gluteal AVM is always sited inside the muscles, involving one or more of them, according to extension. The malformation is mainly unilateral. The feeding arteries are principally the branches of the gluteal artery. In large AVM, dilatation of the draining veins, like the iliac vein, is possible (Figs. 47.11 and 47.12).

Clinically, a pulsating mass may be visible or palpable, sometimes with thrill or vascular souffle.

Duplex scan investigation demonstrates the extension of the defect, muscle involved, and probable site of nidus, if performed by an experienced physician. CT with 3D images shows the extension of the defect, while the different projections indicate the muscle involvement.

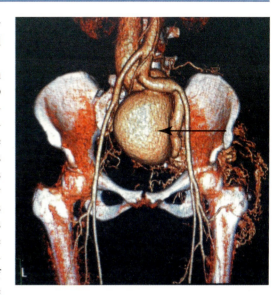

Fig. 47.11 Same case of Fig. 47.10: The frontal 3D CT demonstrates a large aneurysm of the left iliac vein due to the venous high outflow (*arrow*)

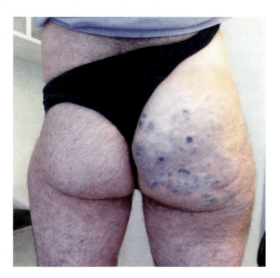

Fig. 47.12 Infiltrating venous malformation of the right gluteus

Catheter embolization and percutaneous alcohol occlusion are both favorable for the treatment of gluteal AVM. A combination of both techniques may be sometimes the best solution, according to the site of the defect and the progression of treatment.

Surgical removal of the malformation can be the first option if the defect is very limited

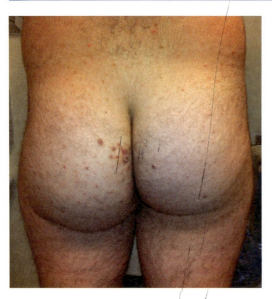

Fig. 47.13 Lymphatic malformation infiltrating left gluteus. Notice small lymphatic cutaneous cysts

and superficial. However, percutaneous alcohol treatment can be also effective and less invasive, even if more than one session may often be necessary. The combination of embolization and surgery has also been proposed [46, 47].

Surgical removal of extended AVM is complex, because of the different orientations of muscle fibers in the three gluteal muscles and complete approach to the malformation requires an invasive procedure. In the pre-catheter embolization and alcohol era, extreme invasive operations were done, but functional and esthetic results were poor [48].

Lymphatic Malformations

LM of the gluteal region may extend variably in the area, from limited and superficial to diffuse infiltrating forms that involve the muscles extensively. LMs are composed of macrocysts (fluid collections > 2 cm diameter), microcysts (<2 cm diameter), or a combination of both [22]. Sometimes, the superficial nevus and/or small lymphatic cysts are visible; in other cases a swell-

ing of the involved buttock is the only visible sign (Fig. 47.13).

The patients complain about episodes of sudden swelling with pain and fever, due to inflammation. By palpation, a consistent mass that may be more or less painful is recognized. Fluid leakage is sometimes possible. Diagnosis is based on a combination of duplex scan which shows liquid no-flow areas and MRI that demonstrates the precise site and extension of the defect.

Treatment by sclerosis (ethanol, doxycycline, OK-432 (Picibanil), or bleomycin) is the less invasive and most effective treatment. We prefer alcohol injections because of the efficacy and the very low complication rate. Interstitial echo-guided laser treatment may be effective in microcystic forms, not responding to sclerosis. Surgical resection is the alternative, more invasive option; a combination of techniques may be sometimes the best solution [21].

References

1. Servelle M, Bastin R, Loygue J et al (1976) Hematuria and rectal bleeding in the child with Klippel and Trenaunay syndrome. Ann Surg 183(4):418–428
2. Azizkhan RG (1991) Life-threatening hematochezia from a rectosigmoid vascular malformation in Klippel-Trenaunay syndrome: long-term palliation using an argon laser. J Pediatr Surg 26:1125–1128
3. Gandolfi L, Rossi A, Stasi G et al (1987) The Klippel-Trenaunay syndrome with colonic hemangioma. Gastrointest Endosc 33:442–445
4. Tamisier D, Melki JP, Cormier JM (1990) Congenital anomalies of the external iliac artery: case report and review of the literature. Ann Vasc Surg 4:510–514
5. Santaolalla V, Bernabe MH, Hipola Ulecia JM, De Loyola Agundez Gomez I, Hoyos YG, Otero FJ, Mendizabal RF, Maldonado FJ, Legrand JL (2010) Persistent sciatic artery. Ann Vasc Surg 24(5):691
6. Knight BC, Tait WF (2010) Massive aneurysm in a persistent sciatic artery. Ann Vasc Surg 24(8):1135. e13–8
7. Tonnessen BH, Sternbergh WC 3rd, Mannava K, Money SR (2007) Endovascular repair of an iliac artery aneurysm in a patient with Ehlers-Danlos syndrome type IV. J Vasc Surg 45(1):177–179
8. Chee YL, Cullighan DJ, Watson HG (2001) Inferior vena cava malformations as a risk factor for deep venous thrombosis in the young. Br J Haematol 114:878–880

9. D'Aloia A, Faggiano P, Fiorina C et al (2003) Absence of inferior vena cava as a rare cause of deep venous thrombosis complicated by liver and lung embolism. Int J Cardiol 88:327–329

10. Ruggeri M, Tosetto A, Castaman G, Rodeghiero F (2001) Congenital absence of the inferior vena cava: a rare risk factor for idiopathic deep-vein thrombosis. Lancet 357:441

11. Pop S, Opincaru I (2012) Anomalies of the inferior vena cava in patients with deep venous thrombosis. Pictorial essay. Med Ultrason 14(1):53–59

12. Malaki M, Willis AP, Jones RG (2012) Congenital anomalies of the inferior vena cava. Clin Radiol 67:165–171

13. Kutsai A, Lampros TD, Cobanogku A (1999) Right iliac vein agenesis, varicosities and widespread hemangiomas: report of a rare case. Tex Heart Inst J 26(2):149–151

14. Onkar D, Onkar P, Mitra K (2013) Isolated bilateral external iliac vein aplasia. Surg Radiol Anat 35(1):85–87

15. Ganguli S, Kalva S, Oklu R, Walker TG, Datta N, Grabowski EF, Wicky S (2012) Efficacy of lower-extremity venous thrombolysis in the setting of congenital absence or atresia of the inferior vena cava. Cardiovasc Intervent Radiol 35(5):1053–1058

16. Sagban TA, Grotemeyer D, Balzer KM et al (2010) Surgical treatment for agenesis of the vena cava: a single-centre experience in 15 cases. Eur J Vasc Endovasc Surg 40(2):241–245

17. Herman AR, Morello F, Strickland JL (2004) Vulvar venous malformations in an 11-year-old girl: a case report. J Pediatr Adolesc Gynecol 17(3):179–181

18. Wang S, Lang JH, Zhou HM (2009) Venous malformations of the female lower genital tract. Eur J Obstet Gynecol Reprod Biol 145(2):205–208

19. Gerald HJ, Steven MS, Charles JD (1997) Surgery of the penis and urethra. In: Patrick CW, Alan BRE, Darracott V Jr, Alan JW (eds) Campbell's urology, 7th edn. Saunders, Philadelphia, 3: 3327

20. Fioramonti P, Maruccia M, Ruggieri M, Onesti MG (2013) A rare case of lymphangioma in the gluteal region: surgical treatment combined with sclerotherapy and laser therapy. Aesthetic Plast Surg 37(5):960–964

21. Burrows P (2008) Vascular malformations involving the female pelvis. Semin Intervent Radiol 25(4):347–360

22. Patel RC, Zynger DL, Laskin WB (2009) Blue rubber bleb nevus syndrome: novel lymphangiomatosis-like growth pattern within the uterus and immunohistochemical analysis. Hum Pathol 40(3):413–417

23. Laor T, Burrows PE (1998) Review congenital anomalies and vascular birthmarks of the lower extremities. Magn Reson Imaging Clin N Am 6(3):497–519

24. Ashour MA, Soliman HE, Khougeer GA (2007) Role of descending venography and endovenous embolization in treatment of females with lower extremity varicose veins, vulvar and posterior thigh varices. Saudi Med J 28(2):206–212

25. Pul-M P-N (1995) Cavernous haemangioma of the penis in an infant. Int Urol Nephrol 27:113–115

26. Keljo DJ, Yakes WF, Andersen JM, Timmons CF (1996) Recognition and treatment of venous malformations of the rectum. J Pediatr Gastroenterol Nutr 23(4):442–446

27. Fishman SJ, Shamberger RC, Fox VL, Burrows PE (2000) Endorectal pull-through abates gastrointestinal hemorrhage from colorectal venous malformations. J Pediatr Surg 35(6):982–984

28. Wilson C, Wong Kee Song LM, Chua H, Ferrara M et al (2001) Bleeding from cavernous angiomatosis of the rectum in Klippel-Trénaunay syndrome: report of three cases and literature review. Am J Gastroenterol 96:2783–2788

29. Hayakawa H, Kusagawa M, Takahashi H et al (1998) Arteriovenous malformation of the rectum: report of a case. Surg Today 28(11):1182–1187

30. Manolitsas T, Hurley V, Gilford E (1994) Uterine arteriovenous malformation–a rare cause of uterine haemorrhage. Aust N Z J Obstet Gynaecol 34(2): 197–199

31. Jain K, Fogata M (2007) Retained products of conception mimicking a large endometrial AVM: complete resolution following spontaneous abortion. J Clin Ultrasound 35(1):42–47

32. Mortensen JD, Ellsworth HS (1965) Internal iliac arteriovenous fistula developing postpartum. Am J Cardiol 16(2):292–296

33. Singh N, Tripathi R, Mala YM, Tyagi S, Singh C (2014) Varied presentation of uterine arteriovenous malformations and their management by uterine artery embolization. J Obstet Gynaecol 34(1):104–106

34. Delotte J, Chevallier P, Benoit B, Castillon JM, Bongain A (2006) Pregnancy after embolization therapy for uterine arteriovenous malformation. Fertil Steril 85(1):228

35. Houbballah R, Mallios A, Poussier B, Soury P, Fukui S, Gigou F, Laurian C (2010) A new therapeutic approach to congenital pelvic arteriovenous malformations. Ann Vasc Surg 24(8):1102–1109

36. Do YS, Kim YW, Park KB, Kim DI, Park HS, Cho SK, Shin SW, Park YJ (2012) Endovascular treatment combined with emboloscleorotherapy for pelvic arteriovenous malformations. J Vasc Surg 55(2):465–471

37. Calligaro KD, Sedlacek TV, Savarese RP, Carneval P, DeLaurentis DA (1992) Congenital pelvic arteriovenous malformations: long-term follow-up in two cases and a review of the literature. J Vasc Surg 16(1):100–108

38. Huang KS, Wang NL, Liu YP (2010) Cystic lymphatic malformation of the pelvis mimicking seminal vesicle cysts. J Pediatr Surg 45(7):1559–1561

39. Kumar S, Sarkar D, Prasad S, Gupta V, Ghosala P, Kaman L, Yadav TD, Ganesamoni R, Singh SK (2012) Large pelvic masses of obscure origin: urologist's perspective. Urol Int 88(2):215–224

40. Häcker A, Hatzinger M, Grobholz R, Alken P, Hoang-Böhm J (2006) Scrotal lymphangioma–a rare cause of acute scrotal pain in childhood. Aktuelle Urol 37(6):445–448

41. Niu ZB, Hou Y, Sun RG, Chen H, Yang Y (2011) Cystic lymphatic malformation of bladder presenting as a pelvic mass. J Pediatr Surg 46(6):1284–1287

42. Burrows PE, Mason KP (2004) Review: percutaneous treatment of low flow vascular malformations. J Vasc Interv Radiol 15(5):431–445

43. Yakes WF (1994) Extremity venous malformations: diagnosis and management. Semin Intervent Radiol 11:332–339

44. Donnelly LF, Bissett GS III, Adams D (1999) Combined sonographic and fluoroscopic guidance: a modified technique for percutaneous sclerosis of low-flow vascular malformations. AJR Am J Roentgenol 173(3):655–657

45. Ishihara T, Hirooka M, Ono T (1997) Arteriovenous malformation in the buttock: treatment with a combination of selective embolization and excision. J Dermatol 24(12):787–792

46. Chien JH, Lee TP, Wang CW, Chen SL, Lin CH (2010) Intramuscular arteriovenous malformation of the gluteus maximus muscle. J Med Sci 30(5):225–229

47. Malan E (1974) Vascular malformations (Angiodysplasias). Carlo Erba Foundation, Milan

48. Loose DA, Faerber G, Weber J (2013) Primäre Varikose und venöse Malformation im Genitalbereich. Phlebologie 5:275–282

Vascular Malformations of the Limbs: Treatment of Venous and Arteriovenous Malformations

48

Raul Mattassi

Introduction

The upper and lower limbs are a very common site of venous (VM) and arteriovenous malformations (AVM) which can be localized in every structure of the limb (skin, subcutis, muscles, joints, and bones) (see Chap. 19). Circumscribed forms, involving only a part of a single structure till extensive infiltrating defects, are possible. Defects of the main arteries or veins, like aplasia, hypoplasia, and dilatation, are another group of malformations. Treatment strategy is strongly dependent on the type and site of the defect. Complete information about the malformation, including involvement of structures, hemodynamic data, and relation with symptoms, should be collected before deciding treatment, avoiding a superficial diagnosis [1] (Fig. 48.1). Diagnostic strategy is discussed in Chap. 22.

Venous Malformations

VM can be divided, according to the Hamburg classification, in truncular (or truncal) forms (defects of the main veins, like aplasia,

hypoplasia, stenosis, or dilatation – aneurysm) and extratruncular defects [2] (see Chap. 21).

Truncular Malformations

Abnormal dilated superficial veins, sometimes including the saphenous vein, are a common type of truncular VM in the lower limbs. It includes diffuse dilated veins and aneurysm of a single vein, like the saphenous vein or others. This anomaly is different from a varicose vein because it is the result of a congenital defect of the superficial veins and not an acquired venous insufficiency. Typical of the truncular superficial dysplastic veins is the early appearance (often in childhood) at an abnormal site (often on the lateral edge of the limb) and the frequent presence of nevus (Fig. 48.2). Duplex ultrasound examination should study the deep venous system to exclude anomalies, like aplasia or hypoplasia [1]. If the deep venous system is normal, the superficial dysplastic veins can be removed surgically. Foam sclerosis is an alternative treatment; however, these veins respond lesser than varicose veins to that treatment.

Congenital aneurysms of the main veins may appear in different vessels; the most frequently involved are the internal jugular vein, the portal vein, the vena saphena magna, the popliteal vein, the azygos vein, and the vena cava superior; pulmonary embolism has been reported in 6.1 % of cases [3–5]. Venous aneurysms of the lower

R. Mattassi
Center for Vascular Malformations "Stefan Belov",
Department of Vascular Surgery,
Clinical Institute Humanitas "Mater Domini",
Castellanza (Varese), Italy
e-mail: raulmattassi@gmail.com

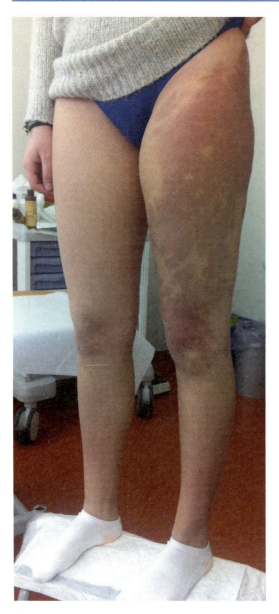

Fig. 48.1 This patient got a diagnosis of "Klippel–Trenaunay–Weber syndrome" when she was 3. As she was told that this is an untreatable disease and because she was free of symptoms, she never had other examinations. A recently new complete study at the age of 20 revealed that she has no vascular anomalies except a cutaneous capillary malformation

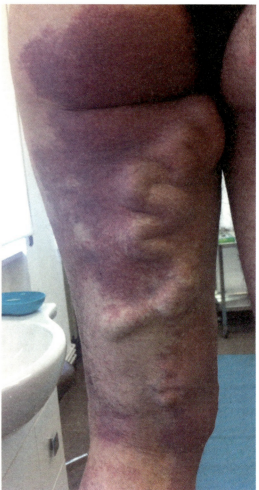

Fig. 48.2 Superficial abnormal veins with diffuse nevus

limbs, like in the popliteal vein, is more likely the source of pulmonary embolism [6]. Surgical treatment with radical resection in vessels like

the saphenous or jugular veins is recommended. In the main vessels, like the popliteal or femoral vein, tangential resection or venous graft implant is the best option [7] (Figs. 48.3, 48.4, and 48.5).

The *persistence of the marginal vein (MV)*, an abnormal, valveless vein sited on the lateral side of the lower limb, is not uncommon [8, 9] (Fig. 48.6). This vein is sometimes evident but in other cases may be not clearly visible because of subcutaneous fat: it can be recognized by palpation or, better, by duplex examination.

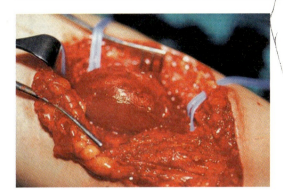

Fig. 48.3 Popliteal vein aneurysm

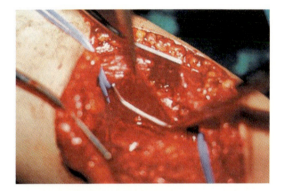

Fig. 48.4 Tangential clamping of the aneurysm by a Satinsky clamp

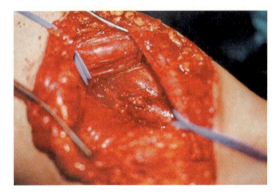

Fig. 48.5 After tangential resection and suture, the popliteal vein is of a normal caliber

This abnormal vessel may create swelling and a sense of heaviness due to the reflux. Limb length discrepancy by overgrowth (angio-osteo-hypertrophy) is sometimes possible because of

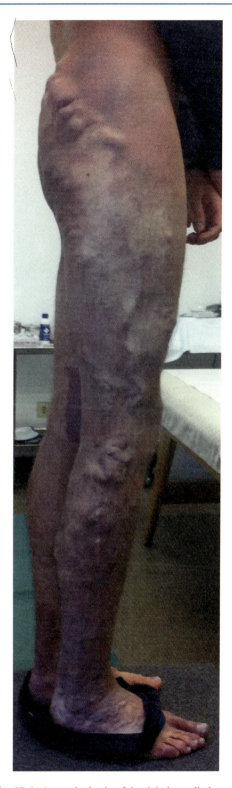

Fig. 48.6 A marginal vein of the right lower limb

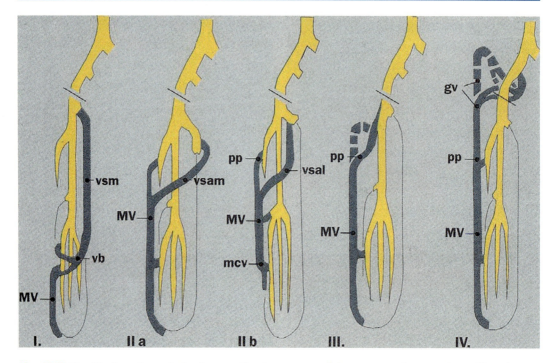

Fig. 48.7 Classification of marginal vein according to Weber: *gv* gluteal vein, *mcv* medial crural vein, *MV* marginal vein, *pp* deep perforants, *vb* anterior arched vein, *vsam* medial accessory saphenous vein, *vsal* lateral accessory saphenous vein, *vsm* main saphenous vein

slight AV communications around or toward the vein. In other, less frequent cases, limb hypotrophy (angio-osteo-hypotrophy) is possible with reduced growth of the limb. In these cases, often masses of pathologic dysplastic veins are associated to the marginal vein. Nevus is not always visible but often exists. The course and extension of the vein are variable: the classification of Weber distinguishes six types [10, 11] (Fig. 48.7). In some cases we found an abnormal lateral lymphatic vessel (the "marginal lymphatic") sited parallel to the marginal vein; more details can be found in Chap. 27.

If an MV with significant reflux is recognized, removal or occlusion is indicated [1, 8, 9]. Surgical resection is the most effective treatment. A correct mapping is required, preferably with duplex aid, in order to recognize site and size and locate perforators [12].

Surgical removal may be sometimes not easy in case of a large MV which may have fragile walls and many collaterals with risk of continuous bleeding, as surgery may be much longer than expected. Temporary ischemia by an Esmark band and a step-by-step planned treatment (avoiding one-step extensive surgery) are effective to reduce blood loss. Huge perforants should be recognized and carefully ligated as their persistence may be the cause of recurrence. Excellent results have been reported by surgical resection of MV [13] (Fig. 48.8).

Foam sclerosis is an alternative treatment which may be effective, especially in small-sized MV [14]. In large vessels with huge perforants, the treatment is less effective and may require several sessions. There exists also the risk of migration of the foam into the deep veins through large perforants.

Endovascular laser occlusion of the MV has been attempted by us with effective closure but with a very uncomfortable scar on the skin. MV is often very superficial and laser heating may affect the skin: saline solution injection between the vein and skin may prevent that complication. Recently this procedure has been reported successfully [15]. Radiofrequency occlusion may be an effective alternative.

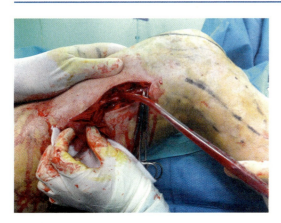

Fig. 48.8 Surgical resection of a marginal vein. Operation revealed long lasting and with significant blood loss due to the fragility of the vein itself and to several, easy bleeding dysplastic veins. Complete resection of the MV was performed in three steps. By removal of the MV at the calf, a tourniquet was applied on the thigh to reduce blood loss. This adjunctive procedure is not always necessary for MV surgery and depends on the characteristics of the vein and of the existence or not of other dysplastic vessels that may bleed

In our opinion, endovascular occlusion and foam sclerosis are effective in small-sized MV; in vessels larger than 1–1.5 cm, surgery is the best treatment option.

The *persistence of sciatic vein* (*PSV*) is a rare venous truncular anomaly in which an abnormal draining vein, located intramuscularly in the thigh near the sciatic nerve, that normally disappears at birth, persists [16]. The vein drains blood from the popliteal area to the gluteal and internal iliac vein system. Sciatic vein is valveless and may create blood stasis in the thigh and in the calf and sometimes have more severe symptoms, like anorectal bleeding if the defect is coupled with AV pelvic malformations. An increased incidence of PSV was found in patients with complex venous malformations of the lower limb, like in the so-called Klippel–Trenaunay syndrome [17]. Diagnosis is not always easy: phlebography was the main diagnostic exam in the past [18]. Duplex ultrasound, phlebo-CT, and phlebo-MR are today excellent diagnostic methods to find out PSV. The treatment of PSV is required only if symptoms are severe. Resection of the distal connection of PSV with the popliteal or calf vein may be sufficient to eliminate distal symptoms; sometimes

extended resection of the vein inside the thigh by a posterior approach has been performed. In a single case, the sural nerve was found inseparably in the wall of the vein, and, after surgical separation of the vein, a sural neuropathy persisted [18].

Hypoplasia of the deep veins, with more or less extended vein segments of a small caliber, is rarely described in literature, except by groups working intensively with CVM [19–21]. Hypoplasias are reported in the femoral, popliteal, and upper limb deep veins. These defects are commonly associated with cutaneous nevus and superficial dilated veins, acting as a collateral pathway. Sometimes, marginal vein may be also present. Limb overgrowth may also be visible. They may be the cause of venostasis and, sometimes, of distal ulcers. Complex cases may also include lymphatic defects of the main trunks which originate a clinical picture that may be denominated as the "Klippel–Trenaunay syndrome," an old term which often is used improperly and creates confusion. This item is discussed in detail in Chap. 36.

Some authors were of the opinion that deep venous hypoplasia is always the result of an abnormal band compression which requires surgical removal [22]. However, other authors do not agree with this concept and believe that the so-called hypoplasia is the result of a defect in the development of the vessel and not an external compression, which has not been clearly demonstrated.

Belov reported that resection of dilated superficial veins may stimulate spontaneous dilation of the hypoplastic deep vein; he called this procedure "rerouting of venous flow" [23]. In extended hypoplasia, a step-by-step resection of the superficial veins is indicated, instead of a single procedure, in order to permit a progressive dilation of the stenotic vessels.

Aplasia of deep veins is well known, even if rare. Aplasia of the inferior vena cava is discussed in Chapter 46.

Aplasia of one common and/or external iliac veins is known, as also absence of the femoral and popliteal veins [24, 25] (Fig. 48.9); bilateral iliac vein aplasia is extremely rare [26], saphenous vein

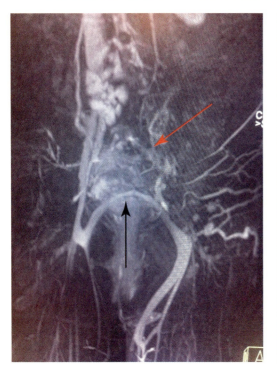

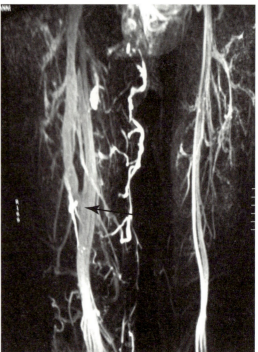

Fig. 48.9 MR angiography demonstrating an aplasia of the left common and external iliac vein (*red arrow*). An evident suprapubic left-to-right spontaneous bypass is visible (*black arrow*)

Fig. 48.10 Angio MR demonstrating avalvulia of the right femoral vein: notice the significant increase of diameter of the deep veins. The patient was treated in the past by ligation of the femoral vein at the connection to the common femoral vein. After a temporary improvement of symptoms, the patient worsens because of the connection of the deep femoral vein, also valveless, with the femoral vein distally (*arrow*)

may also be missed [27]. Combinations of aplasias at different levels are possible. Aplasias of segments of the main veins of the upper limbs are much rarer.

Aplasia of the deep veins of the lower limb may compensate by collateral circulation through normal vessels, like the saphenous vein or profunda femoris, by dilated superficial, varicose-like veins or by persistence of abnormal veins like the marginal or sciatic vein. Different combinations are possible. There is no indication for the treatment of deep vein aplasia. Venous bypass techniques, even if theoretically possible, are not necessary as compensation is normally effective.

Truncular venous defects of the lower limbs may combine, like the marginal and/or sciatic vein and aplasia or hypoplasia of the deep veins. Correct differential diagnosis is crucial, as it conditions treatment [28].

Congenital avalvulia (congenital absence of valves in the deep veins) has been reported several times in the past but lesser in the last years [29, 30]. The common femoral, femoral, and popliteal veins may demonstrate extensive venous reflux due to

the valve absence with calf and ankle swelling and pain (Fig. 48.10). The majority may tolerate the condition with elastic stockings, but in some patients symptoms may worsen till it is impossible to maintain a standing position for a longer time.

In severe cases, treatment by valve reconstruction, like in postthrombotic insufficiency, is not applicable as valves are missing at all. The transplant of a valved vein segment from the axillary vein according to Taheri et al. [31] or a transposition of the femoral to the profunda femoris distally to a normal functioning valve, according to Kistner, is the best treatment option [32]. We treated three cases with the second technique with a good long-term result: all cases are functioning and symptoms improved significantly in two cases after a follow-up of 4 years (Figs. 48.11 and 48.12). The third case complained of a worsening of edema after treatment: examinations demonstrate perfect

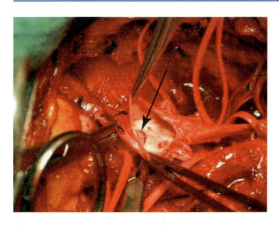

Fig. 48.11 Opened deep femoral vein prior to anastomosis with a valveless femoral vein. The edge of the functioning valve is visible on the left (*arrow*). The common femoral vein is on the left; visible on the right are the bifurcations of the deep femoral vein

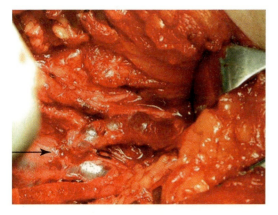

Fig. 48.12 Anastomosis of the femoral vein on the deep femoral vein distally to a functioning valve (*arrow*). The patient was free of symptoms at a follow-up of 4 years

functioning of the transposition. Edema was the result of a lymphatic defect, probably by surgical injury in a case with an unknown primary congenital lymphatic defect (poor lymphatic drainage), that maintained a compensation until surgery.

Extratruncular Venous Defects

Areas of small abnormal veins infiltrating tissues can be found in every part of the limb. The intramuscular site is one of the most common location [33]. Every muscle can be affected; a limited, single muscle-type site can be observed, but extensive infiltration involving several muscles till an almost complete penetration of the whole musculature of a limb segment is also possible.

Extratruncular infiltrating dysplastic veins may also involve the skin, subcutis, bone, joints, and also nerves. Clinically, the limited intramuscular type may show no visible signs, while the more extended forms may manifest with bluish skin and visible masses which are easily compressible and empties spontaneously by limb elevation. Extratruncular venous dysplastic masses which are located around long bones may create bone hypotrophy by compression [34].

Duplex examination and MR are the best tests to find out the defect. However, an experienced examiner in vascular malformations will offer best results, especially in duplex examination, but also in MR [35].

Treatment by foam sclerosis has been attempted in these cases [36]. Foam sclerosis treatment in VM is discussed in Chap. 33.

Alcohol sclerosis by direct puncture of the dysplastic masses has been widely used in extratruncular VM [37, 38]. This technique is effective, allowing complete occlusion of the dysplastic area in many cases, even in extended infiltrating forms (Fig. 48.13). However, the technique should be well known and performed only by experienced physicians to avoid complications. It requires anesthesia (alcohol injection in vessels is very painful), which can be local or truncular, avoiding general anesthesia, if the procedure is limited to the limbs. A multiple-step procedure is often required. It is preferable in our experience to perform treatment every 2–3 months till almost complete occlusion of the malformed vessels, as recurrence is common if treatments happened at too long intervals.

Some significant collateral effects have been described in the past after alcohol treatment of VM, like extensive skin necrosis or nerve palsy [39]. Technique skills, like alcohol reaspiration after injection (alcohol acts by necrotizing the endothelium at first contact: long retention in the vessels is not useful and allows outflow into the main veins), delayed injections, and limited whole dosage (less than 0.5 cc/kg, in our cases), may be effective to reduce complications.

Surgical removal of limited extratruncular venous malformations is possible with excellent

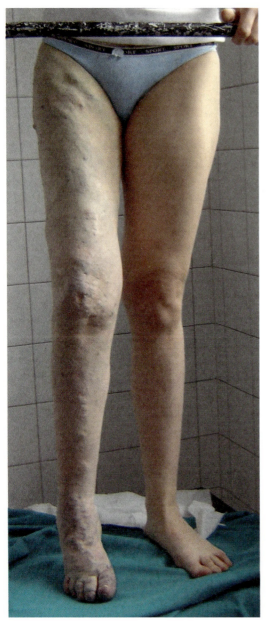

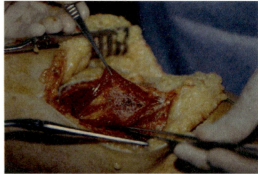

Fig. 48.14 Intraoperative image of an intramuscular venous malformation. The mass has been opened demonstrating a spongelike aspect without visible vessels

Fig. 48.13 Diffuse infiltration of venous malformations of a whole limb, including muscles. The patient complains of pain crisis in some specific areas, due to episodic thrombosis. Treatment by percutaneous alcohol sessions centered on the pain areas improved significantly the conditions by eliminating episodic pain. In these cases complete occlusion of the diffuse infiltration is not possible, but local improvement may be well accepted

results, if the defect is limited and sited in the superficial, subfascial area of the muscle. Limited, deeper-sited defects may be sometimes difficult to recognize during operation. Extensive

infiltrating intramuscular malformations can be a challenge for the surgeon as severe bleeding from all the edges of the defect inside the muscle may be difficult to control during surgery. Large muscles, like those of the thigh (frequent site of these defects), with no possibility to form ischemia, are the most dangerous. To prevent hemorrhage, the technique of tangential clamping of the defect with a Satinsky clamp and application of stitches is effective [40]. The treatment can be completed by alcohol percutaneous procedures and is effective in large, infiltrating intramuscular forms [1].

Interstitial laser treatment of deep limited extratruncular VM is also possible. An ecographic guidance is indicated for these cases. Intramuscular extensive VM treated by laser can be sometimes painful to the patient. Laser treatment is discussed in detail in Chap. 34.

The treatment of venous malformations inside the joints (the knee is the most common site) and also limb length discrepancy management are discussed in Chap. 42.

Recently, we noticed that the morphology of these extratruncular venous defects is not always the same: we could distinguish six different types of extratruncular venous malformations: (1) dilated superficial veins, (2) a mass of small-/medium-sized vessels infiltrating tissues, (3) a spongelike vascular tissue without the aspect of vessels (Fig. 48.14), (4) small dysplastic veins surrounded by an extended fat hypertrophy (Fig. 48.15), (5) a dark compact tissue which includes fibrosis and capillary vessels (Fig. 48.16), and (6) small (few mm),

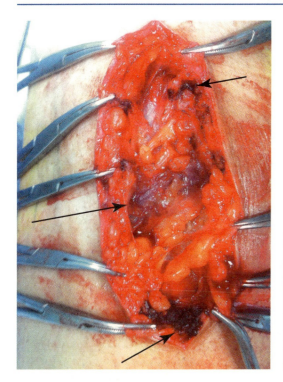

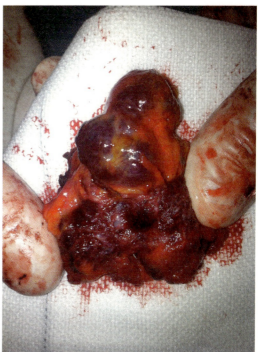

Fig. 48.15 Intraoperative observation of a venous malformation that originates from a swollen, noncompressible area. The mass is formed by some dysplastic vessels (*arrows*) surrounded by a high quantity of fat. This case cannot be treated by sclerosis, as fat does not respond to it and the mass may persist

Fig. 48.16 Removed vascular mass composed of capillary dark areas. No other vessels are visible by opening the mass

round-shaped, intradermic or subcutaneous very painful vascular areas (Fig. 48.17). Some of these last cases have been found to be glomuvenous. Based on these observations, treatment changes because type 1 can be treated surgically or also by sclerosis, types 2 and 3 can be treated successfully by alcohol or foam sclerosis, while types 4 and 5 need surgery to remove the mass as the nonvascular tissues of these types of defects do not respond to sclerosis. Type 6 requires precise recognition and surgical removal. Recently, some of these morphologic peculiarities have been reported in literature, denominating "fibroadipose vascular anomaly" as our type 4 and possibly also type 5 [41].

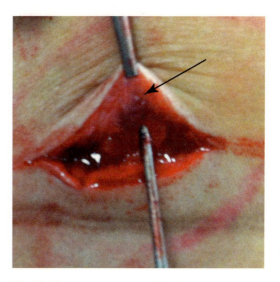

Fig. 48.17 Very small, extremely painful to compression subcutaneous venous malformations. Histology and genetic test demonstrate glomuvenous malformation (*arrow*)

Arteriovenous Malformations

As VM, also AVM may vary extremely in site and extension in the limbs.

Truncular AVM

Truncular AVM (direct communication between the main vein and artery) in the limbs is rare.

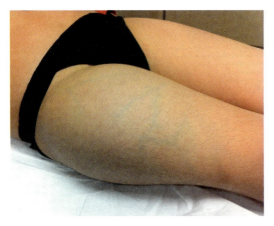

Fig. 48.18 This 12-year-old boy complained of swelling and pain of his right thigh. Clinical examination demonstrated a pulsating area with vascular souffles

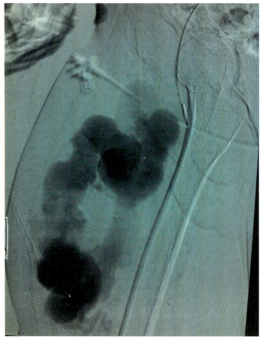

Fig. 48.19 Details of angiography of the case of Fig. 48.11: large intramuscular AV fistulas. Embolization was not possible because of the very large, direct communications between the arteries and veins. It was decided to perform surgery

The most frequent site is the common femoral artery but other arteries may also be involved. Direct AVM at this level may be difficult to recognize, even by angiography, because often a complex system of pulsating vessels may develop, extended far away from the main fistula rendering a precise diagnosis difficult. Angiography needs to be performed with particular skill to find out fistula site (Figs. 48.18 and 48.19). Sometimes, direct communication between the artery and vein may happen at some distance from the main vessel with a large, tortuous artery that passes directly in a large vein.

Truncular AVM is more likely to originate from a secondary cardiac overloading effect, while extratruncular forms, even extended, do not always have an effect on the heart.

Truncular AVM is often not treatable by embolization because of the large size of the communication and the lack of a "nidus." The risk of lung embolization of coils is high. If the precise site of the fistula is known, a covered stent can be deployed. However, as often these patients are young, the procedure should be considered a second option after surgery failure.

Surgical resection and ligation of the communication can be the best choice as it can cure the patient if the surgeon succeeds in occluding the connection (Fig. 48.20). However, the operation could be not simple because of the existence of many very fragile, pulsating vessels

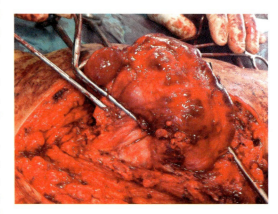

Fig. 48.20 Surgical resection of the fistulous area. Notice the enormous dilated and tortuous vessels. Surgery was successful, even if long lasting (5 h); fistula was completely removed and the patient was cured

in the area and the precise point of connection is not easy to recognize. An aid of an intraoperative Doppler can be crucial. Just after ligation of the fistula, vascular bruits and abnormal pulsation in collateral vessels may disappear. Blood loss can

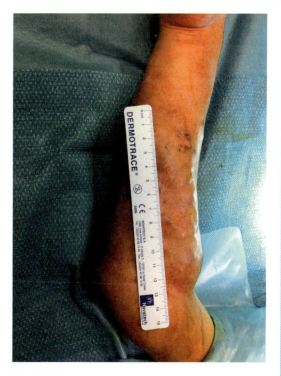

Fig. 48.21 An 11-year-old schoolgirl with an extended infiltrating AVM of the right arm and forearm

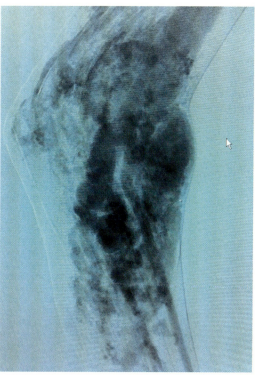

Fig. 48.22 Angiography demonstrating extensive infiltration of AVM. Extensive small fistulas entering very large dilated veins (not the main veins) limited the possibility of embolization as the only treatment technique. The patient was treated step by step with a combination of alcohol treatment, embolization, and surgical resection of the fistulous areas

be conspicuous and should be always prevented. It is recommended to prepare for several blood transfusions, to use a blood recovery system, and to put on a tourniquet [42].

Extratruncular AVM

Extratruncular AVM may develop in all tissues of the limbs, including the bones. Limited forms may be sited in a single muscle; extensive, infiltrating forms may involve several structures and may manifest with pulsating areas, often painful at compression. Diagnosis should be performed by noninvasive techniques, like duplex scan, MR, and CT with 3D images which are very effective to show the site and extension of the malformations. Diagnostic angiography is not recommended as a first step but is preferred after other tests in an intention-to-treat procedure [43].

Extratruncular AVM can be treated often by catheter embolization. However, the final decision of the technique to choose should not be based on

catheter embolization only as the standard therapeutic method, but should be decided on the conditions of the specific case. Besides embolization, surgery, laser, and alcohol percutaneous treatment should be considered in an integrated program which often is a step-by-step procedure [44–47] (Figs. 48.21, 48.22, 48.23, and 48.24).

Based on the angiographic classification of Cho et al., which indicates four types of extratruncular AVM, and the classification of Yakes (see Chap. 32), a decision whether to use catheter embolization, percutaneous alcohol treatment, or surgery should be made [48]. The site of the defect is another useful choosing criterion: limited, superficial, easy accessible malformations can be treated better by surgery or by alcohol techniques rather than by a complex endovascular access. A catheter endovenous approach to the

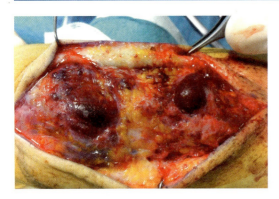

Fig. 48.23 Aspect of the fistulous areas demonstrated during a surgical session

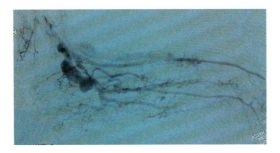

Fig. 48.24 Control angiography at the end of the treatment program (3 years): no fistulas. Some dilated veins, remnant of the high-flow condition, are demonstrated. The patient is free of symptoms. This case is an example of a successful combined treatment by steps

fistulous area and occlusion with alcohol of the venous side of the malformation are other possibilities [49]. Bone involvement by AVM is not rare; percutaneous alcohol treatment, if correctly performed, proved to be very effective [50]. An alternative in bone AVM is the percutaneous puncture of the bone and injection of polymethyl methacrylate (PMMA), which is normally used in percutaneous vertebroplasty. A complete occlusion of the AVM has been reported with this technique [51]. Percutaneous, interstitial laser applications may be effective in limited AVM or as completion procedure.

In a group of 72 cases of AVM treated in the last 2 years, we performed surgery in 16 %, catheter embolization in 23 %, alcohol treatment in 57 %, and laser treatment in 4 % of cases. A combination of procedures was done in 38 % of cases. Sixty-five percent of patients were treated with involvement of two or more specialists in a multidisciplinary approach concept. Results of that approach strategy were complete healing of AVM in 24 %, improvement (residual AVM still present but no symptoms) in 58 %, unchanged condition in 13 %, worsening in 4 %, and only 1 case of amputation (a finger).

However, to be able to approach extratruncular AVM with that strategy, a multidisciplinary stable team is required which is able to perform embolization, surgery, alcohol, and laser technique which the same experience and skill in order to avoid to privilege a single procedure, which may be not the best in the single case, only because the treating physician is not experienced or do not perform one or two of these four methods (52, 53).

References

1. Lee BB, Bergan J, Gloviczki P et al (2009) Diagnosis and treatment of venous malformations. Consensus document of the international union of phlebology (UIP)-2009. Int Angiol 28(6):434–451
2. Belov S (1993) Anatomopathological classification of congenital vascular defects. Semin Vasc Surg 6:219–224
3. Schild H, Berg S, Weber W, Schmied W, Steegmüller KW (1992) The venous aneurysm. Aktuelle Radiol 2(2):75–80
4. Mohanty D, Jain BK, Garg PK, Tandon A (2013) External jugular venous aneurysm: a clinical curiosity. J Nat Sci Biol Med 4(1):223–225
5. Varma PK, Dharan BS, Ramachandran P, Neelakandhan KS (2003) Superior vena caval aneurysm. Interact Cardiovasc Thorac Surg 2(3):331–333
6. Sigg P, Koella C, Stöbe C, Jeanneret C (2003) Popliteal venous aneurysm, a cause of pulmonary embolism. Vasa 32(4):221–224
7. Gillespie DL, Villavicencio JL, Gallagher C et al (1997) Presentation and management of venous aneurysms. J Vasc Surg 26(5):845–852
8. Vollmar J, Voss E (1979) Vena marginalis lateralis persistent- the forgotten vein of the angiologists. Vasa 8:199–202
9. Mattassi R, Vaghi M (2007) Management of the marginal vein: current issues. Phlebology 22:283–286
10. Weber J (1997) Invasive diagnostic angeborene Gefäßfehler (invasive diagnostic of CVM). In: Loose DA, Weber J Angeborene Gefäßmissbildungen. Nordlanddruck Verlag, Lüneburg, pp 127–163
11. Weber J (2009) Invasive diagnostic of congenital vascular malformations. In: Mattasi R, Loose DA, Vaghi M (eds) Hemangiomas and vascular malformations. Springer, Milan, pp 135–143

12. Kim YW, Lee BB, Cho JH, Do YS, Kim DI, Kim ES (2007) Haemodynamic and clinical assessment of lateral marginal vein excision in patients with a predominantly venous malformation of the lower extremity. Eur J Vasc Endovasc Surg 33:122–127

13. Loose DA, Lorenz A (1997) Die Chirurgie der Maginalvene (surgery of the marginal vein). In: Loose DA, Weber J (eds) Angeborene Gefaessmissbildungen (congenital vascular malformations). Nordlanddruck Verlag, Lüneburg, pp 230–244

14. Cabrera J, Cabrera J Jr, Garcia-Olmedo MA, Redondo P (2003) Treatment of venous malformations with sclerosant in microfoam form. Arch Dermatol 139:1409–1416

15. King K, Landrigan-Ossar M, Clemens R, Chaudry G, Alomari AI (2013) The use of endovenous laser treatment in toddlers. J Vasc Interv Radiol 24(6):855–858

16. Kenneth J, Cherry KJ Jr, Gloviczki P, Stanson W (1996) Persistent sciatic vein: diagnosis and treatment of a rare condition. J Vasc Surg 23(3):490–497

17. Trigaux J, Vanbeers B, Delchambre F, de Fays F, Schoevaerdts J (1989) Sciatic venous drainage demonstrated by varicography in patients with a patent deep venous system. Cardiovasc Intervent Radiol 12:103–106

18. Hamilton HEC, Drake SG (1999) Persistent sciatic vein – unusual case of reflux from the popliteal fossa and sural nerve damage. Eur J Vasc Endovasc Surg 17:539–541

19. Servelle M, Babillot J (1980) Deep veins malformations in the Klippel-Trenaunay syndrome. Phlebologie 33(1):31–36

20. Belov S, Loose DA, Müller E (1985) Angeborene Gefäßfehler (congenital vascular malformations). Einhorn-Presse Verlag, Reinbeck

21. Loose DA, Weber J (eds) (1997) Angeborene Gefäßmissbildungen (congenital vascular malformations). Nordlanddruck, Lüneburg

22. Servelle M (1985) Klippel and Trenaunay syndrome. 768 operated cases. Ann Surg 201(3):365–376

23. Belov S, Loose DA (1990) Surgical treatment of congenital vascular defects. Int Angiol 9(3):175–182

24. Onkar D, Onkar P, Mitra K (2013) Isolated bilateral external iliac vein aplasia. Surg Radiol Anat 35(1):85–87

25. Eifert S, Villavicencio L, Kao T, Taute BM, Rich N (2000) Prevalence of deep venous anomalies in congenital vascular malformations of venous predominance. J Vasc Surg 31(3):462–471

26. Doğan R, Doğan OF, Oç M et al (2003) A rare vascular malformation, Klippel – Trenaunay syndrome. Report of a case with deep vein agenesis and review of the literature. J Cardiovasc Surg (Torino) 44(1):95–100

27. Herman J, Musil D (2010) Klippel-Trénaunay syndrome associated with great saphenous vein aplasia. Phlebology 25(1):35–37

28. Mattassi R (1993) Differential diagnosis in congenital vascular-bone syndromes. Semin Vasc Surg 6:233–244

29. Plate G, Brudin L, Eklöf B, Jensen R, Ohlin P (1986) Congenital vein valve aplasia. World J Surg 10(6):929–934

30. Friedman EI, Taylor LM Jr, Porter JM (1988) Congenital venous valvular aplasia of the lower extremities. Surgery 103(1):24–26

31. Taheri SA, Lazar L, Elias S, Marchand P, Heffner R (1982) Surgical treatment of postphlebitic syndrome with vein valve transplant. Am J Surg 144(2):221–224

32. Kistner RL (1978) Transvenous repair of the incompetent femoral vein valve. In: Bergan JJ, Yao JST (eds) Venous problems. Year book medical publishers, Chicago, pp 493–513

33. Mattassi R, Vaghi M (2004) Intramuscular venous malformations. Int Angiol 23(suppl 1):23

34. Belov S (1990) Hemodynamic pathogenesis of vascular-bone syndromes in congenital vascular defects. Int Angiol 9:155–161

35. Kim EY, Ahn JM, Yoon HK et al (1999) Intramuscular vascular malformations of an extremity: findings on MR imaging and pathologic correlation. Skeletal Radiol 28(9):515–521

36. Cabrera J, Loose DA (2009) Sclerotherapy in vascular malformations. In: Mattassi R, Loose DA, Vaghi M (eds) Hemangiomas and vascular malformations. Springer, Milan, pp 171–180

37. Yakes WF, Parker SH, Gibson MD et al (1989) Alcohol embolotherapy of vascular malformations. Semin Intervent Radiol 6:146–161

38. Lee BB, Kim DI, Huh S et al (2001) New experiences with absolute ethanol sclerotherapy in the management of a complex form of congenital venous malformation. J Vasc Surg 33(4):764–772

39. Lee BB, Do YS, Byun A et al (2003) Advanced management of venous malformations with ethanol sclerotherapy: mid term results. J Vasc Surg 37:533–538

40. Belov St (1992) Operative-technical peculiarities in operations of congenital vascular defects. In: Balas P (ed) Progress in angiology 1991. Minerva Mediica, p 379–382

41. Alomari AI, Spencer SA, Arnold RW et al (2014) Fibro-adipose vascular anomaly: clinical-radiologic-pathologic features of a newly delineated disorder of the extremity. J Pediatr Orthop 34(1):109–117

42. Ozcan AV, Boysan E, Isikli OY, Goksin I (2013) Surgical treatment for a complex congenital arteriovenous malformation of the lower limb. Tex Heart Inst J 40(5):612–614

43. Lee BB, Baumgartner I, Berlien HP et al (2013) Consensus Document of the International Union of Angiology (IUA)-2013. Current concepts on the management of arterio-venous malformations. Int Angiol 32(1):9–36

44. White RI, Pollak J, Persing J, Henderson KJ, Thompson JG, Burdge CM (2000) Long-term outcome of embolotherapy and surgery for high-flow extremity arteriovenous malformations. J Vasc Interv Radiol 11(10):1285–1295

45. Kim JY, Kim DI, Do YS et al (2006) Surgical treatment for congenital arteriovenous malformations: 10 year's experience. Eur J Vasc Endovasc Surg 32(1):101–106

46. Do YS, Yakes WF, Shin SW, Lee BB et al (2005) Ethanol embolization of arteriovenous malformations: interim results. Radiology 235(2):674–682

47. Toker ME, Eren E, Akbayrak H, Numan F, Güler M, Balkanay M, Yakut C (2006) Combined approach to a peripheral congenital arteriovenous malformation: surgery and embolization. Heart Vessels 21(2):127–130

48. Loose DA (1993) Combined treatment of congenital vascular defects: indications and tactics. Semin Vasc Surg 6(4):260–265

49. Cho SK, Do YS, Shin SW, Choo SW, Choo IW et al (2006) Arteriovenous malformations of the body and extremities: analysis of therapeutic outcomes and approaches according to a modified angiographic classification. J Endovasc Ther 13(4):527–538

50. Cho AK, Do YS, Shin SW, Kwang B, Park KB (2008) Peripheral arteriovenous malformations with a dominant outflow vein: results of ethanol embolization. Korean J Radiol 9:258–267

51. Do YS, Park KB, Park HS et al (2010) Extremity arteriovenous malformations involving the bone: therapeutic outcomes of ethanol embolotherapy. J Vasc Interv Radiol 21(6):807–816

52. Ierardi AM, Mangini M, Vaghi M, Cazzulani A, Mattassi R, Carrafiello G (2001) Occlusion of an intraosseous arteriovenous malformation with percutaneous injection of polymethylmethacrylate. Cardiovasc Intervent Radiol 34(Suppl 2):150–153

53. Lee BB, Do YS, Yakes W, Kim DI, Mattassi R, Hyon WS (2004) Management of arteriovenous malformations: a multidisciplinary approach. J Vasc Surg 39(3):590–600

Lymphatic Vascular Malformations of the Limbs: Treatment of Extratruncular Malformations

49

Byung-Boong Lee, James Laredo, and Richard F. Neville

Introduction

"Extratruncular" lesion of lymphatic malformation (LM) represents one form of defective development affecting the lymphatic system together with "truncular" lesion [1–3].

Modified Hamburg classification [4–6] subclassified the LM based on the embryological stage when this defect occurred; the outcome of developmental arrest during the "early" stage of lymphangiogenesis was named to "extratruncular" lesion in order to differentiate from those from the "later" stage, named separately to "truncular" lesion.

Such embryological classification provides a critical base to the clinicians to distinguish the morphological differences between two different types of the lesions as well as for proper management of two embryologically as well as lymphodynamically different types of the LM lesions [7–9].

Indeed, all the extratruncular LM lesions, originated from the reticular stage before vascular trunk formation, will appear on birth as the embryonic tissue remnant in amorphous vascular/lymphatic structure with no direct involvement to the lymph-transporting systems – vessels and nodes [10–12].

Therefore, clinically they present as an abnormal tissue cluster infiltrating into the surrounding tissues/organs with the potential risk of compression, known as the "cystic/cavernous lymphangioma" [13–15] (Fig. 49.1a).

Such primitive vascular tissue from the "early" stage of embryogenesis maintains its unique mesenchymal cell characteristics originated from (lymph)angioblast. They have such evolutional potential so that they will never disappear (cf. hemangioma) but continue to grow when stimulated (e.g., female hormone, menarche, pregnancy, trauma, surgery) through the rest of life [1–3].

On the contrary, the truncular lesion is the outcome of defective development along the "later" stage of lymphangiogenesis, while the lymphatic vessel trunk is formed so that it no longer possesses the mesenchymal cell characteristics to grow/progress. But it is directly involved to the lymph-transporting system – vessels and/or nodes – resulting in various defective conditions as aplasia, hypoplasia, and hyperplasia so that the impact to the lymphatic function is more serious, clinically known as a primary lymphedema [16–18] (Fig. 49.1b).

Infrequently, both extratruncular and truncular lesions may exist together; therefore, a clear understanding on this distinctive difference between two different groups (extratruncular versus truncular lesions) from different stages

B.-B. Lee (✉) • J. Laredo • R.F. Neville
Division of Vascular Surgery, Department of Surgery,
George Washington University Medical Center,
Washington, DC, USA
e-mail: bblee@mfa.gwu.edu; bblee38@comcast.net;
jlaredo@mfa.gwu.edu; rneville@mfa.gwu.edu

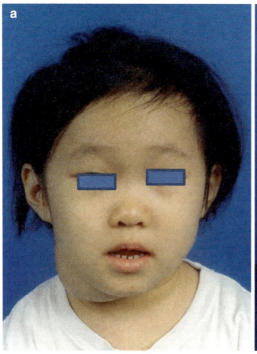

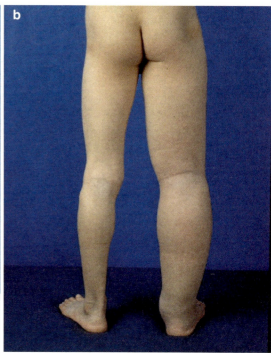

Fig. 49.1 (**a**, **b**) Extratruncular and truncular LM (**a**) depicts a typical "extratruncular" lymphatic malformation (LM) lesion presenting as a localized swelling along the right neck extended to the submandibular region (*left panel*). Such lesion generally presents as a soft boggy mass along the soft tissue plane, but it could be the tip of a quite extensive lesion beneath it infiltrating to deeper tissue/structure, often seen in the head and neck region. (**b**) shows a common clinical condition of "truncular" LM as primary lymphedema (*right panel*), affecting the right lower extremity of a young male patient. It manifests as a diffuse swelling along the entire area affected by lymphatic obstruction/stasis often due to the hypoplasia of the lymph-transporting vessel

of lymphangiogenesis is mandated for safe management of extratruncular LM lesions [5, 7, 9] (Fig. 49.2).

General Principles and Guidelines

The vast majority of extratruncular LMs occur as independent lesions, known as a lymphangioma. Therefore, the treatment decision should follow a complete and appropriate assessment of recurrence risk involved in these unique embryological/mesenchymal cell characteristics, because "recurrence" often follows unnecessary stimulation by ill-planned treatment, especially with incomplete excision [1–3, 19].

But, by the nature/pathophysiology of the CVM development, both extratruncular and truncular LM lesions may further develop together with other CVMs. They could exist with venous malformations (VMs) [20–22] and/or arteriovenous malformations (AVMs) [23–25] further complicating the clinical picture.

These complex lesions are separately classified as hemolymphatic malformations (HLMs) and are also known as vascular malformation components of the Klippel-Trenaunay syndrome [26–28] and Parkes Weber syndrome [29–31]. Knowledge and thorough understanding of these mixed CVMs is required for proper diagnosis and appropriate management of the LM itself (Figs. 49.3 and 49.4).

Nevertheless, compared to other CVMs (e.g., VM and AVM), LMs are rarely life- or limb-threatening and take relatively benign course. They generally remain as the source of compression to the surrounding structure if not as the source of lymphatic leakage and subsequent infection.

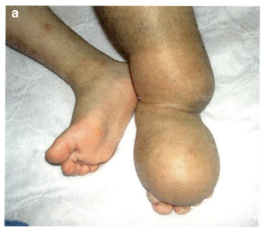
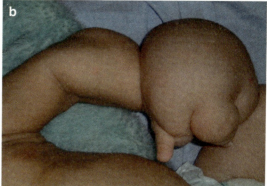

Fig. 49.2 (**a, b**) Mixed condition of truncular and extra-truncular LM lesions (**a, b**), both show massive swelling of the foot (**a**) or hand (**b**) caused by combined condition of truncular and extratruncular LM lesions. A proper combination of various noninvasive and occasionally invasive tests such as direct puncture percutaneous lymphangiography is sufficient for the diagnosis, but if there is any doubt of its status, a tissue biopsy is recommended before the treatment decision is taken

Therefore, not all the (extratruncular) LM lesions are mandated for aggressive care (cf. AVM) and its limited cases are indicated for the treatment.

Further, the treatment modalities associated with high morbidity (e.g., absolute ethanol sclerotherapy) [32–34] should only be considered after lower morbidity treatments have failed. Therapy often begins with safer and less risky treatment methods, such as OK-432 [35–37]. Although these methods carry less risk and morbidity, they are also associated with a higher risk of lesion recurrence. On the other hand, the treatments associated with higher morbidity, such as ethanol, carry a lower risk of lesion recurrence.

LM treatment with sclerotherapy and/or surgical (excisional) therapy should be given to lesions located near vital organs and anatomic structures that threaten vital functions with priority, e.g., respiration, vision, hearing, or eating (Fig. 49.5). Early treatment should also be considered for lesions with accompanying complications, such as lymph leakage, bleeding (LM lesions with a mixed venous component), or recurrent infections or cellulitis (Fig. 49.6). Symptomatic lesions, with or without cosmetically severe deformities or functional disability, such as of the hand, foot, wrist, and ankle, should also be considered for early therapy [38–40].

Definitive treatment in children should be delayed until the child reaches an age at which the risk of therapy is reduced. Unless the lesion is located at a life- or limb-threatening region and requires immediate and/or urgent treatment, conservative management, such as compression therapy, should be continued. Conservative management is usually continued in the young pediatric age group until the age of two or older, when the child can better tolerate the treatment.

Emergency lifesaving measures may be required, especially in neonatal and young pediatric patients where LM lesions cause acute respiratory or alimentary problems (Fig. 49.7).

Treatment Modalities

The treatment strategy for extratruncular LM lesions has changed substantially based on observations regarding their embryology. Incomplete excision is followed by inevitable recurrence, such as cystic hygroma, and often becomes a potential source of significant complications and morbidity. Traditional surgical excision has its role in the treatment of (extratruncular) LM along with a multidisciplinary approach combined with endovascular therapy [19, 41, 42].

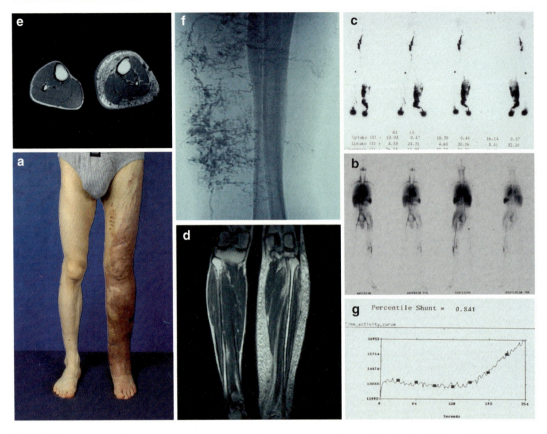

Fig. 49.3 (**a–f**) A complex form of lymphatic/vascular malformation. (**a**) *illustrates* a clinical condition of the swollen left lower extremity by a complex form of vascular malformation that consisted of venous, lymphatic, and capillary malformations. They altogether represent the vascular malformation component of Klippel-Trenaunay syndrome (KTS). Due to the complex nature of vascular malformations, its proper management warrants precise information on each malformation involved, as well as its severity. Generally, noninvasive studies can provide basic information for the diagnosis without difficulty. (**b**) represents whole-body blood pool scintigraphy (WBBPS) showing the exact location and severity of coexisting venous malformation (VM) lesions as an abnormal blood pool

throughout the whole body in addition to the left lower extremity itself. (**c**) displays radionuclide lymphoscintigraphy to identify the accurate condition/severity of lymphatic dysfunction caused by a truncular LM lesion so that lymphedema management can be initiated based on this finding. (**d**) and (**e**) represent MRI study which is essential to assess VM and LM together: a honeycomb-type image of the soft tissue is the hallmark of chronic lymphedema to confirm clinically observed diffuse swelling of the limb as primary lymphedema. (**f**) demonstrates typical percutaneous direct puncture lymphangiography findings of extratruncular LM lesions showing 'lace pattern' structure as its hallmark. (**g**) displays transarterial lung perfusion scintigraphy (TLPS) findings performed to rule out any

Surgical excision is no longer considered as a first-line therapy or as a sole treatment modality because LMs rarely become life-threatening. The combination of conventional surgical excision and endovascular therapy based on sclerotherapy should be considered initially. Endovascular therapy with either OK-432 or ethanol is usually the first treatment option. This is especially true in difficult lesions that are surgically inaccessible [35–37].

OK-432 Sclerotherapy

OK-432 is the preferred initial treatment for LM lesions. OK-432 is a lymphatic sclerosing agent. OK-432 is the lyophilized exotoxin of the low-virulence Su strain of type III group A *Streptococcus pyogenes* and also known as Picibanil. It is produced after removing streptolysin S-producing activity and has a specific

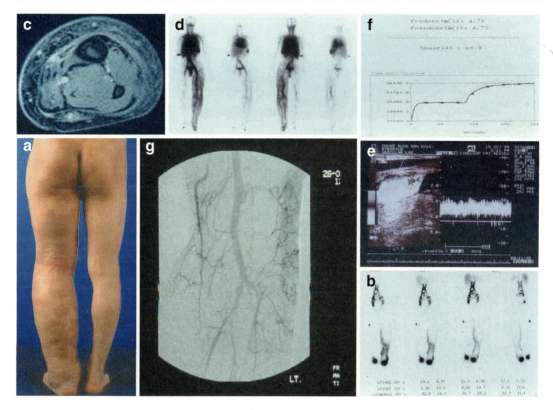

Fig. 49.4 (a–g) (**a**) depicts the clinical feature of Parkes Weber syndrome (PWS) affecting the left lower extremity, which looks similar to common KTS as shown in Fig. 49.3. But PWS has the AVM as an additional vascular malformation component to LM, VM, and CM. Initial evaluation with radionuclide lymphoscintigraphy (**b**) and MRI (**c**) confirmed a truncular LM lesion as the cause of primary lymphedema, while WBBPS (**d**) confirmed the VM component. However, duplex ultrasonography (**e**) shows the evidence of AVM to cause hyperdynamic arterial condition; AVM lesion (**f**) was further assessed to 69.3 % shunting status by the TLPS. Finally, arteriography (**g**) confirmed superficially located multiple microshunting AVM lesions scattered through the lower extremity (From Lee et al. [51])

affinity for lymphatic endothelium resulting in selective injury via a relatively benign inflammatory process [35–37].

OK-432 can easily be injected into a macrocystic lesion or cavity. Outcomes are excellent, with minimal morbidity in the majority of cases (Fig. 49.8) [35–37]. Microcystic cavernous lesions, on the other hand, are virtually impossible to treat/inject so that its efficacy is quite limited with comparatively poor outcomes. In addition, these honeycombed lesions are more likely to communicate with the lymph-transporting system, posing the additional risk of injury to the lymphatic system and perilymphatic tissues (e.g., nerves and blood vessels). Therefore, selective use with precaution is warranted although OK-432 is relatively safe compared to other sclerosing agents even when extravasation occurs.

Multicystic, lobulated lesions are also good candidates for OK-432 therapy. The risk of complication by the extravasation is relatively lower, especially in a mixed lesion with a microcystic component (Fig. 49.9). These lesions, however, require multiple treatment sessions in order to reduce significant local and systemic reactions.

OK-432 is much less effective than more powerful agents, such as ethanol, but carries a lower risk of complications. It is useful even when other conventional sclerotherapies fail. OK-432 has a unique action to thicken the wall of a single-layer endothelial lesion, allowing easier dissection, compared with a primary thin-walled lesion,

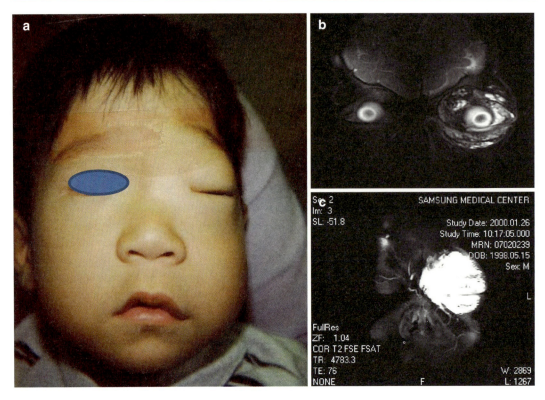

Fig. 49.5 (**a–c**) (**a**) shows a massive swelling of the left eye which was previously known as the condition of moderately puffy eyelids with mild periorbital swelling due to the infiltrating extratruncular LM, as shown in MRI findings (**b**, **c**). Such sudden complete blockage of the vision following mild infection to this LM lesion is as dangerous, if not more, than the VM or AVM lesion in terms of acute/urgent necessity of the immediate treatment which is particularly true to an infant before vision is fully matured

in situations where subsequent surgical excision is necessary.

OK-432 is, therefore, a sclerosing agent with minimal potential for collateral damage and acceptable recurrence rates among many similar sclerosing agents. It is the ideal sclerosing agent for the treatment of LM lesions' relatively benign nature compared to the more virulent VM and AVMs. It is relatively free of significant complications and morbidity that is associated with the more powerful sclerotherapy agents.

When a LM lesion is mixed with a VM lesion (which is easily confirmed by the presence of blood mixed with lymph on the aspiration), OK-432 is totally useless. In these situations, the more powerful sclerotherapy agents such as ethanol are required to control the lesion.

We generally recommend OK-432 for initial treatment of all de novo LM lesions whenever applicable with right indications. Repeating the OK-432 treatment of "recurrent" LM lesions that have failed to OK-432 therapy is also recommended, especially in situations where treatment with ethanol carries unacceptable risk.

Ethanol Sclerotherapy

Ethanol is an excellent sclerotherapy agent for all the varieties of the (extratruncular) CVM lesions [20, 21, 43]; among the LMs, "macrocystic" LM

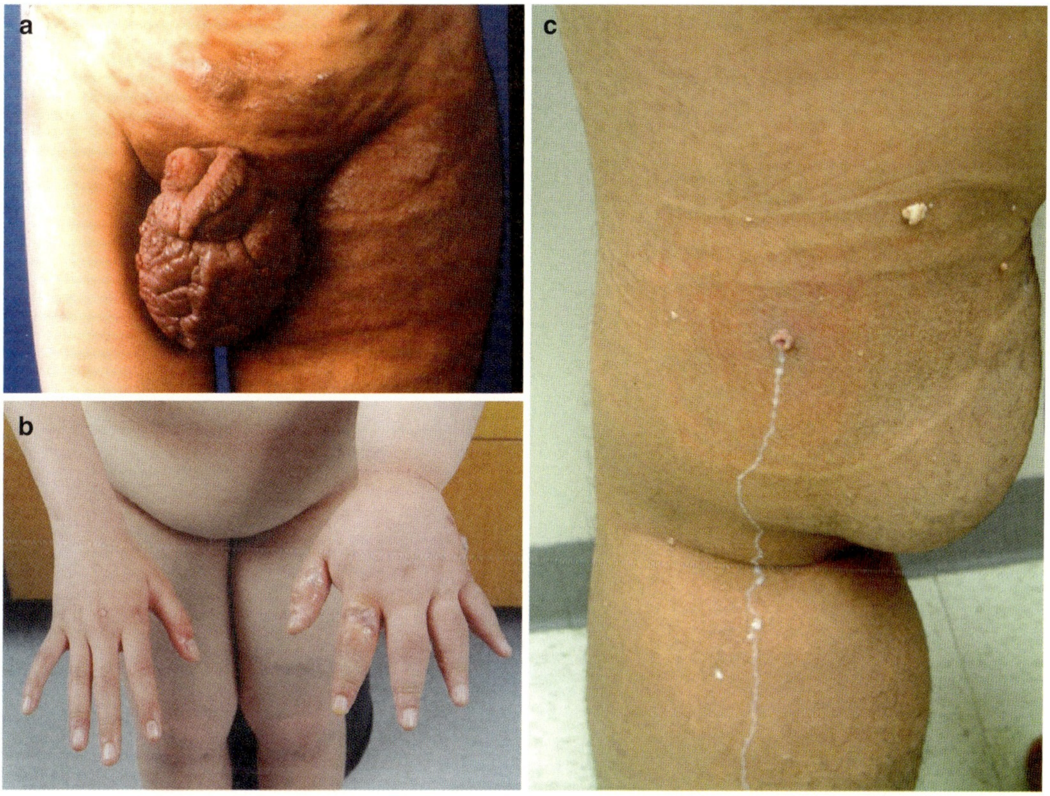

Fig. 49.6 (**a–c**) is the worst combination for the of LM lesions. (**a**) reveals the clinical outcome of chronic infection combined with lymph leakage along the scrotum. The LM lesion itself is relatively benign although it extends into the retropelvic structure as a mixed cystic type, but the infection combined with the lymphatic leakage as its complication remains a poor prognosis as a potentially life-threatening condition which may progress to general sepsis. (**b**) presents a difficult condition with recurrent ruptures of lymph vesicles on the hand/fingers which is already compromised with lymphedema, allowing the progression of acute skin infection. (**c**) shows the leakage of lymphatic fluid from the posterior thigh due to the chylo-reflux from truncular LM lesion; it is further complicated with chylo-ascites by intra-abdominal LM. This patient also has extratruncular LM lesions along the left lower extremity in addition to truncular LM lesion. These complications as well as morbidities indicate early aggressive care with priority

lesion is the most ideal for treatment. In experienced hands, ethanol therapy is associated with minimum morbidity and almost zero recurrence. Therefore, the ethanol is an excellent substitute for OK-432 therapy and has better long-term results for the macrocystic lesions. But, in the treatment of a "microcystic" LM lesion, ethanol sclerotherapy is associated with high complication rates and significant morbidity. Significant collateral tissue necrosis often occurs during treatment of this relatively benign malformation (e.g., nerve damage) (Fig. 49.10).

The general principles of ethanol sclerotherapy should be applied to the treatment of LM lesions: the minimal effective dose of ethanol should be used during each treatment session to minimize the risk of complications [6, 33, 44].

We recommend that ethanol sclerotherapy be limited to the treatment of macrocystic LM lesions occurring in anatomically safe/deep locations. We strongly urge limited use of ethanol for the treatment of microcystic or mixed LM lesions at most. Recurrent symptomatic lesions, failed OK-432 sclerotherapy, LM lesion mixed with VM lesion, and surgically inaccessible lesion are indications for ethanol sclerotherapy [33, 44] (Fig. 49.11).

Post-sclerotherapy Care of the Lesion/Patient

Post-procedure fever is common after OK-432 sclerotherapy and is well managed with antipyretic therapy (acetaminophen or ibuprofen). Pediatric patients often require a short hospitalization post procedure.

Ethanol sclerotherapy patients require close perioperative monitoring for pulmonary hypertension [33, 44]; this is continued postoperatively. These patients also require post-procedure pain control and close observation of the treated areas for local tissue reaction and edema. However, post-procedure compression therapy is controversial at best, with a higher chance of harmful versus beneficial effect following ethanol therapy.

Treatment outcomes are best assessed by duplex ultrasonography performed within a week of treatment and just before additional therapy.

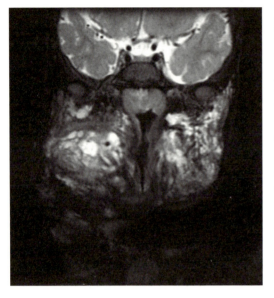

Fig. 49.7 This massive extratruncular LM lesion affecting the entire neck became the source of an acute infection resulting in acute airway obstruction; it required a limited debulking operation to relieve the airway obstruction as an emergency lifesaving procedure. The child subsequently underwent a more radical operation to remove an expanding residual lesion along the left side of the neck

Surgical/Excisional Therapy

Surgical therapy in the treatment of LM lesions is limited due to the significant risk and morbidity associated with the radical procedure

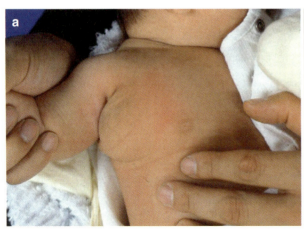
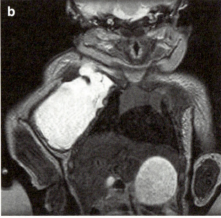

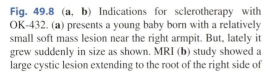

Fig. 49.8 (**a**, **b**) Indications for sclerotherapy with OK-432. (**a**) presents a young baby born with a relatively small soft mass lesion near the right armpit. But, lately it grew suddenly in size as shown. MRI (**b**) study showed a large cystic lesion extending to the root of the right side of the neck with the proximity to the brachial plexus. Therefore, OK-432 was used as scleroagent to control the lesion very effectively since it was a "macrocystic" lesion with minimal septa

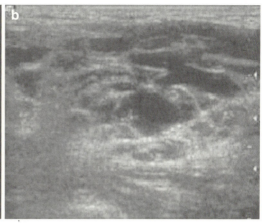

Fig. 49.9 (**a, b**) Microcystic LM lesions. (**a**) depicts extensive multicystic lesions affecting the left groin extended into the retroperitoneal space, mostly consisting of "microcystic" LM lesions. This condition was further confirmed with duplex ultrasonography (**b**). It became the constant source of local cellulitis. In view of the extensive nature of the lesions with proximity to the iliac-femoral neurovascular structures, OK-432 was selected to minimize the potential risk involved in multiple session therapy. However, if the recurrent/residual lesion should become a major problem in the future, a combined approach will be considered with surgical excision limited to the critically located lesion and supplemental ethanol sclerotherapy to other safer parts of the lesion when the child is grown old enough to tolerate such difficult therapy

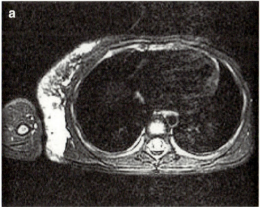
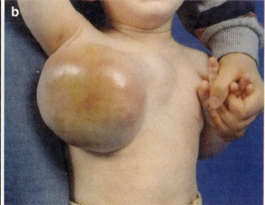

Fig. 49.10 (**a, b**) Microcystic LM lesions. A microcystic LM lesion shown by MRI (**a**) is not a good candidate for ethanol sclerotherapy. However, following repeated failure with OK-432 sclerotherapy, ethanol was carefully combined with OK-432; its injection was carried out under ultrasonographic guidance and limited to the lesion which had best cystic condition to allow safe injection with the least risk of extravasation. However, the outcome (**b**) was alarming with tremendous swelling but without skin necrosis. Following such difficult conditions which cannot be controlled by the conventional sclerotherapy, the lesion was subsequently surgically excised

[13–15]. The majority of LM lesions occur as mixed lesions containing both macrocystic and microcystic components. The presence of the microcystic component limits the effectiveness of OK-432. Ethanol therapy of these mixed lesions is also associated with significant morbidity. In addition, many microcystic LM lesions often exist with VM lesions. In this situation, complications associated with ethanol therapy preclude its use, while OK-432 has no effect on VM lesions. Therefore, this lesion type is best treated with surgical excision with or without preoperative OK-432 sclerotherapy (Fig. 49.12).

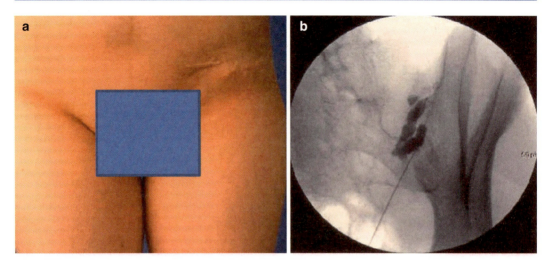

Fig. 49.11 (**a**, **b**) Recurring lesions. (**a**) shows multiple operation scars along the left lower abdomen following surgical excisions of the LM lesions. However, due to their embryologic nature, the extratruncular lesions recurred despite multiple operations to excise them.

Under the fluoroscopic guidance as shown in (**b**), ethanol sclerotherapy was given to these "recurrent" but mostly "macrocystic" and deep-seated lesions; this ethanol therapy potentially cured the lesion (5-year follow-up with no evidence of recurrence on ultrasonography)

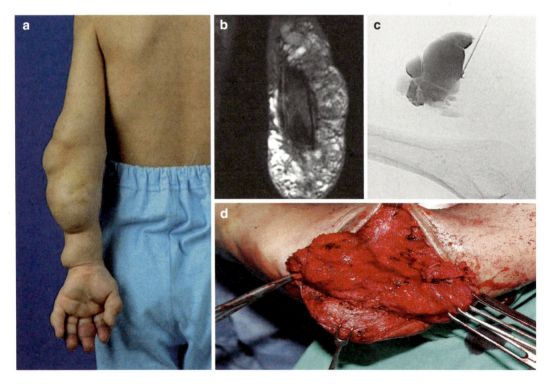

Fig. 49.12 (**a–d**) Mixed LM and VM. (**a**) illustrates a mixed condition of LM and VM, a variant of hemolymphatic malformation, affecting the entire forearm extending to the hand and fingers. Multiple sessions of ethanol sclerotherapy were given first to coexisting VM lesions, as

shown by MRI (**b**), and then, the macrocystic LM lesion was treated with ethanol as shown in (**c**). Finally, the microcystic lesion (**d**) was safely removed surgically following preoperative OK-432 sclerotherapy, delivering a satisfactory outcome

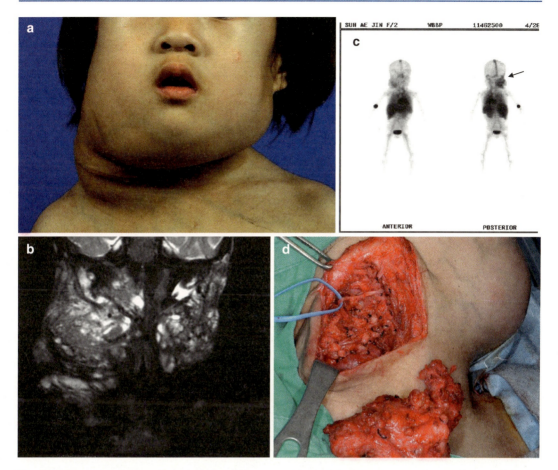

Fig. 49.13 (**a–d**) Rapidly expanding LM lesion. (**a**) shows a young female patient who underwent limited resection of a LM lesion along the right lateral neck, which was rapidly expanding following acute respiratory infection. MRI (**b**) showed expansive lesion with high risk of upper airway obstruction as a potentially life-threatening condition. WBBPS (**c**) showed a significant abnormal blood pool suggesting coexisting VM lesion along this extratruncular LM lesion. Therefore, OK-432 sclerotherapy to this LM lesion was abandoned due to this coexisting VM lesion; surgical excision was carried out as shown in (**d**) to relieve this rapidly expanding LM lesion from the right lateral neck

Certain lesions that cannot be treated effectively with sclerotherapy (such as neck lesions that extend into the deep mediastinal structures) may require surgical excision because of mass effect and extensive involvement of surrounding anatomical structures (Fig. 49.13). The risk of injury to adjacent vessels and nerves during dissection may be prohibitively high and associated with significant lifelong morbidity. This is especially true in the pediatric population [13, 14, 38, 39]. The approach to treatment in these situations has changed over the years. Incomplete excision, sparing vital anatomic structures, is an acceptable alternative to radical resection accompanying with significant morbidity.

The role of surgical therapy in the treatment of LM has been well defined and is now fully integrated with endovascular therapy (sclerotherapy) [7, 19]. Surgical excision is especially useful in the treatment of macro- and microcystic mixed LM lesions. These lesions can be effectively controlled with preoperative sclerotherapy followed by surgical excision.

There is no well-defined optimal time for surgical excision. Surgical resection should be delayed for as long as possible. Partial excision of an easily accessible lesion is acceptable as the first stage of a multistage approach. It allows a better chance for later excision of the residual lesion. Emergency procedures should be limited to decompressing surgery designed to relieve acute symptoms until a later, more definitive treatment can be planned.

Prospects

The future of the clinical management of LM is now brighter than ever, with new concept and approaches based on the correction of defective lymphangiogenesis [45–47]. There has been substantial progress made in the quest to localize and characterize the responsible genes and mutations.

Exogenous growth factor administration will open a new chapter to effective gene and gene product therapy; recently anti-VEGFR-3 neutralizing antibody has been confirmed as having the capacity to completely and specifically inhibit lymphatic vascular regeneration [48–50].

The cloning of the gene responsible for lymphangiogenesis and identification of the defective genes involved in abnormal lymphangiogenesis will eventually lead to prenatal diagnosis and ultimately mutational screening of at-risk populations.

Although therapeutic implementation of the gene modification in embryonic development and also abnormal function in adults is still far from reality, such idea for correcting defective lymphangiogenesis will become major tools for the future management of the LM, and the "molecular antidote" to pathological overgrowth of lymphangiomatosis should become a major player with chance of cure in the near future.

Conclusion

Extratruncular LM lesions can be treated with different sclerotherapy agents. The cystic type is well treated by sclerotherapy with excellent results and minimum risk of recurrence. Surgical excision with and without perioperative sclerotherapy may be considered a better option in the treatment of the localized cavernous-type lesion and carries a reduced risk of recurrence.

References

1. Bastide G, Lefebvre D (1989) Anatomy and organogenesis and vascular malformations. In: Belov S, Loose DA, Weber J (eds) Vascular malformations. Einhorn-Presse Verlag GmbH, Reinbek, pp 20–22
2. Woolard HH (1922) The development of the principal arterial stems in the forelimb of the pig. Contrib Embryol 14:139–154
3. Leu HJ (1990) Pathomorphology of vascular malformations: analysis of 310 cases. Int Angiol 9:147–155
4. Belov S (1989) Classification, terminology, and nosology of congenital vascular defects. In: Belov S, Loose DA, Weber J (eds) Vascular malformations. Einhorn-Presse, Reinbek, pp 25–30
5. Lee BB, Laredo J, Lee TS, Huh S, Neville R (2007) Terminology and classification of congenital vascular malformations. Phlebology 22(6):249–252
6. Lee BB, Baumgartner I, Berlien HP, Bianchini G, Burrows P et al (2013) Consensus Document of the International Union of Angiology (IUA)-2013. Current concept on the management of arterio-venous management. Int Angiol 32(1):9–36
7. Lee BB, Kim YW, Seo JM et al (2005) Current concepts in lymphatic malformation (LM). Vasc Endovascular Surg 39(1):67–81
8. Lee BB, Villavicencio L (2010) Chapter 68. General considerations. Congenital vascular malformations. Section 9. Arteriovenous anomalies. In: Cronenwett JL, Johnston KW (eds) Rutherford's vascular surgery, 7th edn. Saunders Elsevier, Philadelphia, pp 1046–1064
9. Lee BB, Villavicencio JL (2010) Primary lymphedema and lymphatic malformation: are they the two sides of the same coin? Eur J Vasc Endovasc Surg 39:646–653
10. Lee BB (2005) Lymphedema-angiodysplasia syndrome: a prodigal form of lymphatic malformation (LM). Phlebolymphology 47:324–332
11. Lee BB, Andrade M, Bergan J, Boccardo F, Campisi C et al (2010) Diagnosis and treatment of primary lymphedema – consensus document of the International Union of Phlebology (IUP)-2009. Int Angiol 29(5):454–470
12. Gloviczki P, Duncan A, Kalra M, Oderich G, Ricotta J et al (2009) Vascular malformations: an update. Perspect Vasc Surg Endovasc Ther 21(2):133–148
13. Alqahtani A, Nguyen LT, Flageole H et al (1999) 25 years' experience with lymphangiomas in children. J Pediatr Surg 34(7):1164–1168
14. Orvidas LJ, Kasperbauer JL (2000) Pediatric lymphangiomas of the head and neck. Ann Otol Rhinol Laryngol 109(4):411–421
15. Mitsukawa N, Satoh K (2012) New treatment for cystic lymphangiomas of the face and neck: cyst wall

rupture and cyst aspiration combined with sclerotherapy. J Craniofac Surg 23(4):1117–1119

16. Lee BB, Laredo J, Neville R (2011) Primary lymphedema as a truncular lymphatic malformation. In: Lee B, Bergan J, Rockson SG (eds) Lymphedema: a concise compendium of theory and practice, 1st edn. Springer, London, pp 419–426

17. Lee BB, Laredo J, Neville R, Mattassi R (2011) Primary lymphedema and Klippel-Trenaunay syndrome. In: Lee BB, Bergan J, Rockson SG (eds) Lymphedema: a concise compendium of theory and practice, 1st edn. Springer, London, pp 427–436

18. Lee BB (2005) Current issue in management of chronic lymphedema: personal reflection on an experience with 1065 patients. Lymphology 38:28–31

19. Lee BB (2004) Critical issues on the management of congenital vascular malformation. Ann Vasc Surg 18(3):380–392

20. Lee BB, Kim DI, Huh S, Kim HH, Choo IW, Byun HS et al (2001) New experiences with absolute ethanol sclerotherapy in the management of a complex form of congenital venous malformation. J Vasc Surg 33(4):764–772

21. Lee BB, Do YS, Byun HS, Choo IW, Kim DI, Huh SH (2003) Advanced management of venous malformation with ethanol sclerotherapy: mid-term results. J Vasc Surg 37(3):533–538

22. Lee BB (2003) Current concept of venous malformation (VM). Phlebolymphology 43:197–203

23. Lee BB, Do YS, Yakes W, Kim DI, Mattassi R, Hyun WS, Byun HS (2004) Management of arterial-venous shunting malformations (AVM) by surgery and embolosclerotherapy. A multidisciplinary approach. J Vasc Surg 39(3):590–600

24. Lee BB, Lardeo J, Neville R (2009) Arterio-venous malformation: how much do we know? Phlebology 24:193–200

25. Lee BB, Laredo J, Deaton DH, Neville RF (2009) Chapter 53. Arteriovenous malformations: evaluation and treatment. In: Gloviczki P (ed) Handbook of venous disorders: guidelines of the American Venous Forum, 3rd edn. A Hodder Arnold, London, pp 583–593

26. Jacob AG, Driscoll DJ, Shaughnessy WJ et al (1998) Klippel-Trenaunay syndrome: spectrum and management. Mayo Clin Proc 73(1):28–36

27. Lee BB (2005) Statues of new approaches to the treatment of congenital vascular malformations (CVMS) – single center experiences – (editorial review). Eur J Vasc Endovasc Surg 30(2):184–197

28. Gloviczki P, Driscoll DJ (2007) Klippel–Trenaunay syndrome: current management. Phlebology 22:291–298

29. Ziyeh S, Spreer J, Rossler J, Strecker R, Hochmuth A, Schumacher M, Klisch J (2004) Parkes Weber or Klippel-Trenaunay syndrome? Non-invasive diagnosis with MR projection angiography. Eur Radiol 14(11):2025–2029. Epub 2004 Mar 6

30. Wu ZQ (1993) Parkes-Weber's syndrome: report of 5 cases. Zhonghua Wai Ke Za Zhi 31(12):749–751

31. Courivaud D, Delerue A, Delerue C, Boon L, Piette F, Modiano P (2006) Familial case of Parkes Weber syndrome. Ann Dermatol Venereol 133(5 Pt 1):445–447

32. Park JH, Kim DI, Huh S, Lee SJ, Do YS, Lee BB (1998) Absolute ethanol sclerotherapy on cystic lymphangioma in neck and shoulder region. J Korean Vasc Surg Soc 14(2):300–303

33. Do YS, Yakes WF, Shin SW, Kim DI, Shin BS, Lee BB (2005) Ethanol embolization of arteriovenous malformations: interim results. Radiology 235(2):674–682

34. Lee BB (2008) Chapter 4. Lymphatic malformation. In: Tredbar LL, Morgan CL, Lee BB, Simonian SJ, Blondeau B (eds) Lymphedema-diagnosis and treatment. Springer, London, pp 31–42

35. Ogita S, Tsuto T, Deguchi E et al (1991) OK-432 therapy for unresectable lymphangiomas in children. J Pediatr Surg 26:263–270

36. Kim KH, Kim HH, Lee SK, Lee BB (2001) OK-432 intralesional injection therapy for lymphangioma in children. J Korean Assoc Pediatr Surg 7:142–146

37. Luzzatto C, Midrio P, Tchaprassian Z, Guglielmi M (2000) Sclerosing treatment of lymphangiomas with OK-432. Arch Dis Child 82(4):316–318

38. Al-Salem AH (2004) Lymphangiomas in infancy and childhood. Saudi Med J 25(4):466–469

39. Stromberg BV, Weeks PM, Wray RC Jr (1976) Treatment of cystic hygroma. South Med J 69(10):1333–1335

40. Saijo M, Munro IR, Mancer K (1975) Lymphangioma. A long-term follow-up study. Plast Reconstr Surg 56(6):642–651

41. Lee BB, Bergan JJ (2002) Advanced management of congenital vascular malformations: a multidisciplinary approach. Cardiovasc Surg 10(6):523–533

42. Lee BB (2002) Advanced management of congenital vascular malformation (CVM). Int Angiol 21(3):209–213

43. Jeon YH, Do YS, Shin SW, Liu WC, Cho JM, Lee MH, Kim DI, Lee BB, Choo SW, Choo IW (2003) Ethanol embolization of arteriovenous malformations: results and complications of 33 cases. J Kor Radiol Soc 49:263–270

44. Shin BS, Do YS, Lee BB, Kim DI, Chung IS, Cho HS et al (2005) Multistage ethanol sclerotherapy of soft-tissue arteriovenous malformations: effect on pulmonary arterial pressure. Radiology 235:1072–1077

45. Witte MH, Erickson R, Bernas M et al (1998) Phenotypic and genotypic heterogeneity in familial Milroy lymphedema. Lymphology 31:145–155

46. Ferrell RE, Levinson KL, Esman JH, Kimak MA, Lawrence EC, Barmada MM et al (1998) Hereditary lymphedema: evidence for linkage and genetic heterogeneity. Hum Mol Genet 7:2073–2078

47. Michelini S, Degiorgio D, Cestari M et al (2012) Clinical and genetic study of 46 Italian patients with primary lymphedema. Lymphology 45(1):3–12

48. Erickson RP (2001) Lymphedema-distichiasis and FOXC2 gene mutations. Lymphology 34(1):1–5

49. Ghalamkarpour A, Holnthoner W, Saharinen P, Boon LM, Vikkula M et al (2009) Recessive primary congenital lymphoedema caused by a VEGFR3 mutation. J Med Genet 46:399–404

50. Karkkainen MJ, Ferrell RE, Lawrence EC, Kimak MA, Levinson KL, McTigue MA et al (2000) Missense mutations interfere with VEGFR-3 signalling in primary lymphoedema. Nat Genet 25:153–159

51. Lee BB, Mattassi R, Kim BT, Park JM (2005) Advanced management of arteriovenous shunting malformation (AVM) with transarterial lung perfusion scintigraphy (TLPS) for follow-up assessment. Int Angiol 24(2):173–184

Veno-lymphatic Vascular Malformations: Medical Therapy

Sandro Michelini and Marco Cardone

If medical therapy is intended as the set of possible "nonsurgical" treatments reserved for the various clinical forms in which *veno-lymphatic malformations* occur, we can say that today there are a number of therapeutic aids, supported by EBM, which are ideal for many of the clinical problems caused by these malformations.

The *phlebolymphedema* of the limbs is a disorder with frequent occurrence in its various forms, which by its very nature tends to worsen and has a tendency to complications and clinical exacerbation.

Lymphedema is an interstitial edema with high protein concentrations, localized in a limb or part thereof, due to constitutional hypogenesis (often familial) or surgical ablation or destruction and radiotherapy or inflammation of pathways or lymphatic stations [1–4].

Its primary forms are of a hereditary nature and are, in some cases (syndromic lymphedemas), associated with other genetic diseases. The pure forms can be familial (3–5 % of cases) or be in the "sporadic" form (over 95 % of cases). The familial forms are transmitted with an autosomal dominant "variable expressive" character [1, 4].

The diagnosis of lymphedema is based mainly on clinical observations. The edema of the limb (or limbs when the location is bilateral) is hard, whitish, and neither sore nor painful. The fovea is fleeting or absent (an expression of the early overlapping phenomena for the perilymph sclerosis common in the subcutaneous tissue of the affected limb).

Stemmer's sign is always positive in primary forms and negative in the early stages of secondary forms. The edema could pose problems of differential diagnosis with venous edema, cardiac, liver, kidney, and with the lipoedema that, unlike other edemas, never affects the foot or hand.

The diagnostic gold standard is represented by lymphoscintigraphy. This examination compares the two limbs making it possible to view any ipogenesia or agenesia of the paths or lymph nodes along the limb or at the root thereof as well as identify the areas of greatest lymphatic stagnation (dermal back flow) present in the limb. The examination also shows the presence of alternative lymphatic paths, superficial and deep, that can possibly be stimulated with appropriate manual maneuvers and exercises [3, 5].

The high-resolution ultrasonography shows the main lymphatic collectors; their diameter; the presence of "lymphatic lakes," typical of the more advanced clinical stages; and the thickness above and below. The computed tomography, the R.M.N., and laser Doppler complete the diagnostic morphological and functional picture [3, 6, 7].

From the therapeutic point of view, the evolutionary stage of the disease and the type of patient should be noted.

S. Michelini (✉) • M. Cardone
Department of Rehabilitation Medicine,
San Giovanni Battista Hospital –
ACISMOM – Rome, Roma, Italy
e-mail: s.michelini@acismom.it;
m.cardone@acismom.it

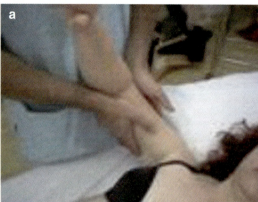
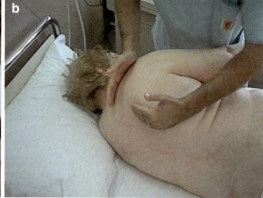

Fig. 50.1 (**a**) Manual lymphatic drainage of the upper limb; (**b**) treatment of posterior lymphatic alternative ways

In the first stage, subclinical (e.g., blood relative to a patient with *primary lymphedema*) primary prevention with the use of compression hosiery in risk conditions (long journeys, heavy work) and periodic medical checks is very important.

In the second phase (presence of edema that spontaneously regresses with nighttime rest), stage III (presence of edema that does not regress spontaneously with rest), and stage IV (imposing edema that deforms the limb, making it similar to an elephant's foot), physical combined with *decongestive treatment* is employed based on:

- Manual *lymphatic drainage* adapted in each case with the stimulation of the possible alternative lymphatic pathways; always performed bilaterally in lymphedema of the lower limbs. Carried out unilaterally in lymphedema of the upper limbs for the distinct "terminus" between the sides [8] (Fig. 50.1a, b).
- Sequential compression (today mostly confined to the self-therapy at home), in which the partial local (lymphangitis, dermohypodermitis, varicophlebitis) and systemic (arterial hypertension and congestive heart failure) contraindication criteria are adhered to; unlike the lymphatic drainage that essentially drains the protein component of edema, this contributes to removing the water component in a short time (Fig. 50.2).
- Isotonic gymnastics with stimulation, through special exercises that activate the muscle pumps of the limbs, both the suprafascial lymphatic pathways and the subfascial to be

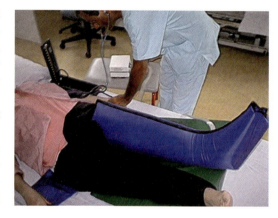

Fig. 50.2 Pressotherapy of the lower limb

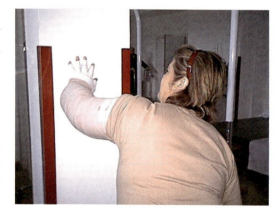

Fig. 50.3 Physical exercise during bandaging for activation of muscular pumps of the upper limb

carried out in groups as well within the structure or on outdoor paths during hospitalization (Figs. 50.3 and 50.4).

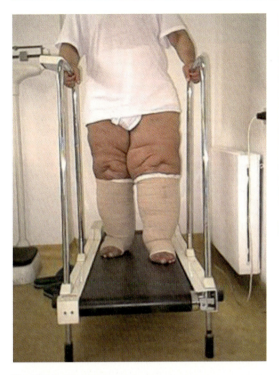

Fig. 50.4 Treadmill under elasto-compression of the lower limbs for specific muscular activation

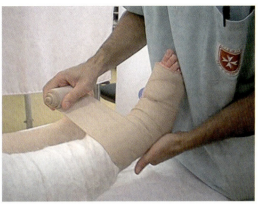

Fig. 50.5 Phases of bandaging of the lower limb

- Personalized *elasto-compression* with multi-layer inelastic bandages on the wound using the "herringbone" or "figure-of-eight" technique in subjects who are able to perform adequate muscle exercise during the various phases of the day; stretch fabric as the first layer and inelastic in the subsequent 2–3 layers in patients able to perform discrete muscle exercise during the day, two-way stretch in a single layer for bedridden, disabled, or elderly patients. After intensive treatment during hospitalization, the operators are in a position to prescribe the definitive elastic garment (standard or "custom-made"), which will provide the primary means of maintaining and consolidating the results obtained with the intensive therapeutic regime (Figs. 50.5 and 50.6).
- Ultrasound, used with a power of 2 W/cm, with good clinical success, is mainly employed, even for prolonged periods of time (30–40 min), in the fibrotic areas (Fig. 50.7). The radial shock waves have important effect on the fibrotic component of the edema and any tissue calcification that is an expression of

past acute lymphatic episodes [3, 9] (Fig. 50.8). In some areas (in case of edema of the face), the only possible physical therapies are the manual lymphatic drainage and the vacuum therapy (Fig. 50.9). In secondary lymphedema, physical protocol must include (above all in some clinical cases) occupational therapy (Fig. 50.10) [10].

The *physical treatment* should always be combined with the pharmacological use of alpha-benzopyrones, especially natural curarine administered for systemic or topical use (including in the form of creams), at a dose of 4–8 mg/day (with titration at 15–18 %) which has a macrophage activation effect, proteolysis, and, simultaneously, prolymphocytic effect (by stimulating the contractility of the lymph collectors with the effect of increasing the lymphatic transport capacity) [11]. The gamma-benzopyrones, as well as the Indian pennywort, also have the effect of reducing capillary permeability (through stabilization of the endothelial membranes) with consequent reduction of the interstitial hydrostatic pressure. The use (oral or parenteral) of active compounds is also effective for the remodeling of the interstitial matrix, mainly reorganizing the coordination functions of the matrix itself. These are made from natural substances (dandelion, calendula, echinacea, condurango, and other substances). In the treatment of infectious complications, or for the prevention thereof, the use of broad-spectrum antibiotics or penicillin for prolonged periods (6–12 months) in susceptible individuals has also been proven to be favorable.

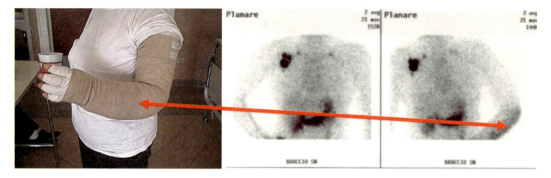

Fig. 50.6 Bandaging in the forearm area increases consistency of the tissue (demonstrated by the lymphoscintigraphy)

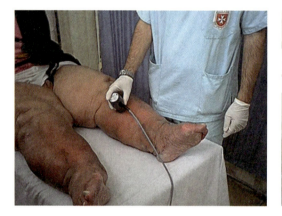

Fig. 50.7 Ultrasound on the fibrosis: 2 W/cm^2 1–3 MHz, 12–15 minutes

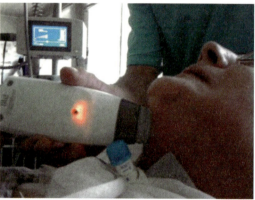

Fig. 50.9 Vacuum therapy on the fibrosis in secondary face lymphedema

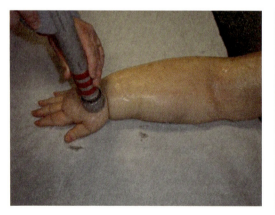

Fig. 50.8 Shockwaves on the fibrosis of the hand

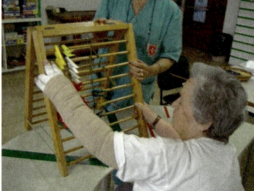

Fig. 50.10 Occupational therapy in secondary lymphedema of the upper limb in an elderly patient

The use of desensitization vaccines with bacterial loads without the pathogenic power is useful for the stimulation and production of specific antibodies for the germs usually implicated in these infectious processes [12].

In the fifth stage where, in addition to the severe deformation of the limb ulcer, fungal or dermohypodermitis complications are also present, particular attention must be paid to local hygiene and the prevention of local infectious and inflammatory complications.

Lymphedema, both in primary familial and sporadic forms as well as syndromic in which it is often associated with malformation venous diseases, is a chronic disease and as such should be classified and controlled over time. It requires full accountability on the part of the patient and consequent adherence to the treatment plan. It requires physical therapy and pharmacological cycles and reconstructive surgery when indicated and, above all, necessitates continuous clinical and instrumental monitoring.

References

1. Connell F, Brice G, Jeffery S, Keele YV, Mortimer P, Smansour S (2010) A new classification system for primary lymphatic dysplasias based on phenotype. Clin Genet 77(5):438–452
2. Pissas A, Albertin J, Dauthevilkle E, Fourquet JP, Castro L (1998) Valutazione clinica del linfedema. Linfologia 1(1):26–29
3. ISL (2009) The diagnosis and treatment of peripheral lymphoedema. Lymphology 42:51–60
4. Michelini S, De Giorgio D, Cestari M, Corda D, Ricci M, Cardone M, Mander A, Famoso L, Contini E, Serrani R, Pinelli L, Cecchin S, Bertelli M (2012) Clinical and genetic study of 46 italian patients with primary lymphoedema. Lymphology 45:3–12
5. Foldi M, Foldi E (2009) Foldi's textbook of lymphology. Elsevier, San Francisco
6. Lee B, Andrade M, Bergan J, Boccardo F, Campisi C, Damstra R, Flour M, Gloviczki P, Laredo J, Piller N, Michelini S, Mortimer P, Villavicencio JL (2010) Diagnosis and treatment of primary lymphedema. Consensus Document of the International Union of Phlebology (IUP)-2009. Int Angiol 29(5):454–470
7. Michelini S, Failla A, Moneta G, Cardone M, Michelotti L, Zinicola V, Rubeghi V (2008) Linee guida e protocolli diagnostico-terapeutici nel linfedema. Eur Med Phys 44(Suppl. 1–3):1–2
8. Leduc A (1980) Le drainage lymphatique: théorie et pratique, Monographie de Bois-Larris. Ed. Masson, Paris
9. Michelini S, Failla A, Moneta G, Cardone M, Antonucci D, Galluccio A (2008) Shockwave therapy in vascular disease rehabilitation: preliminary study. Eur J Lymphol Relat Probl 18(53):16–19
10. Michelini S, Failla A, Moneta G, Rubeghi V, Zinicola V, Cardone M et al (2007) Lymphedema and occupational therapy. Lymphology 55:243–246
11. Casley-Smith JRV (1985) High-protein oedemas and the benzo-pyrones. Ed. Globe Press, Melbourne
12. Michelini S, Failla A, Cardone M, Moneta G, Fiorentino A (2009) Immune stimulation and reduction of infective complications in patients with lymphoedema. Eur J Lymphol Relat Probl 20(56):17–18

Lymphatic Truncular Malformations of the Limbs: Surgical Treatment

51

Corradino Campisi, Melissa Ryan,
Caterina Sara Campisi, Francesco Boccardo,
and Corrado Cesare Campisi

Introduction

While the international scientific community, through its institutional components, most representative of the major societies involved (International Society of Lymphology, ISL;

International Union of Phlebology, UIP; International Society for the Study of Vascular Anomalies, ISSVA; and the newly formed Italian Society for the Study of Vascular Anomalies, SISAV) is fully committed to defining common guidelines for diagnostic-therapeutic considerations based on the official consensus documents, we offer for publication the contributions on the "surgical treatment of lymphatic truncular malformations of the limbs" and "thoracic duct dysplasias with chylous reflux," which we wish to be understood as an attempt to systematically classify a complex pathology of vascular malformation that is still under the "strong influence of subject area," which is often in contrast to a clinical reality, and where there is not a clear and constant academic distinction between diseases and syndromes exclusively attributable to predominantly lymphatic malformations. The contributions will consider lymphatic truncular malformations consisting of primary lymphedema and also the thoracic duct dysplasias and associated syndromes of chylous reflux.

Truncular Lymphatic Malformations

There remains significant confusion about the relationship between primary lymphedema and lymphatic malformations, which is further complicated by disagreements surrounding the definition of primary lymphedema. However, primary lymphedema is regarded as a clinical

C. Campisi, MD, PhD, FACS (✉)
Department of Surgery (DISC),
Operative Unit of General and Lymphatic Surgery,
Section & Research Center of Lymphatic Surgery,
Lymphology, and Microsurgery, IRCCS University
Hospital San Martino – IST National Institute for
Cancer Research, Genoa, Italy

Postgraduate School of Alimentary Tract Surgery,
Siena, Italy
e-mail: campisi@unige.it

M. Ryan, PhD • F. Boccardo, MD, PhD
Operative Unit of General and Lymphatic Surgery,
Section & Research Center of Lymphatic Surgery,
Lymphology, and Microsurgery, Department
of Surgery (DISC), IRCCS University Hospital
San Martino – IST National Institute for Cancer
Research, Genoa, Italy
e-mail: ryame269@hotmail.com

C. Sara Campisi, MD
Operative Unit of Dermatology,
Department of Health Sciences (DISSAL),
IRCCS University Hospital San Martino – IST
National Institute for Cancer Research, Genoa, Italy

C. Cesare Campisi, MD, RAS-ACS
Operative Unit of Plastic, Reconstructive
and Aesthetic Surgery, Department of Surgery
(DISC), IRCCS University Hospital San
Martino – IST National Institute for Cancer Research,
Genoa, Italy

R. Mattassi et al. (eds.), *Hemangiomas and Vascular Malformations: An Atlas of Diagnosis and Treatment*, 451
DOI 10.1007/978-88-470-5673-2_51, © Springer-Verlag Italia 2009, 2015

manifestation of a lymphatic malformation that developed during the later stage of lymphangiogenesis [1, 2]. Lymphatic malformations are low-flow vascular malformations and can be divided into extra-truncular and truncular forms. The truncular lymphatic malformations are further divided into primary lymphedema and visceral forms (those which include lymphangiectasis and lymphangiomatosis). Some truncular and visceral lymphatic malformations have proliferative potential (lymphangiomatosis). Truncular and extra-truncular lymphatic malformations can coexist (ISSVA Classification International Consensus, 11 Workshop, Rome, 1996).

The majority of the clinical conditions that are considered to be primary lymphedema are due to truncular lymphatic malformation that arises during the final stages of the lymphangiogenesis [3, 4], when there is formation of the lymphatic trunks, vessels, and nodes [5, 6]. These malformations result in hypoplasia, hyperplasia, or aplasia of the lymphatic vessels and/or the lymph nodes and may clinically manifest as obstruction or dilatation. When the malformations result in the absence or defectiveness of the endoluminal valves, reflux of the lymph is the primary clinical manifestation. In contrast, the extra-truncular lymphatic malformations develop at an earlier stage of the embryogenesis and are associated with immature embryonic tissue that fails to involute, remaining in the earlier embryonic stages [5, 6].

Some primary or congenital lymphedemas are not true congenital defects but occur due to postnatal destruction of the lymphatic collectors or nodes. These mimic the congenital condition in terms of clinical presentation and are classified as congenital lymphedema because the symptoms are present at birth [7, 8]. Other primary lymphedemas do not have anatomically evident truncular malformations of the lymphatic system but represent a functional defect that is molecular in origin [9, 10].

Primary lymphedemas have typically been classified into three groups, depending on the age of the onset of clinical manifestations: congenital (before age 2 years), praecox (between age 2 and 35 years), and tarda (after age 35 years). However, there is significant criticism of this arbitrary categorization as it is not clinically useful [9].

In addition, the category of primary lymphedema often includes other types of lymphedema of an idiopathic nature without an identifiable etiology (i.e., radiation, surgery, or infection) [11]. Some experts also believe that all lymphedema and lymphatic malformations are genetically derived and have proposed that lymphedema should be considered as an abnormality of lymph drainage and classified only by the tissue territory drained [10]. We prefer to classify the lymphedemas using an etiological basis, as can be seen in Fig. 51.1.

In order to provide a comprehensive classification system of lymphedema that encompasses immunohistopathological criteria, level of clinically evident edema, lymphoscintigraphic findings, and level of physical disability, we developed a three-stage model (Fig. 51.2) [9, 12, 13]. In clinical practice, stages IA, IB, IIA, and early IIB can be considered as early manifestations of disease and late IIB, IIIA, and IIIB stages to be chronic and advanced. It should be noted that lymphedema is a progressive disease and can move rapidly between the stages without adequate treatment [14–17].

General Considerations of the Surgical Treatment of Lymphedema

Refractory lymphedema unresponsive to conservative treatment measures may be appropriately managed by surgical means. Indications for surgery include insufficient volume reduction by appropriate conservative methods (less than 50 % reduction), recurrent lymphangitis or erysipelas episodes, intractable pain or discomfort usually associated with excess swelling and inflammation, loss of limb function and increasing disability, and patient dissatisfaction with previous treatment outcomes and willingness to proceed with surgery.

The initial derivative microsurgical approaches involved lymph node-venous shunts, but, aside from India where these have been used frequently in the treatment of lymphatic filariasis, these approaches have been largely superceded by more refined and effective techniques.

Fig. 51.1 Classification of lymphedema (C. Campisi, 2001)

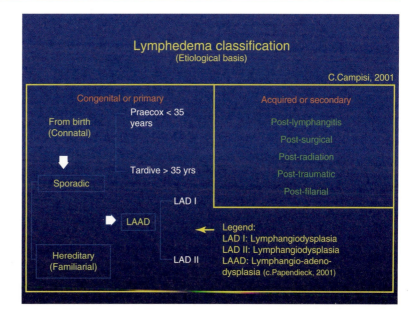

Staging of Lymphedema

Stage I	A. Latent lymphedema, without clinical evidence of edema, but with impaired lymph transport capacity (provable by lymphoscintigraphy) and with initial immunohistochemical alterations of lymph nodes, lymph vessels and extracellular matrix.
	B. Initial lymphedema, totally or partially decreasing by rest and draining position, with worsening impairment of lymph transport capacity and of immunohistochemical alterations of lymph collectors, nodes and extracellular matrix.
Stage II	A. Increasing lymphedema, with vanishing lymph transport capacity, relapsing lymphangitic attacks, fibroindurative skin changes, and developing disability.
	B. Column shaped limb fibrolymphedema, with lymphostatic skin changes, suppressed lymph transport capacity and worsening disability.
Stage III	A. Properly called elephantiasis, with scleroindurative pachydermitis, papillomatous lymphostatic verrucosis, no lymph transport capacity and life-threatening disability.
	B. Extreme elephantiasis with total disability.

Fig. 51.2 Staging of lymphedema, based on immunohistological criteria, lymphoscintigraphic findings, clinical symptoms, and grade of physical disability (C. Campisi, August 2009)

Lymph node-venous shunts had a high rate of anastomotic closure due to the thrombogenic effect of the lymph nodal pulp on the blood and the frequent re-endothelialization of the lymph node surface [18]. Worldwide, surgeons moved to anastomosing lymphatic vessels directly into the veins in order to increase the long-term efficacy of the procedures [19].

The lymphatic-venous anastomosis technique involves joining an appropriate lymphatic vessel to a collateral branch of a main vein, ensuring that the vein has competent valvular function and continence. This is essential to prevent reflux of the blood into the lymphatic vessel and thereby thrombosis of the anastomosis [12].

Clinical Experience and Surgical Techniques

The microsurgical interventions involved multiple lymphatic-venous anastomoses (LVA). Blue patent violet dye (BPV; a sodium or calcium salt of diethylammonium hydroxide) is used intraoperatively to identify properly functioning lymphatic vessels at the surgical incision. Healthy-appearing lymphatic vessels at this site are selected and introduced directly into the vein segment with a U-shaped stitch (using 8/0–10/0 Prolene sutures depending on the caliber of the vessels). These are then secured by additional stitches between the peri-lymphatic adipose tissue and the vein border. The passage of the blue-stained lymphatic fluid into the vein, evident under the operating microscope, verifies the patency of the anastomosis (Fig. 51.3).

For patients with lower-limb lymphedema, multiple LVAs are applied in the subinguinal region. Superficial lymphatic-lymph nodal structures are identified and isolated, and all available and healthy afferent lymphatic collectors are used for the anastomoses. Samples of lymph nodes, vessels, vein segments, and adjacent tissues are subjected to histopathological analyses. Common findings in primary lower-limb lymphedema are significant thickening of the nodal capsule and varying levels of nodal

fibrosclerosis. Afferent lymphatic vessels are usually normal, indicating a proximal obstruction in lymphatic flow.

For patients with upper-limb lymphedema, multiple LVAs are performed at the middle third of the volar surface of the arm. Both superficial and deep lymphatic collectors identified by BPV are used. Deep lymphatics are typically found in the vicinity of the humeral artery, vein, and median nerve. A patent branch of one of the humeral veins is used in the application of microsurgical anastomoses.

Lymphoscintigraphy is performed in all cases as part of the diagnostic workup to select appropriate candidates for surgery based on evidence of proximal obstruction of lymphatic flow. Lymphoscintigraphy is performed with either ^{99m}Tc-labeled antimony sulfur colloid or ^{99m}Tc-nanocolloid human serum albumin (90 % of the particles of >80 nm in size) injected into the interdigital space of the toes or fingers of both limbs in the affected region. It is essential to ensure that the edema is of lymphatic origin. Lymphoscintigraphy also provides important etiological and pathophysiological information about the nature of the disease. In the last 2 years of our experience, evaluation of the superficial lymphatic pathways distal to the surgical site in the affected limb has also been performed using the photodynamic eye (PDE) method with injection of indocyanine green fluorescence. The simultaneous use of PDE with BPV gives two methods of visualizing the lymphatic flow and confirmation of patency of the anastomoses intraoperatively [20, 21]. PDE can also be used postoperatively, in addition to lymphoscintigraphy, to verify the long-term stability of the surgical outcomes.

Primary lymphedemas typically involve lymph node dysplasias (LAD II according to Papendieck's classifications [22]) with hypoplastic lymph nodes associated with sinus histiocytosis and a thick fibrous capsule and microlymphangioadenomyomatosis. In these cases, obstruction to lymphatic flow is evident in the changes in the afferent lymphatic collectors: these are dilated, swollen, and tortuous with thickened walls and reduced numbers

Fig. 51.3 LVA: the passage of blue lymph into the vein branch can be seen under the operating microscope, verifying the patency of the anastomosis

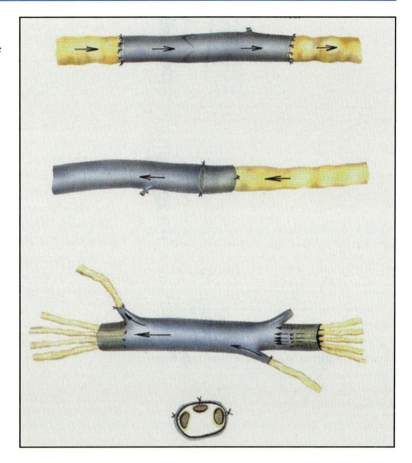

of smooth muscle cells, which are fragmented by numerous fibrotic elements. In our clinical experience, the majority of the peripheral lymphedemas treated by microsurgical means were at stages IIA (39 %) and IIB (52 %), where a minority were at other stages (3 % at stage IB and 6 % at stages IIIA and B; according to the Campisi staging system for lymphedema [9, 12, 13]).

Echo Doppler is performed in all cases to exclude venous-only causes of edema and also to identify any venous anomalies associated with the lymphedema, such as phlebolymphedema. In most cases, the venous anomalies can be corrected contemporaneously, such as valvuloplasty for venous insufficiency. In other cases, venous disease is an indication for performing a venous graft between the lymphatic collectors above and below the site of lymphatic obstruction, as the valvular incompetency of the diseased veins would compromise the efficacy of the anastomoses if LVA was performed instead. This venous bridge type of graft is called a lymphatic-venous-lymphatic anastomosis (LVLA). Competent venous segments are harvested from the same operative site or can be taken from the forearm (usually the cephalic vein). The length of the grafted vein section varies from 7 to 15 cm as required. It is essential to collect several lymphatic collectors to join to the distal end of the vein to ensure that the vein segment is filled with sufficient lymph and to avoid closure due to subsequent fibrosis development. The competent valves of the vein segment are vital for directing the flow of lymph in the correct direction and to avoid gravitational backflow or reflux. As with the LVA, the lymphatic collectors are directly introduced into the vein cut ends by means of a U-shaped stitch, which is then stabilized with additional peripheral stitches (Fig. 51.4).

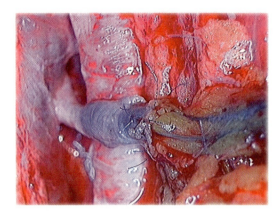

Fig. 51.4 A schematic drawing of the derivative multiple LVA and the reconstructive multiple LVLA technique with the interposition of an autologous vein graft between lymphatics above and below the obstacle to the lymph flow (C. Campisi, 1982)

Results

Clinical outcomes improved earlier that microsurgical techniques are applied in the treatment of peripheral lymphedema, due to the absence of, or minimal, fibrosclerotic tissue changes in the lymph vessel walls and surrounding tissues. Compared to preoperative conditions, patients obtained significant reductions in excess limb volume of over 84 %, with an average of 69 % as measured by limb water volumetry and circumference. These results were stable over an average of 10 years of follow-up. Over 86 % of patients with stages I and IIA gradually stopped using conservative therapies over the length of the follow-up period. In patients with more advanced lymphedema (stages IIB, IIIA, and IIIB), 42 % could decrease the frequency of physical therapies in the long term. In all patients, the frequency of DLA attacks considerably reduced by over 91 %, compared to preoperative conditions.

There were no immediate postoperative complications, such as postoperative infections, postoperative lymphorrhea, or worsening of edema. Most recently, patency verification was also performed postoperatively using the PDE method with indocyanine green fluorescence. This method allows visualization of the superficial lymphatic pathways and is valuable to confirm the significant reduction in dermal backflow of

lymph after microsurgery. When PDE is used immediately after surgery, it is possible to verify the anastomosis patency and provide evidence that no thrombosis has occurred.

Lymphoscintigraphy was used to verify the patency of the microanastomoses in the long term by direct and indirect methods (Fig. 51.5). These included the following:

- Reduced dermal backflow of the tracer and the appearance of preferential lymphatic pathways not evident preoperatively
- The disappearance of the tracer at the site of the lymphatic-venous anastomoses, indicating the passage of lymph into the bloodstream
- Earlier liver uptake of tracer, compared to preoperative parameters, taken as indirect evidence of the passage of lymph in the bloodstream

Additional Considerations

Combined physical therapy should be the initial treatment for peripheral lymphedema and is best conducted in specialized treatment centers. The timing of the surgical intervention is important. In the case of established lymphedema (stages IB and onwards), surgical treatment should be implemented as soon as there is no further reduction in limb volume obtained by conservative methods or earlier if there are recurrent lymphangitic attacks that act to worsen the lymph transport [23]. Microsurgery applied at this point provides further amelioration in the condition [24, 25]. Early application of microsurgery techniques is efficacious in preventing the development of lymphedema in certain cases and is discussed further in a later section.

The ideal indications for microsurgical intervention, in our experience, include relatively early stages of disease (stages IB, IIA, and early IIB); lymphoscintigraphy patterns showing low inguinal or axillary nodal uptake of the tracer and minimal or absent passage of the tracer beyond this proximal area; excellent patient compliance with all treatment aspects; and access to a well-organized lymphedema treatment center where the patient can be referred to a center of lymphatic surgery when a specialized surgery is required.

Fig. 51.5 Preoperative lymphoscintigraphy in a patient affected by primary lymphedema of the left leg (*left*). Postoperative lymphoscintigraphy shows the appearance of preferential lymphatic pathways into the inguinal region (*right*)

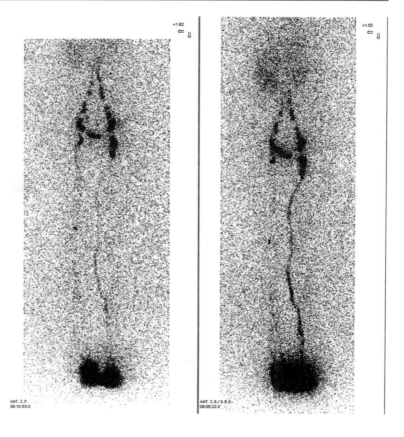

In more advanced cases (late IIB, IIIA, IIIB), where lymphoscintigraphy shows no visualization of lymphatic channels and regional lymph nodes, it is necessary to reduce the stage of lymphedema by intensive conservative methods prior to surgery, in order to reduce the clinical stage of the disease and best prepare the limb for surgery. Lymphatic microsurgery has an important role in the treatment of advanced lymphedema where addressing the chronic lymph stasis helps with edema reduction but also is likely to improve the immune function in the affected limb [15], as recent research indicates that chronic lymph stasis is associated with reduced immune responses to infection. These patients need to be followed closely in the postoperative phase and to adhere to the regimen of complete lymphedema functional therapy, ClyFT [26]; this is essential to maintain the results obtained by the microsurgery and to continue to improve the long-term clinical outcome (Fig. 51.6). As advanced cases of lymphedema are associated with fibrotic adipose tissue deposits due to

chronic lymph stasis and inflammation, an additional surgical approach may be applied and is discussed in a further section.

Regardless of the stage of disease, if patient compliance to the treatment program is poor, then the outcome may be less than satisfactory. Relative contradictions to lymphatic microsurgery are few and are represented by cases of lymphatic-lymph node aplasia (extremely rare), diffuse metastatic disease, and very advanced stage of lymphedema (stage IIIB) totally unresponsive to conservative therapy.

New Directions in Surgical Treatments for Peripheral Lymphedemas

In recent years, primary and secondary peripheral lymphedemas have become better understood, with the recognition of some genes involved in the disease onset and process, and increased awareness and detection of secondary causes

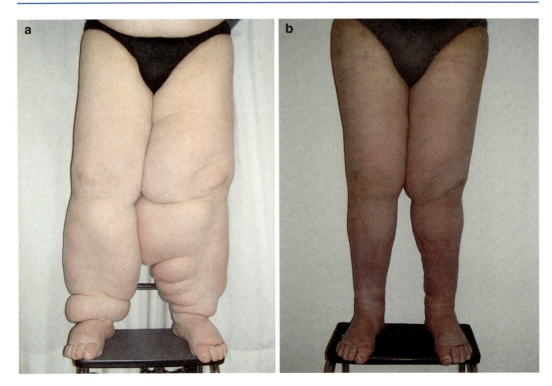

Fig. 51.6 Preoperative photo of a patient with advanced lower-limb lymphedema (**a**). Postoperative photo 1 year from surgery (**b**)

of lymphedema [27–31]. Notwithstanding this, conservative treatments are aimed at minimizing symptoms without addressing the cause of the underlying lymphatic drainage disturbance; which is chronic lymph stasis. Microsurgical derivative and reconstructive techniques are able to restore some, or all, lymphatic circulation in an affected limb by bypassing the obstruction in the lymphatic flow [9, 13, 32, 33]. Short- and long-term restoration of drainage is obtained, and the best results are obtained when the surgery is applied in the early stages of disease and is combined with conservative treatment measures.

In the past few years, we introduced a primary preventive approach using LVA and LVLA at the same time as lymphadenectomy in the surgical treatment of cancer (the lymphatic microsurgical preventive healing approach – LyMPHA [34–36]). Although this research primarily involves secondary lymphedema, which in general is caused by lymphadenectomy for oncological treatment, it is still applicable to a particular group of patients with primary lymphedema, namely,

those undergoing surgery in vulnerable areas – regions involving the axillary/inguinal-crural-iliac-obturator lymph nodes. Initially, this approach was applied in a randomized control trial of patients undergoing axillary lymph node dissection for breast cancer treatment, where pre-surgery measures indicated a risk for lymphedema development (e.g., high BMI or suppressed lymphatic transport evident on lymphoscintigraphy; stage IA or subclinical lymphedema) [34–36]. In the patients who underwent the LyMPHA approach, only a slight transient edema was evident in 4.34 % of cases. In contrast, considering those in the treatment as usual group, 30.43 % developed permanent lymphedema. We have also applied this promising preventive technique to melanoma and vulvar carcinomas with axillary/inguinal-crural-iliac-obturator lymph nodal involvement, with excellent success [37].

Traditional debulking surgeries are currently used much less frequently in the treatment of lymphedema. Total excisional techniques, such as the Charles procedure, when employed as the primary method of surgical treatment for advanced lymphedema have been technically successful in that there is a reduction in the size of the limb, but the results have been also associated with a poor cosmetic result, significant scarring, and sometimes serious complications such as infections [38–40]. Surgical resection of skinfolds and excess tissues can be appropriate in late-stage lymphedemas when there has been marked edema reduction after conservative and microsurgical methods, in body regions relatively inaccessible to conservative measures like the external genitalia, in advanced lymphatic filariasis often treated in combination with LVA or nodal anastomoses when lymphatic channels are widely dilated, or in localized lipolymphedema associated with massive obesity and consequent immobility [41, 42].

Recently, suction-assisted liposuction has been utilized as a less invasive procedure to remove this excess adipose tissue [43, 44]. Given the existing poor lymph drainage in patients with lymphatic diseases, extra caution needs to be taken to avoid damaging the lymphatic vessels further during liposuction. Investigations of lymph vessels in cadavers after dry and tumescent liposuction showed that significant injury to tissues occurred with the movement of the cannula and noted that a tumescent procedure and a parallel approach were necessary to avoid injury in people with normal lymphatic systems [45]. In patients with lymphedema, the lymph vessels and channels are often dilated and tortuous in the advanced stages of disease [46], which is exactly when liposuction is prescribed, and therefore may be more difficult to avoid with the liposuction cannula and more vulnerable to damage. We have recently developed a new lympho-lipo-aspiration technique (fibro-lipo-lympho-aspiration (FLLA) with lymph vessel sparing procedure (LVSP); Corrado Cesare Campisi) to improve the chronic swelling in patients with advanced lymphedema, taking a lymphatic sparing approach. Using blue patent violet (BPV), together with the photodynamic eye (PDE) method with indocyanine green (ICG) fluorescence, to highlight the lymphatic pathways in the limb, the excess adipose tissue is carefully aspirated.

Concluding Remarks

Primary lymphedema is regarded as a clinical manifestation of a lymphatic malformation that developed during the later stage of lymphangiogenesis, where the crucial symptom is chronic lymph stasis. Lymphatic microsurgery provides a means to restore lymphatic drainage, bypassing the obstruction in the lymphatic pathway and directing the flow of lymph into the veins (MLVA) or, in the case of an associated venous pathology, by using an analogous vein graft to bridge the gap in the lymphatic collectors around the obstruction (MLVLA). Lymphatic microsurgery offers excellent outcomes when applied early in the disease process, where a complete resumption of lymphatic flow in the long term is possible, and is a valuable tool in the combined treatment of advanced lymphedema in association with intensive conservative treatments and, when applicable, removal of the fibrotic tissue with an FLLA technique.

References

1. Morgan CL, Lee BB (2008) Classification and staging of lymphedema. In: Tretbar LL, Morgan CL, Lee BB, Simonian SJ, Blondeau B (eds) Lymphedema: diagnosis and treatment. Springer-Verlag Limited, London, pp 21–30
2. Lee BB (2004) Critical issues on the management of congenital vascular malformation. Ann Vasc Surg 18(3):380–392
3. Rutkowski JM, Boardman KC, Swartz MA (2006) Characterization of lymphangiogenesis in a model of adult skin regeneration. Am J Physiol Heart Circ Physiol 291:H1402–H1410
4. Goldman J, Le TX, Skobe M, Swartz MA (2005) Overexpression of VEGF-C causes transient lymphatic hyperplasia but not increased lymphangiogenesis in regenerating skin. Circ Res 96:1193–1199. (Comment: Circ Res. 2005;96:1132–1134)
5. Bastide G, Lefebvre D (1989) Anatomy and organogenesis and vascular malformations. In: Belov S, Loose DA, Weber J (eds) Vascular malformations. Einhorn-Presse Verlag, Reinbek, pp 20–22
6. Leu HJ (1989) Pathoanatomy of congenital vascular malformations. In: Belov S, Loose DA, Weber J (eds) Vascular malformations. Einhorn-Presse Verlag, Reinbek, pp 37–46
7. Witte MH, Jones K, Wilting J et al (2006) Structure function relationships in the lymphatic system and

implications for cancer biology. Cancer Metastasis Rev 25(2):159–184

8. Rockson SG (2008) Diagnosis and management of lymphatic vascular disease. J Am Coll Cardiol 52:799–806

9. Murdaca G, Cagnati P, Gulli R et al (2012) Current views on diagnostic approach and treatment of lymphedema. Am J Med 125:134–140

10. Lee BB, Andrade M, Antignani PL, Boccardo F, Bunke N, Campisi C et al (2013) Diagnosis and treatment of primary lymphedema consensus document of the International Union of Phlebology (IUP)-2013. Published online. http://www.lymphology2013.com/wp-content/uploads/2013/08/IUP-Cosensus-Pr-Lymph-Update-2013-Final-edition-07-10-13.doc

11. Rockson SG (2001) Lymphedema. Am J Med 110(4):288–295

12. Campisi C, Boccardo F (2004) Microsurgical techniques for lymphedema treatment: derivative lymphatic-venous microsurgery. World J Surg 28:609–613

13. Campisi C, Bellini C, Campisi C et al (2010) Microsurgery for lymphedema: clinical research and long-term results. Microsurgery 30(4):256–260

14. Rutkowski JM, Davis KE, Scherer PE (2009) Mechanisms of obesity and related pathologies: the macro- and microcirculation of adipose tissue. FEBS J 276:5738–5746

15. Dixon JB (2010) Lymphatic lipid transport: sewer or subway? Trends Endocrinol Metab 21:480–487

16. Rutkowski JM, Markhus CE, Gyenge CC, Alitalo K, Wiig H, Swartz MA (2010) Dermal collagen and lipid deposition correlate with tissue swelling and hydraulic conductivity in murine primary lymphedema. Am J Pathol 176:1122–1129

17. Schneider M, Conway EM, Carmeliet P (2005) Lymph makes you fat. Nat Genet 10:1023–1024

18. Olszewski WL (1988) The treatment of lymphedema of the extremities with microsurgical lymphovenous anastomoses. Int Angiol 7:312–321

19. Campisi C, Boccardo F (2002) Lymphedema and microsurgery (invited review). Microsurgery 22:74–80

20. Ogata F, Narushima M, Mihara M, Azuma R, Morimoto Y, Koshima I (2007) Intraoperative lymphography using indocyanine green dye for near-infrared fluorescence labeling in lymphedema. Ann Plast Surg 59:180–184

21. Unno N, Inuzuka K, Suzuki M, Yamamoto N, Sagara D, Nishiyama M et al (2007) Preliminary experience with a novel fluorescence lymphography using indocyanine green in patients with secondary lymphedema. J Vasc Surg 45:1016–1021

22. Papendieck CM (1998) The big angiodysplastic syndromes in pediatric with the participation of the lymphatic system. Lymphology 31:390–392

23. Dellachà A, Boccardo F, Zilla A, Napoli F, Fulcheri E, Campisi C (2000) Unexpected histopathological findings in peripheral lymphedema. Lymphology 33:62–64

24. Campisi C, Eretta C, Pertrile D et al (2007) Microsurgery for the treatment of peripheral lymphedema: long-term out come and future perspective. Microsurgery 27:333–338

25. Campisi C, Boccardo F, Tacchella M (1995) Reconstructive microsurgery of lymphatic vessels: the personal methods of lymphatic-venous-lymphatic (LVL) interpositioned grafted shunt. Microsurgery 16:161–166

26. Campisi C, Boccardo F (2008) Terapia funzionale complete del linfedema (ClyFT; complete lymphedema functional therapy): efficace strategia terapeutica in 3 fasi. Linfologia 1:20–23

27. Bellini C, Boccardo F, Taddei G et al (2005) Diagnostic protocol for lymphoscintigraphy in newborns. Lymphology 38:9–15

28. Bourgeois P, Leduc O, Leduc A (1998) Imaging techniques in the management and prevention of posttherapeutic upper limb edemas. Cancer 83:2805–2813

29. Mariani G, Campisi C, Taddei G, Boccardo F (1998) The current role of lymphoscintigraphy in the diagnostic evaluation of patients with peripheral lymphedema. Lymphology 31:316

30. Pecking AP, Gougeon-Bertrand FJ, Floiras JL (1998) Lymphoscintigraphy: overview of its use in the lymphatic system. Lymphology 31:343

31. Witte C, McNeill G, Witte M (1989) Whole body lymphangioscintigraphy: making the invisible easily visible. In: Mitsumas N, Uchino S, Yabuki S (eds) Progress in lymphology XII. Elsevier, Amsterdam/London/Tokyo, p 123

32. Campisi C, Witte MH, Fulcheri E et al (2011) General surgery, translational lymphology and lymphatic surgery. Int Angiol 30:504–521

33. Campisi C, Da Rin E, Bellini C, Bonioli E, Boccardo F (2008) Pediatric lymphedema and correlated syndromes: role of microsurgery. Microsurgery 28:138–142

34. Boccardo F, Casabona F, Friedman D, Puglisi M, De Cian F, Ansaldi F, Campisi C (2011) Surgical prevention of arm lymphedema in breast cancer treatment. Ann Surg Oncol 18:2500–2505

35. Boccardo F, Campisi CC, Molinari L, Dessalvi S, Santi PL, Campisi C (2012) Lymphatic complications in surgery: possibility of prevention and therapeutic options. Updates Surg 64(3):211–216. Epub 2012 Jul. 21

36. Campisi CC, Larcher L, Lavagno R, Spinaci S, Adami M, Boccardo F, Santi P, Campisi C (2012) Microsurgical primary prevention of lymphatic injuries following breast cancer treatment. Plast Reconstr Surg 130:749e–750e

37. Morotti M, Menada MV, Boccardo F, Ferrero S, Casabona F, Villa G, Campisi C, Papadia A (2013) Lymphedema microsurgical preventive healing approach for primary prevention of lower limb lymphedema after inguinofemoral lymphadenectomy for vulvar cancer. Int J Gynecol Cancer 23(4):769–774

38. Fujita T (2013) Optimizing surgical treatment for lymphedema. J Am Coll Surg 216:169–170

39. Mehrara B, Zampell JC, Suami H, Chang DW (2011) Surgical management of lymphedema: past, present, and future. Lymphat Res Biol 9:159–167

40. Ryan M, Campisi CC, Boccardo F et al (2013) Surgical treatment for lymphedema: optimal timing and optimal techniques. J Am Coll Surg 216:1221–1223
41. Narayanarao Y et al (2012) Pseudosarcoma-massive localized lymphoedema in morbidly obese – a rare entity: case report. Int J Surg Case Rep 3:389–391
42. Jensen V et al (2006) Massive localized lipolymphedema pseudotumor in a morbidly obese patient. Lymphology 39:181–184
43. Hoffman JN, Fertmann JP, Baumeister RG, Putz R, Frick A (2004) Tumescent and dry liposuction of lower extremities: differences in lymph vessel injury. Plast Reconstr Surg 113:718–724
44. Brorson H, Svensson H, Norrgren K, Throrsson O (1998) Liposuction reduces arm lymphedema without significantly altering the already impaired lymph transport. Lymphology 31:156–172
45. Schaverien MV, Munro KJ, Baker PA, Munnoch DA (2012) Liposuction for chronic lymphoedema of the upper limb: 5 years of experience. J Plast Reconstr Aesthet Surg 65:935–942
46. Lu Q, Delproposto Z, Hu A, Tran C, Liu N, Xu J, Bui D, Hu J (2012) MR lymphography of lymphatic vessels in lower extremity with gynecologic oncology-related lymphedema. PLos One 7:e50319

Thoracic Duct Dysplasias and Chylous Reflux

52

Corradino Campisi, Melissa Ryan,
Caterina Sara Campisi, Francesco Boccardo,
and Corrado Cesare Campisi

Introduction

Thoracic duct dysplasia refers to the relatively rare clinical picture that in the vast majority of cases is already manifest neonatally or in infancy with regard to the extent and severity of the

C. Campisi, MD, PhD, FACS (✉)
Department of Surgery (DISC), Section & Research Center of Lymphatic Surgery, Lymphology, and Microsurgery, Operative Unit of General and Lymphatic Surgery, IRCCS University Hospital San Martino – IST National Institute for Cancer Research, Genoa, Italy

Postgraduate School of Alimentary Tract Surgery, Siena, Italy
e-mail: campisi@unige.it

M. Ryan, PhD • F. Boccardo, MD, PhD
Department of Surgery (DISC), Section & Research Center of Lymphatic Surgery, Lymphology, and Microsurgery, Operative Unit of General and Lymphatic Surgery, IRCCS University Hospital San Martino – IST National Institute for Cancer Research, Genoa, Italy
e-mail: ryame269@hotmail.com

C.S. Campisi, MD
Department of Health Sciences (DISSAL), Operative Unit of Dermatology, IRCCS University Hospital San Martino – IST National Institute for Cancer Research, Genoa, Italy

C.C. Campisi, MD, RAS-ACS
Department of Surgery (DISC), Operative Unit of Plastic, Reconstructive and Aesthetic Surgery, IRCCS University Hospital San Martino – IST National Institute for Cancer Research, Genoa, Italy

lymphangio-chylous dysplastic malformations. These malformations are, at the very foundation, complex clinical pictures with dysplasias and ectasias of the lymphatic and chyliferous collectors, parietal-valvular insufficiency of these vessels, and gravitational chylous reflux and also associated with severe lymph-nodal dysplasia. In contrast, when due to a secondary or acquired basis, this may be due to complications of lesions acquired posttraumatically or iatrogenically, usually following oncological surgery with retroperitoneal lymphadenectomy, or to accidental ligature or laceration of the thoracic duct or its tributaries from the cisterna chyli up to the outlet in the left supraclavicular fossa in the subclavian-jugular vein junction. These complex clinical conditions (Table 52.1) can manifest as chyloperitoneum, chyledema of the lower limbs or external genitalia, chyluria, chylothorax, chylorrhea, chylous arthritis, and variations of the above and pose a diagnostic and therapeutic challenge. A severe hypoproteinemia

Table 52.1 Clinical manifestations of chyliferous vessel pathology

Clinical manifestation
Chyloperitoneum or chylous peritonitis
Chyledema of the lower limbs
Chyledema of the external genitalia
Chyluria
Chylothorax
Chylorrhea
Chylous arthritis

is the main consequence, on a general metabolic level, of this pathology, manifesting as an exudative protein-losing enteropathy, with serious episodes of diarrhea, the development of which often characterizes the clinical exacerbation of the disease.

Remarks on the Thoracic Duct Anatomy

In the embryo, the thoracic duct originates from six lymphatic sacs, two of which arise from the internal jugular and subclavian veins. The right and left lumbar lymphatic channels stem from several branches and eventually converge to form the thoracic duct [1]. Multiple variations in the thoracic duct anatomy exist in the general population, as is evident in Fig. 52.1. Kato et al. [2] examined the anatomical course of the thoracic duct in 8 patients noting 1 with a right-sided thoracic duct that flowed into the right venous angle, 4 patients had divergences, 1 patient showed an "island" thoracic duct that splits partially into

two channels, and 2 patients had variants that flowed through the left subclavian artery into the left venous angle. The outlet of the thoracic duct empties into the great veins of the neck on the left side in approximately 95 % of cases, into the right side of the neck in 2–3 % of cases, and bilaterally in 1.0–1.5 % of cases [3]. The marked variation from the "normal" thoracic duct described in anatomical textbooks evident in a significant amount of the general population may also be due to basing anatomical studies on cadavers, whereas the thoracic duct in living subjects is swollen with lymph, and this may displace it slightly [4].

Thoracic Duct Malformations and Related Chylous Reflux Syndromes

Aside from anatomical variations within the general population, the thoracic duct can also be congenitally malformed. Malformations may include ectasia, agenesis, dysplasia, and/or cysts.

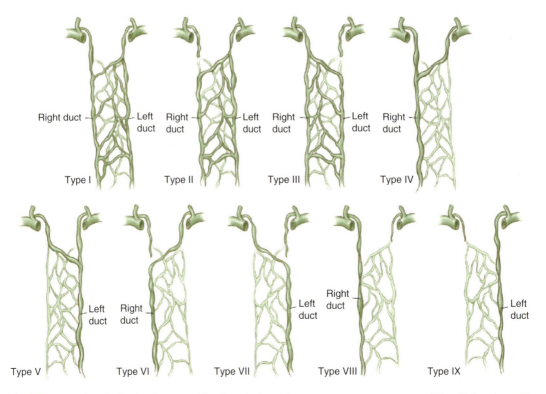

Fig. 52.1 Variations in the development of the thoracic duct. The most common types are type VI at 63 % and type II at 27 % (Reproduced with permission from [1])

Thoracic duct cysts generally develop in the cisterna chyli, the mediastinum, or occasionally in the neck. Congenital weakness, incompetence, or absence of valves lead to obstruction at the lymphatic-venous junction, thus allowing reflux of blood into the thoracic duct. Such cysts usually present with left-sided supraclavicular swelling. Preyer et al. [5] reported that noninflammatory supraclavicular tumors were likely due to chronic localized lymph stasis provoking lymphangiectasia. This lymph stasis was probably due to an anatomical variation that allowed the intermittent occlusion of the duct by the internal jugular vein. They also postulated the role of female hormones in exacerbating the growth of the tumor. Other thoracic duct malformations such as lymphangiomatosis or diffuse lymphangiectasia or thoracic duct atresia, aplasia, hypoplasia, or dysplasia may all cause chylous disorders, such as chylothorax. These may allow the effusion of chyle into the pleural cavity. But there may also be variations within the thoracic duct that do not cause overt chylous symptoms. For example, Hara et al. [6] demonstrated the presence of thoracic duct abnormalities in patients with only primary lymphedema of the extremities.

A malformation of the thoracic duct, cisterna chyli, Pecquet cyst, and/or chyliferous vessels creates a significant obstacle to the lymphatic flow, sometimes presenting as a downstream leakage, uni- or bilateral chylothorax, lymphocele, chylous cyst, mediastinal chyloma, chylomediastinum, and chylopericardium [7–9]. The loss of the chyle leads to nutritional deficiencies, dehydration, electrolyte disturbance, and lymphocyte leaks. This leads to increased risk of infection and eventually respiratory dysfunction [10]. If the obstruction in lymphatic flow persists, there may be an eventual effect on intestinal drainage. The chyliferous vessels of the small intestine become dilated from chyle stasis. This can lead to chylous ascites, chylorrhea in the genitalia, and chylous edema of the lower limbs. Patients may also present with protein-losing enteropathy symptoms due to the failure to absorb proteins by the intestinal lymphatic system. Dual diagnoses are often present; in a sample of patients with primary chylous disorders, 30 % had both chylothorax and chylous ascites,

and 70 % of these also had chylous reflux into the lower limbs [11]. In addition, thoracic duct malformations [12] and the possible coexistence of normal variations within the thoracic duct anatomy [1, 2, 4, 6, 12, 13] present an unknown risk for surgery, particularly that involving the head and neck, that is difficult to plan for. The resulting complex clinical picture can be challenging to manage and often requires a multidisciplinary approach with a coordinated treatment plan.

Clinical Diagnosis

The existence of a malformation of the chyliferous vessels and of the Pecquet cyst considerably obstructs the intestinal lymphatic drainage. The lymphatic collectors along the walls of the small intestine and mesentery dilate, filling with chyle. Considering their position just subperitoneal, they are prone to breakage, resulting in the leakage of chyle into the peritoneal cavity (chylous ascites). Sometimes the breaking of the chyliferous vessels occurs in two stages; chyle escapes from the broken lymph collectors in the peritoneum, which then results in the formation of a chyloma that subsequently opens around the abdominal cavity. The finding of localized dilation of a chyliferous vessel is defined as a chylous mesenteric cyst (Fig. 52.2).

Given the complex clinical presentation of these cases, a thorough diagnostic assessment is recommended [8, 14, 15]:

- Blood tests: serum protein, albumin, triglyceride, cholesterol, calcium, and hemoglobin levels; lymphocytes and immunoglobulins can leak into the ascites fluid. Lymph in the thoracic duct contains from ~2,000 to 20,000 lymphocytes per mm^3, that is, a concentration of lymphocytes two to ten times higher than in the blood.
- Thoracocentesis or paracentesis: chyle is evident by its distinctive milky color but also by chemical analysis demonstrating raised triglyceride levels (generally greater than 110 mg/dl is considered diagnostic) and the presence of lipoproteins and chylomicrons. Thoracocentesis or paracentesis may, in themselves, provide symptomatic relief.

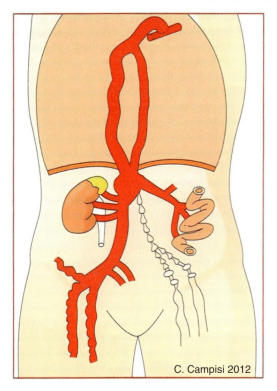

Fig. 52.2 Schematic design concerning the pathophysiological and relevant clinical characteristics of disorders of the chyliferous vessels, cistern chili, and thoracic duct

- Thoracoabdominal CT scan and MRI can exclude malignancies. A recent study has demonstrated that unenhanced MRI can visualize the thoracic duct and tributaries to identify leakage sites [16].
- Lymphoscintigraphy can be useful to demonstrate lymphatic dysplasia involving all compartments of the body, including the peritoneal, external genitalia, and lower limbs. Lymphoscintigraphy allows excellent confirmation of the patency of lymphatic-venous anastomoses post-surgery. Lymphoscintigraphy with 99mTc-filtrated sulfur colloid has recently been reported to visualize the thoracic region and lymphatic leakage into pleural cavities [17].
- Lymphangiography: after isolation and cannulation of the lymphatics, standard lymphangiography is conducted by means of microsurgically injected liposoluble ultrafluid contrast medium. If coupled with a CT scan, lymphangiography allows a more accurate assessment of the extent of disease, as well as the site of the obstacle and source of chylous leak.
- In order to demonstrate concurrent protein-losing enteropathy, albumin-labeled (99 m Tc) scintigraphy can be used to show the enteropathy inside the intestinal lumen in scans taken 1–24 h after intravenous administration of 740 mBq.
- Videothoracoscopy or videolaparoscopy: as an initial approach, videothoracoscopy and videolaparoscopy are preferred for correct placement of drains. Smaller drains placed by an ultrasound or CT-guided approach tend to occlude as chyle is viscous. Sclerosing agents, such as povidone-iodine, and antibiotics may be introduced via these drains. Lavage with a Trémolliéres sterile solution (concentrated lactic acid) combined with an antibiotic (250–500 mg of sodium rifampicin) associated with a rigorous total parenteral feeding has proved to be successful in chyloperitoneum in 2 or 3 weeks maximum.

Therapeutic Procedures

Regarding the therapeutic approach, these complex clinical cases, also in the case of an acute onset (e.g., chylous peritonitis), should not be treated too early by surgery, at least not until the patients have been adequately metabolically stabilized with an appropriate diet. This diet is based on the reintegration of protein and lipid uptake, by limiting only to medium-chain triglycerides (MCT) that, instead of being absorbed by the intestinal chylo-lymphatics, are cleared through the portal venous system. Notably, in order to achieve the most rapid state of metabolic control, an initial regimen of total parenteral nutrition (TPN) can be initiated in order to significantly reduce the source of the chylous leak.

Nonsurgical Procedures

Conservative management of chylous leaks remains the first choice of intervention. There remains some controversy about the timing of surgical intervention, as discussed below, but the general consensus is that the patient should be stabilized first and a proper diagnostic evaluation conducted to identify the source of the chylous leak. Conservative measures include nutritional management, administration of somatostatin analogs, and drainage of the leak.

Nutritional options consist of a low or fat-free diet, enteral nutrition including the use of medium-chain triglycerides (MCT) solutions, or total parenteral nutrition without oral intake. Necessarily, patients should be individually evaluated to determine the most effective type of regimen. As noted by Campisi et al. [18] in their review of chyle leaks in head and neck surgery, all patients must be closely monitored for clinical response irrespective of the nutritional approach employed. This includes nutritional status and protein levels, essential fatty acids and fat-soluble vitamins, and the electrolyte balance to avoid nutritional deficiency or further complications.

Somatostatin is a peptide that acts as a neurohormone as well as a paracrine agent, acting on both the endocrine and paracrine pathways. Octreotide is a synthetic octapeptide that mimics the action of somatostatin, and both have significant action on the gastrointestinal tract. Although the mechanism(s) of action of these peptides remains unclear, it is likely that they cause a reduction of the gastrointestinal blood flow and therefore indirectly reduce lymphatic flow from these areas. Octreotide is also reported to work directly on the somatostatin receptors, minimizing lymphatic secretion [19]. Initially used in pediatric cases of chylous disorders, there are emerging cases of somatostatin and octreotide being used successfully in the suppression of chylous leaks in adults. The efficacy of these peptides in the treatments of high-output chyle flow (more than 1 l per day) is yet to be established [20].

Surgical Procedures

Retrospective accounts indicate that approximately 60 % of patients with chylous disorders will undergo surgical intervention. There is no clear treatment algorithm to guide surgical planning, and general consensus remains that surgery is required in refractory chyle leaks that fail to respond to conservative measures. Definitions of "refractory" chyle leaks are based in the literature on the output of chyle leaks (above 500 or 1,000 ml per day recommending surgical treatment) or a specific time interval (2 weeks of conservative treatment prior to surgery resulted in lower overall morbidity than only 48 h of treatment) [21].

Thoracic Duct Ligation

Thoracic duct ligation is often undertaken to disrupt the flow of chyle. Given the extensive network of lymphatic anastomoses and lymphaticovenous anastamoses between the thoracic duct and the azygos and the intercostal and lumbar veins, it is assumed that occluding the thoracic duct will allow safe rerouting of the chyle flow [22]. Thoracic duct ligation can be performed through an open thoracotomy, but, more recently, a thoracoscopic approach has been successfully used for the treatment of chyle fistulas. Usually, the thoracic duct is identified via a right-sided approach, but of course, natural anatomical variations must be taken into account. Occlusion of the duct occurs by mass ligation of the tissue above the supradiaphragmatic hiatus between the azygos vein and the aorta. This procedure is effective, avoiding the significant morbidity of major thoracic access [23–30]. Intrapleural fibrin or biological glue has also been used to occlude the duct [31, 32].

Some concern has been raised that significant occlusion of the thoracic duct may lead to the redistribution of the chylous flow, such as leg swelling and chylous ascites [18, 33–35]. The development of protein-losing enteropathy, chronic diarrhea, and lower limb swelling has also been demonstrated in experimental studies after thoracic duct ligation [36]. Of note, one case study implicated a thoracic duct ligation performed for idiopathic chylopericardium in the development of chyloptysis 7 years later. The authors suggested that the high-pressure lymphatic flow through the rerouted channels gradually dilated the lymphatic valves, eventuating in retrograde flow of chyle into the peribronchial pulmonary lymphatics. Prospective follow-up studies are needed to confirm the associated risks of thoracic duct ligation [18].

Surgical/Microsurgical Approaches

Surgical decisions should be based on the severity of the case, number of chylous leaks, whether there is a primary or secondary cause for the chylous effusion, and the success of previously implemented nonsurgical methods in slowing or stopping the leak. Depending on the specific clinical picture, the following types of surgical/microsurgical procedures can be performed:

- Identification of the sites(s) of chylolymphorrhea, chyloperitoneum, and chylothorax drainage.
- Thoracoscopic pleurodesis and decortication.
- Ruptured lymphatic vessels can be ligated, oversewn, or clipped as necessary.
- Removal of lymphocele, chylous cysts, and/or chylomas.
- Resection of the lymphangiectasic-lymphangiodysplasic tissue if present.
- "Spaced-out" antigravitational ligatures of lymphatic-chylous vessels:
- The use of carbon dioxide laser which, when applied at low power, has a welding effect on lymphatic vessels, as well as on many other tissues and blood vessels, up to 1 mm in diameter.
- For a better recognition of the chyliferous collectors (Fig. 52.3), the administration of a "fatty meal" is recommended by Servelle, consisting of 60 g of butter in a glass of milk, 4–5 h before surgery.
- A videolaparoscopic approach to support the laparotomy, often in combination with laser-assisted microsurgical procedures, is the therapeutic approach most associated with the greatest number of successes.
- A difficult to control chylothorax may require a pleura-venous/pleura-peritoneal shunt. With the shunt, it is assumed that chyle finds a new outflow path, which may explain the long-term reduction of pressure in the lymphatic system and peritoneal cavity. These shunts can be susceptible to thrombosis or occlusion due to the density of the chyle; however, Tasnádi et al. [37] reported successfully dissolving an occluded shunt with streptokinase.

- Resection of the intestinal tract most affected by dysplasia in cases in which the lymphangiectasia is severe.

In addition to the above procedures, derivative lymphatic-venous anastomosis (LVA) or reconstructive lymphatic-venous-lymphatic anastomosis microsurgery, when technically applicable, can be very effective. These techniques offer a functional repair, depending on the individual case, of lymphatic-chylous leaks by restoring the existing lymphatic pathways and creating new routes in close proximity to the natural pathways [38–43], [44]. A reconstructive approach is in contrast to thoracic duct embolization or ligation that obliterates the thoracic duct or lymphatic-chylous pathways, as this has been associated with unwanted distal complications.

Lymphatic-venous anastomoses can be created at the internal or external jugular vein for chylothorax. Noel et al. [11] reported that by making a right posterolateral thoracotomy, anastomoses can be created between the lower tributaries of the thoracic duct and the azygos vein. In our experience, using the jugular veins, which have larger caliber, is more helpful given the pressure gradient between the lymphatic and venous systems. In the case of chylous ascites or further downstream lymphatic dysplasia, suitable lymphatic or chylous vessels can be used to perform lymphatic-venous shunts on mesenteric or iliac veins.

Regarding the LVA technique we use, the procedure involves the creation of multiple lymphatic-venous microanastomoses. Healthy-appearing lymphatics found at the site of the surgical incision are selected and introduced directly into the cut end of a recipient vein (usually the internal or external jugular vein) by a U-shaped stitch and then fixed by additional stitches between the vein border and the perilymphatic adipose tissue. Using blue patent violet

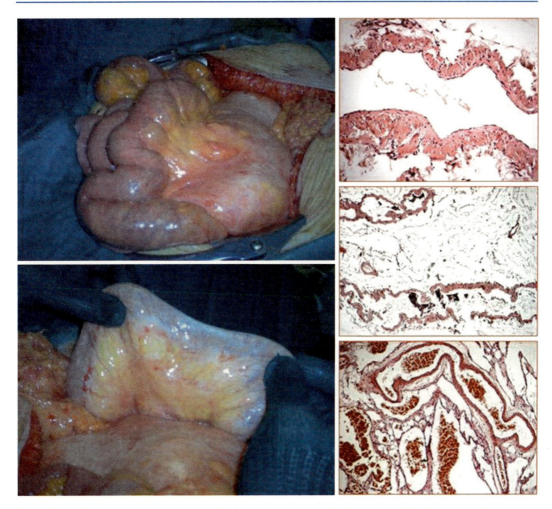

Fig. 52.3 Clinical case of primary intestinal and mesenteric lymphangio-chylous dysplasia. The chyliferous vessels of the intestinal wall are dilated and evident from the "fatty meal." The mesenteric chyliferous leaks are responsible for the free chyle in the abdominal cavity

dye, properly functioning lymph vessels are identified, and the passage of blue-colored lymph into the vein segment, seen under the operating microscope, verifies the patency of the LVA when anastomoses are completed [38–44].

Clinical Case Examples

1. A 45-year-old patient presents a picture of abundant chylous ascites apparent for several years, with a progressively worsening trend, in the absence of other symptoms and clinically relevant signs. The imaging techniques (ultrasound, lymphoscintigraphy, lymphangio-CT) confirmed the picture of chylous ascites and showed the dysplastic nature of the disease. Surgical treatment consisted of drainage of the ascites and the removal of mesenteric lymphangio-chylous dysplasia, which were of microcystic aspects that as a result of spontaneous rupture gave rise to the peritoneal effusion. Multiple antigravitational ligatures of the ectatic and

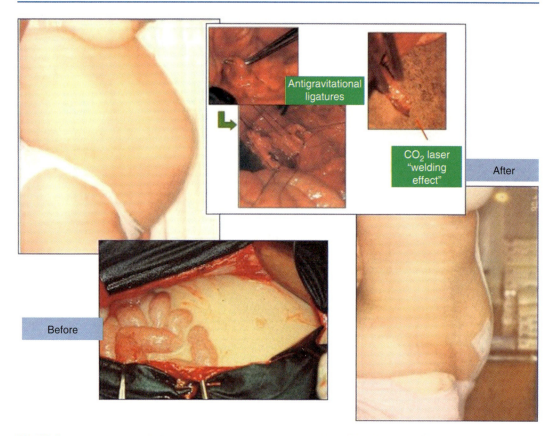

Fig. 52.4 Case of abundant chyloperitoneum on a base of congenital dysplasia, before and after adequate integrated medical and surgical treatment

incompetent lymphatic and chyliferous collectors were also carried out. The postoperative follow-up, of over 3 years, demonstrated the absence of recurrence of ascites (Fig. 52.4).

2. A 51-year-old patient presents with swelling of the left supraclavicular region, the size of a large orange with the consistency of stretched elastic and a smooth surface, which had appeared several months before without any apparent cause. The lesion presented a slow but progressive growth, causing no particular symptoms, with the exception of occasional painful episodes associated with a sense of tension and tenderness to compression. The instrumental investigations (ultrasound,

lymphoscintigraphy, lymphangio-CT) demonstrated the presence of a cystic dysplastic neoformation with multiple cavities containing lymphatic-chylous fluid. The patient had previously presented with bilateral chylothorax, of a dysplastic malformation basis, treated by pleural decortication and talc. The left supraclavicular tumor was surgically removed and found to be a chylocele, adherent to the surrounding tissues and in communication with lymphatic-chylous branches of little functional significance, which were appropriately closed. The postoperative course was favorable, and the follow-up, of more than 7 years, showed no recurrence of the disease (Fig. 52.5).

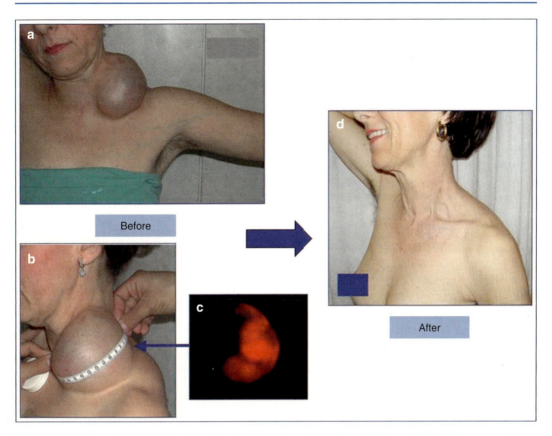

Fig. 52.5 Left supraclavicular chylous lymphangioma on a base of lymphangio-chylous dysplasia. Long-term follow-up after surgical removal

Summary and Conclusion

Complex clinical pictures can develop in patients with lymphatic dysplasia, given the multitude of possible normal variations and malformations of the lymphatic and chyliferous vessels. Most of the diseases of the chyliferous vessels with gravitational lymphatic-chylous reflux are related to dysplasia of the lymphatic and chyliferous collectors with parietal-valvular insufficiency. Sometimes these are pathological and may be iatrogenic, related, for example, to the ligature of the thoracic duct or injury to the retroperitoneal lymphatic and chyliferous vessels. Adequate diagnosis of the nature and site(s)

of the chylous leak is essential to a successful long-term outcome. The choice of technique and timing of the surgical intervention in these complex cases requires the skill of experienced teams with suitable technology and equipment. Various surgical procedures, made after an adequate metabolic control, may include the following:

- Identification of the sites(s) of leakage.
- Ruptured lymphatic vessels can be ligated, oversewn, or clipped as necessary.
- Removal of lymphocele, chylous cysts, and/or chylomas
- Resection of the lymphangiectasic-lymphangiodysplasic tissue if present.

- "Spaced-out" antigravitational ligatures of lymphatic-chylous vessels.
- The use of carbon dioxide laser.
- Derivative lymphatic-venous anastomosis (LVA) or reconstructive lymphatic-venous-lymphatic anastomosis microsurgery.

References

1. Hematti H, Mehran RJ (2011) Anatomy of the thoracic duct. Thorac Surg Clin 21:229–238
2. Kato T, Takase K, Ichikawa H et al (2011) Thoracic duct visualization: combined use of multidetector-row computed tomography and magnetic resonance imaging. J Comput Assist Tomogr 35:260–265
3. Gottwald F, Finke C, Zenk J (2005) Thoracic duct cysts: a rare differential diagnosis. Otolaryngol Head Neck Surg 132:330–333
4. Okuda I, Udagawa H, Hirata K et al (2011) Depiction of the thoracic duct by magnetic resonance imaging: comparison between magnetic resonance imaging and the anatomical literature. Jpn J Radiol 29:39–45
5. Preyer S, Kaiserling E, Heinle H, Foldi E, Zenner HP, Foldi M (1995) Benign supraclavicular tumorous lymphangiectasia: a new disease? Lymphology 28:118–125
6. Hara H, Mihara M, Okuda I, Hirota A, Narushima M, Iida T, Yamamoto T, Todokoro T, Koshima I (2012) Presence of thoracic duct abnormalities in patients with primary lymphoedema of the extremities. J Plast Reconstr Aesthet Surg 65:e305–e310
7. Boccardo F, Bellini C, Eretta C et al (2007) The lymphatics in the pathophysiology of thoracic duct and abdominal surgical pathology: immunological consequences and the unexpected role of microsurgery. Microsurgery 27:339–345
8. Boccardo F, Campisi CC, Molinari L, Dessalvi S, Santi PL, Campisi C (2012) Lymphatic complications in surgery: possibility of prevention and therapeutic options. Updates Surg 64:211–216
9. Boccardo F, Campisi C, Murdaca G et al (2010) Prevention of lymphatic injuries in surgery. Microsurgery 30:401–404
10. Addas R, Thumerel M, Jougon J, Delcambre F, Lelly J-F (2013) Are there early clinical factors to decide early surgical management for secondary chylothorax? A review of 32 cases. Open J Thorac Surg 3:30–36
11. Noel AA, Gloviczki P, Bender CE, Whitley D, Stanson AD, Deschamps C (2001) Treatment of symptomatic primary chylous disorders. J Vasc Surg 34:785–791
12. Hara H, Koshima I, Okuda I et al (2012) Assessment of configuration of thoracic duct using magnetic resonance thoracic ductography in idiopathic lymphedema. Ann Plast Surg 68:300–302
13. Offiah CE, Twigg S (2011) Lymphocoele of the thoracic duct: a cause of left supraclavicular fossa. Br J Radiol 84:27–30
14. Boccardo F, Campisi CC, Molinari L, Dessalvi S, Santi PL, Campisi C (2012) Diagnosis and treatment of chylous disorders. Lymphology 23:15–19
15. Campisi C, Bellini C, Campisi C et al (2010) Microsurgery for lymphedema: clinical research and long-term results. Microsurgery 30:256–260
16. Yu D, Ma XX, Wang Q, Zhang Y, Li CF (2013) Morphological changes of the thoracic duct and accessory lymphatic channels in patients with chylothorax: detection with unenhanced magnetic resonance imaging. Eur Radiol 23:702–711
17. Lee RKL, Wang K (2013) Technetium-99 m filtrated sulfur colloid lymphoscintigraphy for assessment of the site of lymphatic leakage in chylothorax post-oesophagectomy. Hong Kong J Radiol 16:e5–e8
18. Campisi CC, Boccardo F, Piazza C, Campisi C (2013) Evolution of chylous fistula management after neck dissection. Curr Opin Otolaryngol Head Neck Surg 21(2):150–156
19. Sharkey AJ, Rao JN (2012) The successful use of octreotide in the treatment of traumatic chylothorax. Tex Heart Inst J 39:428–430
20. Rosti LD, Battisti F, Butera G et al (2005) Octreotide in the management of postoperative chylothorax. Pediatr Cardiol 26:440–443
21. Li W, Dan G, Jiang J, Zhao Y, Deng D (2013) A 2-wk conservative treatment regimen preceding thoracic duct ligation is effective and safe for treating post-esophagectomy chylothorax. J Surg Res 185:784–789
22. Lyon S, Mott N, Koukounaras J, Shoobridge J, Hudson PV (2013) Role of interventional radiology in the management of chylothorax: a review of the current management of high output chylothorax. Cardiovasc Intervent Radiol 36(3):599–607
23. Merrigan BA, Winter DC, O'Sullivan GC (1997) Chylothorax. Br J Surg 84:15–20
24. Brennan PA, Blythe JN, Herd MK et al (2012) The contemporary management of chyle leak following cervical thoracic duct damage. Br J Oral Maxillofac Surg 50:197–201
25. ChalretduRieu M, Baulieux J, Rode A et al (2011) Management of postoperative chylothorax. J Visc Surg 148:346–352
26. Stringel G, Teixeira JA (2000) Thoracoscopic ligation of the thoracic duct. JSLS 4:239–242
27. Taniguchi Y, Miwa K, Adachi Y et al (2011) Thoracoscopic resection of a thoracic duct cyst that developed during follow-up for a thymic cyst. Gen Thorac Cardiovasc Surg 59:133–136
28. Zoetmulder F, Rutgers E, Baas P (1994) Thoracoscopic ligation of a thoracic duct leakage. Chest 106:1233–1234
29. Ilczyszyn A, Ridha H, Durrani AJ (2011) Management of chyle leak post neck dissection: a case report and literature review. J Plast Reconstr Aesthet Surg 64:223–230

30. Lapp GC, Brown DH, Gullane PJ et al (1998) Thoracoscopic management of chylous fistulae. Am J Otolaryngol 19:257–262

31. Abdel-Galil K, Milton R, McCaul J (2009) High output chyle leak after neck surgery: the role of video-assisted thoracoscopic surgery. Br J Oral Maxillofac Surg 47:478–480

32. Anestis N, Christos FC, Ioannis P, Christos I, Lampros P, Stephanos P (2012) Thoracic duct injury due to left subclavicular vein catheterization: a new conservative approach to a chyle fistula using biological glue. Int J Surg Case Rep 3(7):330–332

33. Christodoulou M, Ris HB, Pezzetta E (2006) Video-assisted right supradiaphragmatic thoracic duct ligation for non-traumatic recurrent chylothorax. Eur J Cardiothorac Surg 29:810–814

34. Raguse J, Pfitzmann R, Bier J et al (2007) Lower-extremity lymphedema following neck dissection – an uncommon complication after cervical ligation of the thoracic duct. Oral Oncol 43:835–837

35. Le Pimpec-Barthes F, Pham M, Jouan J et al (2009) Peritoneoatrial shunting for intractable chylous ascites complicating thoracic duct ligation. Ann Thorac Surg 87:1601–1603

36. Laslett D, Tretorola SO, Itkin M (2012) Delayed complications following technically successful thoracic duct embolization. J Vasc Interv Radiol 23:76–79

37. Tasnádi G, Bihari I, Bihari P (2010) Peritoneo-venous shunt implantation as a therapy for chylous ascites. Phlebologie 1:24–27

38. Campisi C, Boccardo F (2004) Microsurgical techniques for lymphedema treatment: derivative lymphatic-venous microsurgery. World J Surg 28:609–613

39. Campisi CC, Larcher L, Lavagno R, Spinaci S, Adami M, Boccardo F, Santi P, Campisi C (2012) Microsurgical primary prevention of lymphatic injuries following breast cancer treatment. Plast Reconstr Surg 130:749e–750e

40. Campisi C, Boccardo F, Campisi CC, Ryan M (2013) Reconstructive microsurgery for lymphedema: while the early bird catches the worm, the late riser still benefits. J Am Coll Surg 216:506–507

41. Ryan M, Campisi CC, Boccardo F et al (2013) Surgical treatment for lymphedema: optimal timing and optimal techniques. J Am Coll Surg 216:1221–1223

42. Morotti M, Menada MV, Boccardo F, Ferrero S, Casabona F, Villa G, Campisi C, Papadia A (2013) Lymphedema microsurgical preventive healing approach for primary prevention of lower limb lymphedema after inguinofemoral lymphadenectomy for vulvar cancer. Int J Gynecol Cancer 23(4):769–774

43. Campisi CC, Ryan M, Boccardo F et al (2014) Ly.M.P.H.A. and the prevention of lymphatic injuries: a rationale for early microsurgical intervention. J Reconstr Microsurg 30:71–72

44. Boccardo F, Dessalvi S, Campisi C, Molinari L, Spinaci S, Talamo G, Campisi C (2014) Microsurgery for groin lymphocele and lymphedema after oncologic surgery. Microsurgery 34:10–13

Conclusions

53

Raul Mattassi, Dirk A. Loose, and Massimo Vaghi

This is the end of a long journey through the wonderland of vascular tumors and malformations. Along the way, many attempts were done to detect the intrinsic properties of these pathologies, their physiologic and anatomical properties, to highlight the clinical pictures and the modalities of imaging and at least to present the therapeutic options.

In the last years, a dramatic improvement in the pathophysiologic and genetic knowledge of these diseases was achieved. We are spectators and actors of an increasing interest in the medical world on the approach to these diseases. We are aware that there are a great number of unanswered questions, but, to this point, we can rest on this milestone, waiting to go back to that land of wonders in future times, while scanning for any improvement in knowledge regarding this challenging area of medicine.

We hope that this book will be a useful vade mecum for the knowledge, diagnosis, and treatment of these pathologies.

R. Mattassi (✉)
Center for Vascular Malformations "Stefan Belov",
Department of Vascular Surgery,
Clinical Institute Humanitas "Mater Domini",
Castellanza (Varese), Italy
e-mail: raulmattassi@gmail.com

D.A. Loose
Section Vascular Surgery and Angiology,
Facharztklinik Hamburg, Hamburg, Germany
e-mail: info@prof-loose.de

M. Vaghi
Department of Vascular Surgery,
A.O.G. Salvini Hospital,
Garbagnate Milanese, Italy
e-mail: vaghim@yahoo.it

R. Mattassi et al. (eds.), *Hemangiomas and Vascular Malformations: An Atlas of Diagnosis and Treatment*, 475
DOI 10.1007/978-88-470-5673-2_53, © Springer-Verlag Italia 2009, 2015

Index

A

Acebutolol, 99
Acroangiodermatitis, 199–201
Activin receptor-like kinase 1 (ALK1), 23, 31
Airway hemangiomas, 70, 72, 137, 157, 158, 160, 333, 343
Airway occlusion, 338, 340
Airway venous malformations, 332, 346–353
Allergic reactions, 279, 281
Amblyopia, 71, 98, 155
Amplatzer plugs, 273, 275
Amputation, 253, 385, 428
Aneurysm, 40, 49, 183–185, 194, 201, 213, 251, 264, 268, 275, 361, 407, 408, 413, 417, 419
Aneurysmal vein, 263–266, 273–275
Angioblasts, 4, 9–11, 431
Angiodysplasias, 182, 371, 394
Angiogenesis, 7, 9–11, 21, 28, 50, 59, 103, 146, 156, 309
Angiography, 41, 79, 132, 166, 188, 234, 235, 237, 240, 241, 243, 244, 256, 280, 330, 338, 347, 361, 387, 394, 426–428
Angiokeratoma of Fordyce, 205
Angiokeratomas, 204–205, 293, 316, 319
Angio-osteo-hypertrophy, 194, 317, 370, 420
Angio-osteo-hypotrophy, 194, 314, 419
Angiosarcoma, 46, 48, 59, 63–64, 79, 174, 181, 182, 204
Ano-genital region, 91, 93, 113, 151, 152, 281
Anorectal malformations, 75, 151
Antiangiogenesis, 94
Antiproliferative drugs, 92, 94
Aplasia and hypoplasia, 166, 183, 194, 201, 239, 240, 251, 417, 422, 431, 465
Aplasia of the inferior vena cava, 407, 421
Arteriogenesis, 9, 11–12
Arteriographic classification, 263
Arteriovenous fistulae, 83, 132, 133, 182–184, 243, 256, 263, 264, 277, 281, 303, 390, 405, 408
Arteriovenous hemangiomas, 171, 176, 182
Arteriovenous malformations (AVMs), 23, 30, 49, 82, 158, 160, 166, 171, 175–177, 181–184, 199–201, 209, 215–217, 225, 238, 247, 249, 250, 256, 263–275, 295, 303–304, 308, 319, 328, 333–334, 353–354, 357–361, 366, 381, 383, 384, 387, 389–391, 405, 410–414, 417–428, 432

extratruncular, 427–428
truncular, 425–427
Arteriovenous shunting, 77, 82, 85, 132, 133, 158, 172, 176, 184
Aspirin, 48, 50
Auricle, 333
Autosomal-dominant hereditary, 22
AV shunts, 41, 176, 208–211, 234, 284, 288, 296, 297, 316, 318, 319, 393, 394
Axial proptosis, 362

B

Backflow, 191, 230–232, 455, 456
Benign neonatal hemangiomatosis, 72, 160
Benign vascular tumors, 21, 46, 61, 149
Betablockers, 97–100, 104, 131, 145, 147, 149
Bevacizumab, 49, 319
Bleomycin, 246, 277, 338, 346, 349, 350, 364, 365, 389, 414
Blue rubber bleb nevus syndrome (BRBNS), 23, 27, 28, 146, 173, 174, 214, 302, 309, 313, 317, 395–397, 409
Bone, 22, 25, 27, 31, 40, 41, 47, 64, 104, 106, 177–179, 187, 210, 211, 213, 214, 219, 237, 238, 313, 317, 318, 325, 333, 360, 371–374, 376, 379, 381–383, 386–388, 417, 423, 427, 428
Bone scanogram, 187
Bonnet-Dechaume-Blanc syndrome, 295, 313, 319
Bony hypertrophy, 199
Borderline vascular tumors, 59
Bowel hemorrhages, 318
BRBNS. *See* Blue rubber bleb nevus syndrome (BRBNS)
Bruit, 39, 118, 120, 184, 298, 334, 357, 359, 361, 363, 426
Bypass, 176, 235, 245, 251, 344, 403, 407, 422

C

Capillary-lymphatic malformations, 205, 293, 295
Capillary malformations (CM), 22, 23, 77, 159, 166, 167, 182–184, 189, 191, 194, 199, 204–205, 217, 291–297, 303, 314, 315, 334, 343, 353, 396, 418, 434

Cardiac failure, 71, 77, 81, 92, 131, 132, 137, 147, 184, 296, 327, 334, 389
Cavernous hemangioma, 171, 173, 185, 190, 362, 394
CCM. *See* Cerebral cavernous malformation (CCM)
CD31, 174, 178
CD34, 11, 174
Central facial lesions, 137
Cerebral cavernous malformation (CCM), 23, 25–26, 28
Chemosis, 358, 359, 361
Chimney effect, 115
Chocolate cysts, 364
Cho-Do classification, 263–265
Chyledema, 463
Chyloperitoneum, 463, 466, 468, 470
Chylorrhea, 463, 465
Chylothorax, 13, 300, 463, 465, 468, 470
Chylous arthritis, 463
Chylous ascites, 29, 284, 403, 465, 467–469
Chylous reflux, 451, 463–472
Chyluria, 463
Chylus ascites, 403
Clopidogre, 48
CLOVES syndrome, 25, 32, 319
Cobblestoning, 173
Cobb syndrome, 319
Coils, 132, 238, 246, 255, 257, 265, 273–275, 284, 426
CO₂-laser, 112, 142, 292, 294, 295, 344, 346, 347, 349, 350
Colonoscopy, 146, 394, 406
Combined form of CVMs, 194–195
Common IH, 123, 160
Complete excision, 277, 334, 432, 433, 441
Complications, 56, 70–71, 73, 89, 91, 93, 94, 124, 132, 134, 137, 147, 151–152, 157, 160, 193–195, 228, 239, 245, 257, 261, 279, 293, 296, 297, 307, 308, 317, 318, 335, 337–340, 344, 374–376, 385, 389, 391, 398, 405, 407, 423, 433, 435–437, 439, 445, 447–449, 456, 459, 463, 467, 468
Composite hemangioendothelioma, 59, 63
Compression pressure, 114
Compression therapy, 308, 433, 438
Compressive optic neuropathy, 362
Computed tomography (CT), 82, 85, 148, 187, 213–221, 225, 226, 228, 237, 238, 280, 317, 358–361, 394, 400, 404, 408, 412, 413, 427, 466
Congenital angio-osteohypotrophy, 370
Congenital avalvulia, 422
Congenital hemangioma, 21, 59–61, 77, 79, 81, 84–85, 124, 131, 132, 145, 147
Congenital sarcoma, 79
Congenital vascular malformation (CVMs), 39, 165–168, 181, 187, 189–195, 199, 234, 237, 239, 245, 249, 277, 309, 313–319, 337–341, 369, 379, 381, 383–387, 432
Congestion, 219, 257, 359, 363, 397
Conservative approach, 194
Consumption coagulopathy, 61, 147, 395–398
Consumptive coagulopathy, 45, 48, 50, 104, 173
Continuous wave (cw-Nd:YAG) Lasers, 112

Contrast medium, 132, 223, 225, 228, 229, 338, 388, 466
Cooling cuvette, 109, 112, 114, 115, 292–294
Cutis marmorata, 205, 317
Cutis marmorata telangiectacia congenita (CMTC), 205, 296
Cyst diameter, 177, 209
Cystic hygromas, 41, 177, 179, 297, 389, 433

D
Dacron, 251
Dandy-Walker complex, 74, 158
Dark blue keratotic spots, 317
D-dimer, 27, 45, 48–50, 104, 246, 307, 396, 397
De-congestive treatment, 446
Deep and superficial circulation, 229
Deep hemangiomas, 67, 68, 159
Deep lymphatic trunk, 231
Deep vein hypoplasia, 168, 195
Detachable balloons, 256, 273
Devascularization, 131, 245, 246, 249
Diagnostic and therapeutic algorithm, 372
Diameter of bubbles, 279
Differential diagnoses, 49, 60, 75, 77, 79, 84–87, 119, 146, 190, 227, 317, 362, 376, 400, 403, 422, 445
Diffuse infiltrating iH, 92
Diffuse lymphatic vascular malformations, 277
Diffuse neonatal hemangiomatosis, 72, 146, 147, 149, 156, 160
Dilated lymphatic channels, 394
Diplegia, 47, 106
Direct bone puncture, 381
Direct percutaneous venography (DPV), 238–240
Direct puncture, 42, 226, 238, 239, 256, 259, 260, 266, 274, 275, 298, 299, 337, 340, 349, 350, 352, 388, 390, 391, 412, 423, 433
Direct puncture angiography, 387
Doxycycline, 177, 338, 389, 403, 404, 414
Duplex ultrasonography, 187, 190, 279, 281, 435, 438, 439
Dye laser, 152, 153, 293
Dysphagia, 333, 343, 346

E
Echoguided lasertherapy, 383, 414
Edema post-sclerosis, 338, 340
Ehler–Danlos type IV defect, 407
Elasto-compression, 447
Elevated D-dimer, 48–50, 246, 307, 396
Embolization, 41, 79, 92, 93, 131–134, 147, 177, 213, 244, 246, 254, 256–259, 295, 303, 304, 316, 325, 333, 334, 353, 354, 361, 379, 386, 390, 394, 405, 407, 409–414, 426–428, 468
Embolotherapy, 192
Embryonal vein, 209
Embryonic tissue remnant, 189, 431
En bloc-resection, 249, 381
Encephalotrigeminal angiomatosis, 314

Enchondromas, 61, 174, 237, 318
Endoglin (ENG), 23, 30, 31, 176, 318
Endoscopic
    coagulation, 299–300
    sclerotherapy, 397, 398
Endoscopic argon diathermia, 396
Endoscopy, 118–121, 146, 317, 394, 396, 403, 406
Endothelial cells, 3–6, 9, 11, 12, 14, 21, 24, 25, 27, 28,
        31, 32, 48, 50, 62, 70, 73, 80, 97, 106,
        172–174, 177, 178, 200, 314, 339, 360
    sprouting, 10, 13
Endothelial mitotic activity, 171, 177
Endovascular
    embolization, 255, 258–259, 364
    technique, 245
Enophthalmos, 363–365
Enoxaparin, 50
Epidemiologic data, 165
Epilepsy, 25, 314
Epiphysiodesis, 253, 316, 371
Epistaxis, 30, 176, 309, 318, 319, 405, 406
Epithelioid hemangioendothelioma (EHE), 59, 63, 64
Eponyms, 165, 190, 293, 313
Esophago-gastro-duodenoscopy, 394, 396, 406
Estrogen, 29, 308, 309
Ethanol, 209, 210, 244, 246, 257, 266, 272, 274, 275,
        277, 279, 318, 337–341, 388, 389, 391, 410,
        412–414, 433–440
Exophthalmos, 158, 357, 363, 364
Extracutaneous hemangioma, 155
Extratruncular forms, 182, 183, 192, 194, 195, 209,
        225, 245, 249, 251, 341, 389, 391, 426
Ex utero intrapartum tracheotomy, 346

F
Facial nerve, 141, 325, 332, 340
Facial nerve mapping, 332
Familial mucocutaneous disorder, 173
Fast-flow malformation, 49, 213
Fatty meal, 468, 469
Female genital VM, 409
Fiberoptic laryngoscopy, 348
Fibrin degradation products (FDP), 45–47
Fibrinogen, 27, 45, 48–50, 104, 307, 395–397
Fibrofatty tissue, 82, 98, 123, 124, 140
Fibrolipomatous tissue, 95
Fistula, 30, 39–41, 83, 131–133, 152, 176, 179, 182–184,
        201, 234, 243–245, 250, 252, 253, 256, 259,
        264, 277, 281, 288, 303, 304, 318, 325, 358,
        361, 371, 381, 383–385, 390, 403, 405, 408,
        411, 412, 426–428, 467
Flash lamp pumped pulsed dye laser (FLPDL),
        291, 293, 295
Fluid cooling cuvette, 109, 112, 114, 115, 292–294
Follow-up, 47, 60, 61, 125, 192, 209, 211, 223, 235, 240,
        289, 309, 314, 334, 341, 391, 404, 422, 423,
        440, 456, 468, 470
FOXC2, 14, 24, 29, 203
Frequency doubled Nd:YAG laser, 110–111

G
Gastrointestinal (GI) bleeding, 48, 146, 173, 174, 176,
        296, 309, 394, 395, 397, 405
Gastrointestinal tract, 59, 75, 155, 160, 173, 296, 309,
        393, 395, 467
Genetic bases, 22, 25, 30
Glaucoma, 205, 314
Glomangioma, 175, 302–303
Glomulin (GLMN), 23, 26, 27, 281
Glomus tumor, 175, 302
Glomuvenous malformation (GVMs), 23, 26–28, 49,
        175, 202, 203, 302–303, 425
Glottis, 344–346
GLUT1, 172, 174, 177
Gluteal area, 407, 412
Gluteal VM, 413
GNAQ gene, 23, 25, 172, 314
Gorham Stout, 178, 219, 238, 300, 309, 313, 318, 330
    disease, 178
    syndrome, 219, 238, 300, 309, 318, 330
GVMs. See Glomuvenous malformation (GVMs)

H
Hauert disease (HD), 369, 370, 372, 376
Headache, 25, 157, 361
Head and neck, 69, 71, 137–143, 166, 167, 172, 255,
        257, 277, 300, 325, 327–335, 337–341, 344,
        398, 432, 465, 467
Hemangioendotheliomas, 61, 75, 81, 85–87, 91, 93,
        104, 107, 117, 118, 132, 181, 182
Hemangioma
    anogenital, 151, 152, 154
    duplex sonography, 151
    facial, 74, 152
    liver, 81, 92, 146–148
    non-involuting congenital hemangioma (NICH), 21,
        60, 61, 77, 80, 84, 91, 95, 118, 123, 124
    PHACE, 67, 69, 71, 74, 81, 98, 99, 155–160
    physical examination, 75, 77
    problem zones, 91
    rapidly involuting congenital hemangioma (RICH),
        21, 59–61, 77, 79–81, 84, 86, 91, 95, 112,
        131, 133, 147, 148
    regression, 89–92, 103, 109–111, 131, 147, 151,
        156, 189
    spontaneous course, 89–92
    subglottal and tracheal, 118, 119
    ulceration, 71, 75, 137, 145, 151, 152, 155, 184
Hemangioma of infancy (HOI), 55, 59–60, 327
Hemangiomatosis, 89, 145, 149, 182, 288
Hemodynamic
    assessment, 192
    techniques, 251
Hemolymphatic malformation (HLM), 166, 167,
        192–195, 287, 432, 440
Hemorrhages, 25, 27, 39, 63, 104, 147, 176, 194, 199,
        214, 216, 219, 221, 284, 298, 333, 337, 353,
        354, 359, 361–396, 403, 405, 412, 424
Hemosiderin, 86, 200, 297, 372, 373

Hepatic hemangioma, 59, 131, 132, 147, 149, 156
Hereditary hemorrhagic telangiectasia (HHT), 23, 30–31,
          176, 296–297, 308, 309, 318, 393, 405
High flow malformations, 213, 225, 264, 393
HLM. *See* Hemolymphatic malformation (HLM)
HOI. *See* Hemangioma of infancy (HOI)
Homograft, 251
Hormonal change, 329, 334
Hydrocolloid, 152, 153
Hyperkeratotic, 25, 26, 63, 178, 203, 205, 292–294, 299
Hypertrophy, 24, 40, 41, 158, 181, 194, 202, 214,
          230, 293, 295, 297, 314, 315, 319, 334,
          353, 396, 424
    somatic, 40
Hypopigmentation, 90, 93, 154
Hypoproteinemia, 399, 400, 463

I
Ice cube cooling, 114–117, 292, 295, 297, 302
Igloo effect, 115
Ilizarov technique, 253
Impression technique, 117–119, 292, 301, 304
Indeterminate hemangiomas, 69
Induced regression, 92, 95
Infantile haemangiomas (IH), 21–22, 46, 48, 55, 57,
          59–60, 67, 70, 72, 75, 77, 79–87, 89–91,
          93–95, 97–100, 103–107, 109, 110, 116–119,
          121, 123, 131, 132, 137–143, 145, 147,
          151–160, 171, 176, 177, 185, 189, 190, 295,
          301, 343–345
Infected cysts, 399, 403
Infections, 28, 29, 40, 63, 71, 92, 99, 104, 107, 110, 117,
          126, 152, 153, 177, 203, 247, 266, 272, 308,
          332, 335, 337, 364, 376, 403, 405, 432, 433,
          436–438, 441, 452, 456, 457, 459, 465
Infiltrating extratruncular, 192, 251, 337, 436
Integrin, 13, 14, 21, 25
Interfascicular
    neurolysis, 383
    treatment, 383
Interferon, 49, 106, 147, 149, 309, 318
    alpha, 47, 106, 309
Interstitial laser coagulation, 298–299
Interstitial puncture technique, 117, 118, 303
Intestinal lymphangiectasia, 177, 399, 403
Intra abdominal cysts, 393
Intraconal, 71, 72, 77, 360, 362, 364, 365
Intralesional hemodynamics, 172, 226
Intraosseous AVM, 334
Intravascular papillary endothelial hyperplasia, 174, 176
Intussusceptions, 146, 317, 393, 395
Involution, 55, 60, 69, 77, 79, 84, 92, 115, 116, 123,
          124, 128, 137, 140, 147, 341
Iron deficiency anemia, 395, 396, 405, 406
ISSVA classification, 160, 166, 183, 184, 452

J
Joint, 60, 211, 227, 237, 319, 325, 369–376, 380, 417,
          423, 424

K
Kaposiform hemangiendothelioma (KHE), 45–48,
          50, 59, 61, 79, 91–95, 104, 118, 120, 131,
          132, 309
Kaposi sarcoma, 59, 63
Kasabach Merritt phenomenon (KMP), 45–48, 50, 61,
          92, 104, 105, 107, 132
Kasabach Merritt syndrome (KMS), 60, 61, 92, 94,
          118, 307
KHE. *See* Kaposiform hemangiendothelioma (KHE)
Klippel Trenaunay syndrome (KTS), 24, 25, 27, 49, 167,
          174, 179, 185, 190, 193, 195, 202, 205, 217,
          237, 238, 286, 293, 295, 313–317, 395–398,
          407, 421, 432, 434, 435
KRIT1, 23, 25

L
Laparoscopy, 394, 396, 403
Laser
    CO_2-laser, 112, 142, 292, 294, 295, 344, 346,
          347, 349, 350
    intravascular absorption, 109
    specific absorption, 93, 109, 112, 114
    therapy, 90, 92–94, 109, 111, 117, 120, 152, 291,
          293, 295–297, 299, 300, 303, 304, 333, 383
    tracheotomy, 121
    treatment, 90, 93, 109–121, 123, 124, 138–141, 152,
          153, 246, 291–304, 316, 317, 333, 334, 344,
          347, 348, 350, 360, 364, 379, 414, 424, 428
    wavelength, 93, 109, 110
Leakage of cerebrospinal fluid, 329
Leptomeningeal vascular anomalies, 314
Limb length discrepancy, 40, 166, 237, 238, 253, 419, 424
Limitations of classic Sclerotherapy, 279
Liquid embolic materials, 255–257, 259
Liver hemangioma, 81, 92, 146–148
Localized hemangiomas, 56, 68, 126
Localized intravascular coagulation/coagulopathy (LIC),
          27, 45, 46, 49–50, 301, 307, 395–398
Low fibrinogen levels, 49, 396
Low flow masses, 225
Low molecular weight heparin (LMWH), 50, 307, 308
LUMBAR/PELVIS/SACRAL syndrome, 156, 159–160
LVA. *See* Lymphatic-venous anastomoses (LVA)
Lymphangiectasias, 203–204, 465, 468
Lymphangiogenesis, 12–14, 21, 29, 398, 431, 432, 442,
          452, 459
Lymphangiography, 228, 433, 434, 466
Lymphangiomas, 13, 40, 41, 171, 177, 298, 303, 364
    circumscriptum, 204, 293
Lymphangiomatosis, 106, 178, 182, 442, 452, 465
Lymphatic drainage, 29, 195, 423, 446, 447, 458, 459, 465
Lymphatic lakes, 230, 445
Lymphatic malformations, 22, 23, 28, 41, 49, 79, 166,
          171, 172, 177–179, 183, 191, 194, 199, 200,
          203–204, 209, 213, 217–221, 227, 237, 247,
          259, 277, 291, 297, 300, 301, 309, 314, 318,
          319, 327–333, 343–345, 357, 364–366, 382,
          387, 389, 394, 396, 398, 399, 412, 414, 431,
          451, 452, 459

Lymphatic-venous anastomosis (LVA), 454–456, 458, 459, 468, 469, 472
Lymphedema, 13, 28–30, 195, 199, 203, 204, 210, 217, 228, 229, 233, 247, 308, 314, 434, 437, 445–449, 452–459
Lymphedema distichiasis syndrome, 203
Lymphography, 188
Lymphoscintigraphic, 230–233, 452, 453
Lymphoscintigraphy, 187, 191, 228–233, 315, 434, 435, 445, 448, 454, 456–458, 466, 469, 470
Lymphovenous abnormalities, 223, 225
Lymphovenous shunt, 226, 228, 229, 231, 233
Lymph stasis, 457–459, 465

M

Macrocystic, 167, 172, 177, 178, 203, 204, 217, 297, 300, 332, 338, 346, 364, 389, 398, 400, 412, 436, 437, 440
Macrocystic lesions, 28, 203, 221, 435, 437, 438
Macroglossia, 332, 345, 346, 348
Maffucci syndrome, 49, 61, 174, 288, 313, 318
Magnetic resonance (MR), 85, 87, 133, 187, 213–221, 233, 238, 346, 358, 374, 409, 421–423, 427
Magnetic resonance angiography (MRA), 133, 213, 216, 217, 422
Magnetic resonance imaging (MRI), 25, 60, 61, 70, 78, 79, 81, 82, 84, 85, 87, 104, 105, 120, 133, 149, 151, 156, 160, 166, 167, 190–193, 213–215, 217, 219, 233, 237, 280, 288, 330, 338, 346, 347, 352, 354, 358–363, 365, 366, 372, 374, 375, 387, 394, 395, 398–401, 403, 404, 409, 412–414, 434–436, 438–441, 466
Malcavernin, 23, 25
Malignant vascular tumors, 46, 182
Marginal lymphatic, 233, 235, 420
Marginal vein, 168, 193–195, 202, 217, 225, 233, 239, 240, 250, 252, 253, 280, 300, 307, 316, 418–421
Meckel's diverticulum, 394, 396
Mediastinal involvement, 389
Medium-chain triglycerides (MCT), 466, 467
Mesentery, 398, 399, 403, 465
Metalloproteinases, 97
MGC4607, 25
Micelles of purified human albumin, 229
Microcatheters, 132, 255–260
Microcystic, 28, 177, 178, 200, 203, 204, 209, 217, 219, 298–299, 303, 332, 338, 345, 346, 364, 398, 399, 403, 412, 414, 435, 437, 439–441, 469
Microcystic lesions, 203, 440
Microfistulae, 263, 264, 272, 274
Micro-foam technique, 280–289
Microphthalmia, 74
Microscope, 380, 381, 386, 454, 455, 469
Microspheres, 234–235, 391
Microwires, 256
Mixed hemangiomas, 67, 68
Morphologic study, 187
Mosaicism, 172

MR angiography. *See* Magnetic resonance angiography (MRA)
MR imaging. *See* Magnetic resonance imaging (MRI)
Multidisciplinary team, 77, 137, 191–193
Multifocal hemangiomas, 50, 67, 69, 72–73
Multifocal lymphangioendotheliomatosis, 45, 48–49, 73, 160
Multihead gamma camera, 228
Multistaged surgical removal, 389
Muscle, 22, 27, 28, 30, 41, 46, 67, 71, 85, 104, 173, 174, 177, 178, 210, 213, 214, 216, 230, 277, 309, 325, 332, 340, 360, 362, 375, 376, 379, 381, 383, 386–389, 395, 409, 410, 412–414, 417, 423, 424, 427, 446, 447, 455

N

Nerve, 3, 22, 27, 74, 118, 141, 158, 172, 210, 213, 247, 258, 279, 298, 325, 332–334, 340, 358, 360, 362, 364–366, 375, 379–381, 383, 384, 386, 389, 391, 410–412, 421, 423, 435, 437, 441, 454
Nerve damage, 340, 383, 389, 437
Neuritic pain, 247
Nevus, 40, 151, 166, 185, 205, 314, 316, 319, 412, 414, 417, 418, 420, 421
Nidus, 30, 210, 217, 219, 227, 243, 244, 248, 250, 252, 253, 256–260, 263–266, 268, 303, 334, 338, 361, 390, 391, 411–413, 426
Non-pulsatile, 327, 363
Not encapsulated, 362
Nutcracker syndrome, 409

O

Occluders, 273
Occluding mechanical devices, 273
Occlusion of vessels, 246
Octreotides, 317
Ocular motility, 357, 358
OK-432, 177, 277, 338, 365, 389, 403, 404, 412, 414, 433–439
OK-432 sclerotherapy, 401, 403, 404, 434–441
Omentum, 146, 149, 398, 400
Ophthalmic branch of the trigeminal nerve, 172
Optic nerve, 74, 158, 340, 358, 360, 362, 364–366
Optic neuropathy, 358, 362, 364
Oral contraceptives, 308
Orbital compartment syndrome, 365
Orbital vascular malformations, 357, 358, 366
Oropharynx, 178, 299, 301, 302, 343, 345, 346, 353
Osler-Rendu-Weber syndrome, 176, 296–297
Osteolysis, 178, 219, 237, 238, 318, 369

P

Pain, 48, 50, 62, 71, 105, 115, 146, 175, 210, 246–247, 258, 261, 292, 307, 308, 319, 327, 333, 335, 337, 339, 341, 345, 357, 362–364, 369, 370, 372, 374, 376, 383, 385, 396, 398–401, 403, 409, 410, 412, 414, 422, 424, 426, 438, 452

Papillary intralymphatic angioendothelioma, 62–63
Paranasal hemangiomas, 138–143
Parkes Weber syndrome (PWS), 22, 24, 49, 167, 172,
        173, 179, 184, 185, 190, 199, 205, 291–293,
        295, 314, 316, 432, 435
Pascual-Castroviejo type II syndrome, 156
Patch plastic, 251
PDCD10, 23, 25
Pecquet cyst, 465
Pelvic cavity AVM, 411
Pelvis, 75, 151, 156, 159–160, 228, 238, 314, 325, 375,
        396, 408–410, 412
PELVIS syndrome, 75, 151, 159
Percutaneous direct puncture, 256, 259, 260, 434
Percutaneous sclerotherapy, 337, 338, 388, 389
Perineal hemangiomas, 75, 151, 156
Periocular/orbital hemangiomas, 98, 137, 357, 364, 366
Periocular pain, 357
Persistence of sciatic vein (PSV), 239, 421
Persistent fetal circulation, 132
Persistent sciatic artery, 407
Phace, 73, 74, 156
Phace syndrome, 67, 69, 71, 74, 81, 99, 155–160
Phakomatosis pigmentovascularis, 205
Pharynx, 329, 340, 346
Phlebographic study, 238–240
Phlebography, 188, 214, 239, 240, 388, 421
Phleboliths, 41, 49, 173, 175, 210, 213–216, 237, 238,
        327, 347, 363, 372, 409
Phlebolymphedema, 445, 455
Phlebolythes, 246, 247, 317
Phlebotonic drugs, 247
Physical treatment, 447
Pingyangmycin, 338, 389
Podoplanin, 13, 48, 178
Polydocano, 256, 388
Popcorn effect, 293, 296, 299–302
Portable Doppler, 210
Port-Wine stains (PWS), 22, 24, 25, 77, 109, 172–173,
        179, 184, 185, 291–293, 295, 334, 353
p120RasGAP (RASA1), 22, 23, 25, 176
Prednisolone, 47, 92, 103
Prenatal diagnosis, 60, 210, 442
Preoperative
    devascularization, 131
    embolization, 257, 334
    tracheostomy, 338, 339
Preoperative endovascular embolization, 192, 364
Primary lymphedema, 23, 29, 166, 167, 191, 193, 203,
        204, 431, 432, 434, 435, 446, 451–454,
        457–459, 465
Problem hemangiomas, 89
Progesterone, 56, 57, 309
Proliferative phase, 22, 67, 69, 70, 81, 82, 124, 127,
        189, 344
Propranolol, 47, 49, 78, 93, 97–100, 103, 104, 106, 123,
        124, 127, 137, 138, 140–142, 145–149, 152,
        159, 160, 344
Protein loosing enteropathies, 394

Proteus syndrome, 24, 31, 32, 217, 295, 313, 317
Pseudoangiosarcomatous, 176
Pseudo-KS, 200
PTFE, 251, 408
Pulmonary embolism, 49, 132, 194, 195, 279, 281,
        307, 339, 397, 417, 418
Pulmonary perfusional scintigraphy, 234
Pulsatile proptosis, 358, 361
Pulsed Nd:YAG laser, 110–113, 118, 292, 293, 295,
        297, 303
Pupils, 358
Pyogenic granuloma (PG), 59, 61, 63, 73, 79, 177

R
Radiolabelled, 226, 229, 234
    erythrocytes, 225
Rapamycin, 47, 106–107, 309, 317, 396
Rapidly involuting congenital hemangioma (RICH),
        21, 24, 28, 29, 32, 41, 59–61, 77, 79–81, 84,
        86, 91, 95, 112, 131, 133, 147, 148, 165
RASA1, 22–25, 176
Reconstructive lymphatic-venous-lymphatic
        anastomosis, 468, 472
Recurrences, 48, 62, 64, 91, 95, 177, 189, 245, 246,
        252, 291, 297, 334, 341
Rendu Osler, 313, 393
    disease, 318–319
    syndrome, 316, 405
Rendu-Osler-Weber syndrome, 23, 30, 215
Retiform hemangioendothelioma (RH), 59, 61–63
Retrograde
    approaches, 264
    vein approach, 264, 266, 274
Retroperitoneum, 47, 61, 105, 398, 405
Revascularization, 245, 258
Revascularization techniques, 245, 251
RH. See Retiform hemangioendothelioma (RH)
Rhabdomyosarcoma, 75, 77–79, 87, 151, 364

S
SACRAL syndrome, 75, 151, 156, 159–160
Scar, 47, 92, 93, 110, 113, 117, 119, 123, 124, 126, 138,
        141, 153, 154, 285, 286, 294, 301, 302, 304,
        325, 379–381, 420, 440
Sciatic
    artery, 209, 407
    vein, 209, 239, 250, 421, 422
Scintigraphy, 187, 191, 223–229, 234–235, 394,
        434, 466
Sclerotherapy, 93, 175, 177, 192, 194, 195, 214, 226,
        239, 254, 277–289, 291, 298–301, 317,
        332–333, 337–341, 346–350, 352, 363–365,
        379, 383, 386, 388–390, 394, 397, 398, 401,
        403–405, 409, 433–442
Sclerotherapy, requirements of, 279
See-and-wait, 89
Servelle-Martorell syndrome, 202, 316–317

Shunt, 41, 79, 132, 147, 176, 182, 183, 185, 208–211, 226–229, 231, 233–235, 243, 258, 263–265, 270, 272, 275, 284, 288, 296, 297, 316, 318, 319, 361, 393, 394, 405, 452, 454, 468
Sildenafil, 309
Sirolimus, 47, 309, 396
Skeletonization, 251, 252, 390
  of feeding arteries, 390
  of marginal vein, 252
Skin sparing technique, 380, 381
Slow-flow malformations, 26, 213, 214, 313
Sodium tetradecyl sulfate, 277, 279, 338, 388
Soft tissue
  hypertrophy, 173, 199, 295, 353
  mass, 81, 82, 85–87, 216, 394
Somatostatin, 309, 467
Sonography, 87, 91, 151, 295, 341
SOX18, 13, 14, 24, 29
Spider veins, 296, 297
Spindle-cell hemangioma (SCH), 59, 61, 63, 174
Spontaneous regression, 89, 91, 92, 95, 98, 103, 109, 110, 147, 156, 189
Sporadic venous malformation (VM), 23, 26, 28, 174
Stenosis, 39, 41, 74, 158, 183, 194, 208, 251, 344, 346, 409, 417
Steroid therapy, 153
Stewart-Bluefarb syndrome, 200–201
Stewart-Treves syndrome, 204
Strabismus, 362
Stridor, 72, 333, 343
Sturge Weber syndrome, 23, 24, 172, 173, 205, 293, 295, 314, 315, 334
Subdermal undermining, 380, 386
Subglottal, 118, 119
Subglottic stenosis, 344
Subglottis, 72, 343–346
Superficial hemangiomas, 67–69, 100, 132, 159
Superselective kaser systems, 109
Superselective microcoil embolization, 394, 405
Supportive treatment, 160
Support therapy, 246–247
Supraglottis, 344–346, 349
Surgery, 39, 41, 48, 98, 104, 112, 123–128, 138, 139, 143, 159, 175, 184, 192, 233, 245, 246, 249–251, 254, 277, 279, 286, 297, 300, 307, 325, 332–334, 337, 348, 353, 363, 369, 371, 375, 379–381, 383, 385–387, 390, 391, 396, 397, 400, 403–405, 408, 411, 414, 420, 421, 423–428, 431, 442, 449, 451–459, 463, 465–468
Surgical excision, 47, 49, 62, 123, 124, 127, 141, 147, 154, 177, 192, 193, 195, 291, 297, 317, 333, 334, 339, 344, 346, 348, 349, 353, 361–365, 389, 390, 433, 434, 436, 438–442
Syndrome of
  Bean (blue rubber bleb nevus), 23, 27, 28, 146, 173, 174, 214, 302, 309, 313, 317, 395–397, 409
  Kasabach-Merritt, 60, 61, 92, 94, 118, 307
  Klippel-Trenaunay, 24, 25, 27, 49, 167, 174, 179, 185, 190, 193, 195, 202, 205, 217, 237, 238, 286, 293, 295, 313–317, 395–398, 407, 421, 432, 434, 435
  Maffucci, 49, 61, 174, 237, 288, 313, 318
  Parkes-Weber, 22, 49, 167, 185, 190, 199, 205, 217, 314, 316, 432, 435
  Proteus, 24, 31, 32, 217, 295, 313, 317
  Sturge-Weber, 23, 24, 172, 173, 205, 293, 295, 314, 315, 334
Synovectomy, 384, 385

T
Tangential clamping, 251, 252, 419, 424
Telangiectases, 109, 111
Thalidomide, 308, 309, 317
Thermography, 91, 295
Thoracic duct, 12, 451, 463–472
  anatomy, 464, 465
  ligation, 467–468
Thoracocentesis, 465
Thorax wall, 325, 387–391
Thrombin, 45, 50, 364
Thrombocytopenia, 45, 47, 48, 50, 60, 61, 73, 103–105, 132, 160, 307
Thrombus, 45, 174, 178, 301
Ticlopidine, 48
TIE2 (TEK), 13–15, 23, 27, 28, 63
Tissue echogenicity, 209
Tongue, 177, 214, 282, 296, 330, 339, 345, 346, 348, 350, 351, 353, 354
Topical pharmacotherapy, 93
Total parenteral nutrition (TPN), 466, 467
Tournique, 126, 239, 275, 381, 382, 386, 421, 427
Tracer, 225–227, 231, 232, 235, 456
Tracheal, 118, 119, 121, 301, 345
Transarterial lung perfusion scintigraphy (TLPS), 187, 234–235, 434, 435
Transcatheter embolization, 131, 390
Transconjunctivally, 362
Transcutaneous direct application, 112–114
Transcutaneous ice cube-cooled, 295, 301, 303, 304
Transfix suture, 246
Transfix trespassing stitches, 251
Transrectal ultrasonography, 411
Treatment of hemangiomas
  antiangiogenic drugs, 307
  antiproliferative drugs, 92
  bleeding, 92, 95, 118, 123–127, 131, 132, 145, 146, 160
  compression, 92, 93, 104, 111, 112, 114, 115, 145
  corticosteroids, 97, 99, 103–107, 123, 137, 141, 344
  cryotherapy, 92, 93, 153
  cyclophosphamide, 106
  dosage, 98, 99, 103, 104, 107
  embolization, 92, 131–134, 337
  imiquimod, 93, 99

Treatment of hemangiomas (*cont.*)
    indications, 89, 90, 92–95, 109–111, 118, 124,
        132, 137
    interferon, 49, 106, 147, 149, 309
    interstitial corticoid crystals, 93
    interstitial magnesium seeds, 93
    laser therapy, 93, 109, 111, 117, 120, 152, 299
    ligation, 92
    neurotoxicity, 105, 106
    prednisone, 49, 103, 121
    scarification techniques, 92
    sclerotherapy, 93
    side effects, 89, 93, 94, 98, 99, 104–107
    surgical excision, 62, 123, 124, 127, 141, 147, 154
    vincristine, 98, 104–105, 107, 147, 149
    X-ray therapy, 93
Treatment of vascular malformation
    direct puncture, 238, 239, 256, 259, 260, 266, 274,
        298, 299, 337, 340
    sclerotherapy
        ethanol, 279, 433, 436–440
        OK-434, 401, 403, 404, 432–441
        sclerosing agents, 277–279, 434–436
    strategy, 191–193, 339, 341, 417, 428, 433
    surgery, resection, 441
Truncular vascular dysplasia, 245
Tufted angioma, 45, 46, 59, 61, 79, 86, 103
Tumor suppressor gene PTEN, 31
Turner's syndrome, 179

U
Ulcer, 40, 49, 59, 67, 71, 75, 89, 90, 92, 93, 95, 98–100,
    110, 117, 123, 124, 137, 138, 141, 143, 145,
    151–155, 177, 184, 193, 200, 201, 205, 296,
    317, 325, 337–339, 391, 413, 421, 448
Ulcerated hemangiomas, 71, 92, 95, 98, 138, 143,
    153, 154
Ulceration, 49, 59, 71, 75, 89, 90, 92, 93, 98, 110, 137,
    141, 145, 151, 152, 154, 155, 184, 201, 205,
    296, 317, 337–339, 391
Ultrasound, 3, 22, 60, 70, 78, 79, 81–83, 85–87, 89, 91,
    98, 132, 133, 147, 149, 160, 167, 207–211,
    237, 239, 246, 280, 294, 338, 362–364, 371,
    375, 389, 400, 408, 409, 417, 421, 447, 448,
    466, 469, 470
Ultrasound-guided injection, 389
Upper airway, 177, 329, 333, 338, 339, 343–354, 441
    obstruction, 177, 343, 441
Upper trachea, 343
Uterine AVM, 411

V
Valsalva, 239, 357, 363
Vascular-bone syndrome, 194, 369

Vascular endothelial growth factor (VEGF), 10, 97
Vascular malformations
    classification
        congenital vascular malformation (CVM), 39,
            165–168, 181, 187, 189–195, 199, 234, 237,
            239, 245, 249, 277, 309, 313–319, 337–341,
            369, 379, 381, 383–387, 432
        embryological development, 182
        hemolymphatic, 166, 192
        high flow, 175, 183, 192, 213, 219, 225, 226, 237,
            258, 313, 337, 339, 354, 393, 405, 411
        Mulliken and Glowacki, 171, 183
        slow flow, 22, 26, 183, 214, 307, 313, 314,
            372, 395
        truncular, 288, 417
    complications and side effects, 339–340
        cutaneous necrosis, 279
    diagnostic
        arteriography, 240–244
        invasive diagnostics, 394
        lymphoscintigraphy, 187, 228–234, 435
        MRI, 213, 214, 237, 280, 359–361, 365, 366,
            374, 394, 401, 404, 409, 411–414, 434–436,
            438–441, 466
        phlebography, 188, 214, 239, 240, 421
        transarterial lung perfusion scintigraphy (TLPS),
            187, 234–235
        ultrasound, 22, 60, 207, 211, 237, 246, 280,
            294, 338, 362–364
        volumetric asymmetry, 232
        whole body blood pool scintigraphy (WBBPS),
            191–193, 223–228, 434, 435, 441
    incidence, 22, 165, 167, 291, 292, 407, 413, 421
Vascular tumors, 21, 41, 45–47, 50, 59–64, 77, 80, 81,
    89, 92–94, 103–107, 125, 126, 132, 145–147,
    149, 155, 156, 165, 166, 171, 172, 178, 181,
    182, 184, 189, 205, 291, 300–302, 307,
    327–329, 343, 394, 475
Vasculitis, 112, 116, 117
Vasculogenesis, 4, 7, 9, 11, 21, 156, 171
VEGFR-3/FLT-4, 10, 11, 13, 14, 29
Vein valves, 251
Venogenesis, 11–12
Venography, 160, 237–240, 340
Veno-lymphatic malformations, 445
Venous malformations (VM)
    extratruncular, 423–425
    truncular, 417–423
Verrucous, 178, 203–205
Videolaparoscopy, 466
Videothoracoscopy, 466
Vincristine, 47, 49, 98, 104–105, 107, 147, 149
Visceral hemangioma, 71, 73, 79, 81–87, 145–149,
    156, 160
Visual compromise, 71–72
vWF, 174

W

"Wait and see", 89, 152, 156, 189

Werner procedure, 301

Whole blood pool scintigraphy, 187

Whole Body Blood Pool Scintigraphy (WBBPS),
        191–193, 223–228, 434, 435, 441

Whole body tomographic study, 226

Wireless capsule endoscopy, 394, 396, 403, 406

Wound healing, 61, 126, 152, 153, 382

Wyburn-Mason syndrome, 295, 319

Y

Yakes classification system, 264, 267–268

Printing and Binding: Stürtz GmbH, Würzburg